P9-EEG-564

Environmental Health Science

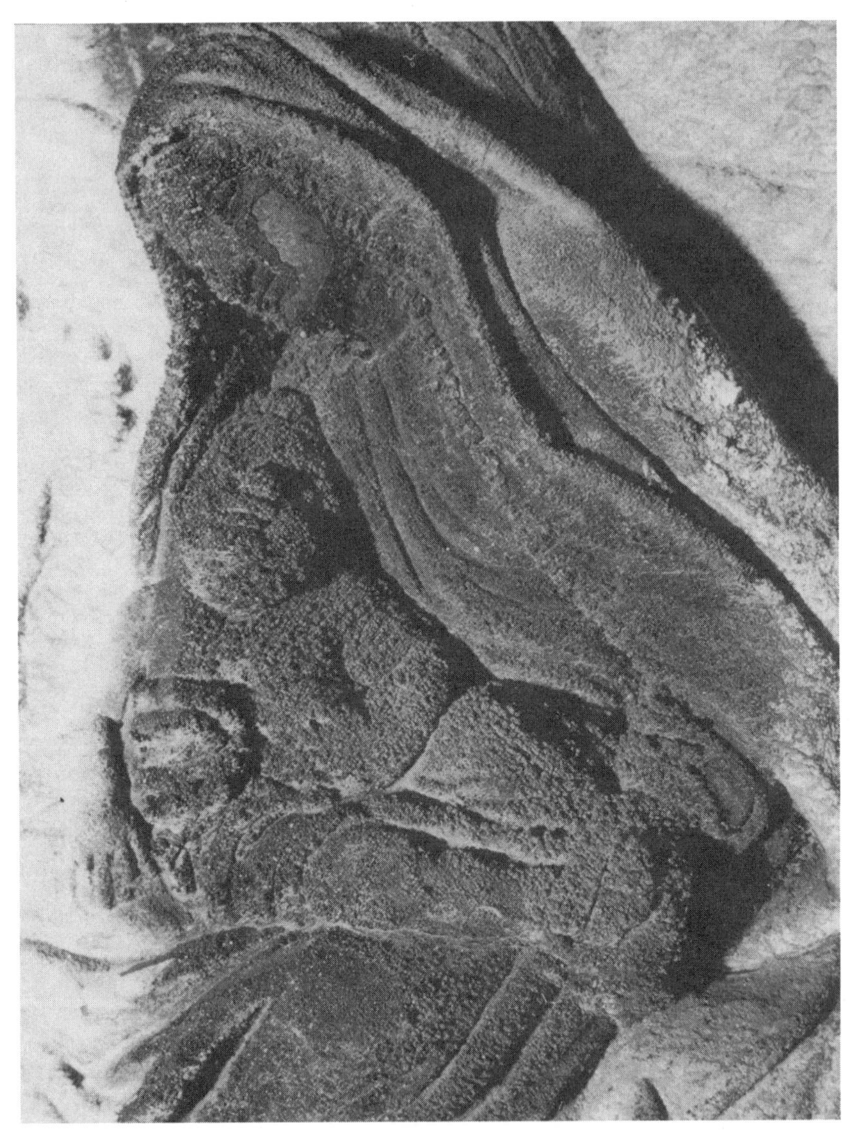

FRONTISPIECE. The marble Madonna in this photograph was carved about 1650 beneath a buttress of the Cathedral of Milan, Italy. The combustion of high-sulfur oil and coal in this industrial area of Italy, as in many cities, results in the generation of sulfur dioxide. This combines with rain water to produce sulfuric acid, which, in turn, reacts with the marble, eventually disintegrating it after prolonged exposure. The lighter areas show less severe damage. *Source*: Young, G., Pollution, Threat to Man's Only Home. *National Geographic* 138 (No. 6):738–81, 1970. © National Geographic Society.

ENVIRONMENTAL HEALTH SCIENCE

Recognition, Evaluation, and Control of Chemical and Physical Health Hazards

MORTON LIPPMANN, Ph.D.
New York University
School of Medicine

BEVERLY S. COHEN, Ph.D.
New York University
School of Medicine

RICHARD B. SCHLESINGER, Ph.D.
Pace University
Dyson College of Arts and Sciences

OXFORD
UNIVERSITY PRESS
2003

OXFORD
UNIVERSITY PRESS

Oxford New York
Auckland Bangkok Buenos Aires Cape Town Chennai
Dar es Salaam Delhi Hong Kong Istanbul Karachi Kolkata
Kuala Lumpur Madrid Melbourne Mexico City Mumbai Nairobi
São Paulo Shanghai Singapore Taipei Tokyo Toronto

This book is a revision and expansion of
Chemical Contamination in the Human Environment
by Morton Lippmann and Richard B. Schlesinger,
published by Oxford University Press in 1979.

Published by Oxford University Press, Inc.
198 Madison Avenue, New York, New York, 10016
http://www.oup-usa.org

Library of Congress Cataloging-in-Publication Data
Lippmann, Morton.
Environmental health science : recognition, evaluation, and control of chemical and physical health hazards /
Morton Lippmann, Beverly S. Cohen, Richard B. Schlesinger
p. cm.
"This book is a revision and expansion of Chemical contamination
in the human environment by Morton Lippmann and Richard B. Schlesinger,
published by Oxford University Press in 1979"—T.p. verso.
Includes bibliographical references and index.
ISBN 0-19-508374-1 (cloth)
1. Environmental health. 2. Pollution.
3. Hazardous substances. 4. Chemicals—Safety measures.
I. Cohen, Beverly S. II. Schlesinger, Richard B. III. Title.
RA566.L55 2003 615.9′02—dc21 2002041

9 8 7 6 5 4 3 2 1
Printed in the United States of America
on acid-free paper

Preface

This book is a revision and extension of *Chemical Contamination in the Human Environment* (1979), which served for two decades as the text for an introductory course at New York University's Graduate Program in Environmental Health Sciences, and for similar courses in other graduate programs elsewhere. The new title reflects the broadened scope of the course, and the fact that we have included chapters on ionizing and nonionizing radiation and noise as well as chemical toxicants. We have also added chapters on modern risk assessment, risk management, and our environmental future.

The basic structure of each updated chapter is essentially the same as in the original text, and most of the basics from that book have been retained. The broad purpose of this revised text is to provide a cohesive, up-to-date overview of the elements of environmental health science, with an emphasis on prevention of the spread of harmful agents and exposures that can cause adverse health effects. As a text for an introductory graduate level course, this book uses scientific notation and nomenclature familiar to those who have completed introductory courses in the basic sciences. Where a greater degree of sophistication is needed in order to adequately discuss a specific issue, it is provided within the discussion.

Most of the chapters focus on the extent and significance of chemical contamination and physical agents in our environment. This information is presented in terms of the underlying physical, chemical, and biological processes that determine the behavior, fate, and ultimate effects on human health and welfare of the multitude of chemicals and radiant fluxes dispersed into the environment. The book thereby provides a comprehensive overview of health risks posed by physical agents and chemical contaminants in the total environment in a way that has seldom been attempted. Many books with overlapping content have concentrated either on one medium (i.e., air, water, food, occupational environment) or on a single element or group of compounds (e.g., mercury, lead, pesticides). Of those books that have attempted to provide comprehensive coverage, most have been multiple-author compilations that lack uniformity in style or depth of coverage.

Our concentration on human health is not meant to belittle additional aspects of the overall environmental stress that are also of great concern, such as disease transmission by infectious agents through air, water, and animate vectors. The human environment is also clearly shaped by social and economic factors, and the health effects of chemical contaminants and physical agents may be greatly influenced or even overwhelmed by the effects of tobacco smoke, alcohol, and drugs. Finally, there is currently great concern about the possible development and inadvertent release of potent mutants produced in research with recombinant DNA. Each of these areas is sufficiently different and complex to warrant separate treatments. They are brought into this book only where they interact with the effects of chemical contaminants and physical agents.

Our main focus is on the potential for effects on human health and welfare. Relatively little space is devoted to disturbances within the environment that have little direct or indirect impact on humans. This is not to say that such disturbances may not eventually be shown to have such effects, or that they are not important in themselves. It is simply not possible to spread the focus of this book to include them while still providing the depth of coverage desired on each topic. An extensive supplementary bibliography is provided in the Appendix for those readers who wish to delve into specific topics in greater depth than we were able to in this book.

In fields as broad and controversial as environmental contamination and environmental health, the perspective offered here will undoubtedly disappoint many. We have attempted to avoid presenting attractive hypotheses and plausible assumptions as proven facts. This may lead to conclusions that differ from some current consensus views on particular issues, and it may upset those who approach specific issues with an advocacy perspective. The current state of knowledge in our field is almost always inadequate in scope and depth, and available data are often unreliable. The uncritical or selective use of these data by individuals with different perspectives accounts for the frequent incidence of scientists coming to diametrically opposed conclusions at public hearings on specific issues. Thus, our major objective in this book is to provide the reader with the technical background needed to intelligently evaluate the scientific issues, and thereby be able to develop informed judgments when sufficient reliable information is available.

In preparing this book, we benefited from the constructive criticisms and comments of numerous people. Of special value were the careful reviews by some of our colleagues at NYU's Nelson Institute of Environmental Medicine. We also gratefully acknowledge the assistance of Toni Moore and Francine Lupino who typed several drafts of the manuscript, and Gordon Cook, who prepared most of the illustrations.

New York

M.L.
B.S.C.
R.B.S.

Contents

Abbreviations

ACGIH	American Conference of Governmental Industrial Hygienists
ACS	American Cancer Society
ADI	acceptable daily intake
ALARA	as low as reasonably achievable
AM	amplitude modulated
ANSI	American National Standards Institute
ASA	American Standards Association
ASHRAE	American Society of Heating, Refrigeration, and Air Conditioning Engineers
BACT	best available control technology
BACTEA	best available control technology economically achievable
BADCT	best available demonstrated control technology
BCC	basal cell carcinoma
BEIR	biological effects of ionizing radiation
BEIs	biological exposure indices
BMDL	benchmark dose level
BMP	best management practices
BOD	biochemical oxygen demand
BPCTCA	best practical control technology currently available
BWR	boiling-water reactors

CAA	Clean Air Act
CAAA	Clean Air Act amendments
CAE	carbon alcohol–extract
CCE	carbon chloroform–extract
CED	critical effect dose
CES	critical effect size
CF	concentration factor
CFC	chlorofluorocarbons
CME	cystoid macular edema
CMN	cutaneous malignant melanoma
CN	condensation nuclei
COD	chemical oxygen demand
CPSC	Consumer Product Safety Commission
CW	continuous wave
CWA	Clean Water Act
dB	decibel
DC	duty cycle
DES	diethylstilbestrol
DHEW	Department of Health, Education and Welfare
DHHS	Department of Health and Human Services
DIH	Division of Industrial Hygiene
DMSO	dimethyl sulfoxide
DO	dissolved oxygen
DOD	Department of Defense
DOE	Department of Energy
DOL	Department of Labor
EEC	European Economic Community
EPA	Environmental Protection Agency
ERC	Educational Resource Centers
ESU	electrosurgical unit
eV	electron volt
FAA	Federal Aviation Administration
FAO	Food and Agriculture Organization
FDA	Food and Drug Administration
FGD	flue-gas desulfurization
FICON	Federal Interagency Committee on Noise
FM	frequency modulated
GI	gastrointestinal
GNP	gross national product
GRAS	Generally recognized as safe
HAPs	hazardous air pollutants
HC	hydrocarbon

HID	high-intensity discharge
HLVs	human limit values
HO	high output
HUD	Housing and Urban Development
IAEA	International Atomic Energy Agency
IARC	International Agency for Research on Cancer
ICRP	International Commission on Radiological Protection
IOD	immediate oxygen demand
IR	infrared radiation
IRIS	Integrated Risk Information System
IRS	Internal Revenue Service
ISO	International Standards Organization
JECFA	Joint Expert Committee on Food Additives
JMEPR	Joint Meeting of Experts on Pesticides Residue
LED	light-emitting diodes
LET	linear energy transfer
LOAEL	lowest observable adverse effect level
MACs	maximum acceptable concentrations
MACT	maximum available control technology
MCLs	maximum contaminant levels
MF	modifying factor
MIC	methylisocyanate
MSHA	Mine Safety and Health Administration
NAAQS	National Ambient Air Quality Standard
NAPAP	National Acid Precipitation Assessment Program
NCHS	National Center for Health Statistics
NCRP	National Committee on Radiation Protection
NEA	Nuclear Energy Agency
NESHAP	national emission standards for hazardous air pollutants
NGOs	non-government organizations
NHANES	National Health and Nutrition Examination Surveys
NHEXAS	National Human Exposure Assessment Survey
NIH	National Institute of Health
NIHL	noise-induced hearing loss
NIOSH	National Institute for Occupational Safety and Health
NIPTS	noise induced permanent threshold shift
NITTS	noise-induced temporary threshold shift
NMSC	nonmelanoma skin cancer
NOAEL	no observable adverse effect level
NORA	National Occupational Research Agenda
NORM	naturally occurring radioactive materials
NPDES	National Pollutant Discharge Elimination System

NRC	Nuclear Regulatory Commission
OD	optical density
OECD	Organization for Economic Cooperation and Development
OMB	Office of Management and Budget
OSHA	Occupational Safety and Health Administration
PABA	para-aminobenzoic acid
PBBs	polybrominated biphenyls
PCBs	polychlorinated biphenyls
PELs	permissible exposure limits
PM	phase modulated
PM_{10}	thoracic particulate matter
$PM_{2.5}$	fine particulate matter
PNdB	perceived noise decibel
ppb	parts per billion
ppm	parts per million
ppm_v	parts per million parts of air, a volume ratio
ppm_w	parts per million parts of water, a weight ratio
PRF	pulse repetition frequency
PVC	polyvinyl chloride
PW	pulse width
PWR	pressurized water reactor
RACT	reasonably available control technology
RADM	Regional Acid Deposition Model
RF	radio-frequency
RfD	reference dose
RIA	regulatory impact analysis
ROS	reactive oxygen species
SAB	science advisory board
SAR	specific absorption rate
SCC	squamous cell carcinoma
SDWA	Safe Drinking Water Act
SF	safety factor
SHO	super high–output
SI	Systeme Internationale
SIL	speech interference level
SLM	sound level meter
SMD	senile macular degeneration
SPF	sun protection factor
SPL	sound pressure level
STEL	short-term exposure limit
SUVs	sport utility vehicles
TDI	tolerable daily intake

TEAM	total exposure assessment methodology
TLVs	threshold limit values
TMDLs	Total maximum daily loads
TOD	theoretical oxygen demand
TSS	total suspended solids
TWA	time-weighted average
U.S. EPA	U.S. Environmental Protection Agency
UF	uncertainty factor
UIC	Underground Injection Control
UK	United Kingdom
UN	United Nations
UV	ultraviolet
VOCs	volatile organic compounds
VSL	value of statistical life
VSLY	value of statistical life-years
WHO	World Health Organization
W-L	Wellman-Lord

Environmental Health Science

1

Introduction

Chemical contamination of the human environment and environmental radiation and noise did not originate at any particular time. Natural processes have been generating noise, heat, and chemical contaminants throughout most of the history of the earth. Some natural waters that are remote from human activities have levels of dissolved chemicals and radionuclides that make them unsafe by today's standards, and the air above swamps and near geothermal springs is contaminated by sulfur gases. There have been some poisonings of humans and grazing animals by natural chemical toxicants in the fruits and foliage they consumed.

Most current problems of chemical contamination, however, arise from anthropogenic sources, i.e., those attributable either directly or indirectly to human activity. In shaping the environment to our needs and convenience, we have used the earth's resources to feed, clothe, and heat us, to power our machines, and to produce material goods. Our ability to mold our environment has enabled us to greatly increase our numbers and improve our standard of living. But in our often careless use of natural resources, we have created contamination. Although the term contamination is often used interchangeably with "pollution," the latter is better defined as contamination to a degree that renders some resource unfit for its desired use.

When early humans discovered how to control and use fire, they must have found that one of its undesirable side effects was exposure to its smoke. When fire was brought indoors to heat caves or shelters, the problem of smoke exposure became more severe, and at least some additional ventilation usually had to be provided in order to enjoy the benefits of the fireplace. However, success in this regard was only partial; mummified human lungs from the preindustrial age show considerable carbonaceous pigmentation. Dwellers in heated caves were undoubtedly exposed to significant levels of carbon monoxide and polycyclic aromatic carcinogens as well as black smoke.

In calling things "clean," "dirty," "contaminated," or "polluted," we are using terms that are subjective or, in specific contexts, have arbitrary meanings. Thus, a human environment can never be absolutely clean because, by definition, it includes at least one contaminant source, a person. An environment passes from clean to contaminated when the source of contamination, relative to its rate of elimination, is sufficiently large, or where there are enough sources whose aggregate output is sufficiently large, to exceed some sensory or predetermined physical concentration limit that is considered acceptable. Thus, practices that are environmentally acceptable in rural areas, such as setting wood fires, discharging sanitary waste liquids into septic tanks or underground drainage fields, and unleashing pet dogs, can become unacceptable in densely populated urban regions.

The degree of environmental contamination that a society finds acceptable is highly variable in both space and time, and depends more on the rate of change in contaminant levels than on their absolute amounts. It also depends on whether there appears to be a realistic alternative. Very high levels of soot from inefficient coal combustion were tolerated for centuries, as long as cleaner combustion alternatives were not available at prices deemed reasonable and the alternative was being cold or worse.

With the large-scale conversion of heating and electric utility boilers to oil and gas combustion in recent decades, there has been a major reduction in sulfur dioxide, dustfall, and suspended airborne particulate matter. As we continue to utilize our vast coal resources in the coming decades, it is not likely that our more affluent and environmentally aware society will permit significantly increased levels of contaminants. We therefore have to pay for the alternate fuels and/or install control technologies needed to prevent the release of air pollutants and greenhouse gases from coal combustion.

Public acceptance of environmental contamination also depends on whether it is perceived to be "natural." Fire and its effluents have been part of the human environment throughout recorded history. Thus, the potential health effects of inhaled combustion products create relatively little concern, even though these effluents contain many readily detectable toxicants.

On the other hand, the nuclear power industry has kept most discharges of radioactive waste products to a very low level, and produces electric power without generating any of the chemical toxicants cited above or carbon dioxide, the major greenhouse gas. But many people prefer greater reliance on fossil fuel–fired power plants than on nuclear-power plants because they associate nuclear power with catastrophic releases of radionuclides, as from the Chernobyl reactor failure, and with bombs, and equate exposure to radioactive wastes with cancer. The fear of bombs and cancer, in effect, leads to public acceptance of increased dependence on fossil fuels, even when their currently documented adverse effects on human health and environmental quality can be shown to be much greater than those from the operation of nuclear power plants.

Similar considerations apply to food safety. Under the Delaney clause of the Food and Drug Act, which was adopted in 1958 and not repealed until 1996, a variety of food additives, colors, and packaging materials were banned because they were demonstrated to have the potential of causing cancer in laboratory animals when administered in high doses. On the other hand, many natural foods contain carcinogens and other toxicants of equal or greater potency, yet neither the Food and Drug Administration nor the general public has shown much interest in banning their distribution.

If the reader is confused about the effects of chemical contaminants on environmental quality and human health, it is not surprising since many reports in the popular media are selective with respect to content and emphasis, the information is fed directly or indirectly to the media for the purpose of advancing a particular viewpoint. In our incomplete state of knowledge about most environmental issues, it is relatively easy to provide plausible documentation for either the pro or con side of almost every issue.

HISTORICAL BACKGROUND

One of the earliest written discussions of the relation between environment and health was the Hippocratic essay *On Airs, Waters and Places,* written around 460 B.C. It advised physicians to consider the winds, seasons, and sources of water when evaluating the health of their patients. Hippocratic works also described lead colic in miners, as well as diseases occurring in other occupational groups.

Other authors of ancient Greece and Rome recognized that some of the materials used in metallurgy were toxic. Pliny the Elder discussed the dangers in handling sulfur and zinc, and Galen recognized the dangers of acid mists among copper miners. Although the ancients were not aware of the possibility, subclinical chronic lead poisoning may have been widespread. Leaded glazes were widely used on kitchen pottery, and acidic wines and foods extracted some of the lead. The Romans also used lead pipes for the delivery of drinking water, and some of the lead was slowly dissolved into the water. The exposures would have been greatest among the more prosperous Romans, who more often had running water and glazed vessels. The decline of the Roman Empire has been partially attributed by some to chronic lead intoxication, on the basis that the recorded decline in fertility among the upper classes was consistent with the effects of ingested lead.

Occupational Diseases

The association between exposure to chemical contaminants and human health effects has been made most often for people with occupational exposures, where the levels of exposure are generally higher than for the general population. Treatises on occupational diseases began to appear in Europe in the Middle Ages. In 1472, Ulrich Ellenbog of Augsburg wrote an eight-page booklet that discussed the toxic actions of carbon monoxide, nitric acid vapors, lead, mercury, and other metals.

A classic description of mining technology and its hazards, *De Re Metallica,* was published in 1556 by the heirs of Georg Bauer, a native of Saxony who was more commonly known by his Latin name of Georgius Agricola. From 1526 to his death in 1555, Agricola had been the official physician of the Bohemian mining town of Joachimstal, a major source of European silver, and more recently of radium and uranium. The silver coins of Joachimstal were known as Thalers, which in English later became dollars. *De Re Metallica* is a scholarly work of 12 books. It was translated from Latin into English in 1912 by an American mining engineer and his wife. (The engineer, Herbert C. Hoover, eventually gave up engineering for public service and was elected President in 1928.) In the last part of the sixth book, Agricola described diseases of the lungs, joints, and eyes that were common among the miners. It appears from descriptions of the diseases that the men had silicosis, tuberculosis, lung cancer, and combinations thereof. The book also contained numerous woodcut illustrations. Figures 1–1 and 1–2 show samples that illustrate means that were used to limit hazardous exposures.

In 1567, a posthumous work appeared with the title *Von der Bergsucht und anderen Bergkrankheiten* (On the Miners' Sickness and Other Diseases of Miners). It was written by Theophrastus Bombastus von Hohenheim, better known as Paracelsus, an itinerant physician and alchemist of Swiss descent. This monograph was devoted to the occupational diseases of mine and smelter workers. Paracelsus did not consider dust exposure to be the causative factor in the lung diseases he observed in miners, but rather explained them in terms of alchemy and the stars. He was considerably more astute in his description of the diseases among smelter workers, however, and differentiated between acute and chronic poisonings. His detailed descriptions of mercurialism covered most of the currently recognized symptoms. Paracelsus is also well-known for his enunciation of a basic tenet of toxicology: "All substances are poisons; there is none which is not a poison. The right dose differentiates a poison and a remedy."

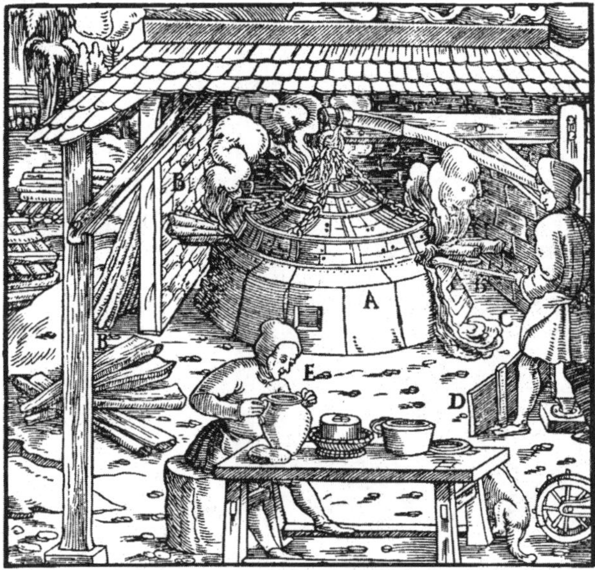

A—FURNACE. B—STICKS OF WOOD. C—LITHARGE. D—PLATE. E—THE FOREMAN WHEN HUNGRY EATS BUTTER, THAT THE POISON WHICH THE CRUCIBLE EXHALES MAY NOT HARM HIM, FOR THIS IS A SPECIAL REMEDY AGAINST THAT POISON.

FIGURE 1–1. Woodcut from Agricola, Book X. The technology of lead smelting was considerably more advanced than the recommended prophylaxis for lead poisoning. Note the barrier plate, D, which protects against splatter burns. (*Source*: Agricola, G. *De Re Metallica,* Basel, 1556. Translated by H.C. Hoover and L.H. Hoover for the *Mining Magazine,* London, 1912. Reprinted by Dover Press.)

The most comprehensive description of occupational diseases of its time, and for well over a century thereafter, was a book of 40 chapters entitled *De Morbis Artificum* (Diseases of Workers), published in 1700 by an Italian, Bernardino Ramazzini, a professor of medicine at the University of Modena and, after 1700, at the University of Padua. Ramazzini is the generally acknowledged "Father of Occupational Medicine." His descriptions of diseases covered most of the trades practiced in his time, including those of dirty and humble trades, such as corpse carriers, porters, and laundresses. He stated: "When a doctor visits a working-class home he should be content to sit on a three-legged stool, if there isn't a gilded chair, and he should take time for his examination; and to the questions recommended by Hippocrates, he should add one more—What is your occupation?" Unfortunately, there is still a great deal of unrecognized occupational disease today because too many physicians still neglect to ask that important question.

Hazardous working conditions and occupational diseases were also common in the more technologically advanced countries in Asia. Extensive descriptions of the operations involved in the mining and refining of metals were provided in the *Atlas of Important Products in Mountains and Sea of Japan* (1754), and

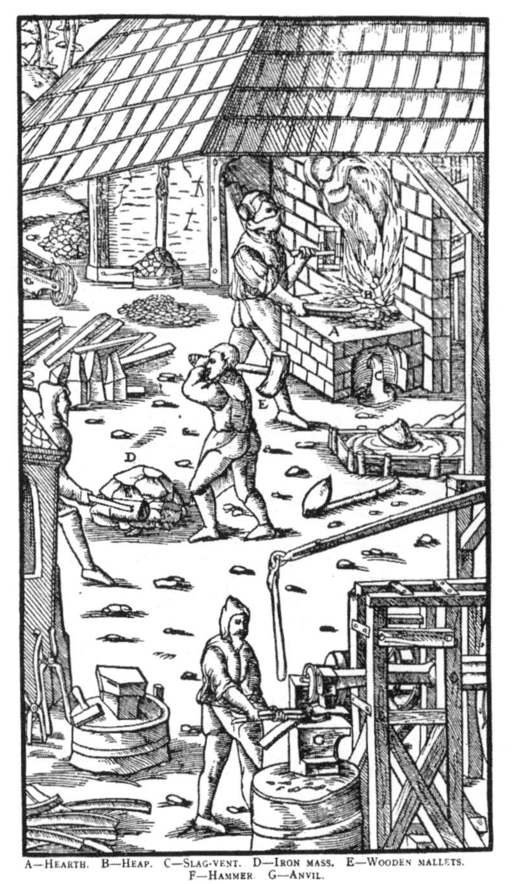

FIGURE 1–2. Woodcut from Agricola, Book IX. Note respiratory protection of the furnace worker. (*Source*: Agricola, G. *De Re Metallica,* Basel, 1556. Translated by H.C. Hoover and L.H. Hoover for the *Mining Magazine,* London, 1912. Reprinted by Dover Press.)

Atlas of Mining and Refining of Copper (1801), and are illustrated by woodcuts, such as the one reproduced in Figure 1–3.

In 1775, an English physician, Sir Percival Pott, provided the first description of occupationally induced cancer, that of scrotal cancer in chimney sweeps.

In 1831, Charles Turner Thackrah made a special contribution to this era by the publication of his 200-page book, *The Effects of Arts, Trades and Professions and All Civic States and Habits of Living on Life and Longevity,* based mainly on his experience in the manufacturing district of Leeds, England.

Scattered reports on occupational diseases appeared in the British, French, German, and American literature through the balance of the nineteenth century. Before the end of that century, it was clear that it was desirable to anticipate problems associated with industrial exposures to toxic chemicals before they happened, rather than after their effects were apparent in workers, and that this could usually be accomplished through the systematic exposure of laboratory an-

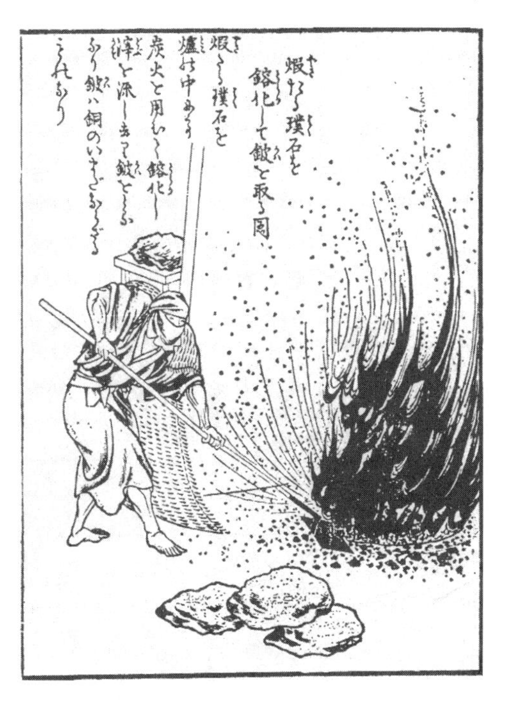

Figure 1–3. The refining of copper in the Besshi Copper Mine in Japan, circa 1800. [*Source*: "Atlas of Mining and Refining of Copper, 1801," Reprinted in: Miura, T.A. Short History of Occupational Health in Japan (Part I). *The J. of Science of Labour* 53:509–25, 1977.]

imals. Pioneering work along these lines began in the 1880s under K. L. Lehmann in Wurzburg, and by 1884 he had published data on the results of toxicological studies with 35 gases and vapors.

With the rapid growth in industrialization in the nineteenth century, more and more workers were being exposed to a broadening spectrum of toxic materials at increasing concentration levels. The obvious effect was a great increase in occupational disease and disability. This was first apparent in England and, by 1833, the first of the English Factory Acts was passed by Parliament. They established the principle that people injured at work are entitled to compensation. While there was no requirement to prevent the conditions that led to the need for compensation, it became more profitable for many businesses to reduce the compensation costs through preventive measures rather than through paying claims. The need for positive preventive measures was recognized later, and the English Factory Act of 1878 created a centralized Factory Inspectorate. Most of the major European countries followed the British lead, but it wasn't until 1911 that Wisconsin became the first U.S. state to establish workmen's compensation, and not until 1948 that the last one did so. The first state programs to inspect industry for occupational exposures began in 1913 in New York and Ohio, but nationwide coverage was not achieved until the passage of the federal Occupational Safety and Health Act of 1970.

The U.S. Federal Government's involvement in occupational health began with the creation of the Bureau of Mines in 1910, and the establishment of an Office of Industrial Hygiene and Sanitation within the Public Health Service in 1914. In that year, they jointly conducted the first of a series of comprehensive studies of certain lung disorders in the dusty trades, under the direction of Dr. Anthony J. Lanza. This was a major activity of the Hygienic Laboratory of the Public Health Service's Office of Industrial Hygiene and Sanitation. With the creation of the National Institute of Health (NIH) in 1937, the Hygienic Laboratory became the Division of Industrial Hygiene (DIH). In 1946, with the increased NIH focus on research, the DIH was transferred to the Bureau of State Services. The research and training activities moved from Washington to Cincinnati in 1950. After several more name changes, the Cincinnati laboratory became the core facility for the National Institute for Occupational Safety and Health (NIOSH), at its creation in 1970. In addition to NIOSH, the Occupational Safety and Health Act of 1970 also created the Occupational Safety and Health Administration (OSHA) to regulate and control occupational health and safety hazards.

In some States, enforcement of OSHA standards is done by state programs that have met OSHA criteria. In others, the OSHA inspectorate is directly responsible. NIOSH continues to be responsible for occupational safety and health research and professional training. Its research is focused in a periodically updated National Occupational Research Agenda (NORA) and it features collaborative sponsorship of research with various NIH Institutes.

Pioneering texts began to appear in 1914 with W. Gilman Thompson's, *The Occupational Diseases*. The first text on industrial toxicology, which appeared in 1925, was *Industrial Poisons* by Alice Hamilton. In 1948, the first edition of Patty's Industrial Hygiene and Toxicology was published. It is now in its fifth edition as two series of volumes, i.e., Patty's Industrial Hygiene[1] and Patty's Toxicology.[2] A current major reference is Rom's 1998 book on *Environmental and Occupational Medicine,* 3rd Edition.[3] It was previously published in 1983 and 1992.

In 1918, Harvard appointed Dr. Hamilton to its faculty of public health, and became the first university to establish a graduate program in occupational health, a program later broadened to environmental health. The faculty at Harvard School of Public Health started the first American scientific journal devoted specifically to occupational health, the Journal of Industrial Hygiene, which first appeared in 1919. In 1947, Dr. Lanza established a graduate and post-graduate program in occupational medicine at the New York University School of Medicine, which became the Department of Environmental Medicine in 1963. In 1977, NIOSH established one or more Educational Resource Centers (ERCs) in each of the ten federal regions. Each provides professional training in at least three of the four core disciplines in Occupational Health and Safety Science, i.e., occupational medicine, occupational hygiene, occupational safety, and occupational health nursing, and can include programs in cognate disciplines such as toxicology and ergonomics.

Air Contamination and Health

Community air contamination arising from the combustion of fossil fuels first received official recognition at the end of the thirteenth century, when Edward I of England issued an edict to the effect that, during sessions of Parliament, there should be no burning of sea coal or channel coal, so-called because it was brought from Newcastle to London by sea transport via ports on the English Channel. Despite a succession of further royal edicts, taxes, and even occasional prison confinements and torture, the use of coal for producing heat continued in London, especially as the increase in population led to a depletion in the availability of wood for fuel. The first scholarly report on the problem: "Fumifugium or the Inconvenience of Aer and Smoak of London Dissipated, together with some Remedies Humbly Proposed" by John Evelyn, was published by the royal command of Charles II in 1661. Evelyn, one of the founding members of the Royal Society, recognized and discussed the problem in terms of the sources, effects, and feasibility of controls.

Unfortunately, no effective controls were instituted until after the report of the Royal Commission on the effects of the "killer fog" of December, 1952, which attributed approximately 4000 excess deaths in London to that pollution episode. Retrospective examinations of vital statistics demonstrated that there had been numerous prior episodes involving excess deaths during periods of air stagnation in London and other British cities. The reductions in smoke levels achieved in Britain since 1952 have eliminated readily observable excess deaths attributable to fossil fuel combustion, and have led to major beneficial changes in visibility and microclimate as well as health.

Excess deaths attributable to coal smoke had occurred elsewhere prior to 1952, but fortunately involved smaller populations. As discussed in Chapter 6, the most notable of these were in the Meuse Valley in Belgium in 1930, and at Donora in Pennsylvania in 1948.

In the 1940s it became apparent that Southern California had an air pollution problem, and that it was a very different kind of pollution from that long known in London and the eastern U.S. The California variety was characterized by oxidant gases, such as ozone, rather than by reducing gases, such as sulfur dioxide. Furthermore, the oxidants were formed in the atmosphere by photochemical processes.

Air pollution research on the federal level began when an occupational health team was sent to Donora, PA to investigate the 1948 pollution disaster. In the mid 1950s, it was decided that a separate federal research program was needed and a separate laboratory program was set up in Cincinnati. However, regulatory aspects of air pollution control were still considered to be the responsibilities of state and local agencies. The Clean Air Act of 1970 established a federal responsibility for air pollution control, and with the creation of the Environmental Protection Agency (EPA) later in 1970, became the responsibility of EPA. This represented a recognition that air pollution had changed from being a local community problem to being a regional problem, and that effective controls had to be taken by national and international authorities, as well as by local authorities and individuals. Oxidant air pollution has now become ubiquitous in regions having a high density of motor vehicles.

By the 1990s, it became evident that fine particles in the ambient air were capable of producing excess mortality and morbidity at contemporary levels of air pollution and a major research effort began to determine the causal components and biological mechanisms for such effects. Also, by the 1990s the international aspects of air pollution had gained widespread recognition. This included not only pollutant transport over the borders between the U.S. and Canada and Mexico, but also stratospheric ozone depletion in the polar regions caused by fluorocarbon emissions, and global climate change caused by secular rises in carbon dioxide and methane releases associated with human economic activities. International agreements have drastically reduced fluorocarbon emissions, and stratospheric ozone depletion should be ameliorated in the next few decades. Effective actions to reduce global climate change remain uncertain as of this writing.

While the focus of this book is on contaminants that are routinely encountered, mention should be made that occasional industrial accidents can be expected to occur. One of the world's worst industrial accidents occurred on December 2, 1984 at the Union Carbide Plant in Bhopal, India, where a release of a gas cloud of methylisocyanate (MIC) killed over 3800 people. It was apparently initiated by the introduction of water into the MIC storage tank, resulting in an uncontrollable reaction, with liberation of heat and escape of MIC and other decomposition products in the form of a gas. Safety systems were either not functioning or were inadequate to deal with large volumes of the escaping toxic chemicals. Among the more than 200,000 persons exposed to the gas, the initial death toll within a week following the accident was over 2000. By 1990, the Directorate of Claims in Bhopal had prepared medical folders for 361,966 of the exposed persons. Of these, 173,382 had temporary injuries and 18,922 had permanent injuries, with the recorded deaths totaling 3828.[4]

Water Contamination and Health

Historically, most contamination problems in water have centered on infectious water-borne diseases rather than on chemical contamination. Furthermore, the growth of cities was historically limited by their ability to prevent contamination of their water supplies by fecal wastes. The more successful ancient cities in the

Roman Empire had their drinking waters supplied from distant sources by aqueducts and enclosed pipes and channels.

In more modern times, the first association between water contamination and human disease was made by John Snow in his classic epidemiologic investigations of the cholera epidemic in London in 1853. It was at about this same time that water pollution was becoming a matter of serious concern in England for esthetic reasons. The rapid growth of London in the first half of the nineteenth century, and the adoption of the practice of discharging the effluent from newly installed water closets into sewers constructed for carrying away storm drainage, led to such an overpowering stench from the Thames at Westminster that Parliament found it difficult to meet in 1858. The solution for that immediate problem was to extend the sewer system, so as to transfer the wastes far enough downstream from Parliament to alleviate the nuisance locally.

The development of bacteriology in the latter half of the nineteenth century provided a scientific basis for understanding the role of water in the transmission of typhoid and other enteric bacterial diseases. Water-filtration processes capable of reducing bacterial concentrations by one or two orders of magnitude were developed. By the turn of the century, these processes were starting to come into widespread use. But in cities such as Pittsburgh and Cincinnati, which still used unfiltered river water, annual death rates from typhoid fever remained around 100 per 100,000 in 1900, and in the U.S. as a whole, the typhoid death rate was about 35 per 100,000. The dramatic effects of filtration and chlorination of a public water supply on the incidence of water-borne disease is illustrated in Figure 1–4, which shows the virtual disappearance of typhoid in Philadelphia during the first half of the twentieth century.

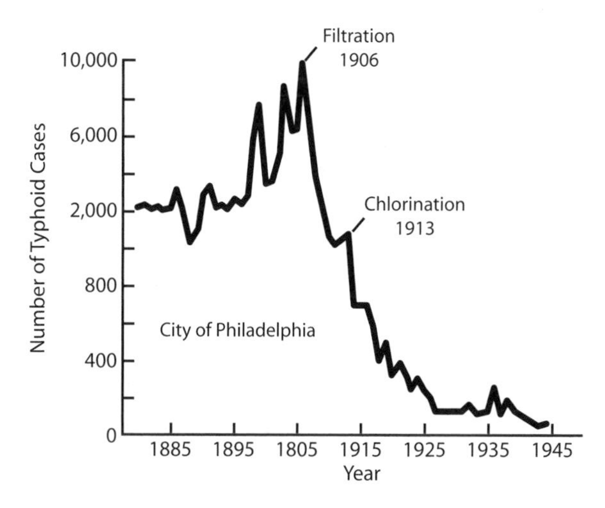

FIGURE 1–4. Reduction of typhoid fever in Philadelphia following treatment of the water supply.

Within the first 30 years of the twentieth century, most of the cities and towns using rivers as sources of water had installed water-treatment plants. In 1908, the use of chlorine as a water disinfectant was introduced, and it became a standard treatment operation. This made possible the production of bacteriologically safe water at very little cost, even when raw water of very poor quality was being treated. However, an epidemic of fatalities associated with cryptosporidium contamination in the public water supply of Milwaukee, WI in 1993 that resulted in about 100 deaths and severe intestinal disorders in about 400,000 people shook the complacency of public health authorities and demonstrated that current water purification technology and monitoring systems need further development to deal with the problem of pathogens resistant to conventional disinfection treatments.

Although much has been done to reduce disease risks from viable agents, very little is known about the possible health effects of the variety of largely unidentified chemical compounds that enter water-supply sources with sewage and industrial wastes. Many of these compounds are not effectively removed by today's water-treatment plants. Recent reports indicating the presence of trace amounts of known carcinogens in most drinking water supplies may lead to a change in the design and performance requirements of our water treatment and waste-disposal facilities.

Food Contamination and Health

The nutritional values and safety of foods have always been important, and the intentional use of chemical preservation techniques, such as salting and smoking, can be traced back to earliest recorded history. Recognition of natural toxicants was often incorporated into dietary laws, which were generally enforced as religious taboos.

Within the last century, modern preservation techniques have made it possible for foods to be processed and distributed for mass markets. It became economically advantageous to make the processed foods attractive in appearance and to keep them that way for extended periods of time. The separation in time and space between production and consumption also created temptations to adulterate the products with fillers and less than wholesome raw materials.

Although the federal government did not begin to enforce food safety regulations until 1906, some individual states recognized their responsibility to provide a safe food supply. As early as 1764, the Massachusetts Bay Colony established a sanitary code for slaughterhouses. California passed a pure food and drug law in 1850, the same year it became a state. In 1856, Massachusetts prohibited the adulteration of milk. Following the enactment of the British Pure Food and Drug Law in 1875, other states passed laws regulating the handling and production of food. By 1900, most states had regulations designed to protect the consumer from unsanitary and adulterated foods.

National recognition of the need for federal regulation in the United States essentially began with the appointment of Dr. Harvey W. Wiley as the chemist for the United States Department of Agriculture in 1883. He campaigned vigorously against misbranded and adulterated foods. Finally, in 1906, the Sherman Act, regulating interstate transportation of food, was passed. But Dr. Wiley resigned from the Department of Agriculture in 1912, embittered by the struggle necessary to pass the legislation.

Most manufacturers observed the Sherman Act, and adulteration with known harmful substances was rare. Economic cheating was widespread, however, and adulterants, sometimes toxic, were common in some foods. Unfortunately, the Act did not provide for legal standards or identification of foods. In 1938, the U.S. Congress passed the Food, Drug, and Cosmetic Act. This law, with its various amendments, is administered by the Food and Drug Administration (FDA), which was also organized in 1938. Some principal amendments relating to foods were the Pesticide Amendment Act of 1954 (revised 1972), the Food Additive Amendment of 1958, and the Color Additive Amendments of 1960 and 1972. These regulations affected about 60% of the food produced in the U.S. The remaining 40% remained under state regulation, which in many cases paralleled federal legislation.

In the 1958 Food Additive Amendment exceptions were made for all additives that, because of years of widespread use in foods, were "generally recognized as safe (GRAS) by experts qualified by scientific training and experience." These exceptions, numbering more than 600 items, comprise the so-called GRAS list, which has been and continues to be a subject of much controversy.

The Food Additive Amendment of 1958 also included the cancer or Delaney amendment, which stated: " . . . No additive shall be deemed to be safe if it is found to induce cancer when ingested by man or animal, or if it is found, after tests which are appropriate for the evaluation of the safety of food additives, to induce cancer in man or animal. . . ." Although the aim of the Delaney amendment was laudable, serious problems arose in the evaluation of data, protocols for testing for carcinogenicity, and the extrapolation of the data to man. These problems polarized scientific and legislative authorities, as well as the consuming public, into proponents and opponents of the measure. The controversy reerupted with each application of the Delaney amendment, such as when cyclamates were banned in 1969, red dye #2 in 1976, and when a proposed ban on saccharin was announced in 1977. The lobby for the diet food industry, and widespread concern about the loss of the only approved nonsugar sweetener among those concerned with obesity as a public health problem, led Congress to approve a specific exemption for saccharin from the provisions of the Delaney amendment. In 1996, the Food Quality Protection Act repealed the Delaney clause and set up an objective limit on lifetime cancer risks at one in a million.

In 1981 the FDA approved certain food uses of the sweetener known as aspartame, and has since permitted additional uses. The compound is a simple monomethylester of a dipeptide; per unit weight it yields about the same number of calories as sucrose (so it is not a nonnutritive agent, like saccharin or cyclamate), but it is 150–200 times sweeter than sucrose.

Recently emerging concerns about food supplies include crops based on genetically modified organisms, contamination of meat products by ingestion of animal by-products in animal feed, such as prions that cause brain wastage (mad-cow disease), residuals of pesticide and growth hormones in animal feeds, and contamination of meat products by persistent organic chemicals produced by combustion, such as dioxin and related compounds. In most cases, the extent of the risks associated with these newer concerns remain unresolved.

SCOPE OF ENVIRONMENTAL HEALTH SCIENCE

Environmental health science has evolved as a multidisciplinary endeavor that applies basic science and engineering knowledge to the recognition, evaluation, and control of physical and, chemical, and biological processes that influence human health and welfare. It is based on the premise that exposures to environmental stressors that adversely affect people can be recognized through observation of environmental quality parameters, and prevented or ameliorated by the application of source controls or, where possible, through pollution prevention.

The field of environmental health science grew and matured greatly during the second half of the twentieth century, especially in the technologically and economically more advanced countries. Objective measures of air, drinking water and food quality have been greatly advanced even while populations have grown, and resource consumption rates have grown even faster. At the same time, evidence for more long-term and potentially serious changes in environmental quality that can have profound effects on human health and welfare have emerged, including stratospheric ozone depletion, global climate change, and species extinctions.

A more thorough understanding of the progress that has been made, the challenges that remain, and the tools that are provided by the environmental health science community can help society in effectively addressing the unfinished business of traditional pollution problems and the new, more global challenges that we face as we enter the new century. The chapters that follow are intended to help graduate students and other interested individuals master the basic concepts and techniques that underlie past and future progress in advances in environmental quality and the quality of life.

For more thorough discussions of the risks associated with current human exposures to environmental chemicals and physical agents, refer to Environmental Toxicants.[5]

REFERENCES

1. Harris, R. L. Patty's Industrial Hygiene, 5th Ed., Volume I. New York: Wiley-Interscience, 2000.
2. Bingham, E., Cohnssen, B., and Powell, C. H. Patty's Toxicology, 5th Ed., Volume 1. New York: Wiley-Interscience, 2000.
3. Rom, W. N. (Ed.) Environmental and Occupational Medicine, 3rd Ed. Philadelphia: Lippincott-Raven, 1998.
4. Dhara, R. and Dhara, V. R. Bhopal-a case study of international disaster. *Int. J. Occup. Environ. Health* 1:58–69, 1995.
5. Lippmann, M. (Ed.) Environmental Toxicants-Human Exposures and Their Health Effects. New York, Wiley-Interscience, 2000.

2

Characterization of Contaminants, Environments, and Human Health

CHARACTERIZATION OF CONTAMINANTS

Concentration Units

In environmental science, confusion often arises from the use of the same or similar sounding terms that have different meanings in different contexts. This is especially true when considering the concentrations of air and water contaminants. Both are frequently expressed in terms of a ratio, such as parts per million (ppm) or parts per billion (ppb). However, when used for air contaminants, the units are molar or volume fractions, while when used for water contaminants, they are weight fractions. In order to avoid unnecessary confusion, the concentration units used in this book have appropriate subscripts: ppm_v to indicate parts per million parts of air, a volume ratio, and ppm_w, to indicate parts per million parts of water, a weight ratio. This problem is often avoided altogether by expressing all fluid contaminant concentrations as the weight of contaminant per unit volume (e.g., cubic meter, m^3, or liter, L) of fluid. In air, the units generally used are mg/m^3 or $\mu g/m^3$, while in water they are most often mg/L or μg/L.

Air Contaminants

Chemical contaminants can be dispersed in air at normal temperatures and pressures in gaseous, liquid, and solid forms. The latter two represent suspensions of particles in air, and were given the generic term *aerosols* by Gibbs[1] on the basis of analogy to the term hydrosol, a term already in use to describe disperse systems in water. On the other hand, gases and vapors, which are present as discrete molecules, form true solutions in air. Particles consisting of moderate to high vapor-pressure materials tend to evaporate rapidly, since those small enough to remain suspended in air for more than a few minutes (smaller than about 10 μm) have large surface-to-volume ratios. Evaporation is also enhanced by the Kelvin effect arising from the interaction of surface tension with the curvature of the droplet surface. Some materials with relatively low vapor pressures can have appreciable fractions in both the vapor and aerosol forms simultaneously, and are sometimes referred to as semivolatiles.

Gases and vapors

Once dispersed in air, contaminant gases and vapors generally form mixtures so dilute that their physical properties, such as density, viscosity, enthalpy, etc., are indistinguishable from those of clean air. Such mixtures may be considered to follow ideal gas-law relationships. There is no practical difference between a gas and a vapor, except that the latter is generally considered to be the gaseous phase of a substance that is normally a solid or liquid at room temperature. While dispersed in the air, all gaseous molecules of a given compound are essentially equivalent in their size and capture probabilities by ambient surfaces, respiratory tract surfaces, and contaminant collectors or samplers.

Aerosols

Aerosols, being dispersions of particles in air, have the very significant additional variable of particle size. Size affects particle motion and, hence, the probabilities for physical phenomena, such as coagulation, dispersion, sedimentation, impaction onto surfaces, interfacial phenomena, and light-scattering properties. It is not possible to characterize a given particle by a single size parameter. For example, a particle's aerodynamic properties depend on density and shape as well as linear dimensions, while the effective size for maximal light-scattering is dependent on refractive index and shape.

In some special cases, all of the particles within an aerosol are essentially the same in size. Such aerosols are considered to be monodisperse. Examples are natural pollens and some laboratory-generated aerosols. More typically, aerosols are composed of particles of many different sizes, and hence are called heterodisperse or polydisperse. Different aerosols have different degrees of size dispersion. It is, therefore, necessary to specify at least two parameters in characterizing aerosol size: a measure of central tendency, such as a mean or median, and a measure of dispersion, such as an arithmetic or geometric standard deviation.

Particles generated by a single source or process generally have diameters following a log-normal distribution, i.e., the logarithms of their individual diameters have a Gaussian distribution. In this case, the most appropriate measure of dispersion is the geometric standard deviation, which is the ratio of the 84.1 percentile size to the 50 percentile size (Fig. 2–1). When more than one source of particles is significant, the resulting mixed aerosol will usually not follow a single log-normal distribution, and it may be necessary to describe it by the sum of several distributions.

Particle characteristics

There are many properties of particles, other than their linear size, that can greatly influence their airborne behavior and their effects on the environment and health. These include:

Surface. For spherical particles, the surface area varies as the square of the diameter. However, for an aerosol of given mass concentration, the total aerosol surface increases with decreasing particle size. Airborne particles have much greater ratios of external surface to volume than do bulk materials and, therefore, the particles can dissolve or participate in surface reactions to a much greater extent than would massive samples of the same materials. Furthermore, for nonspherical solid particles or aggregate particles, the ratio of surface to volume is increased, and for particles with internal cracks or pores, the internal surface area can even be greater than the external area.

Volume. Particle volume varies as the cube of diameter; therefore, the few largest particles in a polydisperse aerosol tend to dominate its volume or mass concentration.

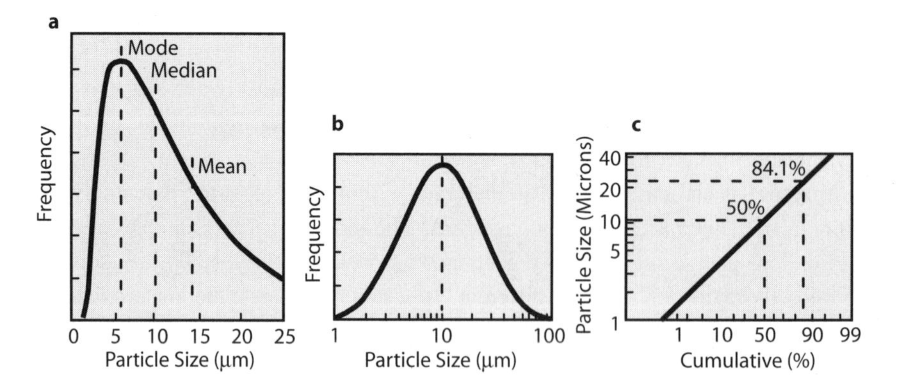

Figure 2–1. Particle size distribution data. **(a)** Plotted on linear coordinates **(b)** Plotted on a logarithmic-size scale **(c)** In practice, logarithmic probability coordinates are used to display the percent of particles less than a specific size versus that size. The geometric standard deviation (s_g) of the distribution is equal to the 84.16% size/50% size.

Shape. A particle's shape affects its aerodynamic drag, as well as its surface area, and therefore its motion and deposition probabilities.

Density. A particle's velocity due to gravitational or inertial forces increases as the square root of its density.

Aerodynamic Diameter. The diameter of a unit-density sphere having the same terminal settling velocity as the particle under consideration is equal to its aerodynamic diameter. Terminal settling velocity is the steady-state velocity of a particle that is falling under the influence of gravity and fluid resistance. Aerodynamic diameter is determined by the actual particle size, the particle density, and an aerodynamic shape factor determined by its drag (fluid resistance).

Types of aerosols

Some of the terminology used for aerosols of various sizes from a variety of sources are indicated in Figure 2–2a, and their concentration ranges are indicated in Figure 2–2b. Aerosols are generally classified in terms of their processes of formation. While the following classification is neither precise, nor comprehensive, it is commonly used and accepted in the industrial hygiene and air pollution fields:

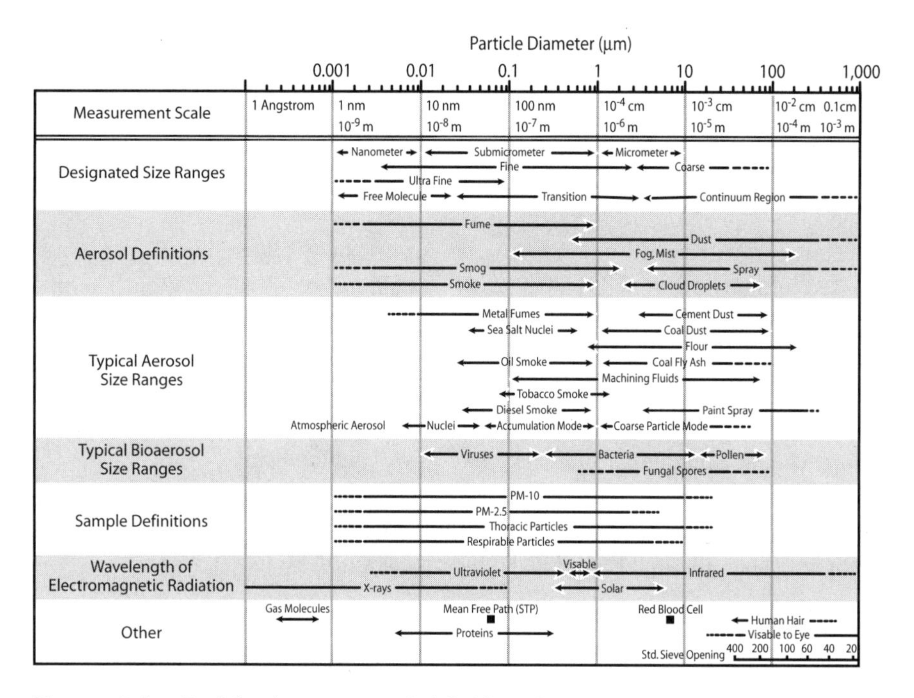

FIGURE 2–2a. Particle size ranges and definitions for aerosols. (*Source*: Hinds, W.C. *Aerosol Technology*, 2nd Ed., New York: Wiley, 1999, p. 9.)

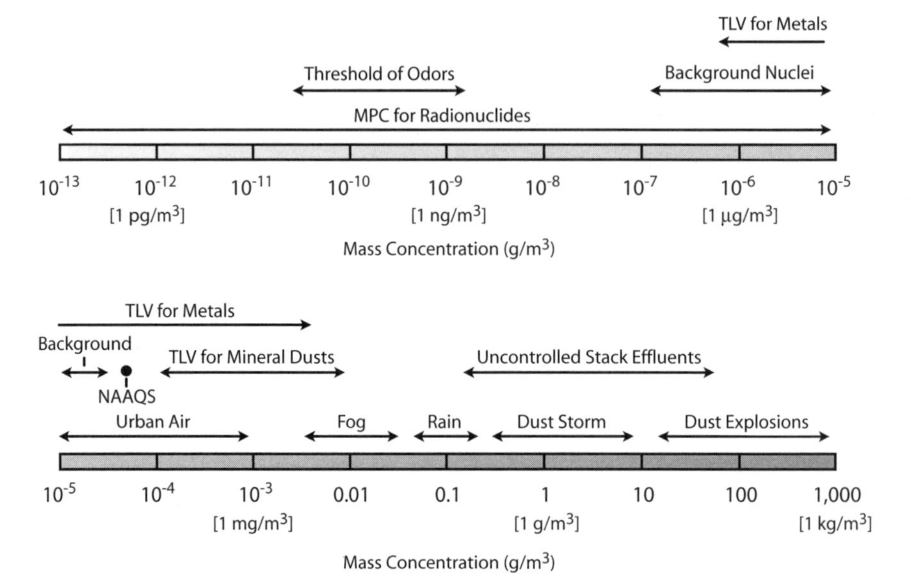

FIGURE 2–2b. Range of aerosol concentrations. (*Source*: Hinds, W.C. *Aerosol Technology*, 2nd Ed., New York: Wiley, 1999, p. 11.)

Dust. An aerosol formed by mechanical subdivision of bulk material into airborne fines having the same chemical composition. A general term for the process of mechanical subdivision is comminution, and it occurs in operations such as crushing, grinding, drilling, and blasting. Dust particles are generally solid and irregular in shape, and have diameters greater than 1 μm.

Fume. An aerosol of solid particles formed by condensation of vapors released into air at elevated temperatures by combustion or sublimation. The primary particles are generally very small (less than 0.1 μm), and have spherical or characteristic crystalline shapes. They may be chemically identical to the parent material, or they may be composed of an oxidation product, such as a metal oxide. Since they may be formed in high number concentration, they often rapidly coagulate, forming aggregate clusters of low overall density.

Smoke. An aerosol formed by combustion of organic materials. The particles are generally liquid droplets with diameters of less than 0.5 μm.

Mist. A droplet aerosol formed by mechanical shearing of a bulk liquid, for example, atomization, nebulization, bubbling, spraying; or by condensation. The droplet size can cover a very large range, usually from about 2 μm to greater than 50 μm.

Fog. A water aerosol formed by condensation of water vapor onto atmospheric nuclei at high relative humidities. The droplet sizes are generally greater than 1 μm.

Smog. A popular term for a pollution aerosol derived from a combination of smoke and fog. The term is also commonly applied to light-scattering aerosols formed by photochemical reactions.

Haze. A submicrometer-sized aerosol of hygroscopic particles that take up water vapor at relatively low relative humidities.

Ultrafine Mode. Also known as Aitken or condensation nuclei (CN), very small atmospheric particles (mostly smaller than 0.05 μm) formed by combustion processes and by chemical conversion from gaseous precursors.

Fine Mode. A term given to the particles in the ambient atmosphere that range from 0.1 to about 2.5 μm. These particles generally are spherical, have liquid surfaces, and form by coagulation and condensation of smaller (ultrafine) particles that derive from gaseous precursors. The characteristics of fine mode aerosols are summarized in Table 2–1 and depicted graphically in Figure 2–3.

Coarse Particle Mode. Ambient air particles larger than about 2.5 μm, and generally formed by mechanical processes and surface dust resuspension. The characteristics of coarse mode ambient aerosols are described in Figure 2–3 and Table 2–1.

Aerosol characteristics

Aerosols have integral properties that depend upon the concentration and size distribution of the particles. In mathematical terms, these properties can be expressed in terms of certain constants or "moments" of the size distribution. Some integral properties, such as light-scattering ability or electrical charge, depend on other particle parameters as well. Some of the important integral properties are:

Number Concentration. The total number of airborne particles per unit volume of air, without distinction as to their sizes, is the zeroth moment of the size distribution. In current practice, instruments are available that can count the numbers of particles of all sizes from about 0.005 to 50 μm. In many specific applications, such as fiber counting for airborne asbestos, a more restricted size range may be specified.

TABLE 2–1. Comparison of Ambient Fine and Coarse Mode Particles

	FINE MODE	COARSE MODE
Formed from	Gases	Large solids/droplets
Formed by	Chemical reaction; nucleation; condensation; coagulation; evaporation of fog and cloud droplets in which gases have dissolved and reacted.	Mechanical disruption (e.g., crushing, grinding, abrasion of surfaces); evaporation of sprays; suspension of dusts.
Composed of	Sulfate, $SO_4^{=}$; nitrate, NO_3^-; ammonium, NH_4^+; hydrogen ion, H^+; elemental carbon; organic compounds (e.g., PAHs, PNAs); metals (e.g., Pb, Cd, V, Ni, Cu, Zn, Mn, Fe); particle-bound water.	Resuspended dusts (e.g., soil dust, street dust); coal and oil fly ash; metal oxides of crustal elements (Si, Al, Ti, Fe); $CaCO_3$, NaCl, sea salt; pollen, mold spores; plant/animal fragments; tire wear debris.
Solubility	Largely soluble, hygroscopic and deliquescent.	Largely insoluble and non-hygroscopic.
Sources	Combustion of coal, oil, gasoline, diesel, wood; atmospheric transformation products of NO_x, SO_2, and organic compounds including biogenic species (e.g., terpenes); high temperature processes, smelters, steel mills, etc.	Resuspension of industrial dust and soil tracked onto roads; suspension from disturbed soil (e.g., farming, mining, unpaved roads); biological sources; construction and demolition; coal and oil combustion; ocean spray.
Lifetimes	Days to weeks	Minutes to hours
Travel Distance	100s to 1000s of kilometers	$<$ 1 to 10s of kilometers

Surface Concentration. The total external surface area of all the particles in the aerosol, which is the second moment of the size distribution, may be of interest when surface catalysis or gas adsorption processes are of concern. Aerosol surface is one factor affecting light-scatter and atmospheric-visibility reductions.

Volume Concentration. The total volume of all the particles, which is the third moment of the size distribution, is of little intrinsic interest in itself. It is however, closely related to the mass concentration, which for many environmental effects is the primary parameter of interest.

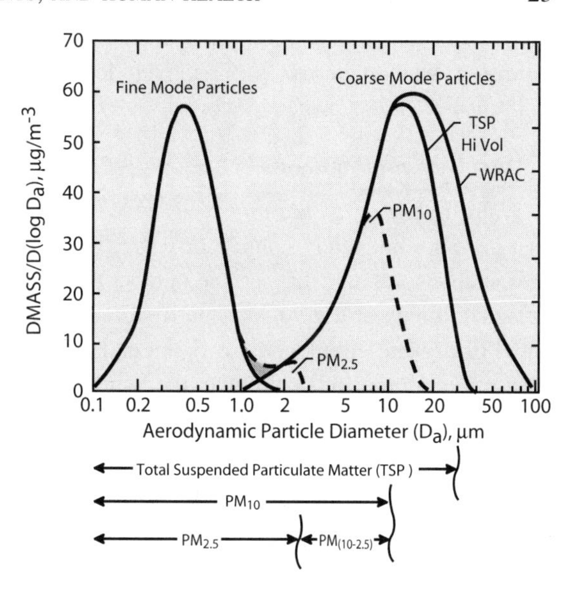

FIGURE 2–3. A multimodal mass distribution of ambient air particulate matter and the components that are collected by size-selective aerosol samplers.

Mass Concentration. The total mass of all the particles in the aerosol is frequently of interest. The mass of a particle is the product of its volume and density. If all of the particles have the same density, the total mass concentration is simply the volume concentration times the density. In some cases, such as "size-selective" dust sampling for health hazard assessments,[2] the parameter of interest is the mass concentration over a restricted range of aerodynamic particle size. In this application, particles too large to deposit in the target region of concern in the human respiratory tract are excluded from the integral.

Dustfall. The mass of particles depositing from an aerosol onto a unit surface per unit time is proportional to the fifth moment of the size distribution. Dustfall has long been of interest in air pollution control because it provides an indication of the soiling properties of the aerosol.

Light-Scatter. The ability of airborne particles to scatter light and cause a visibility reduction is well known. Total light-scatter can be determined by integrating the aerosol surface distribution with the appropriate scattering coefficients.

Water Contaminants

Chemical contaminants can be found in water in solution or as hydrosols; the latter are small immiscible solid or liquid particles with unipolar charges in a stable suspension. An aqueous suspension of liquid particles is generally called an emulsion. Many materials with relatively low aqueous solubility can be found in both dissolved and suspended forms.

Dissolved contaminants

Water is known as the universal solvent. While there are many compounds that are not completely soluble in water, there are few that do not have some measurable solubility. In fact, the number of chemical contaminants that can be detected in natural waters is primarily a function of the sensitivity of the analyses. For organic compounds in rivers and lakes, as the limits of detection decrease by an order of magnitude, the numbers of compounds detected increase by an order of magnitude, so that one might expect to find at least 10^{-12} gm/L (approximately 10^{10} molecules per liter) of each of the million organic compounds reported in the literature. Similar considerations undoubtedly apply to inorganic chemicals as well.

Dissolved solids

Water-quality criteria generally include a nonspecific parameter called "dissolved solids." However, it is customary to exclude natural mineral salts, such as sodium chloride, from this classification. Also, water criteria for specific toxic chemicals dissolved in water are frequently exceeded without an excessive total dissolved-solids content.

Dissolved gases

Compounds dissolved in water may also exist in the gaseous phase at normal temperatures and pressures. Some of these, such as hydrogen sulfide and ammonia, which are generated by anaerobic decay processes, are toxicants.

Oxygen is the most critical of the dissolved gases with respect to water quality. It is essential to most higher aquatic life forms and is needed for the oxidation of most of the organic chemical contaminants to more innocuous forms. Thus, a critical parameter of water quality is the concentration of dissolved oxygen (DO). Another important parameter is the extent of the oxygen "demand" associated with contaminants in the water. The most commonly used index of oxygen demand is the 5-day BOD (biochemical oxygen demand after 5 days of incubation). Another is the COD (chemical oxygen demand). The basic oxygen demand parameters are defined in Table 2–2.

Suspended particles

A nonspecific water-quality parameter that is widely used is "suspended solids." The stability of aqueous suspensions depends on particle size, density, and charge distributions. The fate of suspended particles depends on a number of factors, and particles can dissolve, grow, coagulate, or be ingested by various

TABLE 2–2. Dissolved Oxygen and Oxygen Demand Parameters

BOD	Biochemical or biological oxygen demand. The oxygen consumed by a waste through bacterial action.
COD	Chemical oxygen demand. The oxygen consumed by a waste through chemical oxidation.
TOD	The theoretical oxygen demand required to completely oxidize a compound to CO_2, H_2O, PO_4^{-3}, SO_4^{-2}, and NO_3^-
5-day BOD	The BOD consumed by a waste in 5 days.
Ult, BOD	The ultimate BOD consumed by a waste in an infinite time.
IOD	The "Immediate" oxygen demand consumed in 15 minutes (without using chemical oxidizers or bacteria).
DO	Dissolved oxygen (A "negative" DO is a positive IOD).

BOD, biochemical oxygen demand; COD, chemical oxygen demand; TOD, theoretical oxygen demand; Ult, ultimate; IOD, immediate oxygen demand; DO, dissolved oxygen.

life forms in the water. They can become "floating solids" or part of an oil film, or they can fall to the bottom to become part of the sediments.

There are many kinds of suspended particles in natural waters, and not all of them are contaminants. Any moving water will have currents that cause bottom sediments to become resuspended. Also, natural runoff will carry soil and organic debris into lakes and streams. In any industrialized area, such sediment and surface debris will always contain some chemicals considered to be contaminants. However, a large proportion of the mass of such suspended solids would usually be "natural," and would not be considered as contaminants.

Suspended particles can have densities that are less than, equal to, or greater than that of the water, so that the particles can rise as well as fall. Furthermore, the effective density of particles can be reduced by the attachment of gas bubbles. Such bubbles form in water when the water becomes saturated and cannot hold any more of the gas in solution. The solubility of gases in water varies inversely with temperature. For example, oxygen saturation of fresh water is 14.2 mg/L at 0°C and 7.5 mg/L at 30°C, while in sea water the corresponding values are 11.2 and 6.1 mg/L.

Colloids

Colloids are extremely stable suspensions. They have a very small, uniform particle size and possess unipolar charges that cause the individual particles to repel one another. The particles are so small, on the order of 0.01 μm, that they pass through most filters. For practical purposes, colloids behave like true solutions, and are usually not measured as suspended solids in most assays.

Oil and floating solids

Oil, grease, and other organic immiscible liquids can exist as discrete droplets or globules, or can coalesce on the surface as a film. In extreme cases, they can produce a fire hazard. In lesser amounts, such films can: *(1)* block the absorption of atmospheric oxygen; *(2)* retard photosynthesis in aquatic plants and thereby reduce oxygen production; *(3)* coat and destroy algae and other plankton; and *(4)* make the waters unfit for fish life, swimming, and other recreational uses. Floating solids can simply be an aesthetic blight, or, if they contain oxygen-consuming or toxic materials, can contribute to the degradation of the water quality.

Sediments

Particles that fall to the bottom of a body of water remain accessible to the water for partial dissolution and periodic resuspension during storms and flow surges. If there is enough sedimentary fallout relative to the depth of the overlying water, the sediments can gradually reduce the depth of the water and thereby affect its surface velocity and flow patterns. Finally, the sediment layer can become anaerobic and, therefore, a source of toxic compounds that can diffuse into the overlying water.

Food Contaminants

Chemical contaminants of almost every conceivable kind can be found in most types of human food. Food can acquire these contaminants at any of several stages in its production, harvesting, processing, packaging, transportation, storage, cooking, and serving. In addition, there are many naturally occurring toxicants in foods, as well as compounds that can become toxicants upon conversion by chemical reactions with other constituents or additives, or by thermal or microbiological conversion reactions during processing, storage, or handling.

Each food product has its own natural history. Most foods are formed by selective metabolic processes of plants and animals. In forming tissue, these processes can act to either enrich or diminish incorporation of specific toxicants that are present in the environment. For animal products, where the flesh of interest in foods was derived from the consumption of other life forms, there are likely to be several stages of biological discrimination and, therefore, large differences between contaminant concentrations in the ambient air and/or water, and the concentrations within the flesh of the animals.

Since both natural and anthropogenic toxicants are present in almost all foods, it is important to distinguish between toxicity and hazard. Toxicity is an intrinsic property of the chemical, while hazard is the capacity to produce injury under the circumstances of exposure. A hazard occurs when the inherent toxicity of the chemical is expressed, and is dependent on many factors, especially on the amount ingested.

Natural toxicants

No segment of the environment to which humans are exposed is as chemically complex as food. Food products contain both nutrient and nonnutrient components and, until quite recently, relatively little attention was paid to the latter. The humble potato, a food staple for many millions of people, contains more than 100 nonnutrient chemical substances, including solanine alkaloids, oxalic acid, arsenic, tannins, and nitrates. Table 2–3 lists some of the toxic compounds present naturally in common plant foods.

Despite the presence of a multitude of toxic chemicals in the diets of normal humans, there is usually little hazard because the consumption of each is relatively low. Problems generally arise from an excessive dependence on a limited number of foods during an extended period of time. For example, people consuming large amounts of cabbage have developed goiter, and people with extended daily consumption of a half gallon of tomato juice developed lycopenia, a skin discoloration.

While a balanced diet helps to keep the level of each natural toxicant below hazardous levels, it may also provide opportunities for interactions between toxicants. For example, the toxic effects of cadmium are reduced by an accompanying elevated level of zinc, and copper reduces the toxic effects of molybdenum. On the other hand, not all such interactions may be beneficial.

Natural contaminants

Foods can be contaminated by a variety of natural processes not involving either direct or indirect human intervention. Such processes can result in contamination by: *(1)* products of decay and decomposition that are generated between the growth of the food and its consumption; *(2)* microbiological and animal pests and/or their residues, wastes and metabolites; *(3)* chemical element congeners of normal nutrient materials, which become incorporated into the food during growth, such as excessive levels of nitrates, mercury, selenium, etc., taken up from soils having high concentrations due to geochemical anomalies. As an example of natural contaminants, Table 2–4 lists some mycotoxins that are produced by molds growing on common plant foods.

Anthropogenic contaminants

Human activities can greatly increase the concentrations of the contaminants already present naturally in food, and can also introduce entirely new ones. Some of these latter materials, such as pesticides, are applied intentionally during the growth of the food, and become contaminants to the extent that they persist as residues (within or on the surfaces of foods) long after their intended function has been completed. Others, such as the polychlorinated biphenyls (PCBs), are completely inadvertent food contaminants, since they were never intentionally

TABLE 2–3. Some Intrinsic Components of Food of Known Toxicity

COMPOUNDS	FOOD SOURCES	SUSPECTED OR KNOWN TOXIC ENDPOINTS
Solanine, chaconine	White potato[a]	Nervous system
HCN (hydrogen cyanide)	Many plants, as adducts, released when plant tissue is damaged	Hemoglobin, cyanosis
Vasoactive amines	Pineapple, banana, plum	Cardiovascular system
Xanthines (caffeine, theophylline, theobromine)	Coffee[b], tea, cocoa, kola nut	CNS stimulation, other biochemical changes, cardiac effects
Myristicin	Nutmeg, mace	Nervous system
Carotatoxin	Carrots, celery	Nervous system
Synephrine	Lemons	Vasoconstriction
Hemagglutinins (protein)	Soybeans, other legumes	Agglutination of red blood cells
Norepinephrine	Bananas	Vasoconstriction
Lathyrus toxins	Legumes of genus *Lathyrus*	Lathyrism (neurological disease)
Tannins	Tea, coffee, cocoa	Carcinogenic
Safrole and other methylenedioxy benzenes	Oil of sassafras, cinnamon, nutmeg, anise, parsley, celery, black pepper	Carcinogenic (not all members of the class)
5- and 8-Methoxypsoralen (light activated)	Parsley, parsnip, celery	Carcinogenic, with UV light
Ethyl acrylate	Pineapple	Carcinogenic in animals
Estragole	Basil, fennel	Carcinogenic in animals
Goitrin[c]	Cabbage, turnips	Antithyroid activity

[a]Solanaceous glycoalkaloids are present in other Solanaceae, including eggplant and tomato.

[b]Coffee contains more than 600 compounds in addition to caffeine. This is typical of natural foods. Included are many different classes of organic compounds.

[c]This is not present in the original plant but is formed by enzymatic reactions from nontoxic precursors following harvest, during processing, or following digestion.

CNS, central nervous system.

Table 2–4. Some Mycotoxin Contaminants of Food

MYCOTOXIN	GENUS OF PRODUCING MOLD	TYPICAL SUBSTRATE	TOXIC EFFECT
Aflatoxin B_1	*Aspergillus*	Peanuts, oil seeds, corn	Carcinogen
Ochratoxin A	*Aspergillus*	Grains	Kidney toxin
Sterigmatocystin	*Aspergillus*	Grains	Carcinogen
Patulin	*Penicillium*	Apples	Carcinogen
Cyclopiazonic acid	*Penicillium*	Grains	Tremors, paralysis
Luteoskyrin	*Penicillium*	Rice	Liver toxin
Islandotoxin	*Penicillium*	Rice	Carcinogen

applied to foods. However, they have been widely used in consumer products, have become ubiquitous environmental contaminants, and reached excessive levels in some fish and birds through biological concentration processes.

Air contaminants

Contaminants in the ambient air may produce pervasive contamination of foods, but they are not likely to result in acute intoxications. The atmosphere is a continuous envelope reaching essentially all of the human environment and is capable of rapidly diluting the contaminants discharged into it.

Water contaminants

Contamination of food via water takes place along several distinct pathways. One is by the consumption of fish and shellfish that have taken up chemicals from the water or from lower aquatic life forms. Another is via the consumption of fruits and grains that took up contaminants from irrigation waters. A more indirect path is the consumption of animal products from livestock consuming contaminated irrigation waters, and the crops grown with these waters. Finally, residual contaminants in drinking waters can reach us either directly or through transfers from water used in food processing and/or cooking.

Pesticide residues

Chemical pesticides are applied to crops and soil to increase the quantity and quality of the harvest. They may also be applied to the harvested food during transportation and/or storage to minimize spoilage and losses. Some of the specific residue limits (tolerances) established by the FDA for the major pesticides are listed in Table 2–5. When these limits are exceeded, the foods involved are subject to seizure and withdrawal from the market.

Pesticide residues in and on foods have resulted in readily measurable human body burdens. Since most of the chlorinated hydrocarbon pesticides are known or suspected carcinogens, there is a great concern and effort devoted to the mon-

Table 2–5. Some Food Contaminants of Industrial Origin[a]

CHEMICAL	MAJOR SOURCES	FOODS SUBJECT TO CONTAMINATION
Arsenic	Smelting, mining	Many, including fish[b]
Cadmium	Smelting, sewage sludge	Grains, vegetables, meat
Lead	Smelting, mining, solder in can seams, lead glazed pottery and ceramic ware, automobile exhaust	Several, including acidic foods coming into contact with lead ceramic ware and pottery
Mercury, alkyl mercurials	Chlorine, soda lye manufacturing	Fish
Aldrin, dieldrin, DDT, mirex	Pesticide usage[c]	Fish, milk, eggs
Polychlorinated biphenyls	Electrical industry	Fish, human milk
Polychlorinated benzodioxins	Impurities in certain chemicals; incineration; bleached paper manufacturing	Fish, milk, beef fat

[a]Note that the metals listed are also present in foods because of natural occurrence.

[b]Most of the arsenic in food appears to be organically bound. These forms are substantially less toxic than inorganic arsenic. EPA considers the latter form to be carcinogenic by ingestion.

[c]Pesticide residues in foods for which no official tolerance was ever granted, or was rescinded, are considered contaminants.

itoring and control of their residues in the food supply, and there are continuing efforts to ban more of them from agricultural usage.

Residues of drugs and growth stimulants

Veterinary drugs and growth stimulants are given to domestic fowl and animals to increase the quantity and/or quality of the meat, and to control epizootic disease. They may be applied by injection, implantation, or ingestion, and some fraction may remain as a detectable residue in the flesh, or in the eggs or milk products produced by the animals.

A chemical of particular concern in previous decades was the artificial hormone, diethylstilbestrol (DES), which was a widely used growth stimulant. Its use as a human drug in high doses has been implicated in a higher-than-normal cervical cancer incidence among the daughters of the women treated. Its presence at low levels in meat, therefore, raised the potential of an increase in cancer among the general population.

Concern has also been expressed about residues of antibiotics in meat, resulting from their use to control disease. The residues may be capable of causing adverse reactions among allergic individuals. Also, continued ingestion of low levels in foods may lead to a reduced potency when the antibiotics are used therapeutically in people at a later time, and/or to the selection of drug-resistant strains of animal and human pathogens.

Packaging material residues

Packaged foods can take up chemicals from the materials used to package or contain them. Problems may arise in canned foods; for example, condensed milk was formerly contaminated by lead in the solder used to seal the cans. More recently, most of the focus of concern has centered on plastic packaging materials, especially the polymeric materials such as polyvinyl chloride (PVC) and acrylonitrile. The polymers themselves have long interlocking-chain structures and are not considered toxic. However, the polymers are always contaminated, to some extent, with unpolymerized monomers, and some of these are known carcinogens.

Accidents and misuse

Acute chemical intoxications via food are generally attributable to accidental cross-contamination of foods and industrial chemicals or pesticides in transportation or storage, mislabeling by manufacturers, or by a failure to understand or follow label instructions.

There have been many cases of cross-contamination between bread flour and pesticides, which have led to acute poisonings and some deaths. A notable example of mislabelling occurred in Michigan in 1975, when a fire retardant containing polybrominated biphenyls (PBBs) was mistakenly bagged in containers intended for a cattle feed supplement. The insidious poisoning of the cattle that resulted was not immediately recognized, and a large number of farmers, their families, and people in the general population were severely contaminated and suffered health effects from consuming meat and milk from these animals.

There have been numerous cases of mercury intoxication resulting from the direct consumption of bread made from seed grains treated with mercurial pesticides. Some occurred because the grain was not properly labelled. Others have occurred when the labels were not read, sometimes because they were in the wrong language, or because the people involved were illiterate.

Finally, contamination sometimes has resulted from a major release due to an explosion or other industrial accident. An example is the factory explosion in Seveso, Italy, in July 1976, which spread 2–3 kg of the highly toxic chemical dioxin downwind over a considerable distance. The extent of the contamination was not disclosed to the farmers affected and, therefore, domestic animals grazed on contaminated ground, and contaminated milk and eggs reached many people.

Food additives

Food additives are not contaminants, in the sense that they are intentionally applied to food products for a particular purpose. At the time their usages were approved, there presumably was no evidence that they would produce significant adverse effects. However, in recent years, many food additives have been banned by the FDA, or are being reevaluated because of evidence that they were capable of producing cancer in laboratory animals. Notable examples that attracted considerable public attention in the mid-1970s were the food coloring dye known as red #2, the artificial sweetener saccharin, and the nitrites used to preserve red meat. The latter can combine with secondary amines in the digestive tract to form carcinogenic nitrosamines.

The controversy about food additive safety, and the occasional banning of food additives on the basis of evidence for carcinogenic potential, has led to understandable confusion and concern among the general public about the safety of food additives that are still approved and has resulted, in part, in the proliferation of "natural food" retail stores, cooperatives, and restaurants. It has also led to an increased effort by the FDA to more thoroughly evaluate the safety of commonly used food additives.

Excessive use of food additives may cause increases in diseases other than cancer. Sodium chloride has been associated with human hypertension, while an excessive daily intake of phosphates can lead to premature cessation of bone growth in children.

Many processed foods are fortified with vitamins. When these are added to the vitamins naturally occurring in foods, and to the vitamins ingested in tablets or as liquids, large daily intakes may occur. Excessive intakes of vitamins A and D in particular have caused a variety of acute and chronic health effects. However, it is important to remember that vitamin deficiencies cause many more health problems than does excessive ingestion.

Special problems

Genetic manipulations of plants to introduce more desirable properties and to increase yields may result in alterations of their levels of essential nutrients and natural toxicants. Common plants, such as tomatoes and potatoes, which have toxic foliage, need special attention with respect to altered toxicant levels. On the other hand, selective breeding can be employed to reduce the concentrations of toxic substances in natural foods. For example, lima beans having low cyanogenetic glycoside content have been developed in order to minimize their cyanide-generating capacity.

While toxicants in food represent public health problems, the more important dangers associated with food consumption arise from other considerations. The major problem is undoubtedly overeating, especially of foods rich in fats and sugars, resulting in obesity, cardiovascular disease, hypertension, diabetes, and dental caries. Problems also arise frequently in special populations, such as teenagers, who may consume large amounts of "junk" food, resulting in unbalanced diets that permit the development of deficiency diseases.

CHARACTERIZATION OF ENVIRONMENTS

The abiotic, or nonliving, environment can be divided into three components: *(1)* the atmosphere, or air; *(2)* the hydrosphere, or water; and *(3)* the lithosphere, or earth's crust. The aggregate of all of the life forms within all these three components is termed the biosphere.

Although these components are often separated in terms of many discussions in this book, it is important to realize that transport of contaminants takes place within and between all media. Thus, release of a contaminant into one component does not insure that it will remain there; contamination must be considered in terms of the environment as a whole. Eventually, the contaminants are chemically transformed or are physically trapped into a permanent storage site. The ultimate disposition site or removal mechanism for a contaminant is known as a sink.

Characteristics of the Atmosphere

The earth's atmosphere is simple in some respects, and complex in others. It is relatively uniform in composition with respect to its major mass components (oxygen and nitrogen), yet extremely variable in some minor components, such as water vapor and ozone (O_3), which play major roles in its heat and radiation fluxes. It has a complex structure based on temperature gradients. This structure governs its mixing characteristics and the buildup of contaminants, yet is usually invisible to us, except when light-scattering particles suspended in the air make it visible.

Structure of the atmosphere

The structure of the atmosphere, while largely invisible, is real and of major importance to the dilution and dispersion of contaminants. It is governed by the lapse rate, which is the rate of change of air temperature with height above the ground. The changes in temperature and pressure with height are shown in Figure 2–4.

The lowest of the atmospheric layers is the troposphere. It contains about 75% of the mass of the atmosphere, and almost all of its moisture. It extends to a height that varies from about 9 km at the poles to about 15 km at the equator, and it has an average lapse rate of about −6.5°C/km. The boundary between the

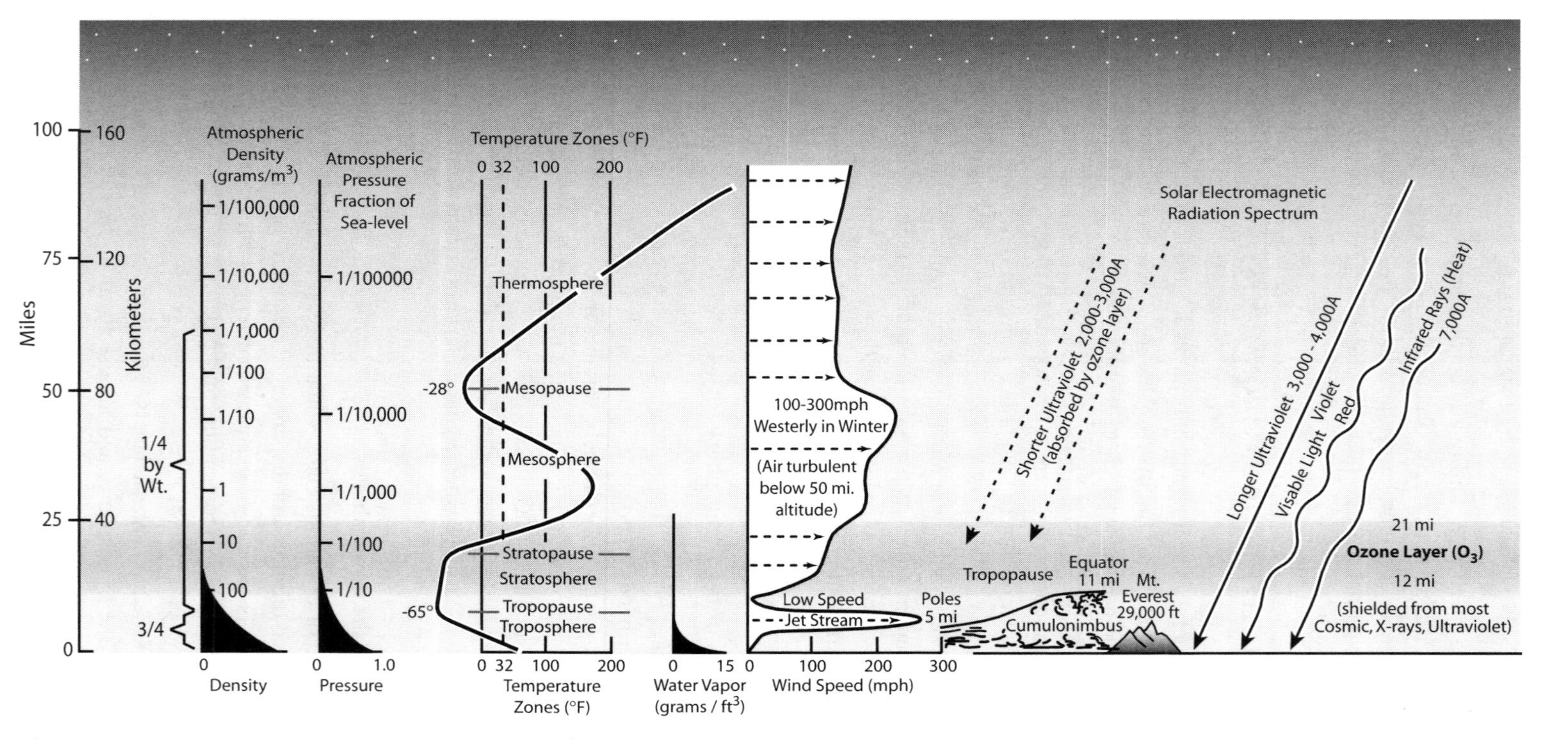

FIGURE 2–4. Physical properties of the atmosphere.

troposphere and the next layer, the stratosphere, is known as the tropopause. The stratosphere contains essentially all of the remainder of the mass of the atmosphere; it is nearly isothermal (the temperature does not change with altitude) in lower regions, and shows a temperature increase with height (inversion) in the upper regions.

Chemical composition

The major constituents of dry air at ground level are nitrogen (N_2) at 78.1% by volume, oxygen (O_2) at 21.0%, and argon (Ar) at 0.9%. Carbon dioxide (CO_2) is present at about 360 ppm_v (0.036%), neon (Ne) at 18 ppm_v, helium (He) at about 5 ppm_v, and methane (CH_4) at about 1.7 ppm_v. All other gases are present at less than 1 ppm_v.

About 2% of the total mass of the lower atmosphere is water vapor (H_2O), but the concentration is extremely variable in both space and time. In general, the warmer portions of the atmosphere contain more water vapor. The water vapor content becomes lower with increasing altitude and with increasing latitude. Water vapor plays a critical role in governing the earth's heat exchange and the motion of the atmosphere, due to its high heat capacity, absorption of infrared radiation, and heat of vaporization. Further effects attributable to atmospheric water result when the air motions create clouds, i.e., aerosols of water droplets, in which the energy received as sunshine in one place is liberated as the latent heat of vaporization in another.

Earth-atmosphere energy balance

The sun is the source of essentially all of the energy that reaches the earth. Radiant energy from the sun covers the entire electromagnetic spectrum. However, most of it occurs in and near the visible portion, i.e., wave lengths from 0.4 μm to 0.7 μm (Fig. 2–5).

Of the incoming radiant energy, about 30%–50% is scattered back towards space, reflected by the atmosphere, due primarily to clouds and to some extent, by solid particles, or by the earth's surface. On a global basis, the average reflectivity, or albedo, of the earth's surface and atmosphere is about 35%. The actual albedo of any specific surface is highly dependent upon the particular area and its characteristics; ice- and snow-covered polar regions have high reflectivity, while the reflectivity of oceans is relatively low, with most incident energy being absorbed.

About 20% of the incident radiant energy is absorbed as it passes through the atmosphere. Stratospheric O_3 absorbs about 1%–3%, primarily in the short-wave ultraviolet (UV) portion of the spectrum; this effectively limits further penetration to those wavelengths greater than 0.3 μm.

In the troposphere, 17%–19% of the incoming radiation is absorbed, due primarily to water vapor and secondarily to CO_2. The total atmospheric absorption

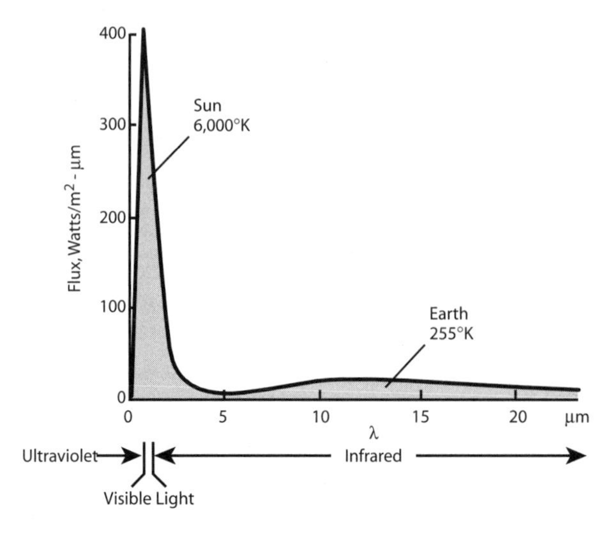

FIGURE 2–5. Emission spectra to and from the earth. The sun and earth radiate as "black bodies" having temperatures of 6000°K and 250°K respectively.

for radiant energy with wavelengths of 0.3–0.7 μm is not very large, and these effectively penetrate an essentially "transparent" atmospheric window.

In total, about 50% of the incoming solar radiation reaches the surface of the earth, and is absorbed. The surface reradiates energy through a broad range of wavelengths, but with a flat maximum in the long-wave, infrared portion of the spectrum at about 10–12 μm (Fig. 2–5). The atmosphere is nearly opaque to this radiation; most is absorbed by water vapor and droplets, and by CO_2. Some is then reradiated back to earth, or out into space. The earth-atmosphere energy balance is summarized in Figure 2–6.

By allowing effective penetration of the short-wave solar radiation, yet retaining a large fraction of the reradiated long-wave radiation, the atmosphere acts as an insulator, keeping heat near the surface of the earth. This phenomenon is known as the "greenhouse effect." The progressive (secular) increase in atmospheric CO_2, an important greenhouse gas, contributes to climate change on a global scale.

The solar flux, which is the intensity of radiation as measured by the amount of energy transferred per unit area per unit time, decreases with increasing latitude. For example, the average mid-winter solar flux is over 800 cal/cm^2/day at the equator, and less than 200 cal/cm^2/day at 50°N. latitude. On the other hand, the flux of infrared radiation from the atmosphere to space only drops from about 470 cal/cm^2/day at the equator to about 400 at 50°N. The average radiation into space must equal that absorbed from the sun. Thus, it follows that a substantial amount of energy must flow from the tropics towards the poles within the tro-

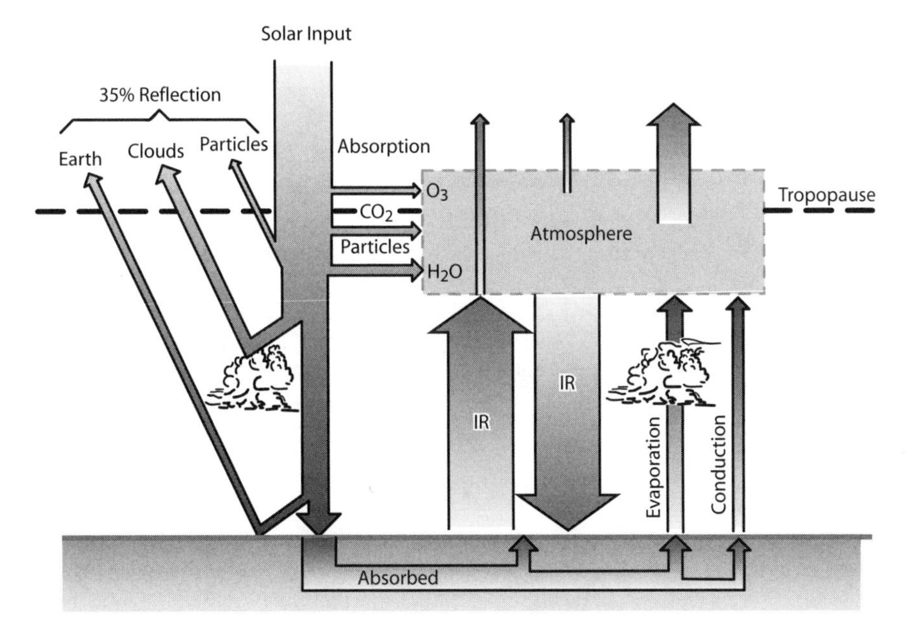

FIGURE 2–6. Earth-atmosphere energy balance.

posphere. This flow of energy is accomplished primarily by systems of warm air currents toward the poles and cool currents toward the tropics, and partially by corresponding ocean currents.

Circulation of the atmosphere

At altitudes above about 500 m, the atmosphere exhibits a general pattern of circulation characterized by several dominant wind systems. These are the trade winds, the jet stream or midlatitudinal westerlies, and the polar easterlies. Below 500 m, the surface of the earth exerts effects of varying degrees upon air circulation. A diagram of the general circulation of the atmosphere is shown in Figure 2–7.

Throughout the troposphere, there is a rapid decrease in temperature towards the poles. One result of this is a high-speed wind known as the subtropical jet stream. As seen in Figure 2–8, the tropopause is discontinuous in the region of the jet stream; it is through these "gaps" in the mid latitudes that much of the circulation occurs between the stratosphere and the troposphere. In addition to this general circulation, the atmosphere has secondary and small-scale circulation patterns. Secondary circulations are exemplified by the migratory high- and low-pressure areas seen in daily weather charts. Examples of small-scale circulations are land-sea breezes, mountain-valley winds, and thunderstorms.

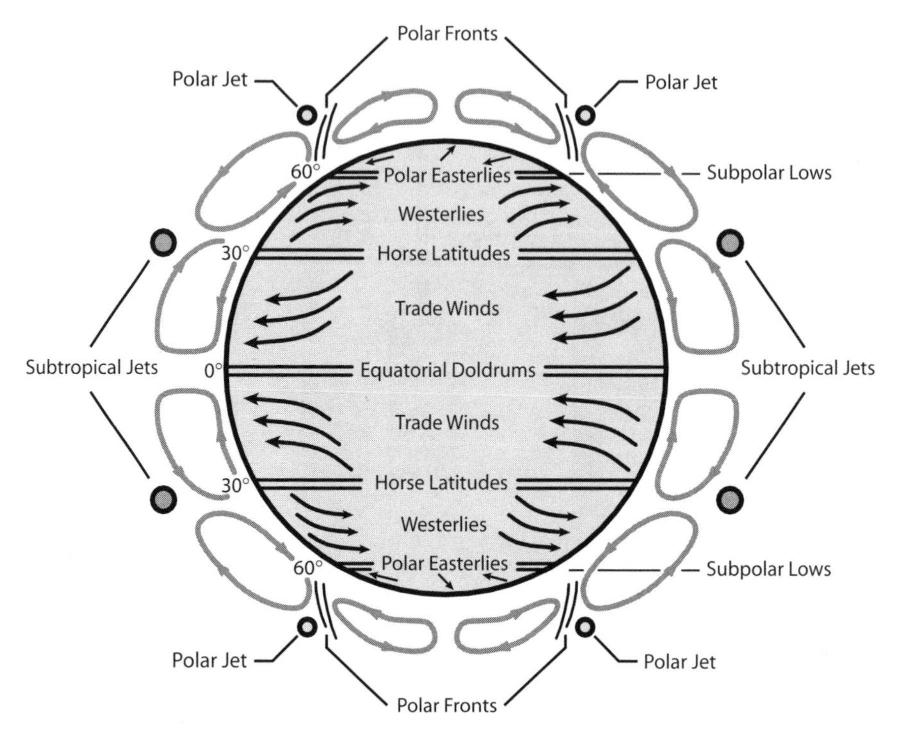

FIGURE 2–7. Schematic representation of the general circulation of the atmosphere.

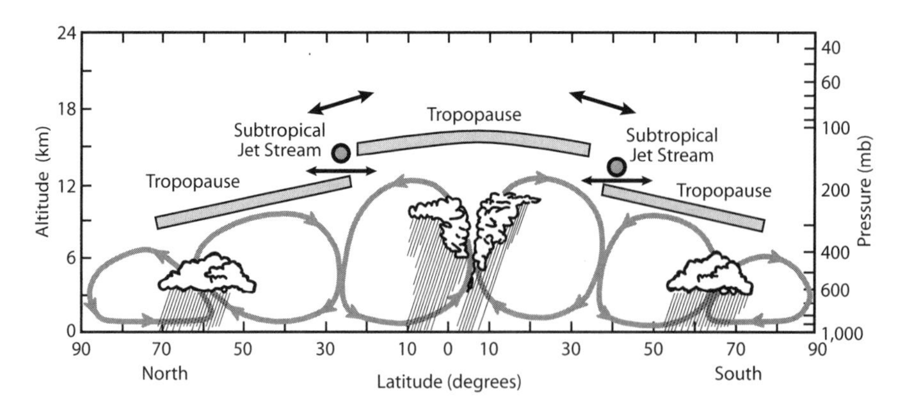

FIGURE 2–8. Schematic representation of the circulatory system in the troposphere during summer in the Northern Hemisphere, showing the discontinuity in the troposphere at the subtropical jet stream.

Characteristics of the Hydrosphere

Hydrologic cycle

The hydrosphere includes a variety of distinctly different aquatic environments that are essential to human life and economic productivity. It is a dynamic system due to the hydrologic cycle, in which liquid water evaporates and is transported through the atmosphere. This cycle is illustrated schematically in Figure 2–9. While the atmospheric water vapor mass constitutes only 10^{-5} of the hydrosphere, it is critical both to the heat balance of the globe, as previously discussed, and to the replenishment of fresh water needed for drinking and for agriculture purposes.

As indicated in Table 2–6, most of the hydrosphere is contained in the oceans, which are saline. Furthermore, most of the fresh water is relatively inaccessible, being in groundwater or in polar ice. Its inaccessibility is indicated by its rate of turnover, i.e., by the time required for each part to be exchanged in the hydrologic cycle.

Fresh surface waters

Chemically pure waters, i.e., containing only H_2O, are not found in nature. Water's great power as a solvent insures that natural waters contain many other substances that are largely derived from the lithosphere. Table 2–7a presents a

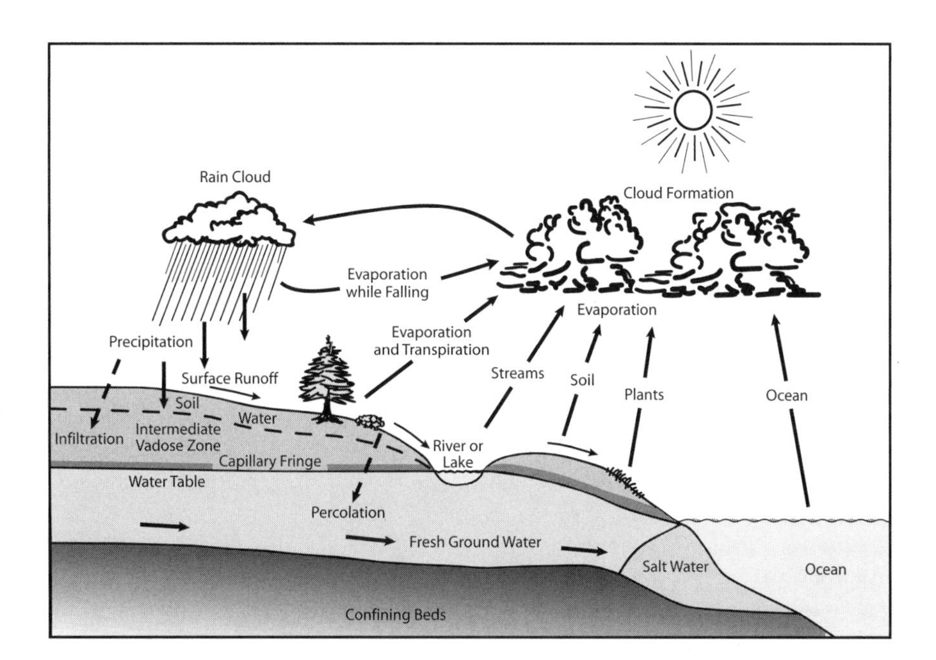

FIGURE 2–9. Schematic representation of the hydrologic cycle.

TABLE 2–6. The Hydrosphere

COMPONENT	APPROXIMATE VOLUME (10^3 km^3)	TURNOVER TIME (YEARS)
Oceans	1,370,000	3000
Groundwater	60,000	5000[a]
(Groundwater zones with active turnover)	(4000)	(300)[b]
Polar ice caps	24,000	8000
Surface waters of land	280	7
Rivers	1.2	0.031
Soil moisture	80	1
Water vapor in atmosphere	14	0.027
Total hydrosphere:	1,454,000	2800

[a]Inclusive of groundwater runoff to oceans, thus bypassing rivers—4200 years.
[b]Inclusive of groundwater runoff to oceans, thus bypassing rivers—280 years.

listing of some major chemicals found in natural, fresh waterways in the United States. The table applies to those waters that support a varied and profuse fish fauna, and are considered nonpolluted. The concentrations of minerals present at lower concentrations, including many of the toxic chemicals of interest, are more variable and cannot readily be summarized. Table 2–7b presents average heavy-metal concentrations in nonpolluted river waters.

Surface runoff into lakes and rivers is used extensively for drinking water supplies. Sometimes it is used with little if any treatment, as in New York City and Boston, which collect their water in distant watersheds that are largely isolated

TABLE 2–7a. Some Average Properties of Natural Waterways in the U.S.[a]

	5% OF THE WATERS CONTAIN LESS THAN	95% OF THE WATERS CONTAIN LESS THAN
Total dissolved solids	72	400
Bicarbonate (HCO_3^-)	40	180
Sulfate (SO_4^{-2})	11	90
Nitrate (NO_3^-)	0.2	4.2
Calcium (Ca^+), Magnesium (Mg^+)	18.5	66.0
Sodium and potassium ($Na^+ + K^+$)	6	85
Free carbon dioxide (CO_2)	0.1	5.0
Ammonia (NH_3)	0.5	2.5
Chloride (Cl^-)	3	170
Iron (Fe)	0.1	0.7

[a]Numbers are in ppm_w (parts per million).

TABLE 2–7b. Trace Metals in River Water

METAL	CONCENTRATION (GLOBAL AVERAGE) (μg/l)
Cd	< 1
Co	0.1
Cr (VI)	1
Cu	7
Hg	0.002
Mo	0.6
Pb	3
V	0.9
Zn	20

[*Source*: Compiled from Miettinen, J.K. Inorganic trace elements as water pollutants. In F. Coulston, E. Mrak (eds.), Water Quality. New York: Academic Press, 1977, pp. 113–136.]

from contaminated runoff. In other cities, located on rivers or lakes with extensive commercial traffic and upstream sources of contamination, the water requires physical and chemical treatment and disinfection before it is safe to use in water-supply systems.

Lakes and other enclosed bodies of water, especially those in temperate zones, show a thermal stratification during different seasons of the year. This pattern is due to the interplay of temperature, water density, and wind, and is shown in Figure 2–10. The maximum density of fresh water occurs at a temperature of about 4°C; density decreases as the temperature is further reduced to the freezing point, 0°C. Thus, in winter a lake surface will be covered by a layer of ice, while waters slightly warmer than 0°C will remain at various depths below the surface. This ice layer prevents wind-induced circulation, suppressing vertical and horizontal movements and further loss of heat to the atmosphere. This situation is known as winter stagnation.

As the weather gets warmer in the spring, and the ice begins to break up, the surface water starts to warm. As its temperature increases towards 4°C, and it becomes denser, this water sinks below the colder, and less dense, layer beneath it. This overturning of the water, which may last several weeks, results in a temperature profile that is essentially uniform at all depths of the lake; as the ice melts, vertical circulation is further aided by wind action. As the weather gets progressively warmer towards summer, the surface water becomes warmer still, and thus less dense than underlying colder waters. The water is directly stratified, in terms of temperature, in the condition known as summer stratification or stagnation. This condition generally persists from April to November in northern latitudes of the Northern Hemisphere. The upper water layer is termed the epilimnion, and has a relatively uniform warm temperature. The bottom layer, the hypolimnion, is characterized by a relatively uniform cold temperature. Be-

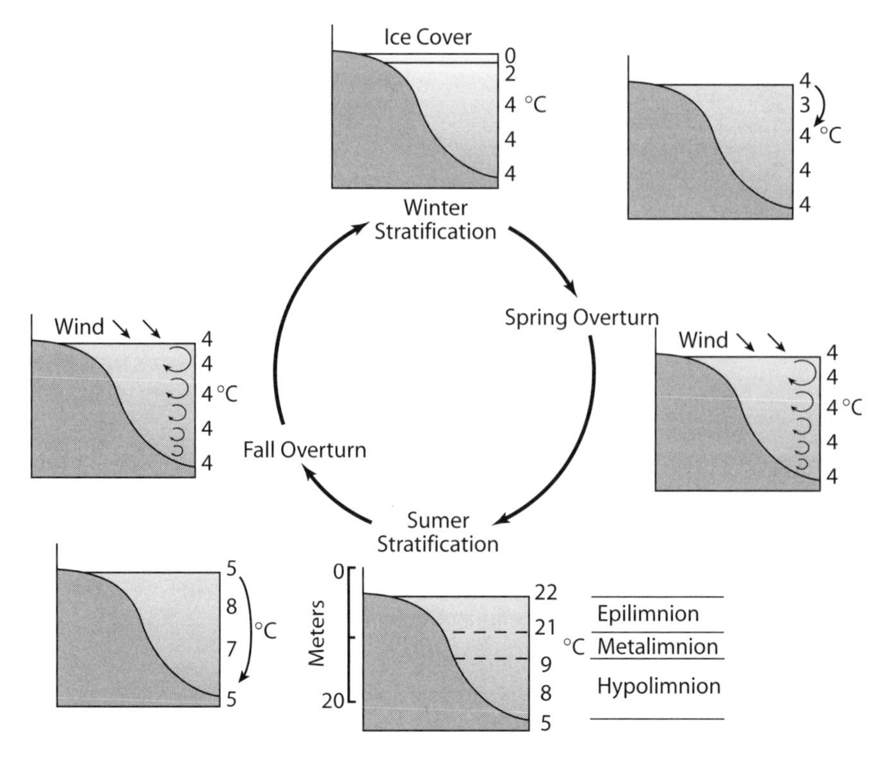

FIGURE 2–10. The seasonal cycle of temperature in a temperate lake.

tween these two layers is the metalimnion, a zone of maximum temperature change. The rapid temperature change itself is termed a thermocline.

As autumn approaches, the surface water layer once again cools and sinks. The water becomes mixed and stirred to increasing depths, and equality of surface and bottom temperatures occur once again, as it did in the spring, in a process termed fall overturn. When the surface freezes, winter stagnation is reestablished.

This temperature cycle has important implications in terms of essential nutrient circulation and contaminant levels in temperate aquatic environments. Thermal gradients are also gradients for concentrations of dissolved gases. Oxygen absorbed at the surface layers is distributed throughout the lake by water circulating within the epilimnion. Waste gases produced during the decomposition of bottom deposits are released by contact with air over surface waters. Within the thermocline, where mixing with surface waters is minimal, there is a sharp drop in DO (and a rise in concentration of gases of decomposition) until DO reaches a minimum below the level of the thermocline. Because the stability of the waters during summer stratification reduces mixing, the hypolimnion tends to become depleted of oxygen. This effect may be enhanced by the discharge of oxygen-demanding contaminants.

As part of the semiannual overturn and mixing of the entire lake, nutrients are mixed and redistributed. Those in lower waters are brought to surface waters, and made available for use in photosynthesis. Thus, overturns may be periods of decreased water quality, as sudden blooms of aquatic plants, such as algae, occur. Lakes, therefore, often exhibit seasonal differences in water quality. In some inland lakes, water in the lower depths remains unmixed, with the main water mass during turnovers, contributing to the stagnation of nutrient cycling. The biological productivity of surface waters depends heavily on temperature, dissolved and suspended nutrients and contaminants, and oxygen concentration. There is continual interchange of nutrients and contaminants between the water, bottom sediments, suspended particles, and various life forms.

Groundwater

While most fresh water is underground (Table 2–6), surface waters supply over 80% of current usage. Thus, as surface water supplies become inadequate, groundwater usage is bound to increase. Groundwater is generally free of significant contamination by bacteria and suspended solids, but will usually contain significant amounts of dissolved solids. These characteristics result from the intimate and extended contact with minerals that constitute the lithosphere. The soil particles filter out the bacteria and suspended particles, and increase the mineral content by dissolution to the point of chemical equilibrium.

As shown in Figure 2–11, groundwater lies in the zone of saturation, where it fills essentially all the voids in the rock stratum. Its upper limit is known as the water table. When usable volumes of water can be extracted from a saturated

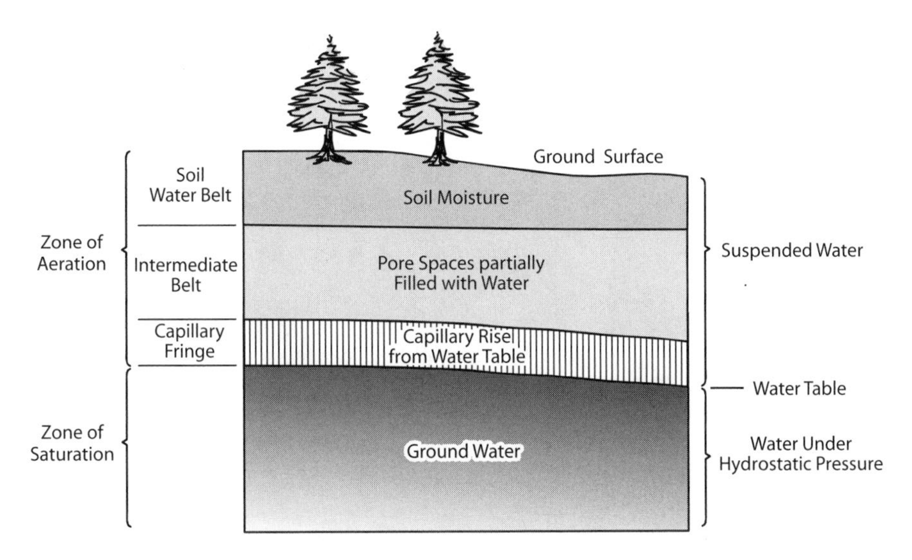

FIGURE 2–11. Groundwater is the part of subsurface water within the zone of saturation.

zone, it is called an aquifer. When the groundwater is under considerable pressure, the water will flow upward without mechanical pumping through a well pipe drilled into it. This is known as an artesian well (Fig. 2–12).

The depth of the water table can be quite variable in time, depending on the rates of water extraction and recharge. Natural recharge through precipitation and infiltration into the ground may be inadequate in areas with heavy use of groundwater, and the resulting fall in the water table may limit the supply and/or cause significant subsidence of the land surface. These problems can be partially or completely overcome in some areas by installing recharge basins or wells. Recharge basins are designed to catch storm water, which percolates through their base to the water table. Recharge wells are used for industrial waste waters and cooling waters, which generally are pretreated to an acceptable quality before being pumped into the groundwater.

Coastal waters and estuaries

The relatively shallow waters of the continental shelves and the estuaries, where tidal action results in mixing of fresh water runoff with saline ocean water, are of particular importance because of their very high biological productivity. They are the major harvest grounds for many commercial shellfish and finned fish. In addition, many ocean fish migrate into estuaries to spawn. Their life cycles can be interrupted by changes in dissolved oxygen, contaminant concentrations, or the benthic environment.

Estuaries are heavily used for marine commerce, and are located within our major population centers. New York, Philadelphia, and Washington, D.C. are sit-

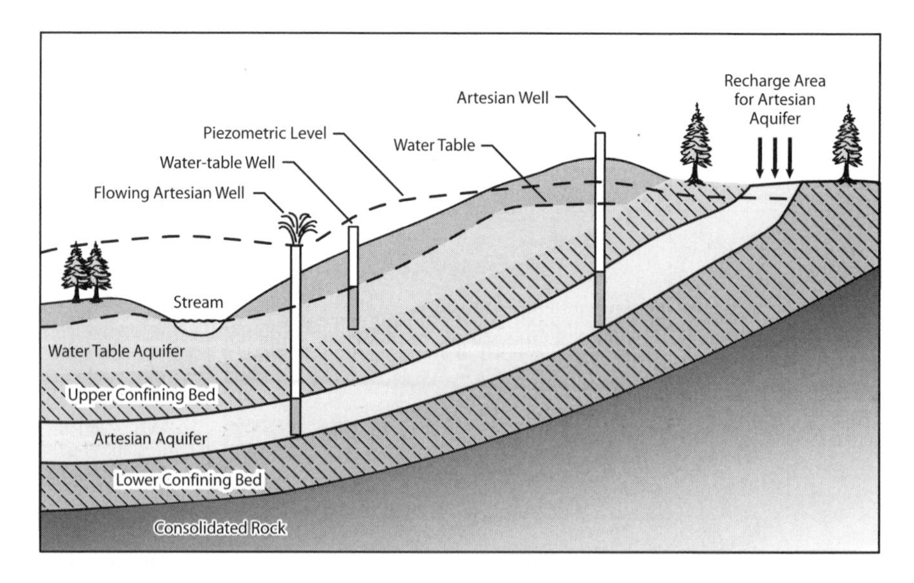

FIGURE 2–12. Subsurface and groundwater phase of the hydrologic cycle.

uated on the estuaries of the Hudson, Delaware, and Potomac Rivers, respectively. The flow in an estuary is cyclic, rising and falling for 6.2 hours from ebb slack (sea-water efflux) to flood slack (sea-water influx) and back to ebb slack. A full tidal cycle is completed in 12.4 hours.

The oceans

The surface waters of the oceans, i.e., those up to 200 m deep, are relatively uniform in temperature, density, and salinity because of mixing due to surface winds. There are characteristic surface currents of the oceans (Fig. 2–13), which largely coincide with surface wind patterns. The intermediate zone, down to a depth of about 1000 m, is characterized by decreasing temperature and increasing density and salinity with depth. This zone has a very low vertical diffusivity and, therefore, acts in effect as a barrier between the surface and deep waters.

The deep ocean waters, with temperatures of 1–4°C, occupy about 75% of the total volume. Thus, most of the ocean waters contribute little to the hydrologic cycle and, in fact, have been relatively inaccessible to human activity.

Characteristics of the Lithosphere

The lithosphere is quite important to our understanding of chemical contamination of the human environment. In terms of contamination, the soil is the most significant part of the lithosphere.

The characteristics of the soil determine the rate of spread of chemical contaminants placed on or in it and, therefore, their access to the ground water. Soil, which is derived from the weathering of rocks, is a very complex system, having solid, liquid, and gaseous phases. Its solids consist of particles of different

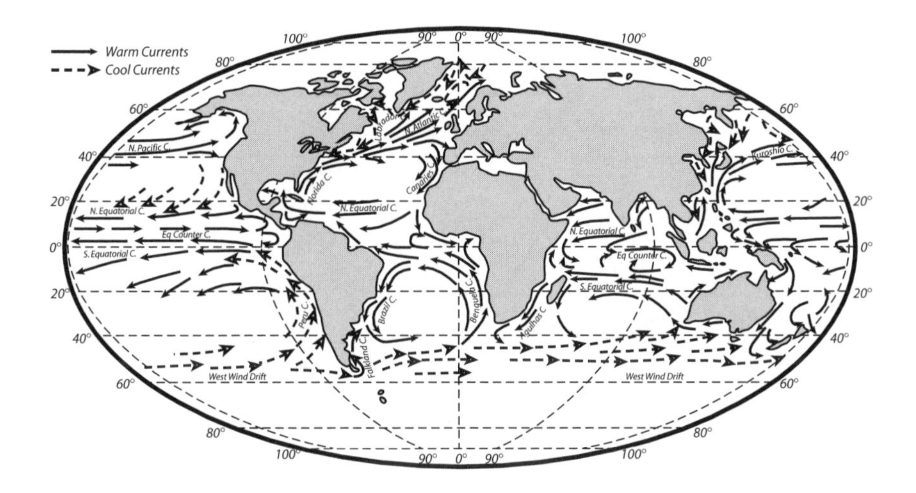

FIGURE 2–13. The principal ocean currents of the world.

chemical and mineralogical composition, and which also vary in particle size, shape, and packing characteristics. The particle configuration determines the characteristics of the channels (pores) that contain air and/or water. The composition of both fluid phases is also variable, both temporally and spatially.

Soils consist of horizons, or layers, which are roughly parallel to the ground surface, with each differing in properties, such as color and texture, from its adjoining layers. A succession of horizons is termed the soil profile. Transfer of minerals and organic material in solution or suspension occurs between horizons via water moving through the pores.

The solid phase of soil may be separated into inorganic and organic components. The inorganic particles are generally classified into fractions, depending on their size. In the U.S. Department of Agriculture classification, particles smaller than 2 μm in diameter are clay, those between 2 and 50 μm are silt, those between 50 μm and 2 mm are sand, and those larger than 2 mm in diameter are gravel. The overall textural designation of a soil depends on the ratio of the masses of the less than 2 mm fractions, and these are generally expressed in terms of a textural triangle, as illustrated in Figure 2–14.

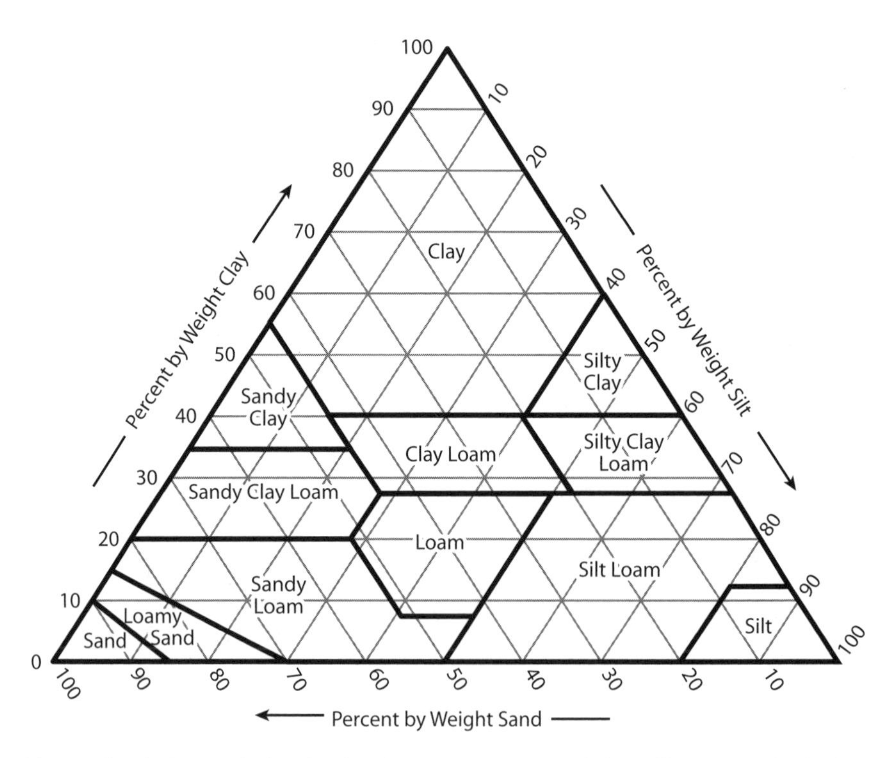

FIGURE 2–14. Textural triangle, showing the percentages of clay, silt, and sand in the basic soil textural classes.

The fraction that largely governs the physical properties and chemical retentions of the soil is the colloidal clay. While sand and silt are composed mainly of quartz and other primary mineral particles, clay is composed of a large group of minerals. Some are amorphous, but many are highly structured microcrystals. The most prevalent of these are the layered aluminosilicates. The clay particles have the highest specific surface. They adsorb water, causing the soil to swell upon wetting and shrink upon drying. Most clays have negative electrical charges, and form electrostatic double layers with exchangeable cations in the water phase.

The quantity of cations adsorbed per unit mass of soil is known as the cation exchange capacity, which may range as high as 0.60 mEq per gram. The attraction of a cation to a negatively charged clay particle increases with increasing chemical valence, while more highly hydrated cations are more easily displaced than less hydrated ones. Thus, the order of preference of the common soil cations would be: $Al^{+3} > Ca^{+2} > Mg^{+2} > K^{+} > Na^{+} > Li^{+}$. When lime is added to an acid soil, Ca^{+2} ions displace many of the hydrogen ions on the surface of the clay particles. Soils with little colloidal materials, such as those consisting largely of sand, have low natural exchange capacities.

Aside from living creatures, the organic fraction of soil consists of plant and animal tissues undergoing decay, plus a relatively chemically stable colloidal fraction called humus. The humic component also plays a part in ion exchange, with the relative role of inorganic vs. organic fractions in total exchange capacity depending upon the soil type; about 20%–70% of the capacity may be due to the humus.

Although ion exchange capacities of soils are usually measured in terms of cations, positively charged soil particles also occur, and soils thus have some degree of anion exchange capacity.

The very large surface area of soil and its great ion exchange capacity permit it to retain nutrient elements to a far greater extent than that retained in the soil moisture.

Characteristics of the Biosphere

All life forms interact with their abiotic and biotic environments. Thus, the biosphere frequently plays a critical role in the spread of chemical contaminants, especially via those forms that undergo transport across or within abiotic components during daily or life cycles. For example, phytoplankton can rise and fall within the aquatic environment in diurnal cycles; many animals can consume their prey in one place, migrate and be consumed by larger predators at another.

The biosphere tends to conserve those chemical elements that are essential to life. This occurs by a process of cycling in characteristic fashion in pathways termed biogeochemical cycles. Very often contaminant residues also cycle, and may thus be retained in the biosphere for long periods of time.

The various biota may also influence contaminant dispersion by their ability to greatly concentrate certain chemical elements or compounds by active metabolic processes. Organic chemicals may accumulate in fatty tissues, while cationic radionuclides of essential elements, or close chemical congeners of these elements (Sr for Ca is an example of the latter case), will accumulate in tissues that store those elements. Metabolic discrimination can work both ways; some chemicals will become concentrated in tissues relative to their environmental levels, while others will be found at much lower levels in biological tissue.

Characteristics of Occupational Environments

Occupational environments have been major sources of excessive exposures of people to toxic chemicals. While the populations exposed are much smaller than those exposed to contaminants in community air, drinking water, and foods, the levels of exposure are potentially much larger. In fact, most cases of chemical intoxication have resulted from occupational exposures, the largest portion from inhalation, but a substantial number have also been due to exposure of the skin. The effects can be localized in the lungs or on the skin, or they can be systemic, after translocation throughout the body via the blood or lymph.

In some ways, the occupational environment is less variable than the community environment outside the workplace walls. The working population is largely limited to healthy adults. The excursions of air temperature, humidity, and air velocity are generally less extreme, and patterns of activity tend to be routine. On the other hand, the spatial variations in air contaminant concentrations may be very large because of the varying proximity to contaminant sources. Also, the workers may be more susceptible to intoxication because of the stresses of the work environment. These include physical exertion with its alterations in the pattern and depth of respiration, and the psychological stresses that may result from keeping up with fixed work schedules. Additional stresses may result from shift work, when work actively conflicts with normal circadian rhythms.

CHARACTERIZATION OF HEALTH, DISEASE, AND DISABILITY

Definitions of Health

There is no universally accepted definition of health. Perhaps the most widely accepted one today is that of the World Health Organization (WHO), which describes health as a state of complete physical, mental, and social wellbeing, and not merely the absence of disease or infirmity. Unfortunately, by a strict interpretation of this rather idealistic definition, very few people would be considered healthy.

The discussion to follow is limited largely to physical well-being. The health effects to be discussed are those that can be recognized by clinical signs, symptoms, or decrements in functional performance. Thus, for all practical purposes, health will be considered as the absence of measurable disease, disability, or dysfunction.

Health Effects

Recognizable health effects in populations are generally divided into two categories: mortality and morbidity. Mortality incidence refers to the number of deaths per unit of population per unit time, and to the ages at death. Data are sometimes available on cause-specific mortality. Morbidity refers to nonfatal cases of reportable disease or dysfunction.

Accidents, infectious diseases, and massive overexposures to toxic chemicals can cause excess deaths to occur within a short time after the exposure to the hazard. They can also result in residual disease and/or dysfunction. In many cases, the causal relationships are well-defined, and it may be possible to develop quantitative relationships between dose and subsequent response.

The number of people exposed to chemical contaminants at low levels is, of course, much greater than the number exposed at levels high enough to produce overt responses. Furthermore, low-level exposures are often continuous or repetitive over periods of many years. The responses, if any, are likely to be nonspecific, i.e., an increase in the frequency of chronic diseases that are also present in nonexposed populations. For example, any small increase in the incidence of heart disease or lung cancer attributable to a specific chemical exposure would be difficult to detect, since these diseases are present at high levels in nonexposed populations. In smokers they are likely to be influenced more by cigarette exposure than by the chemical in question.

Epidemiology is the study of the distribution and frequency of a disease in a specific population. The increases in the incidence of diseases from low-level long-term exposure to environmental chemicals invariably occur among a very small percentage of the population, and can only be determined by large-scale epidemiological studies. The only exceptions are chemicals that produce very rare disease conditions, where the clustering of a relatively few cases may be sufficient to identify the causative agent. Notable examples of such special conditions are the industrial cases of acute and/or chronic berylliosis caused by the inhalation of beryllium-containing dusts, liver cancers that resulted from the inhalation of vinyl chloride vapors, and pleural cancers that resulted from the inhalation of asbestos fibers. If these exposures had produced more commonly seen diseases, the specific causative materials might never have been implicated.

Low-level chemical exposures may play contributory, rather than primary, roles in the causation of an increased disease incidence, or they may not express their effects without the co-action of other factors. For example, the relative risk of lung cancer is very high in uranium miners and asbestos workers who smoke cigarettes, but may only be marginally elevated among nonsmoking workers with similar occupational exposures. For epidemiological studies to provide useful data, they must take appropriate account of smoking histories, age, and sex distributions, socioeconomic levels, and other factors that affect mortality rates and disease incidence.

Mortality

In industrialized societies, there is generally good reporting of mortality and age at death, but with few exceptions, quite poor reporting of cause of death. In studies that are designed to determine associations between exposures and mortality rates, it is usually necessary to devote a major part of the effort to follow-up investigations of cause of death. The productivity of these follow-ups is often marginal, limiting the reliability of the overall study.

Morbidity

Difficult as it may be to conduct good mortality studies, it is far more difficult, in most cases, to conduct definitive studies involving other health effects criteria. While there is generally little significant variability in the definition of death, there is a great deal of variation in the diagnosis of many chronic diseases. There are variations between and within countries and states, and these are exacerbated by the differences in background and outlooks of the physicians making the individual diagnoses. Furthermore, there are some important chronic diseases that cannot be definitively diagnosed in vivo at their early stages, for example, emphysema and Alzheimer's disease.

Many epidemiological studies rely on standardized health status questionnaires, and the success of these studies depends heavily on the design of the questionnaires. Of equal importance in many studies of subtle effects is the training and motivation of the persons administering the questionnaires.

Similar considerations apply to the measurement of functional impairment. The selection of the measurements to be used is very important; those functions measured should be capable of providing an index of the severity of the disease. Equally important here are the skills of the technicians administering these tests, and their maintenance and periodic recalibration of the equipment.

Some studies try to avoid bias from the administrators of the questionnaires and functional tests by having the selected population enter the desired information themselves. They may be asked to make appropriate notations in notebook diaries, or to call a central station whenever they develop the symptoms of interest. Other investigations use objective indices such as hospital admissions, clinic visits, and industrial and/or school absenteeism as their indicators of the health effects to be associated with the environmental variables.

Exposure–Response Relationships

Studies of the specific responses of biological systems to varying levels of exposure can provide a great deal of information on the nature of the responses, their underlying causes, and the possible consequences of various levels of exposure. However, it must be remembered that the data are most reliable only for the conditions of the test, and for the levels of exposure that produced measurable responses.

Generally, in applying experimental data to low-level environmental exposure conditions, it is necessary to extrapolate back to doses that are orders of magnitude smaller than those that produced the effects in the test system. Since the slope of the curve becomes increasingly uncertain the further one extends it beyond the range of experimental data, the extrapolated effects estimate may be in error by a very large factor.

The basic dimensions of the dose–response relationship for populations are shown in Figure 2–15. There are many important factors affecting each of the basic dimensions.

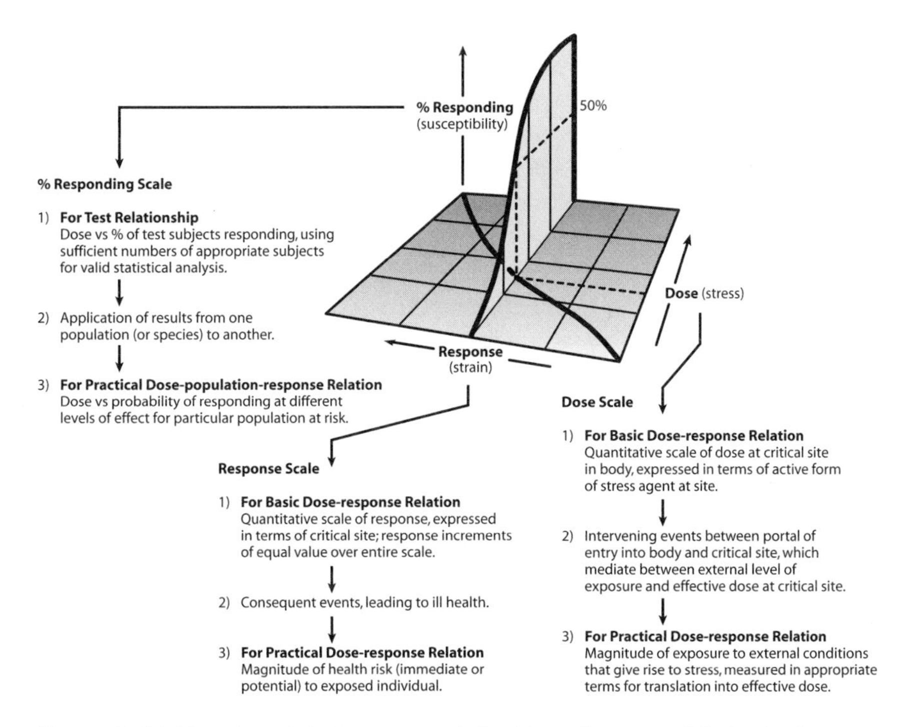

FIGURE 2–15. Dose (population) response relationship with suggested distinction between basic (toxicological) and practical (health) scales on the three axes. The illustrative curve on the horizontal plane portrays the dose-response relationship for the middle (50%) of the exposed population; the curve on the vertical plane shows the percentages of population response of the indicated degree over the whole range of doses. The vertical line from the dose scale indicates the magnitude of dose needed to produce the indicated degree of response at the 50% population level.

Factors affecting dose

The effective dose is the amount of toxicant reaching a critical site in the body. It is proportional to the concentrations available in the environment: in the air breathed, the water and food ingested, etc. However, the uptake also depends on the route of entry into the body and the physical and chemical forms of the contaminant. For airborne contaminants, for example, the dose to the respiratory tract depends on whether they are present in a gaseous form or as an aerosol. For contaminants that are ingested, uptake depends on transport through the membranes lining the gastrointestinal tract, which, in turn, depends on both aqueous and lipid solubilities. For contaminants that penetrate membranes, reach the blood, and are transported systemically, subsequent retention in the body depends on their metabolism and solubility in the various tissues in which they are deposited. In all of these factors, there are great variations within and between species, and therefore great variations in effective dose for a given level of environmental contamination.

Factors affecting response

The response of an organism to a given environmental exposure can also be quite variable. It can be influenced by age, gender, the level of activity at the time of exposure, and the competence of various defense mechanisms of the body. The competence of the body's defenses may, in turn, be influenced by the prior history of exposures to chemicals having similar effects, since those exposures may have reduced the reserve capacity of some important functions. The response may also depend on other environmental factors, such as heat stress and nutritional deficiencies.

REFERENCES

1. Gibbs, W. E. Clouds and Smokes. New York: Blakiston Co., 1924.
2. Vincent, J. H. (Ed.) Particle Size-Selective Sampling of Particulate Air Contaminants. Cincinnati: Am. Conference of Governmental Industrial Hygienists, 1999.

3

Sources of Contaminants

There are a variety of ways to classify the contaminants found in the environment. They can be divided as follows: *(1)* natural and anthropogenic; *(2)* according to the medium in which they are dispersed-air, water, soil, food; *(3)* by specific elements and/or compound classes; or *(4)* by their state of matter-solid, liquid, gas, or dispersion (colloid, suspension, etc.). In this chapter the contaminants are classified according to their sources, and it, therefore, becomes necessary to consider all physical and chemical forms and all media simultaneously. This approach provides the best opportunity to associate specific contaminants with the activities that generate them. Furthermore, it permits an appreciation of the total impact of a given sphere of activity, and of the possible implications of alternative control strategies in those cases where current environmental contamination levels are excessive.

Some contaminants have no known primary sources that could account for their observed concentrations. Ozone (O_3) in urban air and chlorinated hydrocarbons in drinking water are examples of what are termed "secondary" contaminants, those that are formed within the environment by chemical reactions of precursor chemicals derived from primary sources.

PRIMARY CONTAMINANTS IN AIR AND WATER

Natural Contaminants

Chemically pure air and water are not found in nature because there is always an abundance of sources of both chemical and biologically active agents. The life cycles of plants generate pollens, the decomposition of vegetable and animal matter releases various organic and inorganic compounds, and the hydrologic cycle leaches metals from the earth's crust. Thus, unless the compound of interest is unknown in nature, it is generally difficult to apportion measured levels at any particular location to their natural and anthropogenic sources. Table 3–1 shows that on a global basis, the emissions from natural sources for atmospheric particulates can exceed those from anthropogenic sources. However, in any given region, the local sources often have a much greater influence on concentrations, so the increment from natural sources of, for example, gases such as ammonia (NH_3), nitrogen oxides (NO and NO_2), and hydrogen sulfide (H_2S) may be negligible. In order to appreciate when and to what extent natural sources are important to the observed environmental levels, it is necessary to discuss contaminants released by natural processes.

While many "natural" contaminants can be found in areas not significantly influenced by human activity, it does not necessarily follow that the observed levels are independent of human activity. A notable example is air contamination by ragweed pollen. Ragweed grows well in recently disturbed soil, but is at a competitive disadvantage in soils with established covers of natural vegetation. In the sense that it grows best on construction sites, abandoned fields, and urban lots, and coexists with cereal grains on some agricultural fields, more of it is anthropogenic in origin than natural.

Viable particles

A lengthy discussion of viable particles is beyond the scope of this book. However, since the prevalence of some is often largely a function of human activity, and since their impact on human health is greater than all of the other air contaminants combined, they will be discussed briefly in order to place them in perspective with the nonviable chemical contaminants. The size ranges of viable particulates are shown in Table 3–2.

Hay fever severely affects about 10% of the U.S. population, and has been estimated to cause more than 10 million days of lost time from work each year in the United States. Additional costs are attributed to the need for medical consultations and therapeutic drugs. While the dispersion of pollen is seasonal and most of the health effects disappear at the end of the season, some cases of untreated hay fever lead to the development of bronchial asthma.

Airborne microorganisms cause a substantial share of the infectious disease incidence, especially in indoor environments. Pathogenic bacteria, viruses, fungi,

Table 3–1. Aerosol Sources and Source Strengths

	ANTHROPOGENIC		NATURAL	
AEROSOL TYPE	SOURCE STRENGTH (Tg YR^{-1})	MAIN SOURCE ACTIVITIES	SOURCE STRENGTH (Tg YR^{-1})	MAIN SOURCES
Sulfates (as HSO_4^-)	104 (59–182)	Fossil fuels and smelting	49 (24–101)	Dimethylsulfide and H_2S from oceans, land biota, and soils
	3.2 (1.5–9)	Enhanced emissions of dimethylsulfide associated with stronger winds and higher temperature from climate change	18 (8–41)	Volcanic SO_2
Organic carbon	20 (10–30)	Fossil fuels, outdoor cooking	14 (8–40)	Photochemical conversion of terpenes to condensable products and primary biogenics
	6 (3–17)	Enhanced emissions of terpenes from higher temperature due to climate change		
Black carbon	7 (4–11)	Fossil fuels, outdoor cooking	0	No sources
Smoke	70 (50–90)	Biomass burning; smoke is largely composed of organic and black carbon and is therefore often included in those categories	3 (2–4)	Natural fires
Nitrates (as NO_3^-)	14 (10–20)	NO_x from biomass burning, fossil fuel, and aircraft; agricultural soil NO_x	4 (2–8)	Lightning, natural soil, and stratospheric NO_x

(continued)

TABLE 3–1. Aerosol Sources and Source Strengths (*continued*)

AEROSOL TYPE	ANTHROPOGENIC		NATURAL	
	SOURCE STRENGTH (Tg YR^{-1})	MAIN SOURCE ACTIVITIES	SOURCE STRENGTH (Tg YR^{-1})	MAIN SOURCES
Ammonium (as NH_4^+)	19 (11–34)	Enhanced soil emissions from application of nitrogen fertilizer; domestic animals; human emissions; biomass burning; fossil fuel and industry	12 (6–26)	Natural soils, wild animals, and oceans
Sea salt	67 (23–126)	Enhanced wind injections associated with climate change in 2100	88 (30–165)	Formation of jets and bubbles from wind
Dust (r < 1 μm)	200 (100–300)	Agriculturally disturbed lands and increased desertification	200 (100–300)	Wind-blown dust in deserts and other arid, susceptible areas
	20 (10–30)	Dust associated with enhanced winds and arid areas due to climate change in 2100		

Main sources and source strengths of anthropogenic and natural aerosols (r < 1 μm). The source strengths are representative of the mid-1980s except for the changes in natural aerosols (for which the values are estimates for 2100). Uncertainty ranges are given in parentheses.

[*Source*: IPCC 2001: Climate Change 2001; Houghton, J.H.; et al., (eds.), Cambridge, UK: Cambridge University Press, 1996, Chapters 4 and 5.]

TABLE 3–2. Size Range of Viable Particulates

PARTICULATE	STOKES' DIAMETER[a] (μm)
Viruses	0.015–0.45
Bacteria	0.3–15
Fungi	3–100
Algae	0.5
Protozoa	2–10,000
Moss spores	6–30
Fern spores	20–60
Pollen grains (wind-borne)	10–100
Plant fragments, seeds, insects, other microfauna	100^-

[a]The Stokes' diameter for a particle is the diameter of a sphere having the same bulk density and same terminal settling velocity as the particle.

spores, and molds are responsible for a wide variety of diseases. Spores of fungi can become airborne by active processes or by the action of wind, rain, or insects. Bacteria and viruses become airborne in aqueous aerosols formed by a variety of processes, including sneezing and coughing, spraying of sewage in treatment and disposal, and wind action on standing water in ponds and lakes.

The viable contaminants discussed here can, of course, also be ingested in drinking water or with contaminated food products and may produce similar effects following either inhalation or ingestion. The differences will be in the degree of respiratory tract and gastrointestinal tract involvement, the overall pathogenic potential, and the geographic pattern of disease incidence.

Products of plant and animal metabolism

All living organisms create metabolic waste products that are discharged into their environments and normally recycled or neutralized in the immediate vicinity without significant impact on their own or the human environment. Difficulties usually arise when human activities alter the natural patterns of life cycles or the density of the populations. Examples are poultry farms and animal feed lots, where the population density is so great that the volume of waste products cannot be effectively disposed of or recycled on-site by natural processes. These problems will be discussed further under the topic of agricultural wastes.

The respiratory activity of animals and plants and the photosynthetic activity of green plants results in the exchange of O_2 and CO_2. These processes are in approximate balance on a global basis. On a local scale, there is a considerable diurnal variation in CO_2 concentration. It is taken in by plants during daylight at a rate dependent upon the type and density of vegetation, the amount of solar radiation, and the CO_2 concentration. It is released to the atmosphere from decomposing organic material, largely via bacterial activity in the soil. The release rate is dependent on the type of soil, its moisture content, and its temperature. Above a wheat field in sunny weather, for example, the concentration of CO_2 near the ground can reach 500 ppm_v. Much of the CO_2 released is taken up by plants just above the ground and is thus short-circuited. The concentration of CO_2 in soil air can be two orders of magnitude greater than in the surface air.

Vegetation is also responsible for the release of substantial quantities of hydrocarbons. Perhaps the most significant of these is a class known as terpenes. Although released as vapors, they readily condense in the atmosphere to form fine particles. A fairly concentrated light-scattering aerosol may be formed over areas where terpenes are released in significant quantities, such as coniferous forests. These aerosols can be the most characteristic feature of the region, as in the Great Smoky Mountains of North Carolina.

Products of organic decomposition

When living things die, their tissue constituents are recycled to the environment. Some decomposition takes place by physical processes such as evaporation or incineration. However, in the natural state, most organic matter is utilized as an energy and materials source by a succession of microorganisms, and is eventually broken down into simple and stable inorganic chemical entities, such as water and CO_2.

When proteins are broken down in nature by aerobic microorganisms, the process is known as decay. Oxidation continues until stable end products are produced and there are no odorous gases. The nitrogen in the protein undergoes conversion to ammonium, nitrite, and, finally, nitrate. The sulfur compounds are converted to sulfate.

In anaerobic decomposition, or putrefaction, the process of oxidation is incomplete, and the breakdown products include many unstable and odorous gases. The initial products are organic acids, acid carbonates, CO_2, and H_2S. Intermediate products include NH_3, acid carbonates, and sulfides, including mercaptans. The final products include CO_2, NH_3, methane (CH_4), and H_2S. NH_4, H_2S, and the mercaptans have strong and unpleasant odors. H_2S is toxic to many animals, including humans. CH_4 is odorless and nontoxic, but is combustible and can build up to explosive concentrations in underground air spaces.

Erosion

Wind action on land can resuspend settled dust and can erode materials from surfaces. Similarly, wave action and flowing waters can erode the surfaces over which they pass, increasing the dissolved and suspended particulate burdens of the water. While these are natural processes, they can be greatly assisted by human activities. It is much easier to suspend tilled or trampled soil than soil with a natural cover of vegetation, and tilled soil may also be much more susceptible to erosion by storm water. Erosion can also take place with man-made wind or water motion, such as that created by high-speed vehicles, like cars, trucks, and motorboats. Mining and construction activities can also result in heavy local concentrations of dust.

Fire

Lightning strikes and spontaneous combustion of organic matter have always caused and continue to cause fires in forest and brush lands. Such fires generate CO, CO_2, and a wide variety of organic materials that are products of incomplete combustion and/or pyrosynthesis. While most forest fires are attributable to humans in recent years, human intervention has also limited the spread of fires started by natural causes.

Sea spray

The breaking of waves in the oceans creates aqueous aerosols. Most of the droplets fall back into the water, but many of the smaller ones remain air borne long enough for the water to evaporate. A large proportion of the resulting salt particles are sufficiently small to remain airborne for considerable times and distances.

Natural radioactivity

Radioactive isotopes (radionuclides) are continually being released to the atmosphere from two sources. One is the interaction of cosmic rays with atmospheric gases to produce tritium (^3H), carbon-14 (^{14}C), and a variety of other nuclides. Carbon-14, with a half-life ($T_{1/2}$) of 5730 years, is produced from ^{14}N, and is continually incorporated into the biota. The proportion of ^{14}C to ^{12}C, therefore, indicates the elapsed time since the carbon was incorporated into living tissue, and has been used as an index of the age of archeological specimens.

In addition to the nuclides produced continually by cosmic radiation, there are a variety of radionuclides that have been in the lithosphere since it was formed. The ones of greatest interest to humans are ^{235}U ($T_{1/2} = 7.1 \times 10^{10}$ years), ^{238}U ($T_{1/2} = 4.5 \times 10^9$ years), ^{232}Th ($T_{1/2} = 1.4 \times 10^{10}$ years), and ^{40}K ($T_{1/2} = 1.26 \times 10^9$ years). Some radionuclides, for example, ^{40}K, decay directly to stable daughter isotopes. Others, for example, ^{235}U, ^{238}U, and ^{232}Th, decay through complicated chains and have numerous daughters with varying half-lives and emissions. Each chain includes several α emitters, which are of special concern in terms of human carcinogenesis. Certain radionuclides are large contributors to natural atmospheric radioactivity via formation of radioactive noble gases that diffuse from the earth's crust.

When radium-226 (^{226}Ra), a member of the ^{238}U chain, decays, it becomes radon gas (^{222}Rn). Similarly, radium-224 (^{224}Ra), a member of the Th chain, decays to thoron gas (^{220}Rn), another isotope of the element radon. These gases can diffuse into the atmosphere out of the solid matrix holding the parent isotopes. The ^{222}Rn, with a half-life of 3.8 days, is released to a greater extent than the ^{220}Rn, with its much shorter half-life of 54 seconds. The daughter products of radon and thoron decay, which are also radioactive, are molecular-sized particles, and they rapidly diffuse onto available surfaces, primarily other airborne particles. Since most of these airborne particles are very small and remain in the atmosphere for a relative long time, these daughter products can stay airborne for significant time intervals.

The concentration of radon daughters in the atmosphere is quite variable. It depends on the strength of the local sources, i.e., the concentration of radium in the soil and/or building materials, the porosity of the matrix containing the radium, and meteorological factors. Very high concentrations can be found in enclosed spaces, such as mines, caves, and the basements of homes, schools, and commercial buildings where the underlying soil, building materials, or both have relatively high radium contents. On a population basis, radon and daughters account for 50% to 90% of the total background radiation exposure to the lungs.

Vulcanism

Volcanic eruptions occur relatively infrequently and at irregular intervals; those with significant releases to the troposphere occur, on average, only a few times each year. Even less frequently, perhaps once or twice per century, there is a major eruption with sufficient energy to inject ash and SO_2 into the stratosphere. The eruptions of Krakatoa (1883) and Mt. Agung (1963) put enough light-scattering particles into the stratosphere to cause readily observable optical effects which persisted for several years. The sulfur released by volcanoes represents a significant fraction of the total emissions to the atmosphere.

Anthropogenic Contaminants

Fossil fuel combustion for power production and space heating

Over 90% of the current U.S. energy demand is derived from the combustion of fossil fuels, i.e., natural gas, oil, and coal. Approximately 10% of the fossil fuel supply is used as feedstock or raw material for production of products, 25% is used in transportation, and ~60% is burned for space heating (heating of buildings) and to produce electricity. Coal will, most likely, continue to be used primarily for electric power production; oil consumption will decrease somewhat, and natural gas consumption will grow. The fossil fuels contain varying mixtures of hydrocarbons and minerals. Natural gas, as it is commercially distributed, has negligible amounts of sulfur, nitrogen, and noncombustible mineral ash, but may contain noble gases, including radon, and radon daughters. Components of petroleum are classified according to their range of boiling temperatures at atmospheric pressure. The lighter fractions of oil (lower boiling points) will also be low in nitrogen, sulfur, and ash. Coal and the heavier fractions of the oil have mineral contents depending on their source and the amount of pretreatment, if any, they receive. Coal typically contains about 10% mineral ash. It is possible to approach complete combustion of fossil fuels in stationary furnaces. However, this becomes increasingly difficult with the increasing viscosity of fuel oil and the increasing content of volatiles (decreasing fixed carbon content) in coal. The difficulty lies in achieving a sufficiently prolonged contact between the oil droplet or coal surface and the oxygen in the flame.

If combustion is not completed within the high temperature zone of the flame, there will be unburned and/or incomplete products of combustion in the effluent. In an efficient flame, most of the carbon in the fuel will be oxidized to CO_2, the hydrogen to water vapor (H_2O), and the sulfur to SO_2. The source strength depends on the sulfur content of the fuel, and power plants can reduce their SO_2 emissions by switching to desulfurized fuels with naturally lower sulfur content, or by scrubbing the combustion effluents before their discharge to the ambient air. The Federal Clean Air Act Amendments of 1990 mandated phased reductions in sulfur emissions and, as shown in Figure 3–1, the 1995 emissions were substantially below the target. The nitrogen will be released as nitrogen (N_2), nitric oxide (NO), and nitrogen dioxide (NO_2). The amounts of NO and NO_2 are quite variable, and their summed concentration is usually expressed as nitrogen oxides (NO_x). The mineral content of the fuel is converted to an ash composed

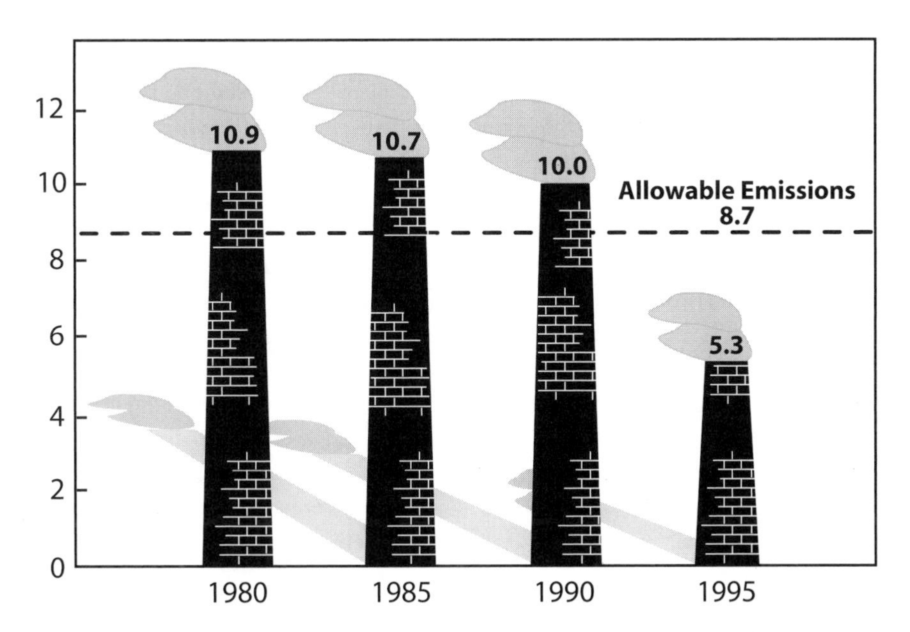

FIGURE 3–1. Annual sulfur dioxide emissions from 445 Phase I electric utility units (1980–1995; in millions of tons).

of mixed oxides. The more volatile materials, such as oxides of lead, cadmium, and mercury, and the radium and polycyclic aromatic hydrocarbons, are released as vapors, but condense as, or on, fine particulates in the stack. Most of the mass of the ash falls to the bottom of the furnace (bottom ash), while the fine particles rise up the stack with the combustion gases (fly ash). Coal-fired utility furnaces generally use various air-cleaning devices to collect most of the fly ash. There is generally much more NO_x in the furnace effluent than could be accounted for by the nitrogen content of the fuel. The excess is formed in the flame by fixation of the N_2 in the air supply, a process whose rate increases rapidly with rising flame temperature. The reaction between atmospheric N_2 and O_2 to form NO is reversible; if the products of combustion were allowed to cool gradually, the NO would decompose. However, since most large furnaces are designed to permit a rapid extraction of heat for useful work, the gases are rapidly quenched, and the NO does not decompose. Beginning in the furnace and stack, and continuing in the atmosphere, it undergoes conversion to NO_2, a brownish-colored and much more toxic gas.

The fate and effects of the effluents from fossil fuel combustion depend on how they are released. Large utility furnaces may discharge effluents through high stacks, diminishing their maximum ground-level concentrations, but increasing their residence times in the atmosphere and increasing their dispersion. Space-heating furnaces usually discharge their effluents at or near roof level. The maximum ground-level concentrations can, therefore, be higher, and thus any effects they produce are more likely to be localized. A potential surface water contaminant produced by electric power generating plants is heat. Spent steam leaving the turbine passes through a condenser, where it is cooled and condensed; the water is then returned to the boiler. The simplest cooling method is to allow cold water from a river or stream to pass through pipes in the condenser. This allows heat exchange between the steam and this cooling water. In a once-through system using river water (the cooling water passes through the condenser only once before returning to the waterway), the discharge water can be much warmer than the intake, affecting the ecology of the river. In some cases, there is inadequate river flow, and structures known as cooling towers are used to discharge the heat to the atmosphere via evaporative cooling. The mists generated by such towers may produce fogs, affecting visibility and traffic safety. These fog droplets will also contain traces of the toxic chemicals that are used to prevent algae growth within the tower. The potential for thermal pollution is greater in nuclear-power electric generating plants, since they release approximately 15% more heat per unit of electricity generated than do fossil-fuel facilities.

Transportation

In a highly mobile society such as ours, a great deal of time and energy is consumed in transporting both goods and people. We purchase products that originate in distant states and countries. The manufacturers, in turn, obtain their raw materials from both local and distant sources. We frequently commute to work at locations far from our residences, and many of us travel great distances on business or vacation trips. As a result, a major portion of our total energy consumption can be attributed to that required for movement. In consuming energy, there is always waste. For transportation, or moving, sources, these are heat, fuel spillage, exhaust products, and various by-products. Fuel combustion that occurs in motor vehicles is generally incomplete, and the exhaust wastes include CO_2, H_2O, SO_2, NO, CO, and a host of organic compounds. They may also include the oxidation products of fuel additives, such as manganese compounds. Some larger ocean-going ships have nuclear propulsion systems, and electrified land transport often uses energy derived, in part, from nuclear power. Waste products of nuclear-power production include various fission products. This topic is discussed more fully in a later section of this chapter.

The use of transportation systems creates additional environmental contamination. Vehicular motion resuspends settled particles. The vehicles rust and wear, spreading iron oxide, rubber particles from tires, and asbestos fibers from clutch and brake linings, along their paths. They leak or vaporize engine oil and other working fluids, elevate noise levels, and contribute to environmental litter, either through the actions of their occupants or by the abandonment of the vehicles or parts thereof. Finally, transportation vehicles alter the environment in very significant, but less obvious, ways. Land transport vehicles need roads, parking areas, and service stations. Major fractions of our urban land surfaces are covered with concrete and asphalt to accommodate the needs of wheeled transport. The mobility that autos provide has led to the rapid growth of the suburbs that, by and large, are less energy-efficient than cities, and has thereby increased the demand and costs of energy for heat and power usage.

Automobile exhaust

A major source of air contamination in the United States is motor vehicle exhaust. Before 1968, there was no intentional control of tail pipe emissions, except in California. With the then constantly increasing numbers of cars in use, the levels of CO, hydrocarbons (HC), NO_x, and lead (Pb) in urban air were high enough to cause concern among health authorities. This led to the passage of the Federal Clean Air Act of 1970. The Act mandated a series of performance goals for automobile engine emissions, with the objective of reducing emissions of CO, HC, and NO_x to the point that they would no longer cause the air quality standards established by the Act to be exceeded. The major auto manufacturers claimed that they could only meet the CO and hydrocarbon emissions limits by the use of catalytic converters in the exhaust system, and their position was accepted by the U.S. EPA. Since catalytic converters are poisoned by lead, which was used as an antiknock additive, they could only be used with unleaded fuel. Thus, lead additives were eliminated from the fuel supply. While catalytic converters increase the extent of oxidation of the hydrocarbons and CO in the exhaust, they also increase the oxidation state of any sulfur in fuel. Historically, the concentration of sulfur in gasoline was relatively low, about 0.03% by weight, and essentially all of the sulfur was emitted from the tailpipe as SO_2. The SO_2 that was released was not generally considered to be a significant problem, since considerably larger amounts of SO_2 were released by fossil fuel combustion in stationary (non-moving) sources. However, in passing through a catalytic converter, some of the SO_2 in the engine exhaust was oxidized to SO_3, which is rapidly hydrolyzed by water vapor in the exhaust to form a sulfuric acid mist (H_2SO_4). Thus, the catalytic converter can be a source of H_2SO_4, a highly irritating chemical. This problem turned out to be self-limiting, at least in part. The initially high rate of formation of H_2SO_4 dropped off markedly as the vehicles aged, and subsequent efforts to control the concentration of ambient air fine particles led to reductions in the sulfur content of motor vehicle fuels.

Other consequences of the reliance on catalytic converters and the modification of engine designs to reduce CO and hydrocarbon emissions in the early 1970s were reductions in performance and fuel economy. To meet the Congressional mandates for improved fuel economy that followed the oil shocks created by the OPEC cartel, the industry developed onboard microchip-based fuel supply and ignition timing controls that optimized emissions, performance, and economy. They also stimulated a minor boomlet in the use of diesel (compression-ignition) engines in automobiles, based on their greater efficiency. However, relatively few diesel-powered cars were sold because of their generally somewhat sluggish performance, black smoke emissions, and the characteristic odor of their exhausts. Thus, the conventional Otto-cycle (spark ignition) internal-combustion engine continued to be used in most automobiles. While it has maximum efficiency and minimal emissions when running at constant power, emissions increase greatly during other operating modes, such as idling, acceleration, and deceleration. At the turn of the twenty-first century, the alternative of hybrid designs became a viable option. The hybrids combine a smaller internal combustion engine with electric motor driven wheels. The internal combustion engine runs at a nearly constant rate (at which it is quite efficient and generates a minimum of pollutant effluents) and the batteries provide peaking power for acceleration. The much smaller battery packs used in these hybrids are recharged by the alternator during cruising and deceleration. Some hybrids are using Otto-cycle engines, while others will use diesel engines of more modern designs. Both these relatively small diesels, and the larger diesels used in trucks and buses made in recent years, produce much cleaner exhausts than those made in earlier years, especially in terms of black carbon particles.

Aircraft exhaust

The black plume exhausts of the early commercial jetliners have been essentially eliminated in the newer engines, as well as retrofitted older engines. However, engine emissions during idling can be a serious problem at airports. All combustion engines, including aircraft jets, generate nitric oxide. The release of NO by jets in the stratosphere has raised the possibility of significant destruction of ozone by interaction with the NO. The fear of a possible reduction in stratospheric ozone, with a projected subsequent increase in human skin cancer, was a significant factor in the decision of the U.S. Congress not to subsidize the production of a U.S. supersonic transport.

Water contamination by boats and ships

A major problem in aquatic environments is oil contamination. There has been considerable attention paid to oceanic oil spills resulting from the breakup of deep-draft oil tankers. However, the oil contamination of the oceans by more mundane sources, such as bilge flushing and leakage, may have greater overall effects. Within coastal and inland waterways, leakage and inadvertent spills create most of the problems related to oil. Another major problem in inland waters is the sanitary wastes which are discharged directly into the water by commercial and pleasure boats. This problem should diminish through the enforcement of holding tank regulations by the U.S. Coast Guard.

Industrial operations

Industrial operations and processes are extremely varied and complex. They involve a diversity of materials in a variety of forms under a broad range of conditions, making it virtually impossible to provide more than a superficial summary of contaminant releases. Tables 3–3 and 3–4 show the diverse types of air and water contaminants that may result from various industrial operations. The contaminants may evolve from the raw materials or processing agents, or can occur during manufacture, shipping, or storage of raw or processed products. Detailed information is available on contaminant releases for most manufacturing industries. Specific industries vary greatly in the types and amounts of their effluents. The approach to contamination from industrial operations that has been adopted for this chapter is to illustrate the extent and diversity of the sources through a brief discussion of environmental releases of chemicals from two specific industries.

Petroleum Refining. The petrochemical industry encompasses processes which range from the manufacture of simple compounds to the production of very complex plastics, all of which are potential sources of contaminant release.

TABLE 3–3. Major Air Contaminants from Some Industrial Sources

Chemical Industry

- Ammonia plant
  - Carbon monoxide
  - Ammonia
- Chlorine plant
  - Chlorine gas
  - Mercury
- Hydrofluoric acid
  - Hydrogen fluoride
  - Silicon tetrafluoride
  - Sulfur dioxide
- Nitric acid manufacture
  - Nitric oxide
  - Nitrogen dioxide
- Paint, varnish
  - Aldehydes
  - Ketones
  - Phenols
  - Terpenes
  - Glycerines
- Petroleum refinery
  - Hydrogen sulfide
  - Selenium
  - Fluorides
  - Hydrocarbons
- Phosphoric acid
  - Silicon tetrafluoride
  - Hydrogen fluoride
- Phthalic anhydride
  - Hexane
  - Maleic anhydrides
- Printing ink
  - Acrolein
  - Fatty acids
  - Phenols
  - Terpenes
- Sulfuric acid
  - Sulfur dioxide
  - Sulfur oxides
  - Nitrogen oxides
- Synthetic rubber
  - Alkanes
  - Alkenes
  - Ethanenitrile
  - Carbonyls

Metallurgical Industry

- Aluminum ore reduction
  - Hydrogen fluoride
  - Particulate fluoride
  - Carbon, alumina
- Copper smelters
  - Carbon monoxide
  - Sulfur oxides
  - Nitrogen oxides
  - Cadmium
- Iron-steel
  - Carbon monoxide
  - Sulfur oxides
  - Iron oxides
  - Fluorides
  - Nickel carbonate
  - Silicates
  - Graphite
- Lead and zinc smelters
  - Sulfur dioxides
  - Fluorides
  - Cadmium
- Magnesium smelters
  - Fluorides chlorine
  - Barium oxide
- Secondary metals industry
  - Nitrogen oxides
  - Metal oxides
  - Hydrochloric acid
- Brass and bronze smelters
  - Zinc oxide
  - Lead oxides
- Secondary aluminum smelters:
  - Fluorides
  - Chlorides
  - Ozone
  - Numerous metals

Construction Industry

- Asphalt roofing
  - Oil mists
  - Benzo(a)pyrene
  - Asbestos
  - Carbon monoxide
- Brick
  - Fluorides
  - Sulfur dioxide
- Calcium carbide
  - Carbon monoxide
  - Acetylene
  - Sulfur oxides
- Cement
  - Various kinds of dust
  - Chromium
- Ceramic and clay processes
  - Fluorides
  - Silicates
  - Ammonia
- Frit (glazing enamel)
  - Fluorides
  - Silica
  - Boron
- Glass
  - Chlorine
  - Fluorides
  - Sulfur oxides
  - Nitrogen oxides
  - Carbon monoxide

Food Industry

- Coffee roasting
  - Smoke
  - Odors
- Fish-metal processing
  - Hydrogen sulfide
  - Trimethylamine

TABLE 3–4. Major Water Contaminants from Some Industrial Sources

INDUSTRY	ORIGIN OF CONTAMINANTS	COMPONENTS AND CHARACTERISTICS OF CONTAMINANTS
Food		
Canning	Fruit and vegetable preparation	Colloidal, dissolved organic matter, suspended solids
Dairy	Whole milk dilutions, buttermilk	Dissolved organic matter (protein, fat, lactose)
Brewing, distilling	Grain, distillation	Dissolved organics, nitrogen fermented starches
Meat, poultry	Slaughtering, rendering of bones and fats, plucking	Dissolved organics, blood, proteins, fats, feathers
Sugar beet	Handling juices, condensates	Dissolved sugar and protein
Yeast	Yeast filtration	Solid organics
Pickles	Lime water, seeds, syrup	Suspended solids, dissolved organics, variable pH
Coffee	Pulping and fermenting beans	Suspended solids
Fish	Pressed fish, wash water	Organic solids, odor
Rice	Soaking, cooking, washing	Suspended and dissolved carbohydrates
Soft drinks	Cleaning, spillage, bottle washing	Suspended solids, low pH
Pharmaceutical		
Antibiotics	Mycelium, filtrate, washing	Suspended and dissolved organics
Clothing		
Textiles	Desizing of fabric	Suspended solids, dyes, alkaline
Leather	Cleaning, soaking, bating	Solids, sulfite, chromium, lime, sodium chloride
Laundry	Washing fabrics	Turbid, alkaline, organic solids

(*continued*)

Table 3–4. Major Water Contaminants from Some Industrial Sources (*continued*)

INDUSTRY	ORIGIN OF CONTAMINANTS	COMPONENTS AND CHARACTERISTICS OF CONTAMINANTS
Chemical		
Acids	Wash waters, spillage	Low pH
Detergents	Purifying surfactants	Surfactants
Starch	Evaporation, washing, etc.	Starch
Explosives	Purifying and washing TNT, cartridges	TNT, organic acids, alcohol, acid, oil soaps
Insecticides	Washing, purification	Organics, benzene, acid highly toxic
Phosphate	Washing, condenser wastes	Suspended solids, phosphorus, silica, fluoride, clays, oils, low pH
Formaldehyde	Residues from synthetic resin production and dyeing synthetic fibers	Formaldehyde
Materials		
Pulp and paper	Refining, washing, screening of pulp	High solids, extremes of pH
Photographic products	Spent developer and fixer	Organic and inorganic reducing agents, alkaline
Steel	Coking, washing blast furnace flue gases	Acid, cyanogen, phenol, coke, oil
Metal plating	Cleaning and plating	Metals, acid
Iron foundry	Various discharges	Sand, clay, coal
Oil	Drilling, refining	Sodium chloride, sulfur, phenol, oil
Rubber	Washing, extracting impurities	Suspended solids, chloride, odor, variable pH
Glass	Polishing, cleaning	Suspended solids

This discussion will be limited to the refining of petroleum. Crude oil, extracted from subsurface wells, is the raw material for a large fraction of our total energy consumption. Most of it is refined into: *(1)* products burned as gasoline or diesel fuel in internal combustion engines; *(2)* light fuel oils used in domestic and industrial furnaces; or *(3)* residual fuel oils used in firing large boilers in power plants, industry, and large housing complexes. Approximately 8% is not burned and is converted into petrochemical products, such as plastics, pesticides, and solvents. Much of the world's crude oil is refined in the United States. Crude oil is a mixture of hydrocarbons of varying chain lengths and varying contents of sulfur, oxygen, nitrogen, and trace elements. In its concept and early practice, refining crude oil into commercial products was relatively simple. When oil is heated to a temperature sufficient to vaporize most of the hydrocarbons, and the vapors are directed into a temperature-controlled column, the vapors condense at different points along the column according to their individual boiling points. Such a "straight-run" distillation yields products defined by boiling-temperature ranges and, in decreasing order of volatility, are given names such as wet gas, gasoline, kerosine, fuel oil, middle distillate (including diesel fuel), lube distillate, and heavy bottom. A schematic design of such a simple refinery is shown in Figure 3–2. Most of the sulfur and trace elements remain in the residual oil at the bottom of the column. The "straight-run" distillation products did not match the consumer demand in terms of quantity or quality, and refineries have accordingly become considerably more complex. When a straight-run product is available in excess of its demand, it is reformed into a needed product, and when there is insufficient product, it is synthesized. The industry has developed a va-

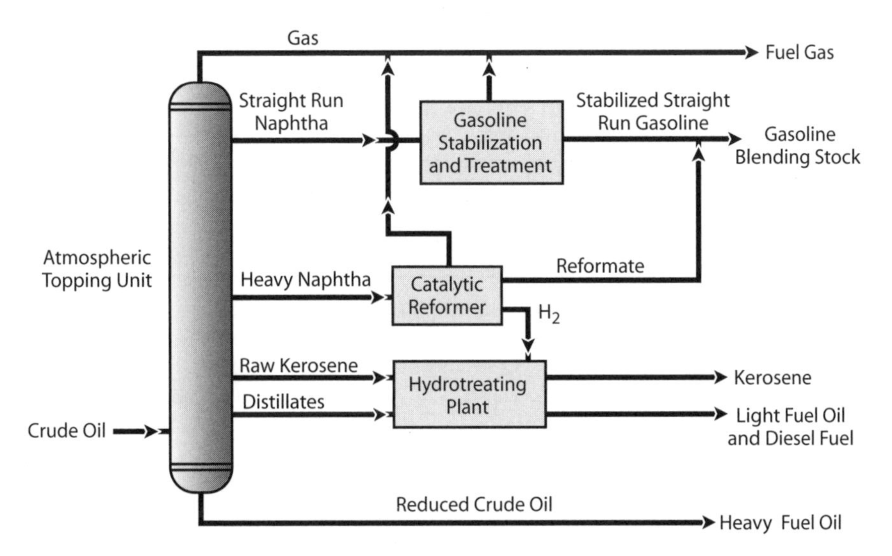

FIGURE 3–2. Processing plan for minimum refinery.

riety of techniques for splitting, rearranging, and combining petroleum molecules to form products meeting customer and/or govern material specifications and a product mix giving maximum economic returns. A simplified schematic diagram of a typical modern refinery is shown in Figure 3–3.

The schematic indicates that crude oil is the only input, and that the commercial products listed on the right side of the diagram are the only output. In practice, however, there are additional inputs, and many waste products are vented into the atmosphere and discharged in waste water. A refinery requires large volumes of steam for heating and distillations, and process water for cooling condensers and process extractions. The various treatment steps require the use of a variety of caustics, acids, and special solvents. All of these can, in part, end up in the waste water, along with process spills and leakages of the various hydrocarbon products and intermediates. The process units of refineries are essentially all outdoors, so that storm-water drainage from the refinery becomes contaminated with materials that have been leaked or spilled into exterior surfaces. Storm and waste waters are, however, generally treated to meet applicable effluent standards for BOD, COD, pH, acidity, alkalinity, suspended solids, oil, phenol, and sulfide. Spills and leaks of liquids also contribute to air contamination if they are volatilized. In addition, there may be leakages of gases and vapors directly into the atmosphere from process equipment.

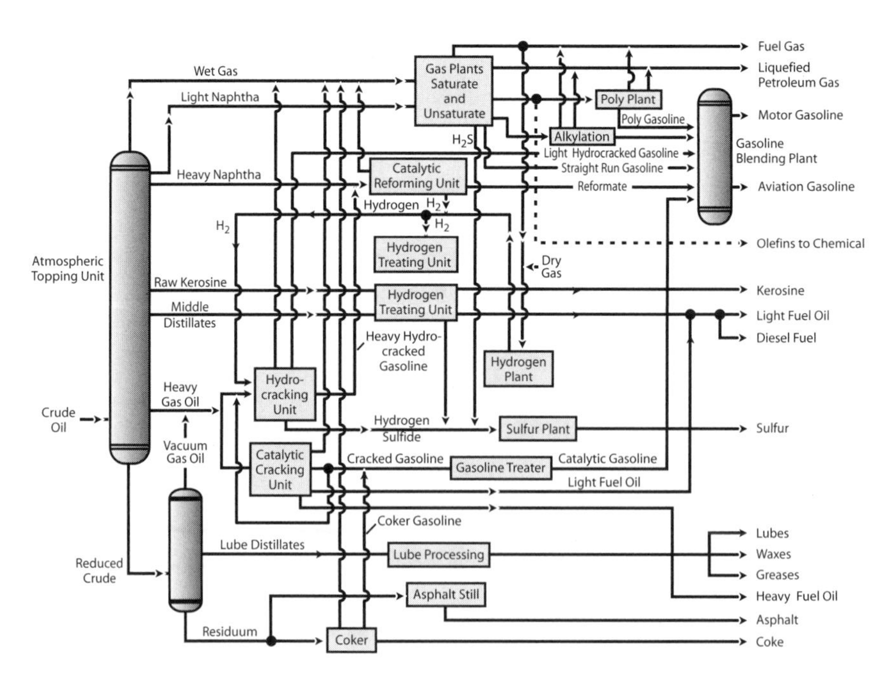

FIGURE 3–3. Processing plan for more complete refinery. Lube: lubricating oil; poly: polymerization.

Total hydrocarbon losses may range from approximately 0.1% to 0.6% of crude throughout, depending on the complexity of the refining and the efforts expended in controlling losses. Some of the crude input ends up within the refinery as fuel to fire boilers and process heaters. Table 3–5 shows the kinds of contaminant emissions into the atmosphere from various sources within refineries.

Pulp and Paper Manufacture. The pulp and paper industry is one of the largest in the United States economy. The manufacture of paper can be divided into two phases: *(1)* pulping the wood; and *(2)* making the final paper product. The raw materials generally used in the pulping phase are wood, cotton or linen rags, straw, hemp, esparto, flax, jute, and waste paper. These materials are reduced to fibers, which are subsequently refined, sometimes bleached, and dried. At the paper mill, which is often integrated in the same plant with the pulping process, the pulps are combined and loaded with fillers and finishes, and transformed into sheets. The fillers commonly used are clay, talc, and gypsum. The four main types of pulp used are: *(1)* groundwood; *(2)* soda; *(3)* kraft (sulfate); and *(4)* sulfite. Fiber industries, therefore, produce two main types of wastes, namely pulp-mill wastes and paper-mill wastes. The major portion of the contamination from papermaking originates in the pulping processes. Raw materi-

TABLE 3–5. Potential Sources of Specific Contaminants from Oil Refineries

EMISSION	POTENTIAL SOURCES
Oxides of sulfur	Boilers, process heaters, catalytic cracking unit regenerators, treating units, H_2S flares, decoking operations
Hydrocarbons	Loading facilities, turnarounds, sampling, storage tanks, waste-water separators, blowdown systems, catalyst regenerators, pumps, valves, blind changing, cooling towers, vacuum jets, barometric condensers, air blowing, high-pressure equipment handling volatile hydrocarbons, process heaters, boilers, compressor engines
Oxides of nitrogen	Process heaters, boilers, compressor engines, catalyst regenerators, flares
Particulate matter	Catalyst regenerators, boilers, process heaters, decoking operations, incinerators
Aldehyes	Catalyst regenerators
Ammonia	Catalyst regenerators
Odors	Treating units (air-blowing, steam-blowing), drains, tank vents, barometric condenser sumps, waste-water separators
Carbon monoxide	Catalyst regeneration, decoking, compressor engines, incinerators

als are reduced to a fibrous pulp by either mechanical or chemical means. Mechanically prepared (groundwood) pulp is made by grinding the wood on large emery or sandstone wheels, and then carrying it by water through screens. This type of pulp is usually highly colored, low-grade, contains relatively short fibers, and is mainly used to manufacture nondurable paper products, such as newspaper. Chemically prepared pulps are produced by reduction to chips, screening to remove dust, and digestion with chemicals. The various processes differ from one another only in the chemicals used to digest chips. Since each type of pulping produces somewhat different wastes, each should be considered separately. The discussion to follow will be limited to sulfate (kraft) pulping. Coniferous woods are used in the preparation of kraft pulps.

A simplified flow diagram for the kraft pulp process is shown in Figure 3–4. In any given pulp mill, a variety of combinations of the various unit processes might be used depending on the product to be produced, the raw material, yield expected, air quality considerations, and the preferences of the manufacturer. The kraft process involves the cooking of wood chips in either a batch or continuous digester, under pressure, in the presence of a cooking liquor containing sodium hydroxide and sodium sulfide. The hydroxide is the reagent that dissolves the

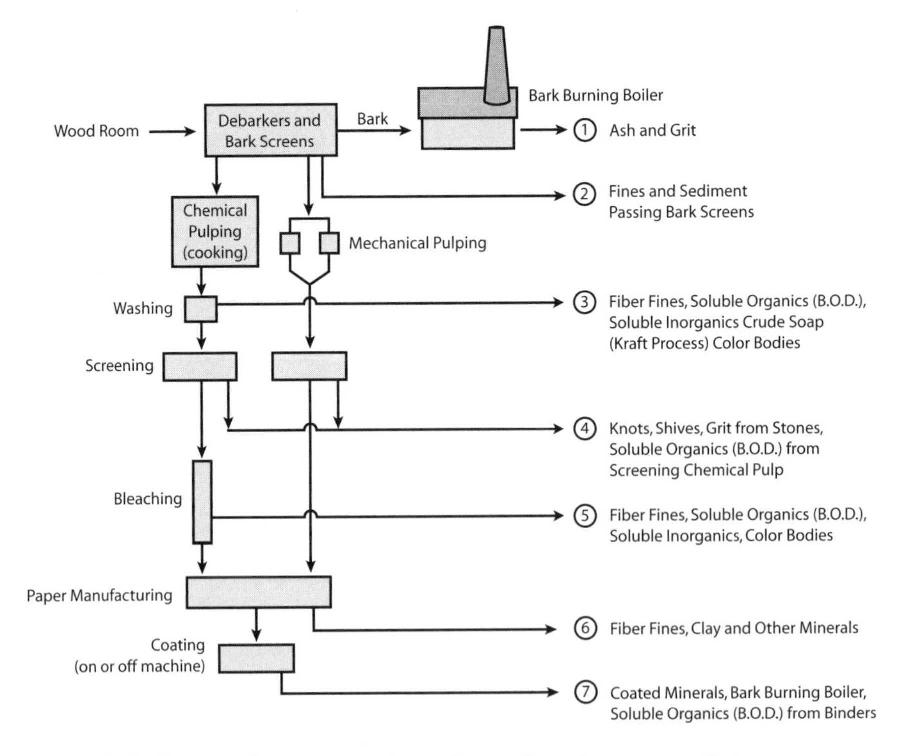

FIGURE 3–4. Sources of water contaminants from pulp and paper manufacture.

lignin in the wood chips. During the cooking reaction, the hydroxide is consumed, and the sodium sulfide serves to buffer and sustain the cooking reaction. At the same time, small amounts of sulfide react with the lignin, giving rise to the odors characteristic of kraft mills (due to hydrogen sulfide and mercaptans). Upon the completion of the cooking reaction, the residual pressure within the digester is used to discharge the pulp into a blow tank. Gases and flash steam released in the tank are vented through a condenser, where heat is recovered and the condensible vapors removed. The noncondensible gases, which are a source of malodors, are either confined and treated, or released into the atmosphere. At the same time, the pulp in the blow tank is being diluted and pumped to washers, where the spent chemicals and the organics from the wood are separated from the fibers. The spent chemicals and the organics, called black liquor, are then concentrated in multiple-effect evaporators and/or-direct-contact evaporators for subsequent burning. The evaporators concentrate the liquor to a solids content of 60%–70%, which is a requirement for combustion in the recovery furnace. During evaporation of the black liquor in the multiple-effect evaporators, volatile odorous gases are released. These gases escape when entrained gases and vapors are drawn off by the vacuum system. In order to eliminate the venting of these gases into the atmosphere, they can be confined and destroyed. The black liquor is generally concentrated further in a direct-contact evaporator using hot flue gases from the recovery furnace. These hot gases, containing CO_2, react with sulfur compounds in the black liquor, leading to the release of gases such as H_2S. Prior oxidation of the black liquor reduces the sulfide content of the liquor and, hence, the amount of H_2S released. Most mills utilize a type of recovery furnace that eliminates direct contact between the flue gases and the black liquor, and are not sources of malodorous emissions. The concentrated black liquor is sprayed into a recovery furnace, where its organic content supports combustion. The inorganic compounds, consisting of the cooking chemicals, fall to the bottom of the furnace where chemical reactions occur in a reducing atmosphere. The chemicals are withdrawn from the furnace as a molten smelt, containing mostly sodium sulfide and sodium carbonate, which is dissolved in water in a smelt-dissolving tank to form a solution called "green liquor." The green liquor is then pumped from the smelt-dissolving tank, treated with slaked lime (calcium hydroxide) in the causticizer, and then clarified. The resulting liquor, referred to as white liquor, is the cooking liquor used in the digesters.

Most kraft mills recover the sludge resulting from causticizing and burn it to lime in a kiln. Pulp-mill wastes are produced at various stages of the pulping process. These wastes contain pulping liquor, fine pulp, bleaching chemicals, mercaptans, sodium sulfides, carbonates and hydroxides, sizing, casein, clay, ink, dyes, waxes, grease, oils, and fiber. Particulate emissions from the kraft process occur primarily from the recovery furnace, the lime kiln, and the smelt-dissolving tank. They are caused mainly by the carry-over of solids plus the sublimation and condensation of inorganic chemicals. The sublimation and condensation normally produces a plume. Little information is available on the actual range of particle sizes from these sources, especially in the recovery furnace, since agglomeration tends to occur readily. In addition, particulate emissions occur from combination and power boilers. The newer plants, with better emission controls, discharge much less contaminants into the atmosphere. Aqueous paper-mill wastes originate in water that passes through the screen wires, showers, and felts of the paper machines, beaters, regulating and mixing tanks, and screens. The paper machine wastes (white waters) contain fine fibers, sizing, dye, and other loading material. Figure 3–4 presents a flow sheet of pulp and paper manufacture in terms of water contamination.

Source inventories and trends

The U.S. EPA periodically publishes detailed anthropogenic activity related source inventory data and analyses of source strength trends to guide decision-makers in formulating control strategies.[1] These data have been summarized in various ways. For example, current sources can be attributed to various economic sectors, as in Figure 3–5, for NO_x emissions (in 1998). Trends data for NO_x, volatile organic compounds (VOCs), SO_2, and PM_{10} are illustrated in Figure 3–6. Inventories of emissions affecting the concentrations of ambient air particulate matter are particularly complex, since they must account for gaseous precursor emissions as well as the direct emission of particles. The secondary particles formed in the atmosphere from gaseous precursors can exceed the primary particle emissions, as illustrated in Table 3–6.

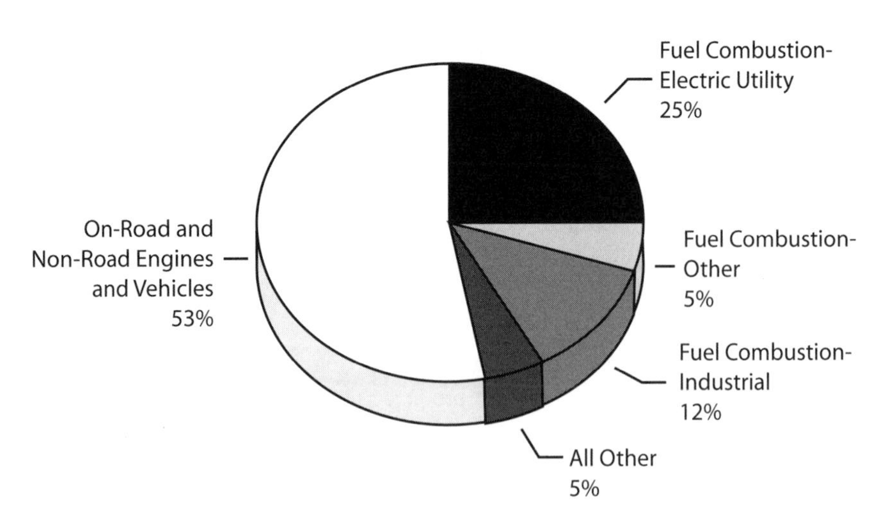

FIGURE 3–5. 1998 National nitrogen oxide emissions by principal source categories. (*Source*: U.S. Environmental Protection Agency.)

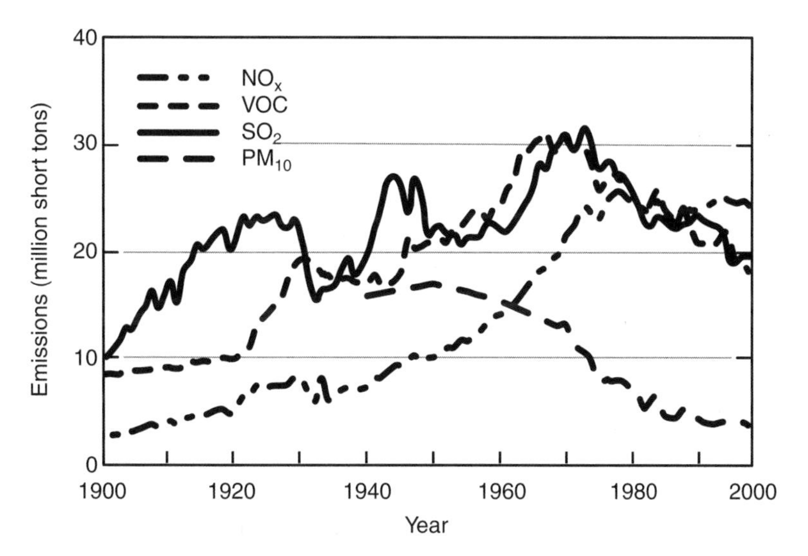

FIGURE 3–6. Trend in national emissions, nitrogen oxides, volatile organic compounds, sulfur dioxide (1900–1998), and directly emitted particulate matter [PM_{10} (nonfugitive dust sources); 1940–1998]. (*Source*: U.S. Environmental Protection Agency.)

Contaminants resulting from unregulated activities

In the U.S., the EPA regulates major categories of anthropogenic pollution, but other significant sources remain unregulated. For example, for thoracic particulate matter, i.e., particles with aerodynamic diameters <10 μm (known as PM_{10}), emission inventories have traditionally been focussed on three categories, i.e., fuel combustion, industrial processes, and transportation (see Fig. 3–7). When considering contributions of sources to ambient air concentrations of PM_{10}, this type of inventory can be misleading in several ways. First, as also shown in Figure 3–7, these three sources contribute only 8.1% of a more complete inventory of PM_{10} source emissions. Second, a significant fraction of ambient air PM_{10} can be attributed to gaseous precursor emissions that combine to form particles downwind of the sources (e.g., sulfate, nitrate, and organic fine particles, which can account for as much as 90% of PM_{10} in the eastern U.S., and ~30% of PM_{10} in some western U.S. locations). By contrast with fine particles, which remain suspended in ambient air for many days, coarse particles in fugitive dust, and dust from wind erosion and agricultural operations, tend to settle out within a few hours.

Agriculture

Modern agriculture is similar to mass-production industry in many respects. It relies heavily on highly specialized automated equipment and the economics of

TABLE 3–6. 1990 U.S. Particulate Matter Emissions[a]

	PM INDICATOR		GASEOUS PRECURSOR EMISSIONS		$PM_{2.5}$ EMISSIONS + SECONDARY AEROSOL
SOURCE CATEGORY	$PM_{2.5}$	PM_{10}	SO_2	NO_x	
Electric utility					
Coal	100,000	270,000	15,000,000	6,700,000	22,000,000
Oil and gas	6000	11,000	600,000	800,000	1,400,000
Fuel use					
Industrial	180,000	250,000	3,000,000	3,000,000	6,500,000
Commercial	15,000	35,000	600,000	700,000	1,200,000
Residential wood	500,000	500,000	9000	66,000	570,000
Chemical manufacturing	40,000	60,000	400,000	400,000	850,000
Metals processing	100,000	140,000	900,000	80,000	1,000,000
Petroleum industry	20,000	30,000	400,000	100,000	500,000
Other industry	250,000	400,000	400,000	300,000	1,000,000
Storage and transport	30,000	60,000	5000	2000	30,000
Waste disposal/ recycle	200,000	230,000	40,000	80,000	300,000
Highway engines	300,000	350,000	500,000	7,000,000	8,000,000
Non-road engines	200,000	220,000	300,000	3,000,000	3,500,000
Agricultural burning	1,000,000	1,200,000	7000	200,000	1,200,000
Wind erosion	800,000	5,000,000	0	0	800,000
Road dust	3,000,000	17,000,000	0	0	3,000,000
Construction	1,600,000	8,000,000	0	0	1,600,000
Agricultural tilling	1,400,000	7,000,000	0	0	1,400,000
Total	10,000,000	42,000,000	22,000,000	23,000,000	55,000,000

[a]In million tons per year.

(*Source*: Wilson, R. and Spengler, J.D. Particles in Our Air. Harvard, 1996.)

high-volume production. In the interests of efficiency, it utilizes man-made fertilizers and pesticides, and concentrates waste products to the point where they create disposal problems. The problems of chemical contamination of the environment by agricultural operations may appear to be remote to urban populations, but the key role of agriculture in the national economy makes it important to understand its total impact on the environment.

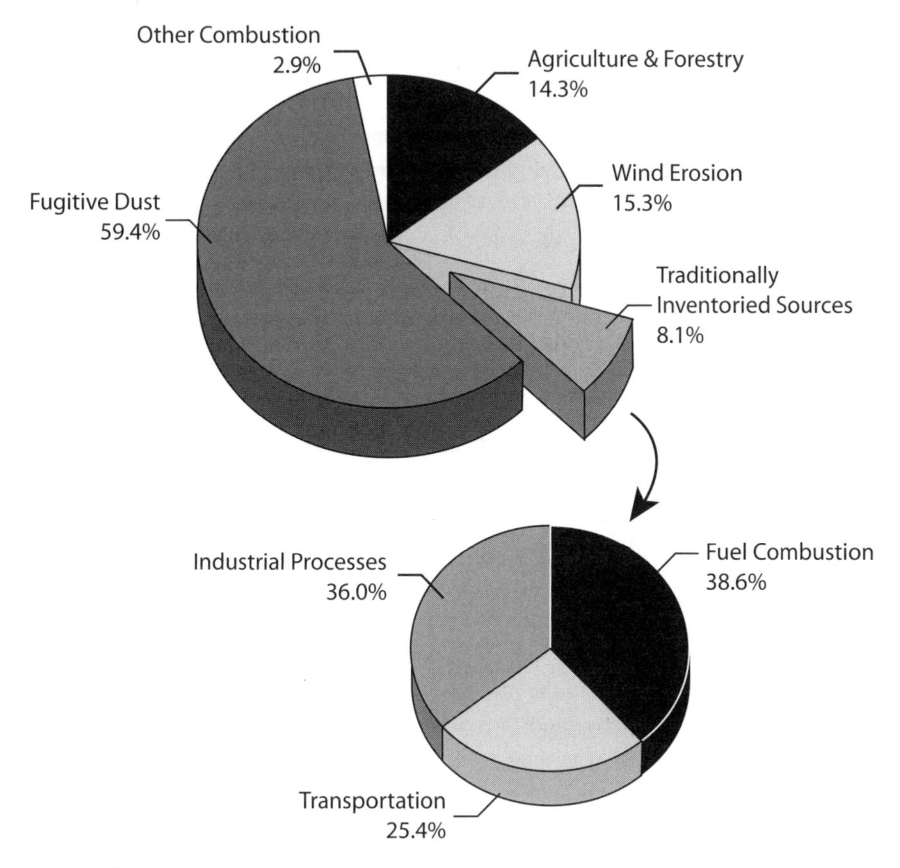

FIGURE 3–7. PM_{10} emissions by source categories, 1998. (*Source*: U.S. Environmental Protection Agency.)

Agricultural Use of Fire. Controlled burning of stubble on harvested fields is a cost-effective means of preparing the soil for the next crop, while simultaneously enriching the soil in nutrients. It also produces large amounts of smoke, which may be objectionable to downwind populations. In many areas, the controlled burning of agricultural fields is allowed only after a permit has been issued, and only under specified meteorological conditions.

Soil Tillage. Mechanical soil tillage, especially when the soil is dry, can result in substantial quantities of dust immediately, or can make it possible for subsequent wind storms to pick up dust from the tilled surfaces. Marginal dry land agriculture has resulted in major dust storms and extensive soil erosion.

Fertilizers and Soil Conditioners. One classic definition of contamination is a resource out of place. Too much inorganic plant nutrient in a waterway is a prime example, since it can cause an undesirable proliferation of rooted aquatic plants and algae, and lead to oxygen depletion and anaerobic decay. The drainage of fertilizers and other soil conditioners from agricultural fields to streams can cause such effects in downstream waters. The main inorganic nutrients used as fertilizers are nitrogen (as nitrate), and phosphorous (as phosphate). The application of fertilizers, manures, and lime as powders or sprays can also create local air contamination problems, which may extend beyond the confines of the farm.

Pesticides. Pesticides are used because their toxic properties reduce or eliminate pest species that consume, destroy, or compete with the efficient production of the product of interest. The ideal pesticide is specific and biodegradable. A pesticide is specific when it destroys the pest without affecting nontarget organisms. A pesticide is biodegradable when it is destroyed or degraded by microorganisms within a reasonably short time after it has fulfilled its intended function. The time frame during which the pesticide should persist without biodegradation depends upon the pest. In some cases, such as rat control, instantaneous killing is adequate, while for insect control, the pesticide may not be effective unless it persists for the full life cycle of the insect. Persistent pesticides, such as DDT and other organochlorines, had practical advantages which led to their widespread use in the mid-twentieth century. They have an extremely low order of acute toxicity, and they were relatively inexpensive. Part of their economic advantage rested in their persistence, since they did not require as frequent reapplication as the more degradable pesticides. Unfortunately, the ability to develop pesticides of sufficient specificity is limited. Frequently, the pesticides used are toxic to species other than the target organisms. The unintended toxicity may be immediate and apparent, such as a fish kill in a farm pond. On the other hand, it may take a long time to develop, and even longer to recognize, such as the effects of the persistent organochlorine pesticides on the reproductive capacities of wild birds in areas removed from the direct applications of the pesticides. Another problem is the potential for human health effects from the ingestion of pesticide residues on or in foods. In summary, agricultural operations with pesticides are sources of environmental effects off the farm in several ways: *(1)* the reduction in populations of desirable mobile nontarget species of insects, birds, and mammals because of exposure on the farm; *(2)* the effects on aquatic organisms resulting from the transport in surface storm drainage; *(3)* the effects on biota in near and remote downwind regions because of the drift of aerosol sprays or from surface deposits which are volatilized by solar heating and are transported long distances as vapors or condensed fine particles; and *(4)* the effects of residues remaining in or on agricultural produce.

Waste Products. In some agricultural operations, such as fruit growing, only marketable products are harvested and there is relatively little waste to dispose of. In other operations, such as the production of rooted crops, i.e., potatoes, beets, carrots, etc., all of the foliage is waste. In animal husbandry, especially on feedlots, the animals generate large amounts of fecal wastes during their growth. In terms of BOD, cattle produce 16.4 times as much waste per capita as people.[2] In the slaughterhouse, large amounts of very rich organic wastes are generated. Such wastes, if not properly processed, can cause significant problems in terms of excessive organic nutrient levels in receiving waters and odor problems in downwind areas.

Domestic activities

The wastes generated in our homes also contribute to the chemical contamination of the environment. Each person disposes of about 500 L per day of waste water, and approximately 1.6 kg per day of domestic refuse. About half of the refuse is paper, and about 10% metal. If buried, the solid wastes can contaminate ground water with dissolved chemicals and oxygen demand. If burned in older municipal incinerators, some of the metals, volatile organics, and products of incomplete combustion will be released into the ambient air. It is extremely difficult to maintain efficient combustion with a material as variable in heating value and moisture content as domestic refuse. Many households minimize the amounts of garbage disposed of as solid wastes by using a garbage grinder on the drain of the kitchen sink. This merely transfers the oxygen demand burden to the sewage treatment facility and/or the receiving waters. The treatment facilities must also cope with the sanitary wastes and laundry wastes from the individual residences, along with the storm waters that pick up some of their waste burdens in passing over the surfaces of residential properties.

Municipal services

Municipal governments are generally responsible for disposing of solid and liquid wastes generated by their residents, and, therefore, reduce the volume and strength of the wastes they collect. For example, an efficient sanitary landfill disposes of the solid wastes without significant reentry to the general environment. In sanitary landfilling, the wastes are spread in thin layers, compacted, and covered with soil each day. In some cases, where wetlands are used as fill sites, there is a negative impact, in the sense that the wetlands environment is destroyed in the landfill process. Many municipalities use large central incinerators to reduce the mass and volume of solid wastes by approximately 90%. The residual ash is a relatively clean fill material, and can be used as a cover for the refuse in the landfill. Unfortunately, as discussed, the incinerators put partially burned hydrocarbons, ash, and trace metals into the atmosphere. Community opposition to new incinerators has frequently been sufficiently intense to prevent their construction. Incinerators can be operated as energy recovery systems, utilizing the heating value of the refuse. Municipal sewage treatment facilities, are, at best, only partially successful in removing wastes and contaminants from the incoming waters. Some operate only primary treatment facilities, consisting of gravity settlement chambers. These remove the more massive suspended solids, but very little of the finer solids, and hardly any of the dissolved solids. Most of the rest of the facilities include secondary treatment involving some kind of biological oxidation. Such plants may remove from 50% to 95% of the oxygen demand from the wastes, but usually have lower efficiencies for the removal of nitrates, phosphates, and trace metals. The large portion of the oxygen demand removed from the incoming sewage by the treatment plant does not disappear. Some is oxidized to harmless end products in the process, but the rest is simply transferred into sewage sludge, which must itself be disposed of.

Sludge disposal remains a major problem for many large cities. For many years, New York City and other coastal cities dumped digested sewage sludge into designated dumping grounds within coastal waters. In New York's case, this was a site approximately 12 miles out to sea. As a result of potential hazards to marine life and the public health, the city terminated such dumping. Land disposal can involve significant problems in odor generation and/or ground-water contamination. Some of the sludge is now being incinerated.

Another municipal activity that generates chemical contamination in some regions is the road and street salting done in the winter to improve traffic safety. The salt corrodes metals, damages plants, shrubs, and trees, and increases the salinity of the receiving waters. However, the environmental contamination from street salting appears generally acceptable in comparison to the alternative, i.e., impassable and unsafe roadways.

Radiological contamination resulting from nuclear fission reactions

This section discusses the types and sources of anthropogenic radioactive contaminants in the environment derived from military and civilian applications of nuclear fission. The sources for these materials are quite different from those that emit the chemical contaminants described in previous parts of this chapter. In general, the mass concentrations of radionuclides released are too low to result in any chemical toxicity following their uptake; the focus of concern is, therefore, on their radiobiological effects. Radiological contamination may be quite pervasive, since radionuclides follow the same environmental and metabolic pathways as do the stable nuclides of the same element. While there is no question that the total amount of radioactive material in the world has been increased by human activity, the radiation dose to the general population from natural sources is much greater than that from anthropogenic environmental releases. Natural sources account for approximately 97% of the per capita annual dose in the United States due to environmental radioactivity (i.e., not including medical diagnostic or therapeutic procedures).[3] However, any exposure above background level is considered deleterious to some degree, since radioactivity can alter genetic materials.

Contaminant radionuclides are generated as fission products and by neutron activation. In the latter process, bombardment by neutrons induces radioactivity in elements in air, water, soil, or in structural materials. The main anthropogenic source of environmental radioactivity during the past 50 years has been nuclear-weapons testing. Use of nuclear energy for electric-power generation has added a relatively small increment, and the industrial and medical uses of radionuclides have added still smaller amounts.

Nuclear-Weapons Testing. The basic fuel for nuclear weapons is either uranium-235 (^{235}U), which is naturally occurring, or plutonium-239 (^{239}Pu), which is produced from ^{233}U by neutron capture. Contamination due to testing involves the release of: *(1)* unfissioned ^{235}U or ^{239}Pu; *(2)* hundreds of different fission-product nuclides having half-lives ranging from fractions of a second to years, the most hazardous of which are iodine-131 (^{131}I), cesium-137 (^{137}Cs), strontium-89 (^{89}Sr), and strontium-90 (^{90}Sr); and *(3)* products formed by neutron activation of air, water, soil, and the metal casings that surround the weapons. The most extensive series of atmospheric tests occurred in the 1950s and early 1960s, and resulted in the release of about 20 megacuries (MCi) of ^{90}Sr, 30 MCi of ^{137}Cs, 5 MCi of ^{14}C, and 3000 MCi of ^{3}H into the environment.[4] Some atmospheric testing has been done by France, China, and India; the contribution since 1972 due to these is about 5% of the amount produced in the earlier test series. A number of proposals have been advanced for the use of peaceful nuclear explosions for various purposes, such as releasing natural gas from underground sources, building harbors, and excavating for canals. If detonated in the atmosphere, these explosions would also release both fission and neutron activation products; the amounts of each would depend upon the particular type of explosive device used and the composition of the soil and rock surrounding the site.

Nuclear-Power Reactors. In power reactors, controlled fission is used to generate electricity. The first nuclear central power station began operation in 1957 in Pennsylvania. At the end of the twentieth century, nuclear power accounted for about 20% of the total U.S. electrical production. However, no new nuclear power reactors have been ordered since 1979, when a reactor failure occurred at one of the units at Three Mile Island in Pennsylvania. While the reactor itself was destroyed, there was no significant release of radioactivity or reactor fission products to the environment because of the effectiveness of the containment structure, which is a feature of all U.S. power reactors.

A quite different exposure scenario occurred when a power reactor failed at Chernobyl in the Ukraine in 1986, which was then in the Soviet Union. This reactor had no containment structure. As a result, about 1000 cases of acute radiation poisoning occurred, including 28 early fatalities. There were approximately 95,000 persons within 3 km of the reactor who were exposed to quite high radiation. About 135,000 people living within 30 km were evacuated about 10 days later. A radioactive cloud moved downwind into central and northern Europe and the fallout from the cloud caused somewhat elevated radiation exposures to many millions. Within the next 10 years, there were several thousand cases of thyroid tumors in downwind populations in Ukraine and Belarus that were attributable to radioactive iodine (in dairy products), that delivers a concentrated radiation dose to the thyroid. The exposed populations are being monitored to determine the extent of the elevation that will actually occur for tumors at other organs of the body with longer lag times.

While there may be future generations of nuclear power reactors in the U.S. at some time, that time is at least several decades in the future. The fraction of the electrical power supply generated by nuclear fission can be expected to decline as some of the older units reach their economically useful lifetime and are retired, decommissioned, and dismantled.

In the meantime, there is a growing inventory of spent fuel rods stored under water in tanks maintained at nuclear power plants. In 2002, the U.S. Congress endorsed the Department of Energy's plan to transfer high-level power plant wastes to an underground storage facility at Yucca Mountain in Nevada as a secure long-term repository. A brief summary outline of the nuclear power industry follows.

Nuclear fuel cycle

All power reactors currently in use in the U.S. use ^{235}U for fuel. Contaminants may be released into the environment at a number of steps in the fuel cycle.

Mining. Uranium is mined both underground and in open pits. In order to protect workers in underground areas, the radioactive radon gas, which diffuses into the mine air, and its daughter products are vented into the atmosphere outside the mine. While locally high radioactivity levels may occasionally result, the releases generally do not contribute significantly to community exposures. Analogous to the case of ragweed discussed earlier in this chapter, anthropogenic activity results in an increase in what is essentially a natural contaminant. In this case, it is radon gas.

Milling. Milling involves crushing of the ore and the use of chemical methods to extract, concentrate, and purify the uranium into a semirefined oxide, U_3O_8. The major contaminant problem in this step is the large amount of residual solids. This waste material, known as tailings, occupies as much volume as the material taken into the mill. These solids contain most of the radium originally present in the ore. There were over 80 million metric tons of tailings occupying over 2100 acres of land in the United States, this inventory that is being reduced by removal to more secure locations. The radiation and radioactive dust from the tailing piles constitute contamination from natural sources that are redistributed and localized in areas that generally are closer and more accessible to human populations than are the ores in the mines. As a result, the radiation levels in cities near piles of tailings may be higher than normal. In addition, in some towns in the western United States, these tailings, which resemble construction sand, were used for landfill and incorporated into construction materials. Their high radium content resulted in high radon levels in many buildings.

Milling operations use large amounts of water, which often became contaminated with nonradioactive chemicals and with small amounts of uranium, radium, and their decay products. Discharges to streams resulted in local contamination problems.

Refining and Conversion. In this step, the uranium concentrate (U_3O_8) is chemically purified. The uranium to be enriched in its ^{235}U content is converted into a volatile hexafluoride, UF_6. Some nonradioactive liquid wastes and acid gases may be released in these chemical conversion processes.

Enrichment. The concentration of ^{235}U in natural uranium is approximately 0.7%. Most reactors operate more efficiently with higher amounts. Thus, in enrichment, the concentration of ^{235}U in the UF_6 is increased to approximately 2%–4%, by multistage gaseous diffusion or centrifugation. Large amounts of electric power and cooling water are consumed in these processes.

Fuel Fabrication. Enriched UF_6 is converted into a dioxide powder, UO_2, made into pellets and loaded into alloy tubing, which is then formed into individual fuel-rod elements. Up to this point in the fuel cycle, environmental contamination problems are minimal, and are similar to those of the chemical industry in general. Although dusts and fumes of natural uranium are mildly radioactive, they have been well controlled. The greatest potentials for general environmental contamination are associated with power production and fuel reprocessing.

Power Production. Various types of reactors may be used to convert heat into electrical power. Modern reactors are primarily of two types: pressurized-water reactors (PWR) or boiling-water reactors (BWR). In both, water is used as both the coolant and the moderator of the fission reaction. In the boiling-water reactor, water is heated as it passes through the reactor core and steam is produced. The steam passes through turbines and is then condensed for return to the reactor. In the pressurized-water reactor, the water pumped through the core is maintained at a high pressure to prevent it from boiling in the core. Rather, the water, which leaves the core at about 318°C, passes through a steam generator unit, where its heat is transferred to the water-steam loop that passes through the turbines. The nature and amount of any atmospheric discharges depend upon reactor type, operating history, and condition of the fuel. Reactor products include products of uranium fission and of neutron activation of coolant water in the core. The latter results in short-lived radioactive gases, such as ^{41}Ar, ^{16}N, and ^{19}O. Radioactive noble gases produced from fission, for example, ^{85}Kr, may diffuse through the fuel-element cladding and be carried by steam to the turbines in a BWR system. Some noble gases may boil off with the steam, and escape into the atmosphere via the condensor air ejector and through a stack. Most of the radiation which would escape through the stack is short-lived. Because of this, a 30-minute delay is maintained between the air ejector and the top of the stack to allow for radioactive decay before emission. Under normal operations, the radionuclide release from power reactors is very low, and is not important as a source of public exposure. Radiation doses are less than 1% of the natural background dose, and usually much less. It is an accidental release of large amounts of radioactive material from these plants that is the focus of public concern. Further discussion of sources of environmental radioactivity can be found in Chapter 11.

Fuel Reprocessing. After some time, the fuel in the reactor must be reprocessed. This involves recovery of the unused uranium, and also of the ^{239}Pu that is produced during reactor operation, from the fission wastes. The recovered uranium is recycled for fuel-element fabrication. Reprocessing was generally performed only at government installations and only for military weapons purposes. One commercial plant operated in the United States. It was located in western New York State and it closed in 1972. Future commercial plants would have to be designed with improved emission controls; the main releases, however, would still be ^{85}Kr and ^{3}H. Until commercial reprocessing resumes, all power-plant spent fuel is being stored. Fuel reprocessing is the phase of the cycle having the greatest potential for significant radionuclide releases under normal operation.

Waste Management. Ultimate disposal of radioactive wastes is a contentious issue. There are low-level (not very radioactive materials) and high-level (highly radioactive substances, primarily fission products produced at the power plant and separated during reprocessing) wastes. The former are buried at commercial sites in the United States. The latter are stored in liquid form in underground tanks. Future disposal techniques remain a subject of much discussion, with high-level wastes likely to be transported to the underground storage site at Yucca Mountain in Nevada.

SECONDARY CONTAMINANTS

Many of the chemical contaminants in the environment, including some of the most important ones, such as O_3 in urban air, chloroform ($CHCl_3$) in drinking water, and aflatoxin in certain foods, are not directly released into the environment by any primary source. Rather, they are formed within the environment by chemical reactions among their precursor compounds, as in O_3 or $CHCl_3$ formation, or by biological processes, as in the formation of aflatoxin by the action of *Aspergillus flavus* mold on stored peanuts and corn. This section presents some of the important mechanisms for forming secondary environmental contaminants, citing a few more notable examples of transformations within the ambient air and surface waters which have affected public health or attracted considerable public attention.

Chemical Transformations in the Atmosphere

Relatively little attention was paid to chemical reactions within the atmosphere until the 1940s, when the characteristic southern California smog, with its visibility reductions and eye-irritation properties, became persistent. It was very different in character from the classic urban air pollution of London or Pittsburgh, which was characterized by its soot and SO_2 content and reducing properties. The Los Angeles smog, by contrast, had oxidizing properties. It was found to contain O_3, which seemed inexplicable initially, since an inventory of known sources did not yield an adequate O_3 source. At the time, it seemed unlikely that atmospheric chemistry would account for the O_3. The available information on reaction kinetics suggested that the concentrations of potential reactants in the air were too low. Reactions require molecular collisions, and there are many fewer collisions per unit time in air than, for instance, in water, where the effective density is more than 800 times greater. However, chemical transformations within the atmosphere, while they initially appeared unlikely, do lead to the formation of O_3 and a host of other reactive species. Advances in atmospheric chemistry not only helped to develop an understanding of the formation of the oxidizing atmospheres of southern California, but also were able to help lead to a better appreciation of the transformations undergone by SO_2 within the atmosphere and, therefore, of our understanding of the modes of action and effects produced by the more classic kinds of reducing contaminants.

An important ingredient in many of the atmospheric transformations is actinic radiation, i.e., sunlight. Reactions depending on light are known as photochemical reactions.

Photochemical reactions in smog formation

Solar radiation consists of a broad spectrum of wavelengths and energies. The higher-energy wavelengths dissociate gas molecules in the upper atmosphere. Photodissociation of O_2 produces a mixture of the highly reactive atomic oxygen (O), the stable diatomic molecular oxygen (O_2) and the relatively reactive triatomic ozone (O_3). There is relatively little O_3 below the stratospheric O_3 layer, except for that formed in urbanized areas. The background tropospheric level of about 0.03 ppm ~ is attributable to the small amount of mixing that occurs between the stratosphere and troposphere. Photochemical reactions are facilitated by the absorption of solar energy, which raises the reactivity of the absorbing molecules to a level enabling them to react with other molecules. Only colored substances can absorb the longer wavelength photons which can penetrate the O_3 layer. In plants, the key substance is chlorophyll. In the atmosphere, the key gas is the brownish-colored NO_2. Absorption of light quanta having sufficient energy (those with wavelengths up to 0.38 μm) will cause photodissociation:

$$NO_2 + h\nu \rightarrow NO + O \qquad (3\text{–}1)$$

where $h\nu$ is an index of the energy of the light, and h = Planck's constant, ν = frequency. Some organic compounds can also undergo photodissociation to form free radicals, for example:

$$R-\overset{\overset{\large O}{/\!/}}{\underset{\underset{\large H}{\diagdown}}{C}} + h\nu \rightarrow \dot{R} + H\dot{C}O \qquad (3\text{–}2)$$

The highly reactive atoms and free radicals formed in these dissociations may combine with their original partners, but will more likely interact with other molecular species in the atmosphere, utilizing the extra energy received from the solar radiation in their dissociation. Free radicals are so reactive that in aqueous systems their lifetimes are measured in microseconds or nanoseconds. However, in the atmosphere they are present in concentrations of less than 1 part per 100 million, and can have half-lives of minutes to hours. Free radicals can also be formed in nonphotochemical reactions, such as the reactions of O_3 with olefins:

$$O_3 + RCH = CHR \rightarrow RCHO + R\dot{O} + H\dot{C}O \qquad (3\text{–}3)$$

Solar energy quanta, which are not sufficiently energetic to dissociate molecules, can excite them, enabling them to react more readily. Oxygen (O_2) absorbs visible light poorly, but there is so much O_2 in the atmosphere that a sufficient number of excited molecules are formed to play a role in reactions with aldehydes and possibly other hydrocarbons.

After the initial steps of photodissociation and excitation, an extremely complex series of secondary and chain reactions can be initiated, depending on the mixture of raw materials available in the atmosphere and on the ambient temperature and humidity. There are so many possible sequences of reactions that the presentation of a particular pathway is highly speculative. Those presented in this discussion are merely some plausible ones.

Some free radicals attach to O_2, forming peroxy radicals (ROO ·). These can react with NO_2 to form peroxyacetylnitrates (PANs), which are responsible for much of the eye irritation and plant damage produced by the smog mixtures. The peroxy radicals can also react with other primary and secondary air contaminants to form alcohols, ethers, acids, etc.

Many of the secondary products are relatively unstable, and undergo further chemical and photochemical reactions, which may generate NO_2, O_3, and a variety of free radicals; these than participate in further chemical and photochemical reactions. The gas-phase photochemistry can continue through many generations of complex chain reactions and has the net effect of converting most of the NO in the atmosphere to NO_2, and of increasing the levels of O_3 and of light-scattering aerosols of sulfur oxides and highly oxidized hydrocarbons.

The net result of the series of complex reactions is illustrated in Figure 3–8. Levels of the primary contaminants, i.e., the hydrocarbons and NO from auto exhaust, rise through morning rush hours. However, the buildup of NO is stopped by its conversion to NO_2. Aldehydes are partly a primary contaminant, but their continued rise through the morning, and the late-morning fall in hydrocarbons, indicates that the aldehyde level is augmented by photochemical formation processes. As the NO_2 levels fall, the O_3 levels rise. It is interesting that the evening rush hour does not produce the same sequence of events. The better ventilation in the evening limits the accumulation of the primary contaminants. Also, the sunlight is not as strong, nor does it last as long as in the morning. Finally,

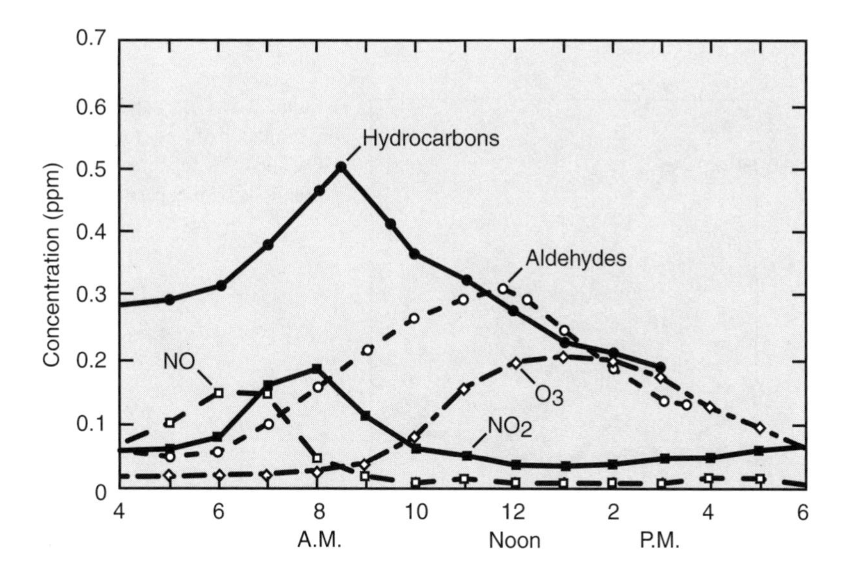

FIGURE 3–8. Average concentration of contaminants during days of eye irritation in downtown Los Angeles, CA. Hydrocarbons, aldehydes, and ozone for 1953–1954. Nitric oxide and nitrogen dioxide for 1958.

the residual O_3 reacts with the NO to form more NO_2, accounting for the late-afternoon rise of the latter. Much of what is known about these complex series of chemical reactions has been learned in smog-chamber tests in which primary contaminants are irradiated by ultraviolet light. The experiment illustrated in Figure 3–9 began with initial concentrations of 2 ppm_v of propylene (C_3H_6), 1 ppm_v of NO, and 0.05 ppm_v of NO_2. The decline in C_3H_6 and NO, and the successive rises of NO_2 and O_3, closely parallel those seen in ambient atmospheres.

Atmospheric transformations of sulfur dioxide and other gas-phase emissions

Sulfur dioxide (SO_2) released to the atmosphere can remain in the air for several days. Some of it, especially when emitted at or near ground level, is taken up by vegetation and materials. It can also be taken up by water droplets in the atmosphere. However, most of it will undergo a series of chemical transformations before it reaches the earth's surface. The first step in the transformation is oxidation to sulfur trioxide (SO_3). This can take place by photochemical oxidation, but the rate is relatively slow and this mechanism does not account for much of the conversion. Most is believed to occur by catalytic oxidation on the surfaces of airborne particles and within droplets. The SO_3 vapor is rapidly hydrolyzed by atmospheric water to form small droplets of sulfuric acid (H_2SO_4). These droplets take on water of hydration, coagulate with other atmospheric particles, and scavenge gas molecules, including more SO_2 and ammonia (NH_3). They thus accumulate trace-metal cations and ammonium ions, and provide a

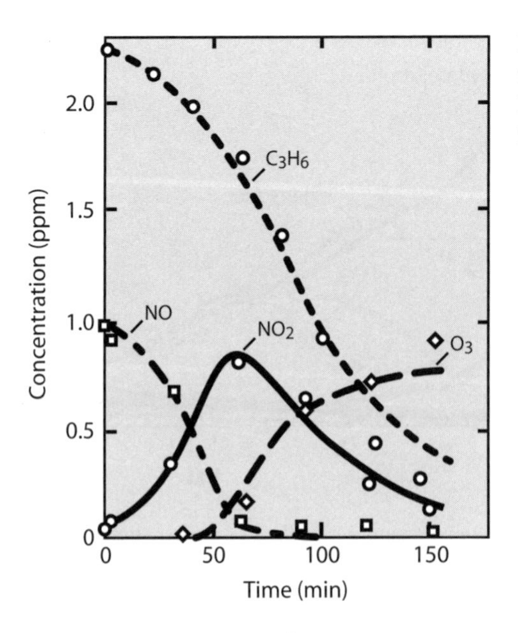

FIGURE 3–9. Concentration changes on irradiation of a mixture of NO, and NO_2, and C_3H_6; comparison of model predictions with experiment.

medium for conversion of the absorbed SO_2 to sulfite and sulfate ions. The end stage of the process is generally an aerosol with a mass median diameter of about 0.5 μm, composed primarily of ammonium sulfate, but also containing traces of other sulfate and nitrate salts. This fine-particle aerosol is very stable in dry conditions, and can travel for hundreds and thousands of kilometers before it is removed from the atmosphere, primarily via precipitation. The processes that determine the composition and characteristics of the ambient air aerosol are summarized in Figure 3–10.

Chemical Transformations in the Aquatic Environment

The primary contaminants discharged into surface waters can be transformed within the aquatic environment into other chemical species. The possibilities for such transformations are virtually unlimited. The examples to be discussed here illustrate two kinds of transformation. One results from human intervention—this is the unintentional production of chlorinated hydrocarbons during the process of disinfection with chlorine. The other involves the intervention of aquatic bacteria, whereby inorganic mercury compounds are converted into much more toxic organic mercury compounds.

Synthesis of chlorinated hydrocarbons in drinking water

Surface waters in the United States are all contaminated, to some degree, with organic compounds. Even natural waters in protected watersheds will have some

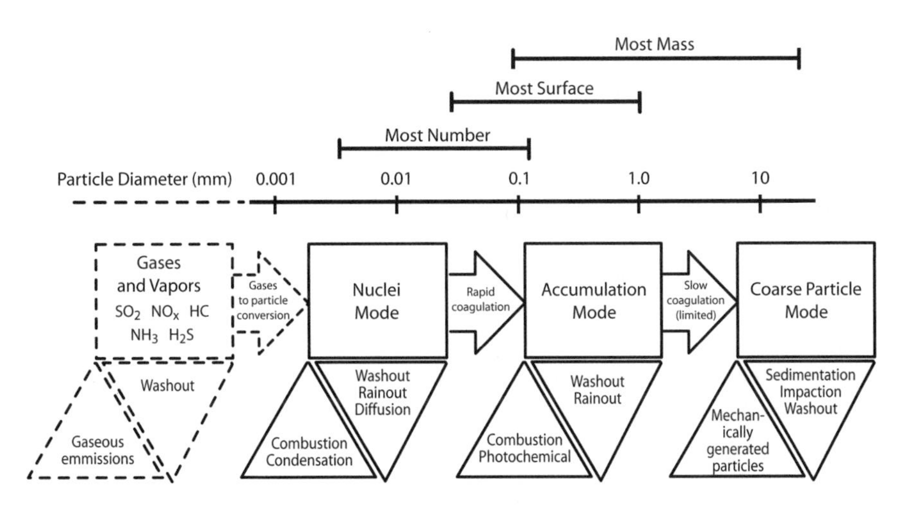

FIGURE 3–10. Schematic representation of the ambient air aerosol and the processes that modify it. (*Source*: Hinds, W.C. *Aerosol Technology*, New York: Wiley, 1999.)

contamination from the natural products and wastes of aquatic life and from the storm-water pickup of land-deposited animal and plant debris and air-contaminant fallout. Many communities produce their drinking water from river water that has been contaminated upstream by agricultural runoff, municipal sewage discharges, industrial wastes and spills. The physical and/or chemical treatments given to these waters to remove their contaminants are never 100% efficient. Thus, when the waters are disinfected, they still contain a variety of organic materials. Some waters are disinfected with O_3, but most are chlorinated. In the process, some of the hydrocarbons react with chlorine to produce chloroform and other trihalomethanes, which are classified as carcinogenic compounds. Many drinking-water supplies also have measurable levels of carbon tetrachloride, methylene chloride, and other halogenated hydrocarbons; but some of these do not appear to be formed to any appreciable extent in the treatment process. Byproducts of drinking water chlorination include various trihalomethanes, haloacids, haloacetonitriles, haloaldehydes, haloketones, halophenols, other aldehydes, and carboxylic acids.

Methylation of mercury by aquatic organisms

In the natural environment, mercury is found in soil, air, and water. The natural level for mercury in water is 0.06 ppb_w in the northeastern United States. Mercury can enter the environment, via a host of sources, either directly or indirectly. There are direct mercury releases in the waste effluents from manufacturing processes. The use of fossil fuels, such as coal (containing approximately 0.5 ppm_w mercury), and the burning of mercury-containing paper constitute indirect means of mercury release. Additionally, accidental misuse must also be considered. The most well-known source of mercury contamination is the chloroalkali industry, which formerly discharged 0.25–0.5 lb of mercury per ton of caustic soda produced. It is important to consider the various forms of mercury present in water. Methyl mercury is the most toxic; other alkyl forms are also toxic but to lesser degrees. Phenyl and inorganic mercury derivatives are also less toxic than the methyl form, but when released into water they can be converted to methyl mercury by a variety of microorganisms. Various factors influence the rate of bacterial methylation in water. Methylation occurs rapidly in the winter and early spring, but slows down during summer and fall. Waters of low pH contain more methyl mercury than those of high pH. Also, aerobic conditions enhance methylation. When exposed to similar concentrations of methyl mercury and inorganic mercury, fish are able to absorb methyl mercury from water 100 times as fast as the inorganic mercury, and are able to absorb five times as much methyl mercury from food as compared to inorganic mercury. Once absorbed, methyl mercury is retained two to five times as long as inorganic mercury. With increased fish size, both the uptake of methyl mercury from the environment and its clearance is decreased. Since methyl mercury is strongly bound

TABLE 3–7. Toxic Food Constituents and Contaminants of Natural Origin

CATEGORIES	SOURCES	EXAMPLES
Intrinsic food components	Natural constituents of plants and animals	Natural pesticides in plants, puffer fish (fugu) toxin
Soil and water constituents	Natural mineral sources	Nitrate; metals such as mercury, arsenic
Microbial metabolites	Toxins from bacteria and fungi growing on food	Aflatoxin B_1, botulinum toxins
Contaminants of natural origin	Toxins accumulating in marine organisms and forage plants	Ciguatera, paralytic shellfish poison
Products of storage or preparation	Toxins arising in aged foods or in food preparation	Oxidized fats, polycyclic aromatic hydrocarbons

to muscle, it accumulates with increased muscle mass and increased duration of exposure. Assuming a steady mercury-containing diet, it takes about a year to establish a balance between mercury intake and mercury excretion. Very high concentrations of mercury have been found in salmon caught in lakes contaminated by industrial discharges. The FDA limit for mercury in fish is 0.5 ppm_w. Among ocean fish, some tuna and most swordfish exceed this limit. However, examination of the tissues of museum specimens captured before the advent of large-scale anthropogenic releases of mercury to the environment show similar levels, suggesting that background sources of mercury still exceed anthropogenic sources.

CONTAMINANTS IN THE FOOD SUPPLY

The chemicals that deposit on soil and vegetation can be taken up in biomass that reaches us via our food supply, where it can add to the toxicity inherent in the foods themselves. Toxicants and allergens can be found in foods even under

TABLE 3–8. Some Mycotoxins of Potential Concern as Food and Feed Contaminants

MYCOTOXIN	HEALTH CONCERN	SOURCE
Aflatoxins	Carcinogenicity	Peanuts, corn, milk
Ergot alkaloids	Neurotoxicity	Grains
Ochratoxins	Nephrotoxicity	Grains
Trichlothecense	GI, blood, and neurotoxicity	Grains
Zearalenone	Interference with reproduction	Grains, corn

ideal conditions, and others can be present because of the spread of anthropogenic pollutants and/or poor handling and storage practices. Examples are illustrated on Tables 3–7 and 3–8.

REFERENCES

1. U.S. EPA. National Air Pollutant Emission Trends, 1900–1998. U.S. Environmental Protection Agency, Research Triangle Park, NC 27711. EPA-454/R-00-002.
2. Wadleigh, C.H. Wastes in Relation to Agriculture and Forestry. Misc. Publ. #1065. Washington, DC: U.S. Dept. of Agriculture, 1968.
3. Eisenbud, M. and Gesell, T. Environmental Radioactivity, 4th Ed. San Diego: Academic Press, 1997.
4. Harley, J.H. Radiological contamination of the environment. In: N.I. Sax (ed.), Industrial Pollution. New York: Van Nostrand Reinhold, 1974 pp. 456–480.

4

Dispersion of Contaminants

The contaminants generated by primary and secondary sources tend to spread continuously within the environment. This chapter reviews how the characteristics of the medium affect the dispersion of contaminants within and between the atmosphere, the hydrosphere, the lithosphere, and the biosphere. Some of the basic transport phenomena are illustrated in Figure 4–1, and these will be discussed in the sections that follow.

CONTAMINANT DISPERSION IN THE ATMOSPHERE

Diffusion in the Atmosphere

The dispersion of contaminants within the atmosphere is generally referred to as diffusion. In still air, the process occurs by molecular diffusion, and can be described by Fick's equation, which was developed in the 1880s for physiological applications. It states that the net rate of flow is directly proportional to the product of the concentration gradient and a constant known as the molecular diffusivity, or coefficient of diffusion. The coefficient decreases with increasing molecular or particle size, since the displacement resulting from a collision of the contaminant molecule or particle with an air molecule decreases as particle size increases.

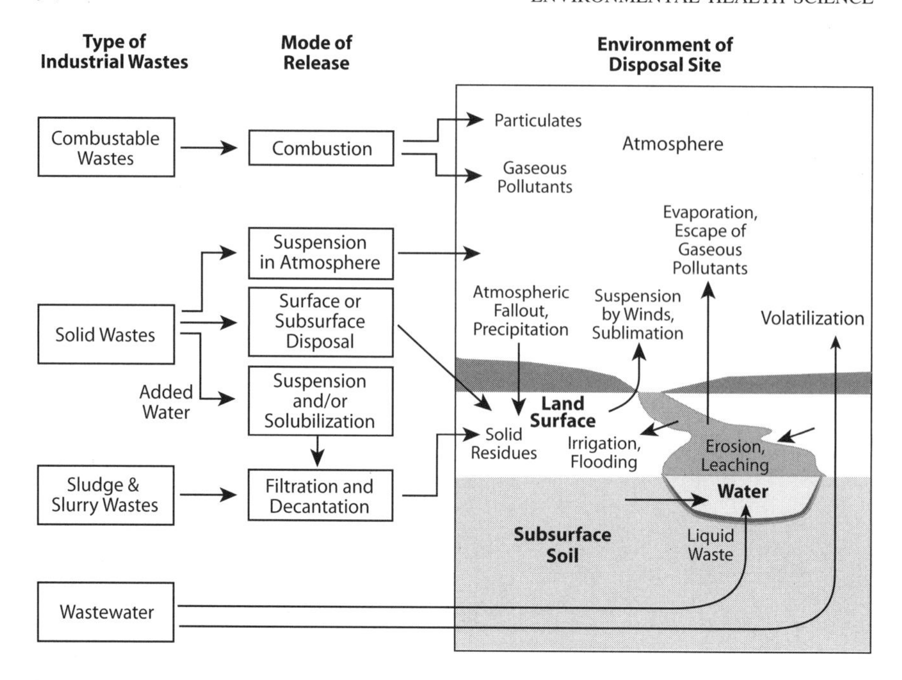

FIGURE 4–1. Sources and modes of releases of pollutants into the environment.

For practical purposes, however, the dispersion of contaminants within the atmosphere by molecular diffusion is negligible, even for gaseous contaminants of small molecular sizes. This is because the displacements are generally infinitesimal compared to the displacements of the air volumes containing them by the turbulent motions of the air. Thus, atmospheric diffusion is synonymous with convective or turbulent diffusion, which may be defined as the random motion and exchange of parcels (small volumes) of air between neighboring parts of the atmosphere. The dispersion of atmospheric contaminants depends primarily on the scale of this turbulence.

Atmospheric Turbulence

Atmospheric turbulence is such a complicated phenomenon that it has defied attempts to describe it in rigorous mathematic terms. In turbulent air, parcels exchange in irregular patterned motions termed eddies. The lack of a general theory of turbulence applicable to the prediction of the eddy diffusion of atmospheric contaminants has led to the development of empirical methods. Even the definition of turbulence remains a matter of debate. For our purpose, it is the almost random variation of the velocity of a fluid, in contrast to the constancy in steady-state streamline flow, or the periodicity of wave motion. In a practical sense, fluctuations about the mean or average wind speed are called turbulence. Such variations are associated with complicated eddy patterns of flow in both the horizontal and vertical directions.[1]

The characteristics of turbulence can depend upon whether the wind velocity component of interest is directed along the average horizontal wind direction, the transverse direction, or the vertical direction. The conventional coordinate system (Fig. 4–2) has the x-axis along the wind direction, the y-axis along the transverse horizontal direction, and the z-axis in the vertical direction. The average wind speed is denoted by $\overline{u}$, and is along the x-axis. The fluctuating components of the wind along the x-, y-, and z-directions are denoted by $u,'$ $v,'$ and $w,'$ respectively.

Actual fluctuations in the wind velocity represent a superposition of a number of different sized turbulent eddies (Fig. 4–3). Some are related to known effects. The intensity of the high-frequency components increases with increasing wind speed and decreases with increasing altitudes, suggesting that they are associated with the friction of the air over the surface terrain. Lower frequency components have been observed to increase with increasing solar flux, suggesting that they are associated with thermal effects. Above about 500 meters, frictional effects from level ground have little effect on the motion of air masses. Over rougher ground, the effects of the surface friction would extend to greater altitudes.

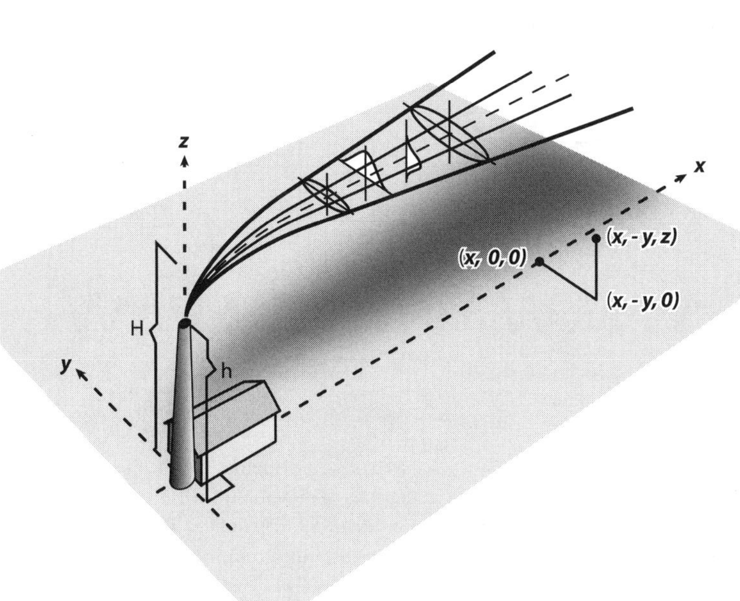

FIGURE 4–2. Conventional coordinate system and basic geometry of plume dispersion. h = geometric (actual) stack height, H = effective stack height.

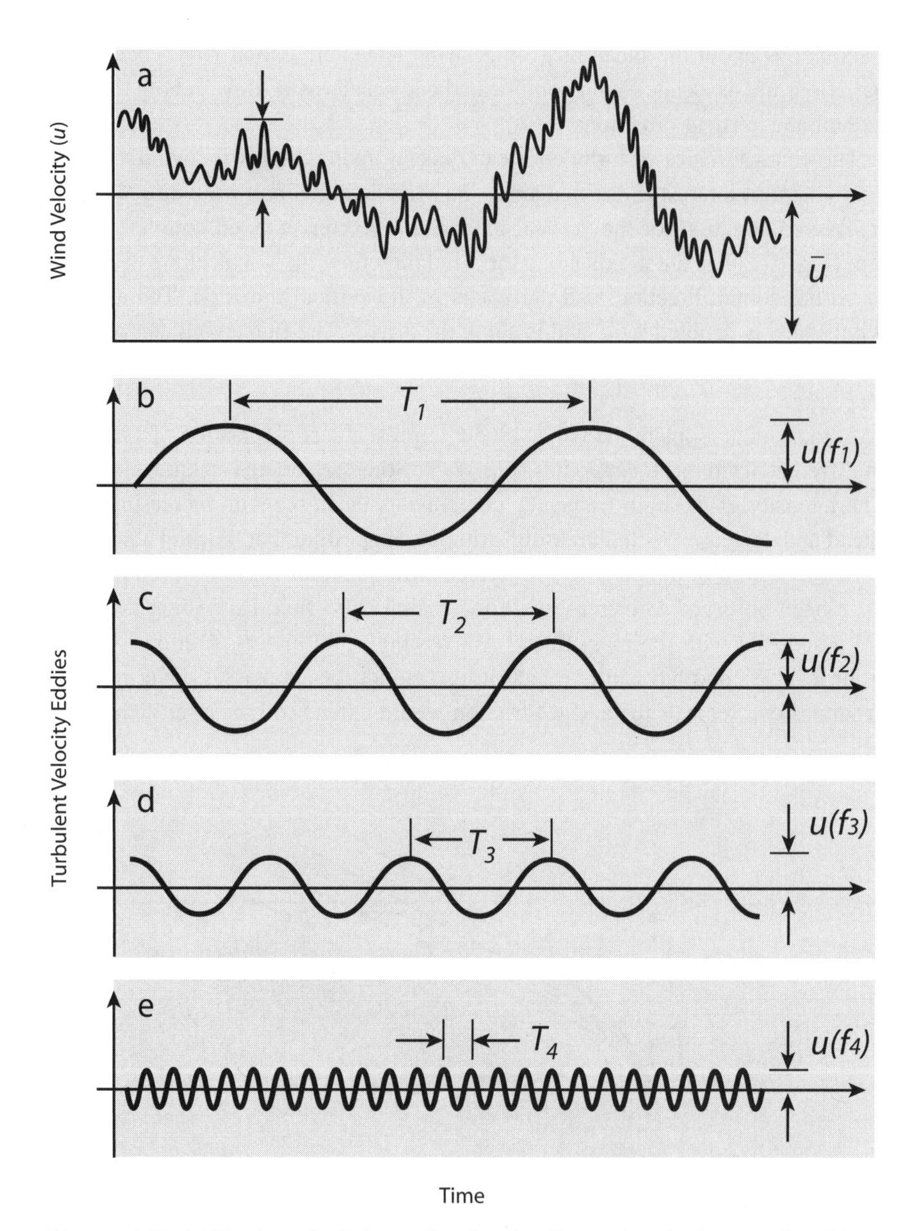

FIGURE 4–3. *(a)* Tracing of wind velocity showing fluctuations in the velocity. *(b)–(e)* The turbulent eddies that cause the fluctuations. The value of u fluctuates about its average, $\bar{u}$, so that u-$\bar{u} = u'$ at any instant in time due to turbulence. The fluctuations are due to the superposition of eddies, each of which has a different frequency and intensity. The contribution due to four eddies is illustrated in *(b)–(e)*. The intensity of each eddy is labeled $u\ (f_n)$ for turbulent components at frequency $f_n = Tn^{-1}$. For example, $u\ (f_2)$ = intensity of component at frequency $f_2 = T_2{}^{-1}$, etc.

Plume Dispersion

When considering the extent and rate of contaminant dispersion, contaminant sources can be divided into three different categories. These are: *(1)* point sources, such as tall stacks; *(2)* line sources, such as highways; and *(3)* area sources, such as whole urban regions. The simplest is an elevated point source, such as a power-plant smokestack. The light-scattering properties of the aerosol in the plume from such a stack, consisting of fly ash and condensed water, provide an opportunity to observe plume dispersion with the unaided eye.

The concentration of a contaminant downwind from a stack will fluctuate with time as turbulence distorts the plume. The plume will meander over the ground, as illustrated in Figure 4–4a. At any given instant, the variation of the ambient contaminant concentration along the y-axis may appear as shown in Figure 4–4b. Over a longer period of observation, the plume will wander to either side of the average direction of the wind velocity, with the result that a one-hour average concentration at each point along the y-axis, as illustrated in Figure 4–4c, has a wider spatial extent but a lower maximum concentration. Thus, as a result of atmospheric turbulence, any one location downwind from the source will be subject to an ambient concentration that strongly fluctuates with time, but the average concentration over a long period of time will be considerably less than the peak values measured during short time intervals. The variation of the plume in

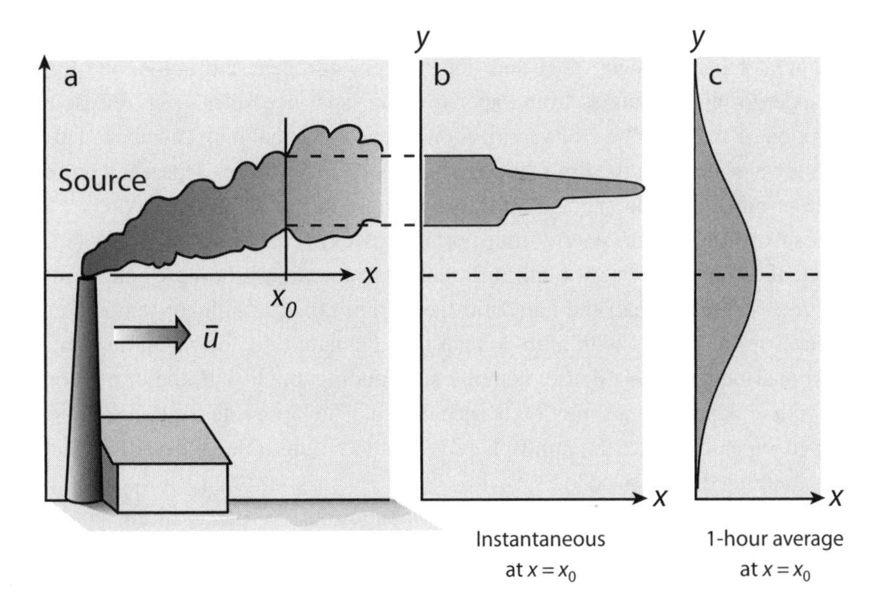

FIGURE 4–4. (a) Instantaneous top view of a plume; (b) instantaneous horizontal profile of the plume concentration x along a transverse direction at some distance downwind from the source; (c) one-hour average profile for the same downwind distance.

the *y*-direction is, therefore, due both to the spread of the plume and to the shifts in the downwind direction. The plume will also spread vertically along the *z*-axis. The vertical mixing of air is dependent upon the temperature profile of the atmosphere, i.e., the lapse rate. The immediate ground level concentrations of air contaminants may be reduced by good vertical mixing, since dispersal into higher regions would tend to dilute the contaminant. Poor vertical mixing may allow contaminants released at low altitudes to remain there in relatively concentrated form.

The simplest way to illustrate vertical mixing is in terms of the concept of a parcel of air. The parcel is a small volume of air having a uniform temperature throughout. Furthermore, if some disturbance causes this parcel to rise or fall in the atmosphere, it generally will do so adiabatically, i.e., with no heat exchange between the parcel and its surroundings.

A rising parcel of air expands and, therefore, according to the gas laws, will cool; a descending parcel will contract and become warmer. If the actual lapse rate of the atmosphere is identical to that of the adiabatically rising or falling parcel, the parcel will neither increase nor decrease its rate of ascent or descent. In other words, the parcel will be in equilibrium with the surrounding air. In this case, the atmospheric lapse rate is known as the adiabatic lapse rate. Since vertical motion is neither encouraged nor discouraged, the atmospheric condition is said to be neutral. Mixing only occurs if the parcel continues to be buoyant as it cools. The exact atmospheric lapse rate depends upon the amount of moisture in the atmosphere. The dry adiabatic lapse rate is approximately 10°C/km. In moist air, water vapor has a greater heat capacity than does the oxygen, nitrogen, and argon, and may also undergo phase changes from vapor to liquid and vice versa, with release or absorption of the latent heat of vaporization. Thus, the actual moist adiabatic lapse rate is always less than the dry rate, ranging as low as 3.5°C/km depending on the degree of moisture. The average tropospheric lapse rate is about 6.5°C/km.

Because of the various energy-transport processes occurring in the atmosphere, the actual lapse rate is very often different from the adiabatic lapse rate. If the lapse rate is greater than the adiabatic lapse rate, i.e., the ambient temperature decreases more rapidly with altitude than the adiabatic rate, the rising air parcel will be warmer, and less dense, than the surrounding air. It will, therefore, continue to rise, since upward motion is accelerated. The lapse rate for this situation is called superadiabatic; the atmosphere is said to be unstable, and vertical mixing is facilitated (Fig. 4–5).

If the actual lapse rate is less than the adiabatic rate, the parcel of air will begin to rise until it reaches a point where its temperature equals that of the surrounding air; upward movement would then cease, opposed by negative buoyancy. This atmospheric condition leads to a stable condition. The parcel rises (or falls) only a short distance until it reaches a point of temperature equilibrium (Fig. 4–6).

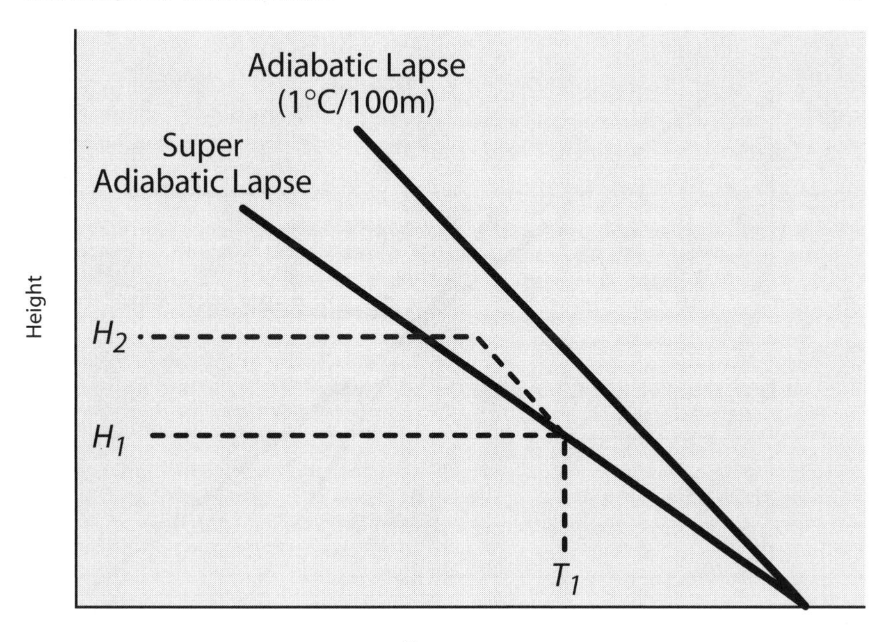

FIGURE 4–5. The instability of the superadiabatic atmosphere. A parcel of air raised in height from H_1 to H_2 cools adiabatically, and its rate of rise is accelerated because it becomes warmer and, therefore, less dense than the ambient atmosphere.

An extreme case of atmospheric stability occurs when the atmospheric lapse rate is negative, i.e., temperature increases with altitude (Fig. 4–7). This condition is known as a temperature inversion. The atmospheric strata within which the inversion occurs is termed an inversion layer. Vertical air movement within inversion layers is essentially nil (low-mixing) and contaminants accumulate within them. These layers are frequently visible because of the light-scattering properties of contaminant aerosols contained within them.

Depending upon how they are formed, inversion layers may have their base on the ground or they may be elevated. Figure 4–8 shows the development of a ground-based inversion, which occurs because the lapse rate near the ground is strongly influenced by radiative heat transfer. This property frequently results in a diurnal variation in lapse rate near ground level.

The effects of lapse rate on the vertical spread of a plume are illustrated in Figure 4–9. In terms of the potential for adverse effects on people, animals, plants, and buildings, we are generally concerned about the groundlevel concentrations rather than the concentrations aloft within the plume, and since most effects are concentration dependent, we are most concerned with the maximum ground-level concentration. Thus, for stack discharges, as illustrated in Figure 4–9, the worst

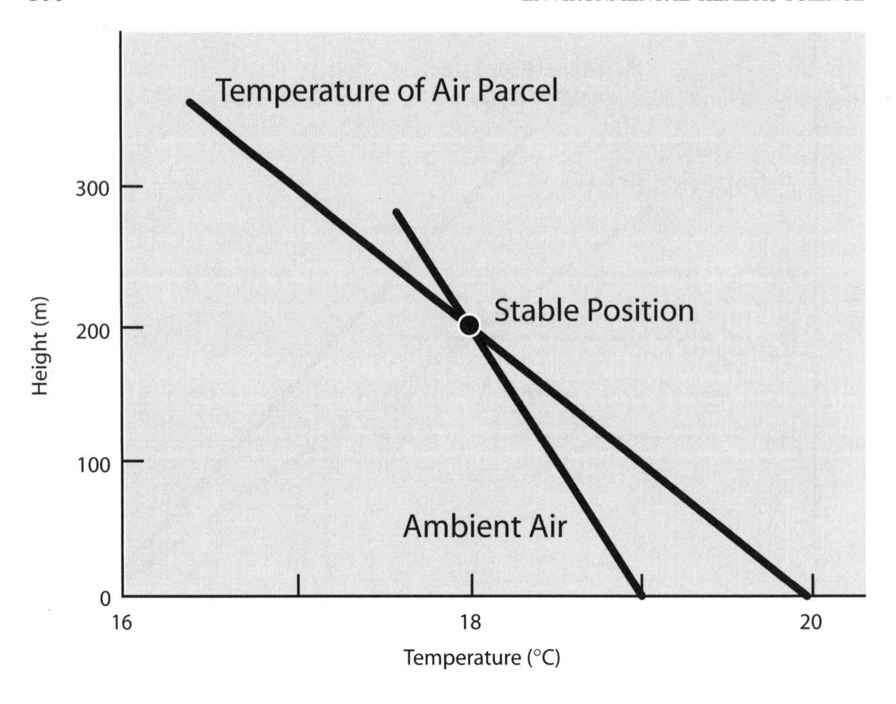

FIGURE 4–6. A rising parcel of air will cease its upward motion if at some point its temperature is identical to the ambient temperature and the ambient lapse is less than the adiabatic rate.

condition is fumigation, where the emissions are all retained within the static inversion layer. At the other extreme, the looping that occurs with a very strong lapse can also bring the plume to the ground close to the stack. However, the time of contact at any one location will be very brief, and the high degree of turbulence will rapidly dilute the contaminant.

Equations have been developed for predicting the downwind concentrations of contaminants discharged from elevated point sources. These are all empirical, since, as discussed earlier, no adequate theory has yet been developed which can cope with the complexity of the atmospheric turbulence. Even those equations based on clearly artificial constraints appear to be formidable to the nonmeteorologist. For example, if we make the simplifying assumption that the average wind speed, $\bar{u}$, does not vary with position, and if contaminants are emitted from an elevated point source, the downwind ground level ($z = 0$) concentration can be approximated by:

$$X\,(x,y,0) = \frac{Q}{\pi \sigma_y \sigma_z \bar{u}}\, e^{-(H^2/2\sigma_z^2 + y^2/2\sigma_z^2)} \tag{4–1}$$

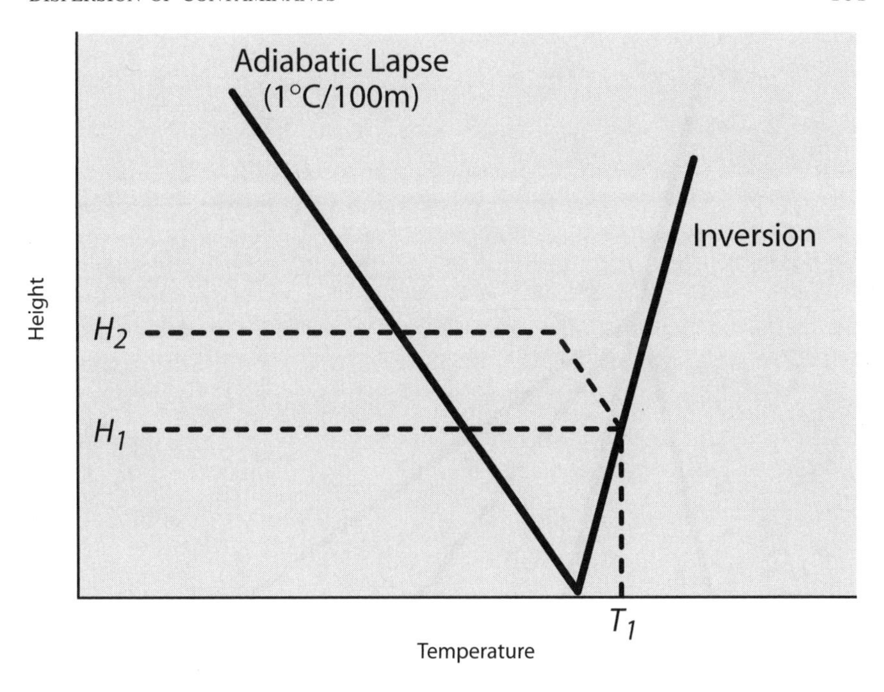

FIGURE 4–7. The inherent stability of the inverted temperature gradient. A parcel of air raised in height from H_1 to H_2 cools adiabatically and sinks to its original position because it becomes more dense than the ambient atmosphere.

where

χ = concentration of contaminant in mass per cubic meter at $(x,y,0)$
Q = emission rate from the source in mass per unit time
σ_y = standard deviation of concentration in y-direction
σ_z = standard deviation of concentration in z-direction
H = effective height of discharge above the ground in meters
y = crosswind distance in meters
x = distance downwind in meters

Power-plant stacks emit hot gases with an upward velocity. These emissions are, therefore, known as buoyant plumes, since they tend to rise until their momentum is spent and they reach thermal equilibrium with the surrounding air. This buoyancy produces an effective increment to the actual physical stack height. The effective stack height (H) used in dispersion equations includes both the actual height and the increment due to buoyancy (Fig. 4–2).

If one's interest is restricted to the ground-level concentration directly downwind of an elevated source, i.e., where $y = 0$, Eq. *(4–1)* reduces to:

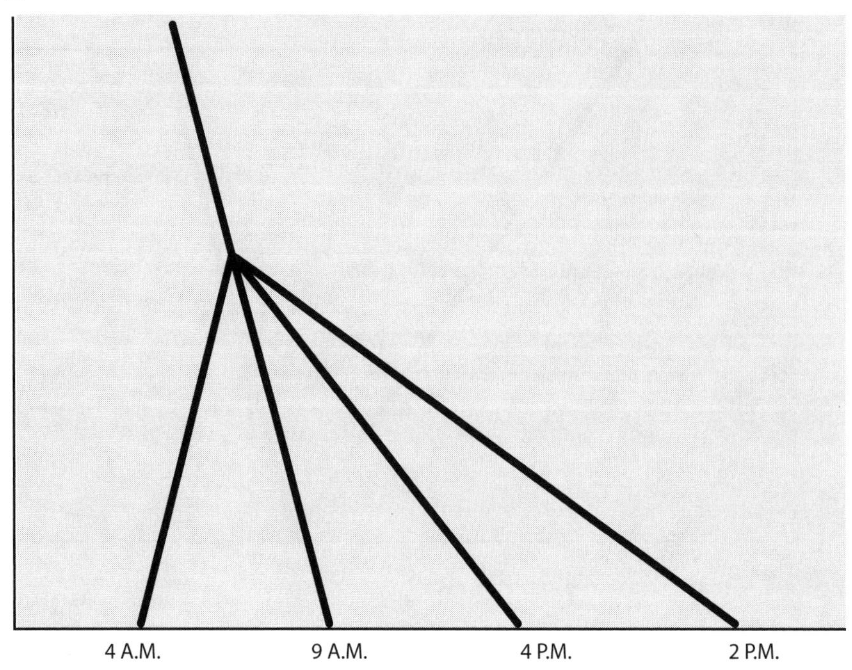

FIGURE 4–8. Typical diurnal variation of temperatures near the ground. *4 A.M.*: Radiation from earth to black sky cools ground lower than air producing a groundbased inversion. *9 A.M.*: Ground heated rapidly after sunrise. Slightly subadiabatic. *2 P.M.*: Continued heating. Superadiabatic. *4 P.M.*: Cooling in the afternoon returns the temperature profile to near adiabatic.

$$X\,(x,0,0) = \frac{Q}{\pi \sigma_y \sigma_z \bar{u}}\, e^{-}(H^2/2\sigma_z^2) \tag{4–2}$$

A feature of Eqs. *(4–1)* and *(4–2)* is the fact that the maximum concentration depends upon the mass emission rate. For a given release height, H, it is independent of the concentration of the contaminant in the exhaust gas. Thus, emitting a more dilute mixture without decreasing the mass emission rate will not reduce the ground-level concentration. The implicit assumption is that only contaminant—and no air—is emitted from the stack, and that dilution in ambient air after emission is the primary means by which the concentration is reduced. If the ambient concentration downwind from an elevated point source is given by Eq. *(4–1)* with empirical values for the x-dependence of (σ_y) and (σ_z), then several statements can be made concerning the magnitude and distribution of the ground-level concentration. The location which received the maximum ground-level concentration will be, of course, on the plume line ($y = z = 0$). This location depends upon the empirically determined dependence of the standard deviation σ_z

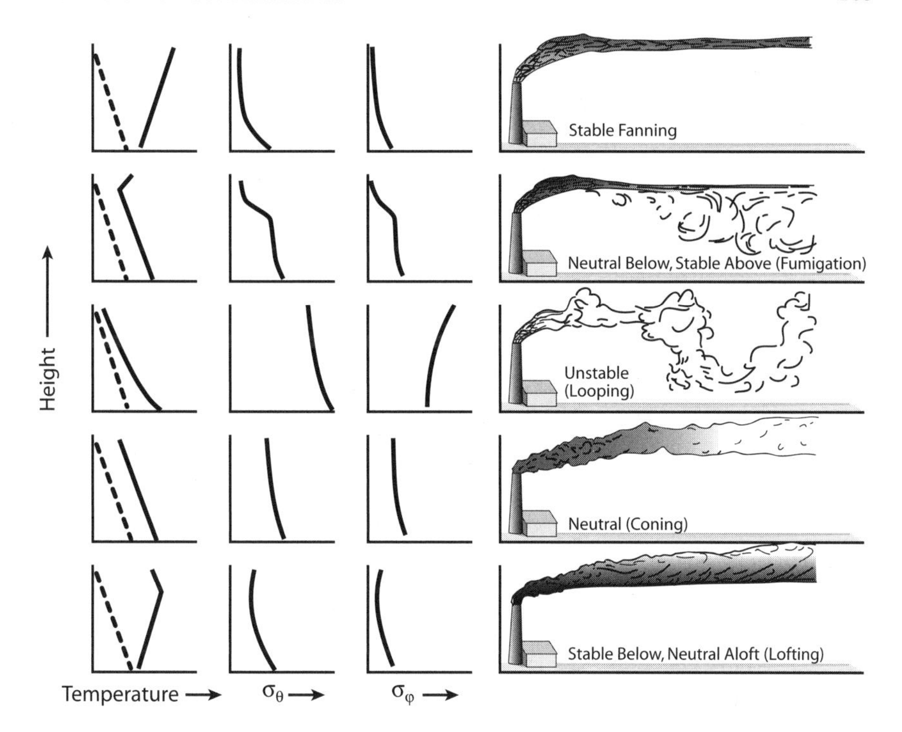

FIGURE 4–9. Various types of smoke-plume patterns observed in the atmosphere. The dashed curves in the left-hand column of diagrams show the adiabatic lapse, and the solid lines are the observed profiles. The abscissas of the columns for the horizontal and vertical wind-direction standard deviations (σ_θ and σ_Ψ) represent a range of approximately 0° to 25°. [*Source*: Slade, D.H. (Ed.) *Meteorology and Atomic Energy*, 1968. U.S. Atomic Energy Commission, TID-24190, Oak Ridge, TN, 1968.]

on the value of *x*. For lack of simpler or more accurate alternatives, a power law dependence is often assumed, whereby:

$$\sigma_y^2 = x^{(2-n)}\, C_y^2/2$$
$$\sigma_z^2 = x^{(2-m)}\, C_z^2/2 \qquad (4\text{–}3)$$

where *n* and *m* are appropriate numbers representing atmospheric stability factors; these numbers, together with the constants *Cy* and *Cz*, are called "diffusion parameters." Thus, for the case where $n = m$, and $Cy = Cz = C$, so that σ_y/σ_z is independent of *x*, the point of maximum ground level concentration is given by:

$$x = (H^2/C^2)\,(1/2 - n) \qquad (4\text{–}4)$$

Under the same conditions, the ambient concentration at this location can be obtained by evaluating Eq. *(4–1)*, with the result:

$$X_{\max} = \frac{2Q}{e\pi\bar{u}H^2} \qquad (4\text{–}5)$$

Representative values of n and C^2 are shown in Table 4–1.

Under these simplifying assumptions, it can be seen from Eq. *(4–5)* that the maximum ground-level concentration is directly proportional to the source strength and inversely proportional to the wind speed. It is also inversely proportional to the square of the effective stack height. Thus, tall stacks, i.e., greater than about 100 m, can greatly reduce local ground-level concentrations due to two factors. One is that the maximum ground-level concentration varies as the inverse square of height. The other is that they generally reach above the morning inversion layer and, as shown in Figure 4–9, this results in the condition known as lofting, where the plume theoretically never reaches the ground.

The preceding brief discussion of dispersion from an elevated point source was limited to the simplest, most basic relations and to their application under many simplifying assumptions. They were developed for applications close to the source. The situation becomes much more complex when considering other types of sources. For example, line sources such as roadways are spatially extended, and the wind direction with respect to source geometry influences the downwind dispersion of contaminants. In area sources, contaminants are received not only from sites directly upwind, but also from those to the sides as well.

Effects of Surface Features

In addition to the imperfections in all of the available empirical relationships for predicting downwind concentrations of airborne effluents, there are a number of other complicating factors that limit their general application.

One key assumption is that there is a free flow field around the top of the stack. This is frequently not the case. Figure 4–10 shows a common complication. Many power plants and factories are built within river valleys because of their need for large volumes of cooling water and/or waterborne transportation.[2] In deep valleys, even a tall stack may not extend above the valley walls. Table 4–2 describes some of the effects of natural surface features upon plume dispersion.

The ability of a stack to disperse contaminants can also be diminished by the presence of a large building in the vicinity. The plume becomes distorted, even

TABLE 4–1. Values of n and C^2 for Several Lapse Conditions

		C^2			
CONDITION	N	AT 25 M	AT 50 M	AT 75 M	AT 100 M
Unstable	0.20	0.043	0.030	0.024	0.015
Neutral	0.25	0.014	0.010	0.008	0.005
Moderate inversion	0.33	0.006	0.004	0.003	0.002
Large inversion	0.50	0.004	0.003	0.002	0.001

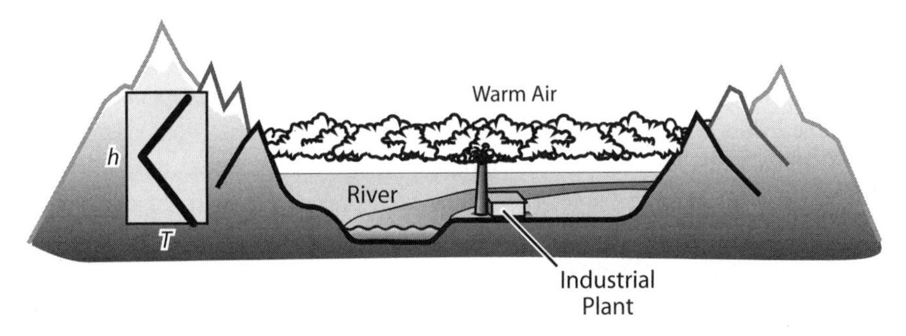

FIGURE 4–10. Fumigation of a valley floor caused by an inversion layer that restricts diffusion from a stack.

TABLE 4–2. Effects of Terrain Features Upon Plume Dispersion

TOPOGRAPHIC FEATURE	EFFECTS
1. Elevated regions	a. Increased wind speed (and increased ventilation) over hill tops. b. Occasional impacting of elevated plumes on ground level.
2. Deep valleys	a. Channeling of wind flow along the valley axis, resulting in higher average concentrations in the valley. b. Development of stable drainage winds during calm, nighttime conditions, resulting in higher concentrations along the valley floor.
3. Undulating regions	a. Increased atmospheric turbulence near the ground level during times of moderate or strong winds. This results in lower pollutant concentrations at locations near sources. b. Accumulation of pollutants in low spots during calm, nighttime conditions (i.e., localized drainage-wind conditions).
4. Regions of tree cover	a. Enhanced turbulence near the ground during moderate or strong winds, resulting in lower concentrations for locations near sources. b. In fully covered regions, blockage of elevated plumes, resulting in lower concentrations at ground level.
5. Bodies of water	a. Increased moisture content in the local atmosphere, favoring fog formation at low-lying spots, and affecting the removal rate of SO_2 and other pollutants from the atmosphere. b. For larger bodies of water, formation of local circulation (lake and sea breezes) which can cause ground-level fumigation on the landward side of sources, during sunny daytime conditions.

if it does not actually contact the building. This effect occurs because the plume is carried in an air stream that accommodates itself to the shape of the building. If the airflow is disturbed locally, that portion of the plume that penetrates the disturbed flow region will also become distorted. Plume distortions near buildings are controlled by the local air motions.

Figure 4–11 shows characteristic flow zones around a sharp-edged cubical building oriented with one wall normal to the wind direction. The background flow, or the flow that would have existed in the absence of the building, is shown at the left, where the streamlines are horizontal. The mean velocity increases upward from zero at the ground, rapidly at first and more slowly at high elevations. In the center of the figure, the building creates a disturbance in the flow, whose main characteristic is the highly turbulent wake.

Within the wake, adjacent to the ground and walls and roof of the building, there exists a region called a cavity; in the cavity, the mean flow is in the direction of the background flow in the outer portion and opposite to the background flow near the axis. Changes in building shape and orientation to the wind affect the cavity dimensions and flow. Rounded buildings have smaller displacement zones and wakes.

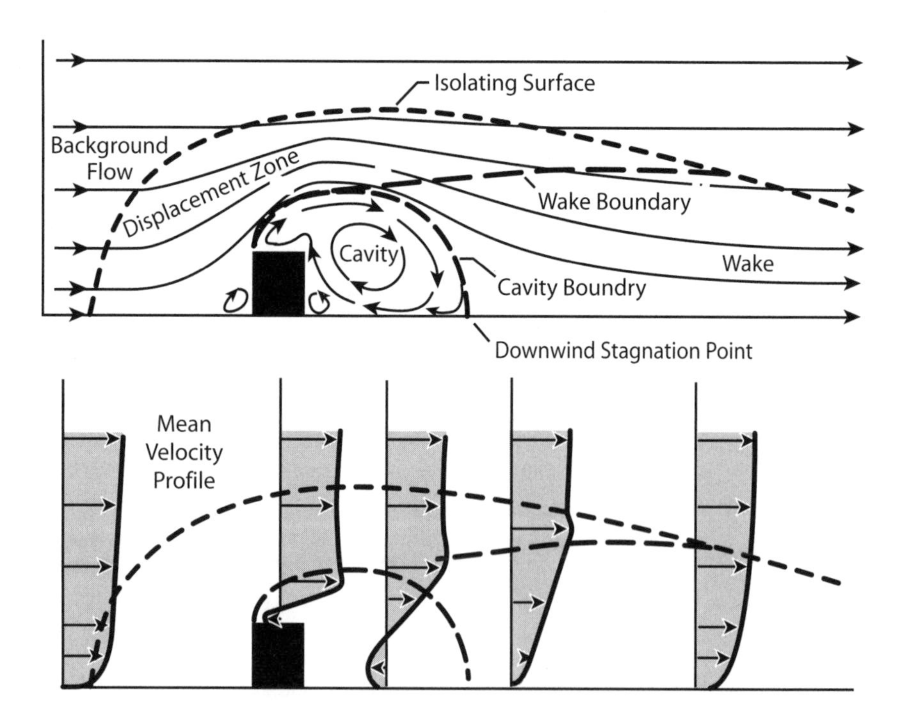

FIGURE 4–11. General arrangement of flow zones near a sharp-edged building.

Contaminant Removal to Surfaces

All of the preceding discussion was based on the behavior of the inert gas within the plume. It does not take into account removal of contaminant by precipitation or by contact with the surface of the ground or vegetation. It also does not take the gravitational sedimentation of particles into account, although the sedimentation rate of particles smaller than 20 μm diameter is so low that there is little significant error introduced when applying the empirical equations to the turbulent diffusion of small particles within the air.

Empirical correction factors for the diffusion formulas have been developed to account for the capture of particles smaller than 20 μm diameter and reactive gases by ground-level surfaces. They employ the concept of deposition velocity (v_g), which is determined experimentally and defined as follows:

$$v_g = \frac{\textit{mass deposited per unit area per unit time}}{\textit{mass concentration above the surface}}$$

The product of the mass concentration given by the diffusion equation and v_g in m/sec will be the deposition in mass/m^2/sec.

The effect of precipitation on the removal of particles and soluble gases can be accounted for using a washout factor rather than a deposition velocity. The washout factor is defined as the fraction deposited per unit time, and some experimental values are illustrated in Figure 4–12. Table 4–3 provides a summary of the effects of various meteorological factors upon plume dispersion.

Dispersion from Ground-Level Sources

In contrast to elevated sources, most of which can be considered discrete point sources whose impacts on the environment are at distant sites, most ground-level sources have their major effects immediately downwind. Furthermore, since such emissions occur within the air most affected by surface roughness, they rapidly become well mixed into the surface air, a layer of varying height which normally extends from about 100 m to 2000 m. As illustrated in Figure 4–11, the effluent from a short stack or roof vent will be influenced by the aerodynamic flow pattern around the building(s) with which it is associated. In estimating the downwind concentration patterns caused by this phenomenon, the most conservative approach is to assume that the effluent is trapped in the wake and brought quickly to the ground without being enveloped and mixed in the cavity directly behind the structure.

If the effluent is trapped in the cavity, it will be mixed rapidly into a volume determined essentially by the cross-sectional area of the structure and wind speed. An appropriate formula for the downwind concentration is:

$$X = \frac{Q}{(\pi\sigma_y\sigma_z + cA)\,\bar{u}}\, e^{-[y^2/2\sigma_y^2]} \tag{4–6}$$

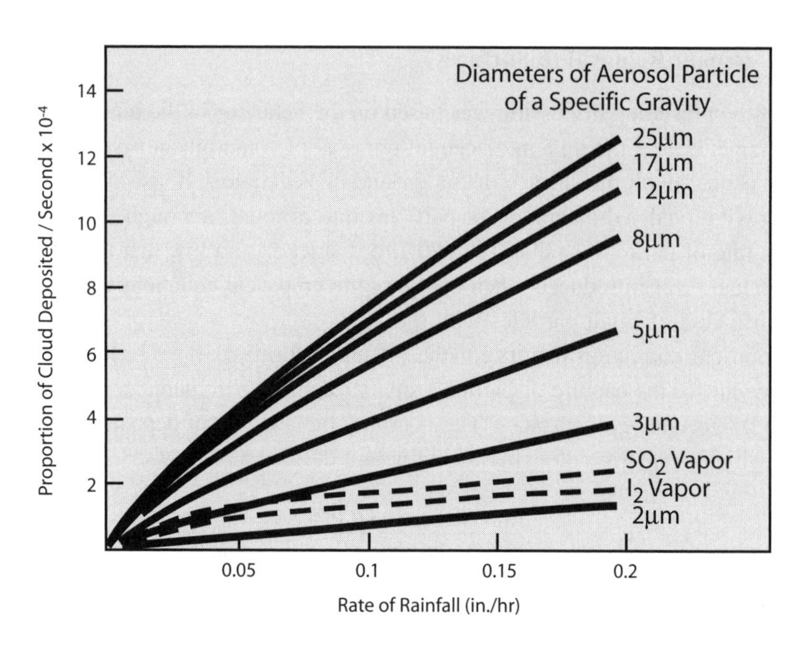

FIGURE 4–12. Percentage removal of particles according to particle size and rate of rainfall.

TABLE 4–3. Summary of Effects of Meteorological Conditions Upon Plume Behavior

CONDITION	EFFECT
Wind speed	Determines initial dilution
Wind direction	Determines downwind geometry
Atmospheric stability category	Determines plume spread associated with turbulent motions in the atmosphere
Mixing layer depth (or height of inversion base)	Determines limit to the vertical spread of the plume-important for downwind flow distances greater than 1000 m
Humidity	High humidity associated with visibility decreases for water-vapor plumes
Surface temperature	Determines possibility of ice formation from water-vapor plumes
Precipitation	Determines possibility of washout of contaminants near the source

where A is the cross-sectional area of the building normal to the wind and c is a shape factor, ranging from 1/2 for a relatively streamlined shape to 2 for a blunt building. This formula gives a maximum concentration directly downwind of the building (σ_y, $\sigma_3 = 0$) of $Q/cA\ \bar{u}$, a simple volume approximation.

In urban areas where there are many buildings with short stacks and roof vents, the situation becomes more complex, but the likelihood of thorough mixing of the various effluents is generally quite high. There is usually relatively little variation of concentration with height for CO and Pb emitted at street level, or for SO_2 emitted from rooftops of private homes or apartment houses.

Long-Range Transport in the Troposphere

While elevated discharges are an effective means of reducing maximum ground-level concentrations, they obviously do nothing to diminish the total amounts of contaminants emitted into the atmosphere. In fact, by minimizing contact between the ground-level surfaces and the contaminants, they actually act to increase the residence times and total atmospheric burdens of the contaminants. The development of a persistent haze layer over the eastern third of the continental United States in recent decades appears to be due in large part to the sulfate particles in the air that are transported in the prevailing winds over many hundreds of kilometers. These, in turn, were formed in the atmosphere from the airborne oxidation and hydrolysis of SO_2, much of which was discharged at elevated levels by the tall stacks of utility boilers. Even in the vast continental atmosphere, dilution is no longer the "solution to pollution."

The spread of environmental contaminants via the air depends upon their physical and chemical forms. Nonreactive and water-insoluble gases, vapors, and submicrometer particles can remain airborne for weeks within the troposphere and can, therefore, spread throughout the world. Evidence for such transport of chemical contaminants via the atmosphere is the presence of lead, nuclear weapons test debris, and various organic pesticides in samples of polar ice collected at locations that are remote from known sources of such contaminants.

Tropospheric-Stratospheric Interchange

The transport of contaminants from near-surface sources covers time scales measured in hours and days. When contaminants were generated by thermonuclear explosions, they were spread throughout the atmosphere on a global scale, following injection of some of the debris into the stratosphere.

Our knowledge of stratospheric dispersion was derived from gas and dust samples obtained by aircraft or balloons at an altitude of about 35 km. On two occasions, nuclear weapons were exploded at unusually high altitudes, and unique tracers were intentionally added to facilitate the dispersion studies. ^{102}Rh was injected into the stratosphere by an explosion at an altitude of 43 km above Johnston Island in the Pacific in August 1958. The cloud from this nuclear explosion was believed to have risen to about 100 km. In July 1962; an explosion conducted about 400 km above Johnston Island contained a known amount of ^{109}Cd.

Stewart et al. developed a model of stratospheric-tropospheric exchange that is consistent with the observed pattern of nuclear weapons fallout.[3] According to this model, air enters the stratosphere in the tropical regions, where it is heated and rises to an altitude of about 30 km, at which level it begins to move toward the poles. As shown in Figure 2–6, the tropopause is lower in the polar regions than at the equator, and tropopause discontinuities in the temperate regions facilitate transfer from the stratosphere to the troposphere. The jet streams, with velocities of 100 to 300 km/hr, occur at these discontinuities. The rate of transfer from the lower stratosphere is most rapid in the winter and early spring.

A summary overview of the transport and fate of atmospheric emissions is provided in Figure 4–13.

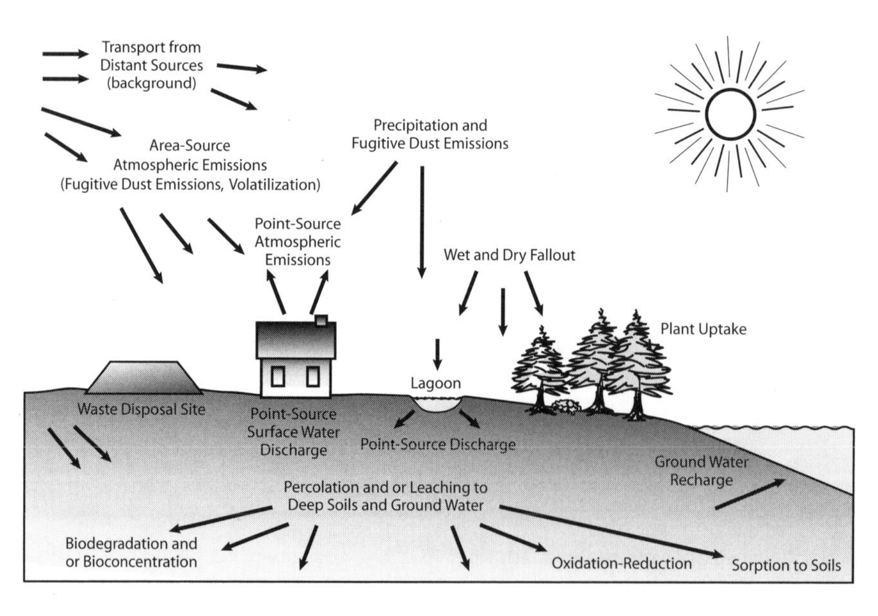

FIGURE 4–13. Schematic illustrating the transport and fate of atmospheric emissions into various parts of the environment. (*Source*: Paustenbach, D. The Risk Assessment of Environmental Hazards, New York: Wiley, 1989.)

CONTAMINANT DISPERSION IN THE HYDROSPHERE

The aquatic environment is considerably more varied and complex than the atmosphere with respect to contaminant dispersion. There are large differences in dilution volumes, mixing characteristics, and transport rates between rivers, lakes, estuaries, coastal waters, and oceans, making a generalized approach to the dispersion of contaminants introduced into bodies of water not possible with the current state of knowledge. Also, there is a much more active interchange of contaminants between the hydrosphere and the biosphere than between the atmosphere and biosphere.

While this section will be concerned primarily with contaminant transport within the abiotic hydrosphere and a subsequent section will be concerned primarily with transport within the biosphere, it is not really possible to treat either in isolation. Some of the possible routes of contaminant transfer between the hydrosphere and the biosphere are shown in Figure 4–14.

Precipitation and Surface Runoff

The atmosphere is a source of chemical contaminants for deposition on the surface of the earth, for example, by gravitational settlement and via precipitation. Precipitation on the land becomes surface runoff, which picks up additional contamination by dissolution and suspension of contaminants deposited on the sur-

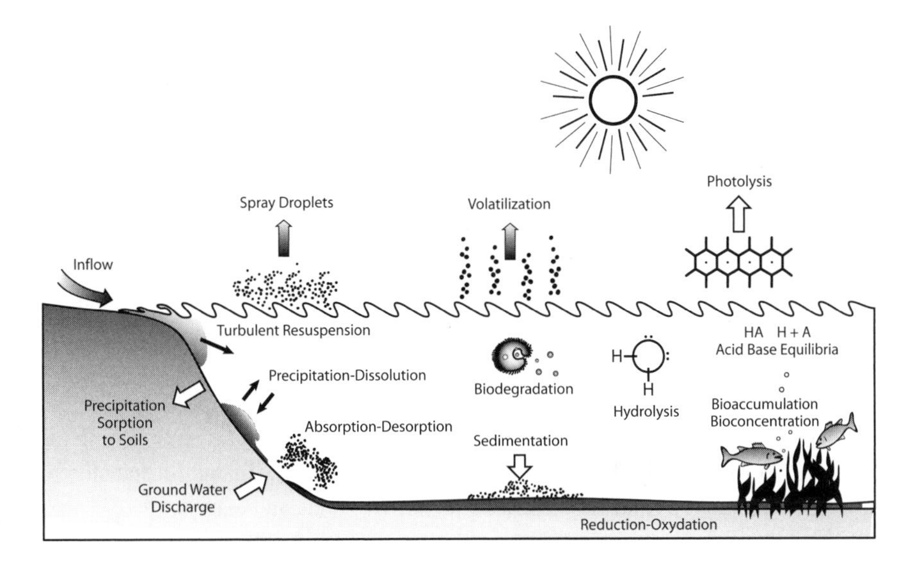

FIGURE 4–14. Schematic illustrating the various avenues for degradation and movement of chemicals and sediments in the environment. (*Source*: Paustenbach, D. The Risk Assessment of Environmental Hazards, New York: Wiley, 1989.)

face since the last rain. On the other hand, the land surface also acts as a filter and chemical buffer to the surface runoff, reducing part of its contaminant load. During light precipitation, the runoff may become relatively concentrated with dissolved contaminants that do not react with nor are readily sorbed by surface soil; at the same time, it would be relatively well filtered of suspended solids. On the other hand, during heavy precipitation the soluble contaminants would be very much diluted, while the turbulent flow would stir up relatively high concentrations of suspended solids.

Streams, Rivers, and Lakes

Rivers and streams vary so much in bed structure, depth, and flow rate that it is not possible to generalize dispersion rates for the contaminants discharged into them. Further complications are added for "managed" rivers. Most of the larger rivers in the United States have been extensively dammed for purposes of flood control, hydroelectric power generation, and navigation, and large stretches of them are really a series of shallow lakes rather than a free-flowing river. There are also major withdrawals of river water for drinking-water supplies, industrial and utility usage, and irrigation of agricultural lands. Some of these waters, especially the industrial and utility process and cooling waters, are largely returned to the river, albeit with added contaminant loads. On the other hand, the irrigation waters are largely lost to evaporation, ground-water recharge, and possibly to drainage into another watershed. In an extreme case, such as the Colorado River where withdrawals by the U.S. and Mexico are equal to the total flow, virtually none of the water leaves the mouth of the river.

Lakes have the additional component of greater depth of water. As discussed in Chapter 2, the water can become thermally stratified, with the lower portion (hypolimnion) becoming isolated from oxygen sources. In nutrient-rich lakes, this results in complete oxygen depletion and anaerobic decay within the hypolimnion. The spring and fall turnovers of the waters in the lake then spread the products of this decay throughout the lake.

The natural dispersion of waste water effluents in lakes is often poor. In the absence of wind and tide, there is little turbulent mixing. Lake waters are normally colder and, therefore, heavier than waste water effluents. Effluents discharged at or near the surface of denser receiving waters are likely to overrun them. Discharged at some depth below the surface, they rise like smoke plumes and, on reaching the surface, fan out radially. Because chemical diffusion is slow, natural dispersion or mixing of the unlike fluids is mainly a function of winds and currents.

Estuaries

The spread of contaminants within estuarine waters depends heavily on the structure of the estuary. In some, the sea water forms a distinct wedge beneath the fresh water. More typically, there is sufficient turbulent mixing to create a more gradual change from fresh to salt water. At the other extreme, there is so much turbulent mixing that both the horizontal and vertical concentration gradients disappear.

Estuary flow is so complicated that there is no generalized dispersion model; the physical characteristics of each estuary must be studied on an individual basis. For example, in a study of diffusion and convection in the Delaware River Basin, Parker et al.[4] constructed a scale model of the Delaware Basin at the United States Army Waterways Experiment Station at Vicksburg, Mississippi. The model was 750 ft long and 130 ft wide, and the expected dilution was studied using dyes. Figure 4–15 illustrates the type of information obtained from a study of the dilution of dye over a period of 58 tidal cycles (approximately 1 month). In this particular study, which involved instantaneous injection of a given dose, the concentration at the end of the 58 cycles remained at approximately 1% of the maximum concentration during the initial tidal cycle. The conditions of the experiment were conservative: There were no losses due to sedimentation or biological uptake. Thus, only the diminution owing to mixing was measured.

The Oceans

Dispersion of contaminants in ocean waters depends primarily on the characteristic physical features discussed in Chapter 2. These are the temperature, density, and salinity gradients with depth, and the surface currents.

Vertical mixing is vigorous within the surface zone due to wind action, but is very poor within the lower parts of the intermediate zone. This is illustrated in

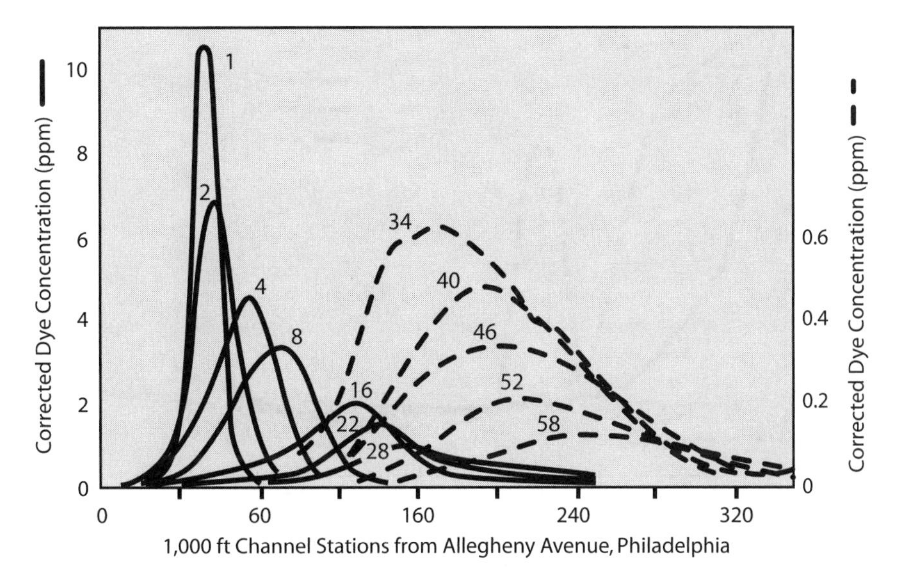

FIGURE 4–15. Longitudinal distribution of contaminants after a designated number of tidal cycles in a scale model of the Delaware River near Philadelphia.

Figure 4–16, which shows the distribution of radioactive debris at 6, 28, and 48 hours after it was deposited on the surface of the water. Since material deposited on the surface of the ocean mixes very slowly into the deep water, it is possible to find measurable amounts of residual material on the surface at a considerable time following deposition. For example, Figure 4–17 shows the first year's path for weapons test debris from a June 1954 test. Comparison of this figure with Figure 2–11 shows that the debris followed the normal circulation of ocean surface water.

While the rate of movement of the bottom water has not been mapped, Koczy[5] estimated rates of vertical diffusion from measurements of radium and other substances dissolved in ocean waters. Dissolved ^{238}U gives rise by radioactive decay to ^{230}Th, which precipitates rapidly to the bottom sediments. The decay of ^{230}Th results in the formation of ^{223}Ra, which tends to return into solution at the ocean bottom. The vertical gradient of dissolved radium is a measure of the rate of movement of bottom water toward the surface. Koczy's model of vertical diffusion is shown in Figure 4–18. Dissolved substances released from the ocean floor diffuse slowly through a friction layer 20 to 50 m in depth, where diffusion rates are on the order of molecular diffusion. Mixing is most rapid (3–30 cm^2/sec) just above the friction layer, and decreases rapidly with height above the ocean floor to a level about 1000 m below the surface, where a secondary minimum (10^{-2} cm^2/sec) is thought to exist. Diffusion rates then increase as one

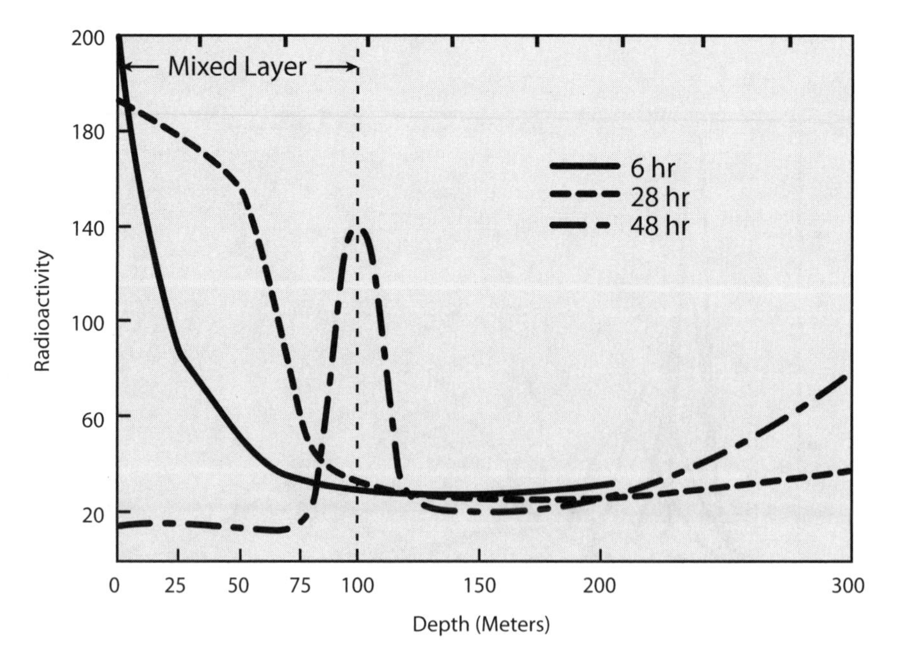

FIGURE 4–16. The vertical distribution of radioactivity in the ocean at selected times after fallout of debris from a nuclear explosion.

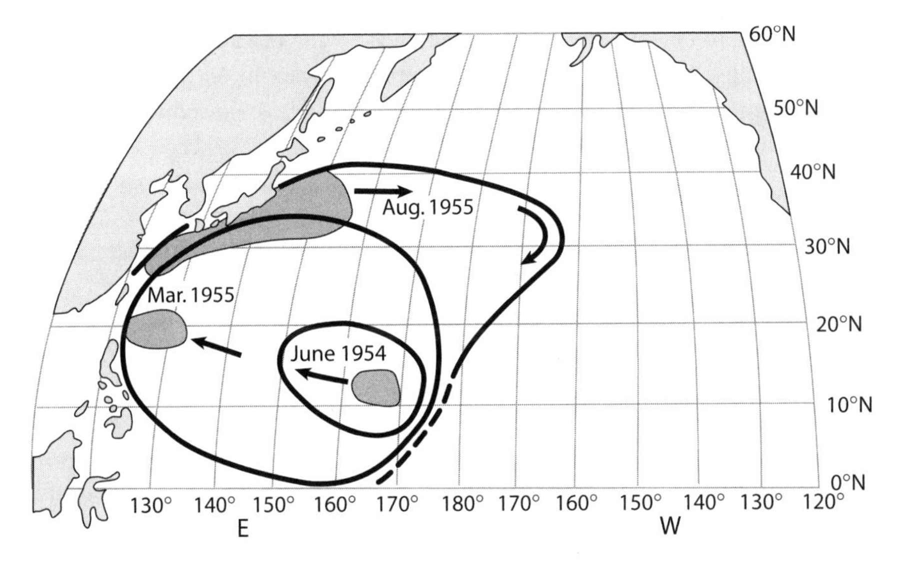

FIGURE 4–17. The horizontal dispersion of nuclear weapons debris in the north Pacific Ocean after tests by the United States in the Marshall Islands, 1951. Striped regions indicate areas of maximum contamination.

approaches the mixed layer, where diffusion coefficients ranging from 50 to 500 cm^2/sec are found.

Koczy's estimate of vertical transport in the Atlantic Ocean is between 0.5 and 2 m/year at depths ranging from 750 to 1750 m. If these values apply at greater depths, a solution placed at a depth of 3000 m would not appear in the surface

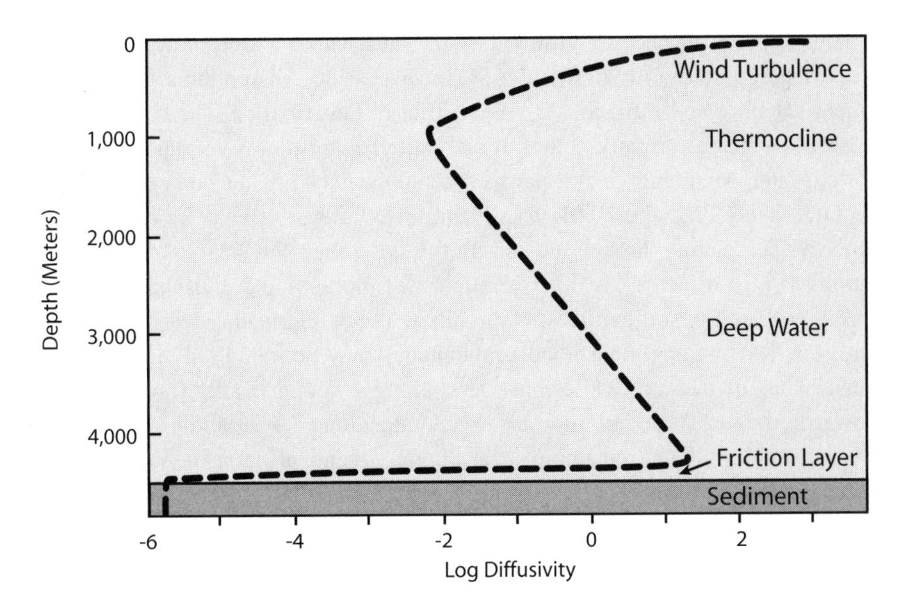

FIGURE 4–18. Vertical diffusion in the oceans.

water for more than 1000 years. Limited areas of the oceans are characterized by upwellings, which carry water from deep regions to the surface via vertical currents having a velocity of a few meters per day. These upwellings could facilitate the vertical transport of contaminants.

CONTAMINANT DISPERSION IN THE LITHOSPHERE: SOILS

Like the hydrosphere, the soil environment is quite complex with regard to contaminant dispersion. The different soil types have individual characteristics that affect the movement of chemicals introduced, intentionally or otherwise, into or onto the soil.

Contaminant dispersion in soil depends upon the specific nature of the chemical, the soil type, and other soil factors such as moisture, pH, and temperature. Except for gases, which readily diffuse through the air channels, most chemical contaminants do not readily move once they enter the soil. The main processes that affect movement of contaminants through soil are adsorption, leaching, and diffusion.

Chemicals may become dispersed in soils via movement with the soil water. The major direction of movement is downward to lower levels (horizons), but it may also be upward, due to evaporation of water, or even laterally, due to surface runoff. Downward movement is, of course, the major direction in soils through which there is rapid percolation of water. As the rate of percolation slows in deeper layers, chemicals may diffuse into the pores between soil particles, and be further dispersed and redistributed.

Many chemicals become adsorbed to soil particles via various processes; these are discussed more fully in Chapter 5. However, since adsorption affects subsequent leaching and diffusion, it may restrict the distribution of a contaminant. Chemicals that are tightly bound to soil particles are poorly leached by percolating water. Many high molecular weight halogenated organic compounds, such as DDT and PCBs, show little movement, even after several years of exposure to water percolating through the soil. In this case, their low degree of water solubility is also a factor. As other examples, ammonium and phosphate ions are strongly bound to soil particles, while nitrate is not and readily leaches through the soil. Thus, strongly adsorbed contaminants may be found only in the upper few inches of the soil, while those less strongly bound readily travel through lower horizons. These are, of course, generalizations, since binding and subsequent leaching of any contaminant is highly dependent upon the specific soil type.

Little is known of the rate at which chemical contaminants migrate through different types of soils under different environmental conditions, i.e., degree of drainage, pH, degree of moisture.

CONTAMINANT DISPERSION IN THE BIOSPHERE: TRANSPORT THROUGH FOOD CHAINS

In the biosphere, essential nutrients and energy are tranferred from organism to organism along pathways called food chains. Very often, single chains are interconnected, resulting in a more complex interlocking pattern termed a food web.

Solar energy is utilized by organisms known as producers, for the assimilation of simple, inorganic chemicals (nutrients) into energy-rich compounds. The primary producers are green plants, whose chlorophyll absorbs solar radiation, and which produce organic compounds from CO_2 and H_2O via photosynthesis. The potential food energy and nutrients within the plants are then transferred to the primary consumers, or herbivores, i.e., organisms that eat plants. By eating the herbivores, carnivorous secondary consumers obtain energy and nutrients indirectly from plants. Food webs can also involve omnivores, organisms intermediate between the primary and secondary consumers, who eat both plants and animals. Carnivorous tertiary consumers feed on secondary consumers, etc., with the number of levels of carnivores varying with the specific biotic community. The organic compounds in waste products and in dead plant and animal bodies provide the substrate for the decomposers, largely bacteria, which break down these compounds, releasing inorganic nutrients. A generalized food chain is shown in Figure 4–19.

Organisms that obtain their nutrients from plants by the same number of steps along a food chain are said to belong to the same trophic level. Green plants are the first level, herbivores the second, and so on. Trophic structure is often graphically represented as an ecological pyramid, with producers comprising the base of the pyramid, and successive trophic levels making up the tiers. Pyramids may be based upon the total number of organisms in each level, their biomass, or their energy content. One such pyramid is shown in Figure 4–20. Humans are generally at the apex of their ecological pyramid, i.e., at the end of the food chain. Thus, we are very dependent upon the natural environment for nutrient needs.

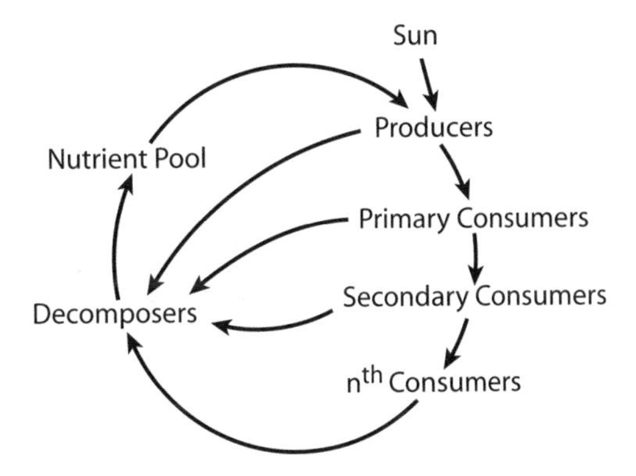

FIGURE 4–19. A generalized food chain.

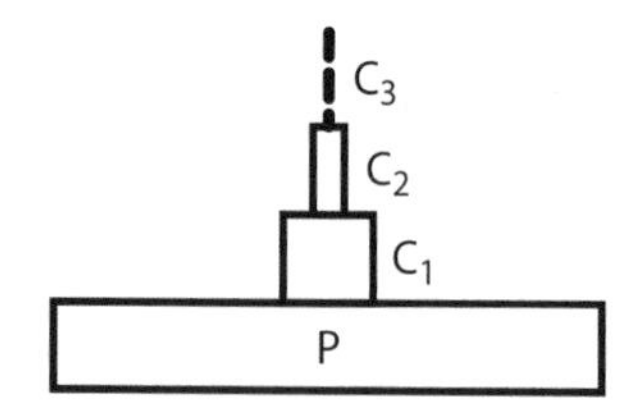

FIGURE 4–20. A trophic pyramid, arranged according to biomass, in an aquatic ecosystem in Silver Springs, FL. The numbers represent gm of dry biomass per m^2. P = Producers; C_1 = Primary Consumers (herbivores); C_2 = Secondary Consumers; C_3 = Tertiary Consumers.

Transport via food chains is an important route by which chemical contaminants may reach us. In addition, damage to the environment may also occur along the transport chain. Contamination of food chains may occur in the aquatic or terrestrial environments. There is, however, never a sharp delineation between these two, and transport of chemicals often occurs between them. For example, carnivorous birds may consume contaminated marine organisms, then deposit their droppings on land. Humans, while being terrestrial organisms, often consume marine creatures directly.

In aquatic environments, contaminants may become adsorbed on solids suspended in the water. The solids may eventually settle to the bottom, deposit on the surfaces of aquatic plants, or be directly taken up by filter feeding marine organisms. Bottom sediments receive the settling remains of dead organisms or deposits of contaminated excreta. Dissolved chemicals may also be directly taken up by plants or animals.

The sediments often provide the organic substrate that supports the benthic organisms. Contaminants taken up by the latter may then be passed to higher trophic levels, and then back to the sediments, or possibly to humans via their consumption of aquatic biota. This chain of contaminant uptake bypasses the primary trophic level, since chemicals may directly enter the food chain at a consumer level.

As in aquatic environments, contaminants generally enter terrestrial food chains through the producers. Incorporation into green plants may occur by root uptake from the soil or by absorption following deposition upon foliar surfaces. Uptake from soil depends upon the amount of time the contaminant remains within the root zone and, of course, whether it is in a form usable by the plant. The structure of a plant is a prime determinant of its ability to act as an efficient trap for contaminant deposition.

In some biota, the concentrations of particular chemicals may be greater than those in the surrounding environment. The process by which this occurs is called biological magnification or bioconcentration. The degree of increase is often indexed by a concentration factor (CF); this is the ratio of the contaminant concentration in the organism to that in its environment. The effects of bioconcentration may lead to reduced populations among members of a food chain. However, when the acute toxicity of a contaminant is low, harmful effects may be delayed until chronic symptoms develop. By this time, damage to the biota may persist long after emissions are curtailed. Bioconcentration poses the greatest threat to those consumers, such as humans, that are at the upper trophic levels. In some cases, a process of biological exclusion may occur, i.e., an organism actually has a lower concentration of a contaminant than is present in its environment.

Examples of Food-Chain Transport of Contaminants

Radionuclides

Most of the basic chemical elements required by plants are obtained from the soil in terrestrial environments, or from the water and sediments in aquatic environments. As these nutrients are taken up, so may contaminants. This is especially true of many radionuclides.

The property of radiation itself does not usually affect the uptake of an element, although once absorbed, tissue damage may ensue. A biological system will incorporate material based solely upon its chemical properties, without discrimination between radioactive and nonradioactive isotopes. The advanced technology available for isotope identification and quantitation has made it possible to do tracer studies with radionuclides, providing some of the best available information on food-chain transport of contaminants.

Studies in the Pacific Ocean atolls performed following nuclear testing in the 1950s showed that a difference existed between the types of radionuclides that enter aquatic and terrestrial food chains. Marine organisms contained highest amounts of radionuclides that either formed strong complexes with organic matter (e.g., ^{54}Mn, ^{59}Fe, ^{65}Zn, ^{30}Co) or which occurred in particulate or colloidal form (e.g., ^{95}Zr, ^{106}Rh, ^{144}Ce, ^{144}Pr). Soluble fission products, for example, ^{90}Sr and ^{137}Cs, were found in highest concentrations in land biota.

In general, the relative proportion of radionuclides that enter food chains, as well as their concentration factors, are greater in nutrient-poor environments. For example, concentration factors tend to be greater in fresh water than in sea water, since the former usually contains lower concentrations of mineral nutrients. Concentration factors in aquatic environments, however, tend to be greater than in terrestrial environments, largely due to more rapid nutrient cycling.

A potential danger to humans is posed by the selective concentration of radionuclides from the soil by food-crop plants. In one analysis,[6] for example, relative concentration factor values (ppm_w. in dry plant material/ppm_w in dry soil) of particular elements were examined, and found to be 10 to 1000 (strongly concentrated) for K, Rb, P, Na, Li; 1–100 (slightly concentrated) for Mg, Ca, Sr, B, Zn; smaller than 0.01 (strongly excluded) for Pb, Pu, Zr, Y. Table 4–4 presents average concentration factors of some elements for the main groups of edible organisms in aquatic environments.

TABLE 4–4. Typical Concentration Factors of Elements for Various Classes of Aquatic Organisms

	CF (CONCENTRATION ORGANISM/CONCENTRATION WATER)					
BIOTA	Co	Cs	I	K	Sr	Zn
Fresh water plants	6760	907	69	—	200	3155
Fresh water molluscs	32,408	—	320	—	—	33,544
Fresh water crustacea	—	—	—	—	—	1800
Fresh water fish	1615	3608	9	4400	14	1744
Marine plants	553	51	1065	13	21	900
Marine molluscs	166	15	5010	8	1.7	47,000
Marine crustacea	1700	18	31	12	0.6	5300
Marine fish	650	48	10	16	0.43	3400

(*Source*: Eisenbud, M. Environmental Radioactivity, 4th Ed. New York: Academic Press, 1997.)

A major route of food-chain contamination by radionuclides is foliar contamination via fallout. For example, during the atomic bomb testing periods in the 1950s and 1960s, approximately 80% of the total ^{90}Sr in British milk was due to foliar contamination.[7] The degree of danger from foliar contamination depends partly upon the half-life of the nuclide. Short lived nuclides (^{131}I) could produce immediate contamination of the food chain following foliar deposition, since the process of uptake from soil would be slow relative to the half-life.

A classic example of food chain concentration involves the Finnish Laplanders and Alaskan Eskimos. The matlike vegetation of the tundra provides a highly efficient collection surface for fallout. Caribou, which feed upon this vegetation, are a staple in the diet of these people. The Eskimos were found to have 2 to 3 times the level of ^{137}Cs present in the caribou.[8]

The potential danger to humans of the bioconcentration of any contaminant is dependent upon whether the particular site of sequestration in the plant or animal is eaten. To use radionuclides as the example, ^{90}Sr is concentrated in shells and bones, while ^{60}Co and ^{137}Cs concentrate in the edible tissues of organisms. In addition, other factors also affect the amounts eaten by humans. Food processing and cooking may result in the reduction of the amounts of many contaminants from levels found in the raw food.

Pesticides

Together with radionuclides, pesticides have provided good examples of contaminant transport along food chains, with the best examples of pesticide transport having been provided by DDT. Although pesticide residues may reach humans directly via the water supply, the greatest danger to both humans and the environment is due to bioamplification along food chains in aquatic environments.

Because it is fat-soluble, DDT is concentrated in the fatty tissue at each link of the food chain. Residues may thus be passed to large game fish and carnivorous birds. For example, a Long Island marsh had been sprayed with DDT for 20 years to control mosquitoes; plankton were found to contain 0.04 ppm_w., minnows 2 ppm_w and carnivorous gulls 75 ppm_w (whole body, wet weight) in their tissues, and eastern U.S. oysters were found to concentrate DDT up to as much as 70,000 times.[9]

Polychlorinated biphenyls, dioxin and dioxin-like chemicals

Polychlorinated biphenyls and dioxins undergo bioconcentration along the aquatic food chain, being concentrated in fatty tissue because of their high lipid solubility. Shrimp exposed to 10 ppb_w for only 48 hours accumulated 1300 ppb_w;[10] large concentrations subsequently occur in fish and carnivorous birds. Peregrine falcons from the coast of California were found to have up to 2000 ppm_w of PCBs in their fatty tissue.[10] With the imposition on controls of PCBs and dioxin and related compounds in recent decades, the levels of these polychlorinated compounds in the environment and in human tissues have declined markedly in recent decades.[11,12]

Mercury

Mercury compounds can undergo bioconcentration in aquatic food chains by up to as much as 10,000 times the concentration in the sea water. The greatest degree of concentration of mercury occurs for its alkyl compounds, such as methyl mercury. In one stream in central Sweden, water was found to contain 0.13 μg/gm H_20, while a 1-kilogram pike had 300 μg/gm body weight. Some degree of bioconcentration may occur in terrestrial food chains. For example, some seed-eating birds were found to have concentration factors of mercury in their livers of only 2 to 3; however, the factors for predatory birds were in the 100's or 1000's.[13] The pathways for mercury bioaccumulation are illustrated in Figure 7–6.

REFERENCES

1. Wallace, J. M. and Hobbs, P. V. Atmospheric Science: An Introductory Survey. London: Academic Press, 1987.
2. Eisenbud, M. and Gesell, T. Environmental Radioactivity, 4th Ed. San Deigo: Academic Press, 1997.
3. Stewart, N. G. et al. World-Wide Deposition of Long-Lived Fission Products from Nuclear Test Explosions. U.K. Atomic Energy Auth. Res. Grp. Rep. MPIR 2354, 1957.
4. Parker, F. L., Schmidt, G. D., Cottrell, W. B., and Mann, L. A. Dispersion of radiocontaminants in an estuary. *Health Phys.* 6:66–85, 1961.

5. Koczy, F. F. The Distribution of Elements in the Sea. Proc. Disposal of Radioactive Wastes, IAEA, Vienna, 1960.
6. Menzel, R. G. Soil-plant relationships of radioactive elements. *Health Phys.* 11:1325–1332, 1965.
7. Russell, R. S. Interception and retention of airborne material on plants. *Health Phys.* 11:1305–1315, 1965.
8. Miettinen, J. K. Enrichment of Radioactivity by Arctic Ecosystems in Finnish Lapland. Radioecol. Proc. Nat. Symp. 2nd, USAEC CONF-670503, 1969.
9. Pimental, D. Evolutionary and environmental impact of pesticides. *Bio. Sci.* 21:109–130, 1971.
10. Gustafson, C. G. PCB's-prevalent and persistent. *Env. Sci. Technol.* 4:814–819, 1970.
11. Winters, D. L. et al. Trends in dioxin and PCB concentrations in meat samples from several decades of the 20th century. *Organohalogen Compounds* 38:75–87, 1998.
12. Liem, A. K. D. et al. Dietary intake of dioxin and dioxin-like PCBs by the general population of ten European countries. Results of EU-SCOOP Task 3.2.5. (Dioxins). *Organohalogen Compounds* 48:13–16, 2000.
13. Borg, K., Wanntorp, H., Erne, K., and Hanko, E. Alkyl mercury poisoning in terrestrial Swedish wildlife. *Viltrevy* 6:301–379, 1969.

5

Fate of Environmental Chemicals: Translocation, Transformations, and Sinks

Following their release, chemical contaminants may be converted to different forms and/or transferred within and between the various compartments of the environment, i.e., the atmosphere, the hydrosphere, the lithosphere, and the biosphere. The transformation, degradation, and sequestration of chemicals in the environment may occur via three processes: *(1)* chemical, for example, atmospheric oxidation by O_2, and its subclass, photochemical reaction; *(2)* biological, the degradation due to the metabolic action of microorganisms, primarily bacteria, which occurs mainly in soil and aquatic sediments; and *(3)* physical, for example, solubility and gravitational settlement.

The ultimate disposition site or removal mechanism for a chemical contaminant is known as a sink. Ideally, the distribution of a contaminant within the environment would be determined by the dynamic steady-state existing between all of its sources, intermediate forms, and sinks. However, many chemicals are not normally in a steady-state, largely because their source strengths vary too rapidly due to economic drivers, seasonal cycles, or climatic and technological changes.

The time between contaminant release and any transformations or entrapment is quite variable, and depends upon the physical and chemical characteristics of the material released, the characteristics of the environmental compartment into which it is released, and the degree to which it crosses between compartments.

There may be several time constants for retention within the various component regions of each compartment. For example, within the atmosphere, the average residence times, i.e., the average time a contaminant remains in the atmosphere, may be very different in the stratosphere and troposphere, while in the biosphere, with contaminants interacting among numerous organisms, the complications increase enormously.

FATE OF AIR CONTAMINANTS

Contaminants emitted into the atmosphere are removed by various natural mechanisms, either while in the primary form in which they were originally released, or following their conversion to other forms. To a large extent, the fate of an airborne chemical depends upon whether it is in the particulate or gaseous phase.

Particles

Airborne particles are removed primarily via natural processes, often after undergoing alterations in size, number, or chemical composition. The principal processes are: *(1)* gravitational settlement; *(2)* impaction on and interception by earth surface objects; and *(3)* rainout and washout. Certain of the mechanisms are more effective for particles of one size range than for those of another, and for particles in specific regions of the atmosphere.

Gravitational settlement, or sedimentation, increases with the aerodynamic diameter of the particle, and is important for those with diameters greater than approximately 20 μm. Below this size, the particle's settling velocity is insignificant compared with its displacement by vertical motions of the atmosphere.

Impaction and interception onto surface objects (buildings, vegetation, etc.) are often effective removal processes for particles suspended near ground level; these particles may be transported to the surface by atmospheric convection. Impaction occurs when the momentum of a particle moves it across flow streamlines, causing it to collide with a surface. Interception refers to contact with a surface because the flow streamline coincident with the center of the particle is less than one particle radius away from the surface. The efficiency of removal by these processes is dependent upon such factors as the rate at which the particles are supplied to the surface and the collection efficiency of the surface features. The former is affected by wind velocity and by the general stability of the atmosphere, the latter by the shape, size, texture, and degree of wetness of the deposition surface. Submicrometer particles, which have high diffusivity, may be removed via diffusion to surface objects.

Sedimentation and surface impaction, which are also known as dry deposition, are the principal removal mechanisms in the lower troposphere. At altitudes above

TABLE 5–1. Mean Tropospheric Residence Times for Nitrogen Gases

CHEMICAL	RESIDENCE TIME
N_2O	4 years
NO	4–5 days
NO_2	3–5 days
NH_3	7–14 days

ble chemically, and, thus, plays an insignificant role in low-level air pollution chemical reactions. Most of the N_2O is removed via its only known atmospheric reaction, which is photolysis occurring in the upper troposphere and stratosphere and resulting in the production of NO and N_2. Some N_2O is also removed from the lower troposphere by soils, plants, and bodies of water.

Nitric Oxide and Nitrogen Dioxide. Nitric oxide is removed largely via oxidation to NO_2. Although this may occur by reaction with O_2, O_3 oxidizes NO much more rapidly. For example, at atmospheric concentrations of ~1 ppm of NO, approximately 100 hours are necessary for conversion of 50% of the NO to NO_2; with O_3, the half-life of NO is only 1.8 sec. In the upper troposphere and stratosphere, photolysis of NO results in the production of atomic nitrogen (N), which may then form N_2 following reaction with other molecules of NO.

The primary mechanism for removal of NO_2 is dissolution in cloud and rain droplets. Although numerous schemes have been proposed for subsequent reactions of NO_2, the end result is always production of nitrous acid (HNO_2) and ni-

TABLE 5–2. Sink Strengths for Nitrogen Compounds

SINK	SINK STRENGTH (10^{10} kgN/YEAR)
N_2O, NO, NO_2	
Rainout/washout	2–7.5
Dry deposition	1.9–7
Stratosphere	0.03–0.2
Gaseous deposition on surfaces	4.5
NH_3	
Rainout/washout	3–19
Dry deposition	5–7
Gaseous deposition	75
Oxidation in troposphere	7
Stratosphere	0.04

tric acid (HNO_3), which may then be converted to nitrite and nitrate salt aerosols by reaction with NH_3 or other atmospheric bases, or become adsorbed onto other particles. These acid or salt particles are then removed by wet or dry deposition mechanisms. Some NO_2 may react with O_3, also producing particulate nitrites and nitrates. Both HNO_2 and HNO_3 may be photochemically decomposed, resulting in the reformation of NO and NO_2. Minor sinks for NO_2 and NO are vegetation and soils, the latter partly by biological means. However, the NO_2 that is absorbed by soils is eventually oxidized to nitrate which, upon oxidative decomposition, produces NO_2 once again. Nitrogen dioxide is important because of its involvement in atmospheric photochemical reactions. It absorbs solar energy over the entire visible and UV range of the spectrum in the troposphere. At wavelengths less than 0.38 μm, NO_2 is photodissociated into NO and O; the latter reacts with O_2 to produce O_3. (The photochemical reactions of NO_2 have been discussed in detail in Chapter 3). In the stratosphere, NO and NO_2 form nitrogen pentoxide (N_2O_5), which combines with water vapor to produce HNO_3 vapor.

Ammonia. Although most sources of NH_3 are natural, it plays a major role in the formation of particulate matter in the atmosphere. In fact, the main sink for NH_3 is aerosol formation. This occurs by reaction with acids or acid-forming oxides in the gaseous phase or after dissolution in rain water; the latter process also enhances the oxidation of dissolved SO_2 and NO_2. The main aerosol species produced are ammonium bisulfate (NH_4HSO_4), ammonium sulfate ($[NH_4]_2SO_4$) and ammonium nitrate (NH_4NO_3).

Because of its high water solubility, NH_3 may be removed from the troposphere by absorption onto wet surfaces such as vegetation, bodies of water, and soils. Some ammonia may also be removed by reaction with hydroxyl radicals to form NO.

Carbon-containing gases

The main carbon-containing gases in the atmosphere are carbon monoxide (CO) and carbon dioxide (CO_2).

Carbon Monoxide. With the exception of CO_2, more CO is released into the atmosphere than any other contaminant. The major removal pathways of CO are via the soil and gas-phase reactions in the troposphere and stratosphere.

Many soils have been found to be able to remove CO from the atmosphere, releasing CO_2, likely the result of biological activity. Greatest activity is shown by organically rich tropical soils, and organically poor desert soils have the least.

There are two atmospheric sinks for CO. One involves the reaction of CO with hydroxyl (•OH) and hydroperoxyl (•OOH) radicals in the troposphere, producing CO_2 and H atoms. The other involves reaction with hydroxyl radicals in the

TABLE 5–3. Sink Strengths for CO

SINK	SINK STRENGTH (10^9 kg/YEAR)
Soil	67–1400
Gas phase oxidation in stratosphere	52–71

stratosphere, following CO migration through the tropopause. The importance of the stratosphere as a sink is dependent upon ambient CO levels, rate of transport into the stratosphere and hydroxyl levels in the stratosphere. Sink strengths for CO are presented in Table 5–3.

Carbon Dioxide. Approximately 30%–50% of the CO_2 released into the atmosphere, largely due to combustion of fossil fuels, stays within the atmosphere. The remaining 50%–70% enters sinks in the hydrosphere and biosphere.

Green plants may be a temporary sink for CO_2; although they take it up in photosynthesis, the CO_2 ultimately returns to the atmosphere during respiration and upon oxidative decomposition of dead plants. The largest natural influence upon CO_2 levels in the atmosphere is the exchange with the oceans, which contain approximately 60 times as much CO_2 as the atmosphere. The average residence time of CO_2 in the atmosphere before it transfers to ocean waters is around 10 years, but the actual approach to equilibrium levels between atmosphere and oceans may be much slower, inasmuch as atmospheric CO_2 levels are increasing.

Carbon dioxide is destroyed by photochemical decomposition in the mesosphere.

Sulfur-containing gases and vapors

The primary gaseous compounds of sulfur present in the atmosphere are hydrogen sulfide (H_2S) and sulfur dioxide (SO_2). Another sulfur species of importance is sulfur trioxide (SO_3).

Hydrogen Sulfide. Hydrogen sulfide is produced primarily from natural sources and is not an important general air contaminant in terms of anthropogenic emissions. Its only significant mode of removal from the atmosphere is oxidation to SO_2. Although the reaction proceeds fairly slowly in the gas phase, it may be catalyzed by the presence of particulate matter, which provides reaction surfaces. Most of the oxidation of H_2S occurs by O_3. Reaction with atomic oxygen may be significant in the stratosphere and under conditions of photochemical smog, where significant quantities of atomic oxygen are produced by the photolysis of O_3. The reaction system in this latter case results in the production not only of SO_2, but also SO_3 and H_2SO_4. Tropospheric residence times for H_2S range from hours to days.

Sulfur Dioxide. The sinks for SO_2 are precipitant scavenging, diffusion to and absorption onto earth-surface features, and chemical conversion into other sulfur species.

Washout and rainout are the major mechanisms for removal of atmospheric SO_2, largely because SO_2 is very soluble in water. Scavenged SO_2 undergoes a series of chemical reactions, ultimately forming sulfuric acid (H_2SO_4) and its ammonium salts.

Under conditions of high relative humidity, and in the presence of catalytic surfaces on particles, SO_2 may undergo oxidation. Salts of certain metals, for example, iron and manganese, serve as the catalysts, either by acting as condensation nuclei or by undergoing hydration; both actions result in the production of liquid droplets. Both SO_2 and O_2 readily dissolve in these droplets, producing sulfite (SO_3^{-2}) and eventually strong acid droplets. The H_2SO_4 may react with other atmospheric constituents to produce ammonium, sodium, and calcium salts, and numerous other sulfate species.

The presence of NH_3 in water droplets also enhances the oxidation of SO_2 in solution. As a droplet becomes highly acidic, the rate of SO_2 oxidation decreases, due to the decreased solubility of SO_2 in acid solutions. Ammonia dissolved in the droplet increases SO_2 solubility, and if sufficient levels of NH_3 are present, oxidation is not impeded by accumulation of H_2SO_4, since conversion to $(NH_4)_2SO_4$ occurs. Calcite dust and other airborne alkalis besides ammonia are also involved in the rapid oxidation of SO_2 to sulfate. The rate of catalytic oxidation of SO_2 decreases if the water concentration in the atmosphere falls below the level necessary to maintain catalyst droplets, ~70% relative humidity.

In clean, dry air, SO_2 is only very slowly oxidized via homogeneous reactions (gas phase) to SO_3 vapor. The most important transformation of SO_2 under low-humidity conditions is photochemical oxidation. Photochemical reactions have been discussed in Chapter 3, and only a general description will be presented here.

In the initial photochemical event, the absorption of light results in activation of a molecule of SO_2 which then proceeds to react with O_2 or O_3 at a faster rate than would unactivated SO_2 molecules. The resultant SO_3 reacts almost immediately with water vapor to produce H_2SO_4.

The rate of photochemical oxidation of SO_2 is fairly slow; estimates range from 0.006%/min to a theoretical maximum of 0.03%/min.[1] However, the rate may be greatly accelerated by the co-presence in the air of certain reactive intermediate species in the photooxidation of hydrocarbons under the influence of NO_x, for example, NO and olefins.

In the stratosphere, SO_2 reacts with atomic oxygen, resulting in the formation of SO_3 vapor, which reacts with water vapor to form H_2SO_4 vapor. The latter combines with more water to produce H_2SO_4 droplets, which are removed by precipitation.

Aside from atmospheric sink reactions, SO_2 may also be removed by other mechanisms. Some plants may absorb SO_2. Soils are also able to absorb significant amounts of SO_2; the SO_2 may then be oxidized to sulfate. Other sinks are absorption by the hydrosphere, and uptake by carbonate stones, for example, buildings, in moist atmospheres. Sink strengths for SO_2 are presented in Table 5–4.

Hydrocarbon gases and vapors

A broad range of gaseous hydrocarbons are emitted into the atmosphere. Certain of these may be taken up via soil microbial action. Most organic molecules are oxidized only very slowly in clean atmospheres. The mechanism involves reaction chains that are initiated by removal of a hydrogen atom from the molecule, producing a radical that combines with an oxygen molecule to form a peroxide. The latter, being reactive, may go on to remove a hydrogen from another organic molecule.

In the presence of light sensitizers or initiators, hydrocarbons may be degraded by photochemical reactions. These initiators provide the energy necessary for radical production from the organic molecule. Photochemical reactions are the primary degradation processes for reactive hydrocarbons, for example, olefins and polycyclic aromatic hydrocarbons. These molecules rapidly undergo transformations under the influence of sunlight and in the presence of atomic oxygen, O_3, SO_2, and NO_2. The result is conversion to other organic molecules. The reaction rates for various hydrocarbons are quite different, and there are few data on the rates for many species or for the products formed.

Up to about 10% by weight of the reactive hydrocarbons emitted into the atmosphere eventually is converted to or adsorbed onto particles that are then removed by wet or dry deposition processes. The remainder of the hydrocarbons eventually undergo chemical degradation, becoming oxidized to other hydrocarbons, and if oxidation is complete, to CO_2 and H_2O. For substituted hydrocarbons, the noncarbon constituents are found in various salts.

Methane (CH_4) is the predominant atmospheric hydrocarbon; however, the paraffin group, of which CH_4 is the first member, is much less reactive than other

TABLE 5–4. Sink Strengths for Sulfur Compounds

SINK	SINK STRENGTH (10^9 kg/YEAR)
Gaseous absorption, SO_2	
Vegetation	15–75
Ocean	25–100
Washout/rainout (land)	70–85
Dry deposition (land)	10–20
Wet and dry deposition, SO_4^{-2} (oceans)	70–100

hydrocarbons. The main sink for CH_4 is oxidation to form CO and CO_2, through the action of hydroxyl radicals in the troposphere.

Except for CH_4, the lack of precise estimates of emissions and ambient levels of hydrocarbons prevents an accurate estimation of atmospheric residence times. The residence time of CH_4 in the troposphere is 1.5–2 years; that for higher molecular–weight hydrocarbons is on the order of days to months. In the stratosphere, many hydrocarbons react with atomic oxygen, and may eventually be oxidized to CO_2 and H_2O.

Ozone

Ozone is a constituent of photochemical smog atmospheres. A major O_3 sink is the surface of the earth, primarily soils and vegetation; absorption by oceans may also occur to some extent.

Ozone is a powerful oxidizing agent. It is involved—especially in contaminated atmospheres—in many reactions, such as photooxidation of hydrocarbons in atmospheres containing NO_2.

FATE OF WATER CONTAMINANTS

Chemical transformations and physical or biological removal of contaminants from the atmosphere may be thought of as natural purification processes that produce nonreactive (both physiologically and chemically) products and/or otherwise result in removal from the atmosphere of the chemical agent. Analogous self-purification processes occur in aquatic environments.

The self-purification processes by which natural waters tend to rid themselves of contaminants involve physical, chemical, and biological mechanisms that occur simultaneously and interact with each other. At one time, these processes were sufficient to prevent permanent effects on many bodies of water, but now this is not always the case.

Self-purification processes in aquatic environments are quite complex, especially due to the interaction of the biota. Each specific waterway, be it estuary, stream, river, lake, or ocean, has its own capacity for self-purification and recovery due to its unique combination of physical, geochemical, and biological characteristics. Nevertheless, the main processes in all environments are basically the same. This section will deal with these general processes.

Physical Self-Purification

The physical mechanisms involved in self-purification of water are the processes of dilution, mixing, sorption (adsorption and absorption) and sedimentation. Dilution of chemicals occurs due to diffusion, advection (movement of one parcel of water with respect to another), and turbulence (eddy diffusion). Mixing is primarily due to turbulence, which results from temperature gradients in large bodies of water, and from bed friction in rivers and streams. In coastal areas and estuaries, the action of tides also helps in the mixing of contaminants.

Sorption of chemicals may alter their behavior and often results in a purification of the water. Particles are quite ubiquitous in natural waters, occurring in a wide assortment of sizes, shapes, chemical compositions, and concentrations. In terms of sorption and binding of chemicals, the colloidal particles are the most important, with clay being the most significant class of common mineral that occurs as colloidal matter in natural waters. Because of their strong tendency to sorb chemicals from the water, clays may effectively immobilize dissolved chemicals, purifying the water. In addition, some microbiological degradation processes for organic wastes may also occur at the clay-particle surfaces, giving clay a role in biological purification.

A wide variety of dissolved chemical effluents may be sorbed and bound by suspended particles. This includes various organic chemicals, such as herbicides and nonvolatile organics, as well as dissolved inorganic materials, such as trace metals.

Particulate matter, either natural or that discharged into water, along with any sorbed chemicals, may eventually be removed from suspension by sedimentation. This process depends upon the particle size, shape, and density, and the mixing and flow characteristics of the waterway. In turbulent streams, suspended particles may be carried for long distances before they settle.

The sedimentation of the small colloidal particles may be enhanced by aggregation, which involves the processes of coagulation and flocculation. Coagulation is the aggregation of colloidal particles of the same material. Flocculation is dependent upon the presence of bridging compounds that form chemically bonded links between the colloidal particles and enmesh the particles in large floc networks.

Movement of suspended particles into different waters may affect their sedimentation. The size of colloidal particles may change due to coagulation when they travel from fresh water into salt water; the salt ions act to reduce the normal electrostatic repulsion between the particles. This process may be accompanied by the uptake and/or loss of some of the sorbed contaminations.

Particles that deposit on the sediments may remain there, undergoing no removal processes. However, very often accumulation and precipitation processes are reversible. Bottom sediments undergo a continuous process of leaching and ion exchange with the overlying water. For example, trace metal ions sorbed on particles deposited in the sediments may be released by ion-exchange mechanisms. Sediments that move from aerobic to anaerobic environments may undergo changes in sorbed chemical species.

Nevertheless, bottom sediments are often the ultimate sinks for many contaminants. The deposition may occur in the waterway into which the contaminant discharge occurred, or in downstream areas. In this regard, oceans are an enormous sink, often representing the ultimate "downstream" locale for flowing waterways. Rivers deliver billions of tons of dissolved and suspended matter each year to the oceans and seas; much of this is subsequently deposited in the sediments, often in coastal regions.

Chemical Self-Purification

Specifics of the chemical reactions of many contaminants in aquatic environments are unknown; the nature of chemicals is often influenced by the biota. In addition, chemical reactions are also affected by water temperatures and pH. It is beyond the scope of this book to discuss the fate of specific chemicals in water. However, certain types of chemical reactions are often involved in the self-purification of inorganic contaminants, and these will be presented. Purification of many organic contaminants involves biological processes, and these are discussed in a subsequent section.

Acid–base reactions are important in the assimilation of acid and alkaline wastes discharged into water. Acids may react with numerous minerals, such as those in crystalline rocks, clays and other silicates, limestone and other carbonate rocks. The capacity of a waterway to neutralize acid is primarily a function of the bicarbonate, carbonate, and hydroxide ions. Alkaline contaminants are purified mainly via reactions with silica, bicarbonate, and free carbonic acid in the water, resulting in the production of silicate and carbonate salts. The rates of acid–base reactions differ in different aquatic systems, and are important determinants of the area of the waterway over which unassimilated acids and alkaline wastes traverse.

Nonbiologically mediated oxidation-reduction reactions are also of great significance in the purification of aquatic environments; many hydrocarbons and heavy metals undergo these types of reactions.

Metal ions may be removed from solution by the formation of insoluble complexes known as coordination compounds. Some naturally occurring organic complexing agents, for example, humic and fulvic acid, are found in certain aquatic environments, and these agents strongly bind heavy metals. Synthetic chelating agents (e.g., NTA, EDTA) are used in detergents and industrial processes, and are often discharged into surface waters where they may form complexes with metals. On the other hand, metal ions may also be solubilized by formation of complexes.

Some dissolved chemicals may be precipitated under the influence of other agents in the water (coprecipitation), while some may leave by volatization. Others may be hydrolyzed in the aquatic environment. For example, hydrolysis of esters results in products that may then be degraded by biological processes. Some organic chemicals may undergo light-induced transformation reactions in water.

In aquatic chemistry, interactions occurring solely in solution are of less significance than those that occur at solid–water and gas–water interfaces. In this regard, colloidal solids are of great significance in chemical interactions in the aquatic environment.

Biological Self-Purification

Although some chemicals may undergo a limited number of reactions that may serve to remove them from the water, others, for example, nitrate (NO_3), undergo few reactions without the action of microorganisms.

Biological purification processes generally involve the assimilation of putrescible organic wastes entering waters. The process involves the transformation of the chemicals into innocuous products due to action of the aquatic biota, primarily microorganisms; it usually occurs at the expense of dissolved oxygen and of some species which normally are present in the biota of the uncontaminated waterway.

Because of the multitude of microbial types that exist in aquatic environments, the overall process is quite complex. However, most aquatic environments show, to some extent, common biological reactions, which may vary due to differences in flow and mixing characteristics and according to the concentration and composition of the specific contaminant.

As an example of biological self-purification, consider the case of a discharge of organic matter into a stream. The discharge initially results in an increase in the BOD; the levels of DO in the stream below the point of discharge, therefore, decrease. Depending upon the initial waste load, a certain time and distance of flow downstream are necessary before stream reaeration processes return the DO to near air-saturation levels. By considering factors of BOD loading, reaeration processes and rate of flow, an oxygen sag curve may be developed (Fig. 5–1).

Suspended organic solids eventually settle out to the bottom. These may be subject to microbial decomposition, although the processes differ from those occurring in flowing water. Decomposition in bottom sediments varies, with the depth of deposit, from aerobic to anaerobic.

Dissolved solids are also removed or diluted as the stream flows. As the various nutrient cycles occur, organic compounds are broken down, and levels of inorganic nutrients (ammonia, nitrate, phosphate) are increased. This results in changes in biota, since species differ in their ability to tolerate increased nutrients (some are favored and others are disadvantaged). Bacteria and sewage fungi predominate in the zone where oxygen becomes a severely limiting factor. Further downstream, these decline and algae may bloom, benefiting from the increase in mineral nutrients. Eventually, these also decline. Low oxygen levels cause reduction in the number of species of larger invertebrates; highly specialized sewage organisms, for example, tubificid worms, midge larvae, and other

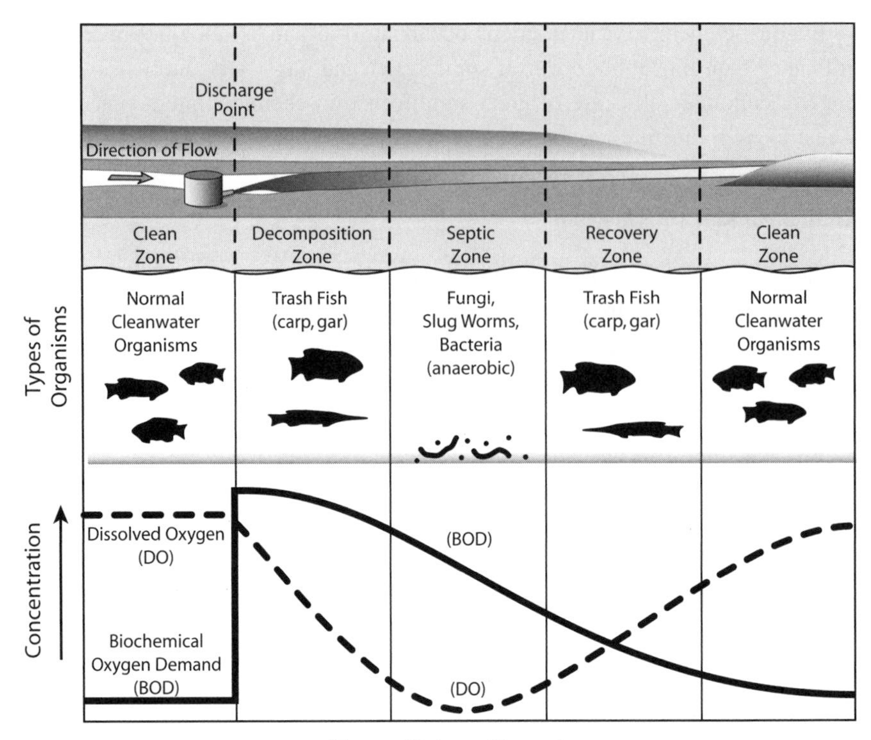

FIGURE 5–1. The oxygen sag curve (- - -) versus oxygen demand (———). The rate of recovery depends on flow rates and the amount of pollutants.

undesirable forms that can tolerate these conditions increase in number due to the large supply of food and little interspecies competition. Increasing dilution occurs with flow downstream and, as the river oxygen and minerals return to normal, the number of species able to survive increases and the strong numerical predominance of particular species tends to disappear. A gradual return to the community found upstream of the discharge occurs. The water has purified itself and has recovered from the discharge. The entire scheme of biological purification is shown in Figure 5–1.

Natural microbial purification is not a fast process, and heavily contaminated streams may have to travel fairly long distances before any significant degree of purification occurs. Exact rates are quite difficult to estimate because of the compositional and mixing complexities of most waterways and the interaction of biological, chemical, and physical processes.

There are generally significant differences in biological reactions between flowing waterways and enclosed bodies of water. Flow and mixing in the former systems make them less susceptible to permanent damage by a given concentration of organic wastes. For example, an increase in the decomposition of sewage acts to reduce DO in the bottom waters of a lake. In flowing waters, the constant mixing acts to hinder establishment of such distinct surface-to-bottom gradients in the entire waterway. Under severe conditions, however, streams can be completely changed, returning to normal only after long distances downstream from the point of contaminant discharge.

Ground water also has some capacity for self-purification, although the mechanisms differ from that in surface waters. Because of certain limiting factors, such as darkness, the variety of microbes in ground waters is restricted. However, the reduction in biological self-purification is offset by the process of physical purification via filtration through the soil and rocks. Soils may remove particles by physical means and chemicals by various means, as discussed in a subsequent section. But, there is a limited ability to remove many chemical compounds that commonly occur in industrial waste waters.

Aside from sewage, other organic contaminants may be subject to microbial attack. For example, the degradation of many hydrocarbons, such as those in fuel oils, proceeds primarily via microbial utilization of the constituent alkanes.

Residence Times

Residence times for chemical contaminants in the hydrosphere are extremely difficult to determine because of the various types of aquatic environments, and the complex physical, chemical, and biological factors that determine the fate of the contaminant, which differ to some degree in these different environments.

The oceans often represent the ultimate sink for contaminants contained in flowing waterways. Unless they are removed into the atmosphere, the ultimate fate of chemical contaminants entering the oceans is usually removal to the sea floor. Thus, the residence time in the marine environment is generally considered to be the time the contaminant remains in the ocean water between its introduction and its incorporation into the sediments.

Residence time depends upon the degree of reactivity of the specific contaminant, a factor that also determines the region in the marine environment in which the chemical reaches its sink. As a generalization, chemically reactive elements, for example, iron and aluminum, and those involved in biological cycles, for example, phosphorus and nitrogen, have shorter residence times then do those contaminants that tend to be less reactive or inert in solution, for example, alkali metal ions. The first two groups tend to become associated with particulate matter and/or biota prevalent in the coastal ocean regions, and are largely removed there by deposition processes. The latter group tends to reach the open ocean waters, where they accumulate until they eventually undergo downward transport in the waters. Contaminants that do not undergo biological degradation may have residence half-times in the ocean of thousands of years.

FATE OF CONTAMINANTS IN SOIL

Soil may be a sink for numerous chemicals. The fate and persistence of chemicals in soil is a complex function of physical, chemical, and biological factors, the main ones being the specific chemical and its formulation, soil type and specific physicochemical properties, type of cover vegetation, degree of soil cultivation, and nature of the microbial population. The major routes of removal of contaminants from soil are: *(1)* degradation via microbial action, which is discussed in the next section; *(2)* chemical degradation, for example, hydrolysis; *(3)* evaporation and volatilization from the surface; and *(4)* uptake by vegetation. Most contaminants are not effectively removed by leaching.

Uptake by plants may only be a temporary sink, since the contaminant may return to the soil in plant litter. Temporary removal may also be afforded by microbial assimilation without degradation, which may immobilize the contaminant until the death of the microorganism. Chemicals may also be immobilized in soil via various adsorption processes.

Colloidal soil particles adsorb various chemicals. Neutral organic molecules, for example, may be adsorbed by physical mechanisms, such as via van der Waals forces. Polar or polarizable organic ions, especially cations, and inorganic metallic ions, such as Pb^{+2}, Hg^{+2}, $^{90}Sr^{+2}$, may be adsorbed via ion exchange. Other processes implicated in adsorption of contaminants, particularly pesticides, are hydrogen bonding and coordination, the latter being formation of a complex between the chemical and an exchangeable ion on the soil particle. Some metals, such as Cu and Zn, may become tightly bound to soil organic matter by chelation. Other soluble inorganic chemicals may precipitate out of solution in soil water as oxides or hydroxides.

Thus, a wide variety of immobilization processes may involve all types of chemicals. Immobilization affects the subsequent fate of the contaminant in the soil in any number of ways. It may hinder volatilization and leaching, act to catalyze chemical degradation, prevent biological degradation by sequestering the contaminant from the microbes, enhance biological decay by concentrating the chemical near microbes, etc.

Specific components of certain soils may affect the fate of contaminants. For example, part of the humic fraction in many agricultural soils is composed of lipids; contaminant-lipid interactions in these soils often serve to immobilize fat-soluble pesticides.

There are few reliable data on the residence times of chemicals in soils, since these depend upon so many physicochemical and biological factors. Type of soil is, of course, a major factor. For example, many pesticides tend to persist longer in soils with higher organic matter than in sandy soils, since the former tend to bind the residues much tighter.

FATE OF CONTAMINANTS IN THE BIOSPHERE

The discussion in this chapter has concentrated on the physicochemical processes by which contaminants are removed from air, water, and soil environments. In this section, we discuss microbially mediated transformations and their relation to the biodegradability of chemicals.

Biogeochemical Cycles

The biological cycles for carbon, nitrogen, and sulfur are discussed in the following sections. Bear in mind that they are not independent of each other, but, as with most environmental processes, they interact.

Carbon cycle

The biological carbon cycle is shown in Figure 5–2. There are two main reservoirs for inorganic carbon: the atmosphere and the hydrosphere. In both, carbon naturally exists in the form of CO_2; interchange occurs via diffusion, evaporation, and precipitation.

The atmospheric or hydrospheric CO_2 is fixed into organic carbon as biomass via photosynthesis, primarily by green plants on land and by phytoplankton in the sea. The organic carbon then moves through various trophic levels and is eventually released back to the reservoir as CO_2, via the respiratory activity of plants and animals, in the processing of waste products and remains of dead biota by decomposers, and via the process of combustion.

Some carbon is trapped in deposits of the remains of plants and animals and becomes peat, coal, and oil, some in the shells of aquatic organisms, and some in formation of carbonate rocks in the oceans. The weathering of these rocks and the combustion of oil and coal release this formerly trapped carbon into the cycle once again.

Nitrogen cycle

The nitrogen cycle is shown in Figure 5–3. Although nitrogen is the dominant gas in the atmosphere, very few living organisms are able to use gaseous nitrogen. Rather, nitrogen must first be fixed into an inorganic compound for utilization by the producers in biological processes. The primary compound for such utilization is nitrate, and the primary mechanism for fixation is biological. Various groups of free-living aerobic and anaerobic microorganisms, primarily bacteria, and also certain symbiotic microorganisms, for example, the root-nodule bacteria of legumes, are able to fix atmospheric nitrogen. Fixation occurs primarily in terrestrial ecosystems, although certain organisms in aquatic ecosystems, for example, blue-green algae, are also capable of nitrogen fixation. Physicochemical processes in the atmosphere may

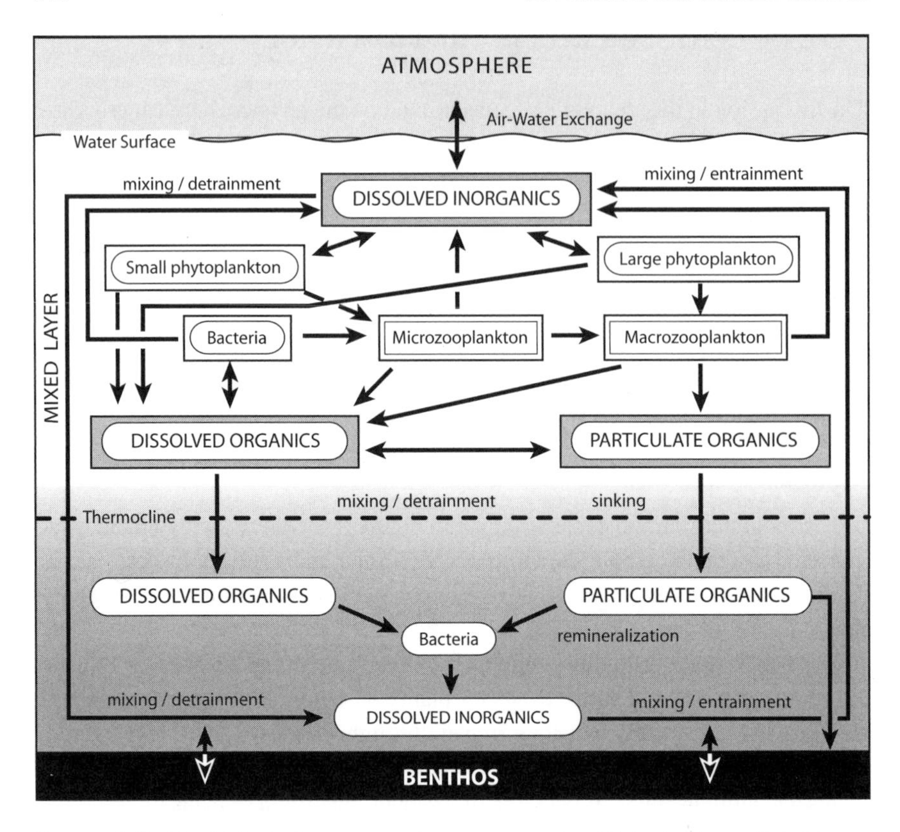

Figure 5–2. The biological carbon cycle in ocean water. Biologically mediated transformations of carbon in ocean water begin with the small plankton, which primarily recycle CO_2 within the euphotic zone, and the larger plankton, which generate most of the flux of organic carbon in particulate and dissolved form from the deep ocean. Some of the carbon that reaches the deep ocean is remineralized into dissolved inorganic form, some is consumed at the benthic surface, and a small portion is buried in the sediments of the ocean floor.

also result in fixation; these include electrification (lightning) and cosmic radiation.

The nitrogen contained within the bodies of plants and animals exists as ammonium ions, in amino-compounds, such as proteins, and in nucleic acids. Mineralization of this nitrogen occurs via the processes of ammonification and nitrification.

In the process of ammonification, numerous aerobic and anaerobic microorganisms metabolize bound nitrogen, releasing NH_3 gas or ammonium (NH_4^+) compounds. The subsequent conversion of the NH_3 and NH_4^+ salts back to ni-

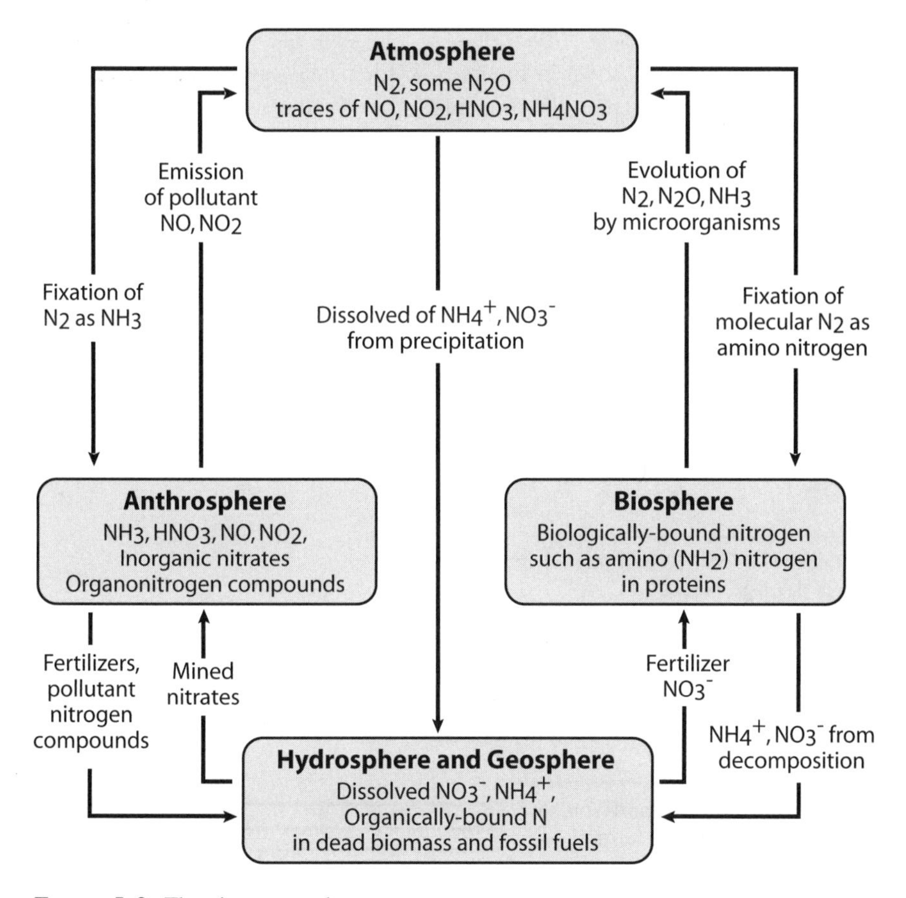

FIGURE 5–3. The nitrogen cycle.

trate (NO_3^-) is called nitrification. This occurs in two stages, and involves two classes of aerobic bacteria. The first step is oxidation of ammonia to nitrite (NO_2^-) by nitrite bacteria; the nitrite is then converted to nitrate (NO_3^-) by nitrate bacteria.

Under total or partial anaerobic conditions in soils, various microorganisms convert nitrate into nitrite, various nitrogen oxides, NH_3, and gaseous N_2, in processes collectively termed denitrification. Some of these products remain in the soil and others are released into the atmosphere. Under certain soil conditions, such as high acidity, chemical denitrification of nitrate may also occur, resulting in production of NO_2, N_2O and, eventually, HNO_3.

Some nitrogen is trapped in the deep ocean sediments and in sedimentary rocks.

Sulfur cycle

The sulfur cycle is shown in Figure 5–4. Elemental sulfur is not utilized by producer organisms. Rather, the principle form of sulfur used in biological systems is inorganic sulfate (SO_4^{-2}), although some organisms may obtain their sulfur from certain organic compounds. Microbial decomposition results in mineralization of sulfur bound in biomass.

Under anaerobic conditions, especially in swamps, marshes, and soils, various bacteria reduce sulfate, producing sulfides, such as H_2S, or elemental sulfur. In aerobic environments, microorganisms oxidize H_2S to elemental sulfur, H_2S to SO_4^{-2}, or elemental sulfur to SO_4^{-2}. Sulfur may be removed from active cycling by precipitation in neutral or alkaline water under anaerobic conditions by

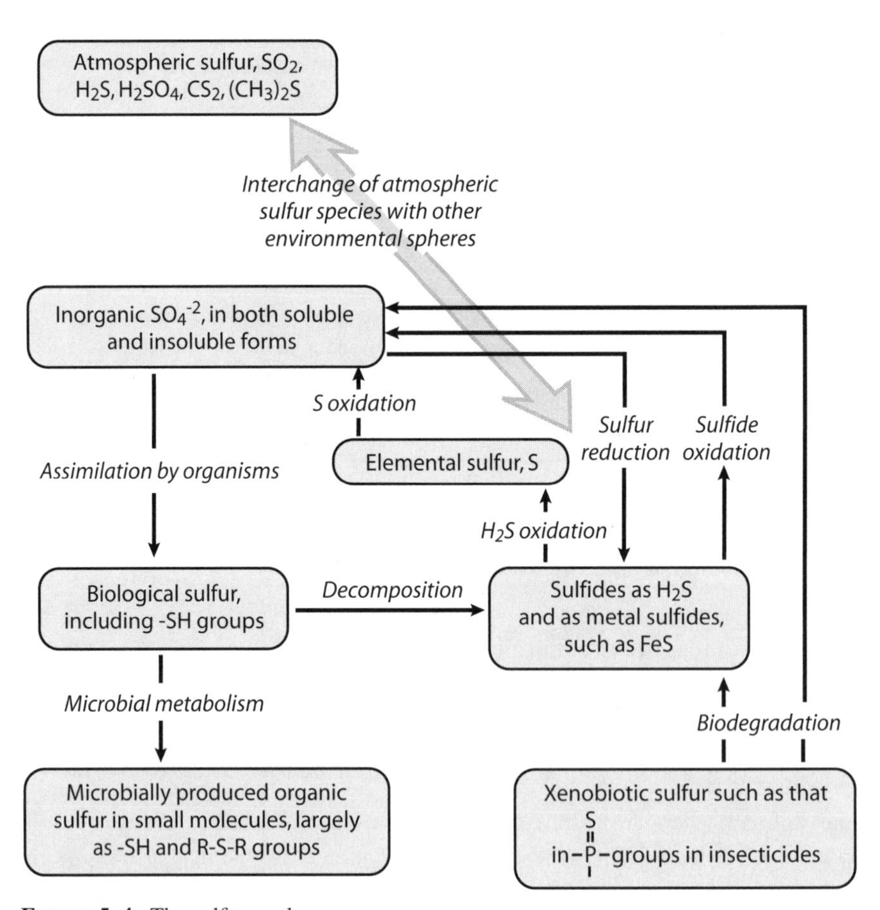

FIGURE 5–4. The sulfur cycle.

formation of ferrous and ferric sulfide. The sulfur may be trapped to the limits of the amount of available iron present.

Biodegradability of Chemical Contaminants

It should be clear from the previous discussion that the ultimate mineralization and degradation of a chemical in any biogeochemical cycle is dependent upon microorganisms, primarily bacteria. Microbial metabolism is, therefore, responsible for the mobility, or lack of it, of chemicals in the biosphere. These microbes purify streams into which organic contaminants are dumped, degrade pesticides in soil, decompose sewage sludge, and even have a role in the degradation of oil spilled into waterways. Contaminants that may be degraded by microbes are termed biodegradable. Although these chemicals are primarily organic in nature, they yield inorganic end products. It should, however, be mentioned that microbial conversion may result in products that are more hazardous than the original material.

On the other hand, certain chemicals released into the environment are resistant to microbial decomposition or else are degraded at such slow rates that they build up in the environment. These types of contaminants are termed nonbiodegradable, refractory, or persistent, and include many chemicals. Notable examples are organochlorine insecticides, such as DDT, and numerous synthetic polymers, such as PCB, PVC, teflon, polyethylenes, and mylar. The residence times in soil for selected biodegradable and persistent pesticides are presented in Table 5–5.

Various reasons for resistance of chemicals to microbial degradation have been proposed. They include the inability to be attacked by a microbe having an enzyme capable of producing degradation, or the complete absence of an essential microbial enzyme.

Table 5–5. Residence Times of Selected Pesticides in Soil

DESIGNATION	CHEMICAL GROUP	RESIDENCE HALF-LIFE (YEARS)
Degradable	Organophosphate insecticides	0.02–0.2
	Carbamate insecticides	0.02
Moderately degradable	Urea herbicides	0.3–0.8
	2,4-D; 2,4,5-T herbicides	0.1–0.4
Persistent	Organochlorine insecticides	2–5
Permanent	Lead, arsenic, copper pesticides	10–30

CONTAMINANT RESIDUES

Following their release, contaminants may be dispersed throughout the environment until they reach a sink. The dispersal may result in global distribution, as well as high levels on a local or regional scale.

The actual concentrations of contaminant residues in the air, water, soil, and biota vary greatly in different parts of the world due to differences in dispersion patterns and source strengths and characteristics. Based upon the discussions in this and the previous chapters, it should be clear that the distribution and, therefore, resultant residue levels are a complex function of physical, chemical, and biological processes acting on the contaminant and within the components of the environment. Thus, it is difficult to generalize as to global residue levels.

The long-range transport of chemical contaminants often results in their presence in regions far removed from any known anthropogenic source. This is especially true for those refractory chemicals that do not degrade and may, therefore, travel long distances before reaching some ultimate sink.

For example, DDT has been found in Antarctic snow, and one estimate is that approximately 2.4×10^6 kg were collected in the snow over a 22-year period.[2]

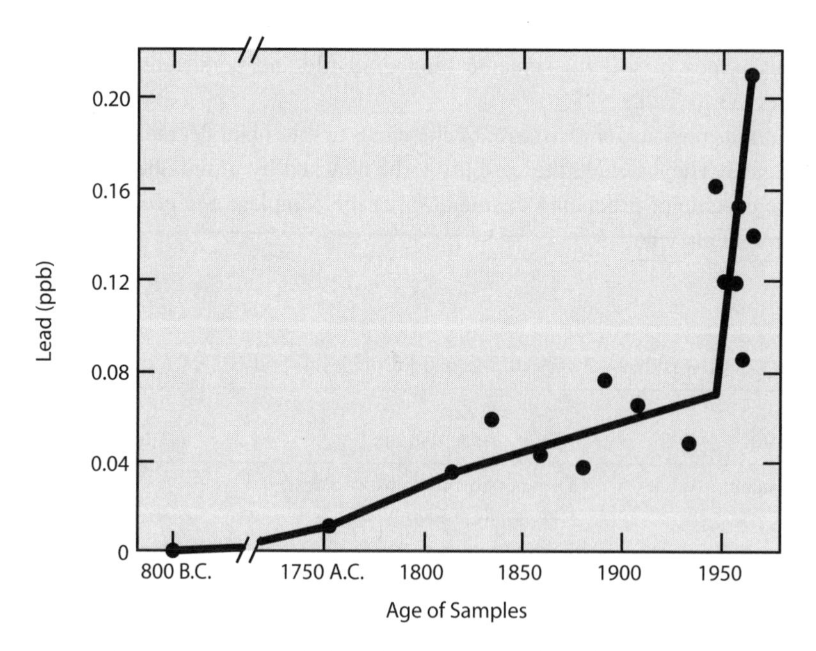

FIGURE 5–5. Lead concentration in dated levels of a Greenland glacier. (*Source*: National Academy of Sciences. Lead: Airborne Lead in Perspective. p. 7. Washington, DC, 1972.)

These residues were probably transported from Europe and North America via northeasterly trade winds and were removed by wet deposition.

Another classic example is lead, which has been analyzed in chronologic layers of snow strata in Greenland.[3] Annual ice layers from the interior of northern Greenland show a rise in lead concentration (Fig. 5–5). The layer corresponding to 1750 represents the lead concentration at the beginning of the Industrial Revolution. The concentration at that date was already 25 times greater than the natural level. In the early 1970s, the lead concentration in Greenland snow was approximately 400 times the natural level.

Additional evidence reflects increasing lead concentrations in other regions. For example, the preindustrial lead content for marine water is estimated at 0.02–0.04 μg/kg.[4] However, ocean surface waters in many areas away from anthropogenic sources show lead concentrations as high as 0.20–0.35 μg/kg, and only deep waters (below 1000 m) remain relatively uncontaminated.

REFERENCES

1. Seinfeld, J. H. Atmospheric Chemistry and Physics of Air Pollution. New York: Wiley, 1986.
2. Peterle, T. J. DDT in Antarctic snow. *Nature* 224:620–623, 1969.
3. Nraigu, J. O. Tales told in lead. *Science* 281:1622–1623, 1998.
4. Chow, T. J. Isotope analysis of seawater by mass spectrometry. *J. Water Poll. Control Fed.* 40:399–411, 1968.

6

Effects of Chemical Contaminants on Human Health

The first indications that environmental chemicals could affect human health were associations between certain diseases and occupational exposures. It is now clear that chemicals in the ambient environment can also influence the health of the general population. This chapter presents a broad overview of the health effects of chemical contaminants in the environment. The emphasis is on general aspects of environmental toxicology and epidemiology. For consideration of the specific effects of individual chemical contaminants, the reader is referred to various books listed in the Appendix. Some of the chemicals cited in this chapter are of primary concern within the occupational environment. However, the effluents from industrial operations can also pose similar hazards to the general community. There have been numerous incidences of disease in neighborhoods downwind or downstream from certain industries.

Human exposures to chemicals are often mediated by complex environmental pathways, and uptake may occur via more than one route. People may be exposed to a chemical via the air they breathe, the water and food they ingest, or by skin contact with air, water, or solid surfaces. Once exposure does occur, depending upon its specific nature, a chemical contaminant may exert its toxic action at various sites in the body. However, the first contact is at a portal of entry: the respiratory tract, gastrointestinal tract, skin, or eyes. At the portal, a chemical may have a topical effect. However, for actions at sites other than the portal, the agent must be absorbed through one or more body membranes and enter the general circulation, from which it may become available to affect internal tissues (including the blood itself). The initial distribution of any chemical contaminant in the body is, therefore, highly dependent upon its ability to traverse biological membranes. There are two main types of processes by which this occurs: passive transport and active transport. Figure 6–1 outlines the pathways for lead and its effects on biological systems.

Passive transport is absorption according to purely diffusional processes in which the cell has no active role in transfer across the membrane. Since biological membranes contain lipids, they are highly permeable to lipid-soluble, nonpolar, or nonionized agents, and less so to lipid insoluble, polar, or ionized materials. Many chemicals may exist in both lipid-soluble and lipid-insoluble forms; the former is the prime determinant of the passive permeability properties for the specific agent.

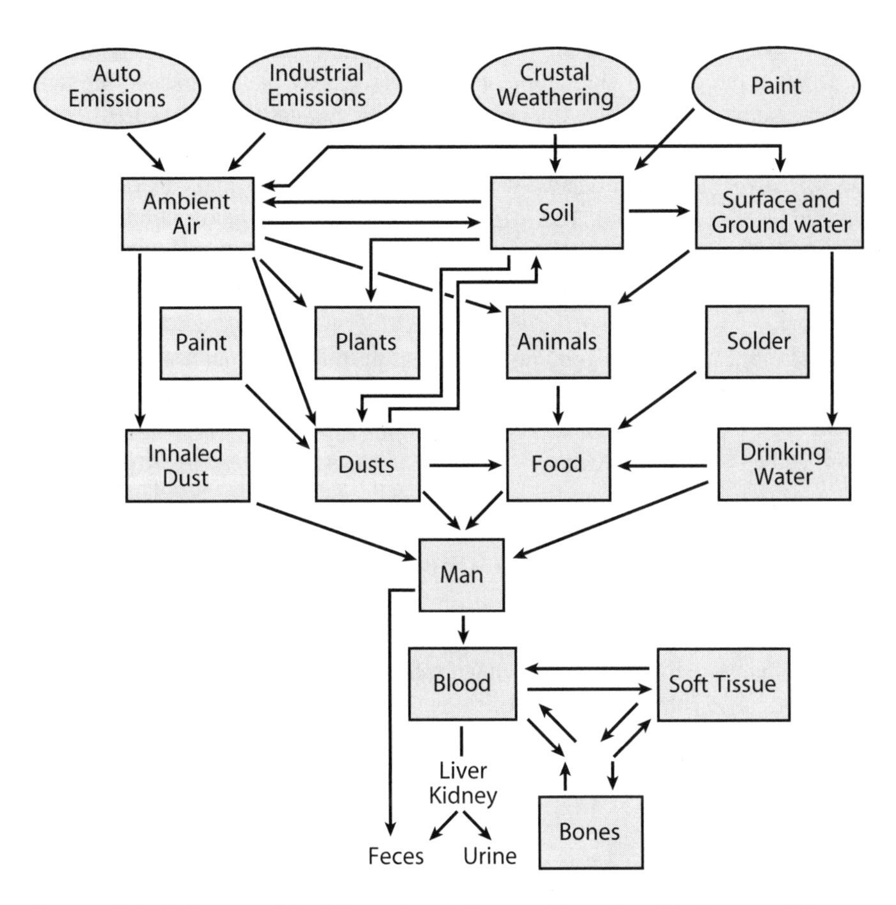

FIGURE 6–1. Pathways of lead from the environment to and within humans. (*Source*: EPA, 1986.)

Active transport involves specialized mechanisms, and in these the cell actively participates in transfer across the membrane. These mechanisms include carrier systems within the membrane and active processes of cellular ingestion, i.e., phagocytosis and pinocytosis. Phagocytosis is the ingestion of solid particles, while pinocytosis refers to the ingestion of fluid containing no visible solid material. Lipid insoluble materials are often taken up by active-transport processes. Although some of these mechanisms are highly specific, if the chemical structure of a contaminant is similar to that of an endogenous substrate, the former may be transported as well.

In addition to its lipid-solubility characteristics, the distribution of a chemical contaminant is also dependent upon its affinity for specific tissues or tissue components. Internal distribution may vary with time after exposure. For example, immediately following absorption into the blood, inorganic lead is found to localize in the liver, the kidney, and in red blood cells. Two hours later, approximately 50% is in the liver. A month later, approximately 90% of the remaining lead is localized in bone.[1]

Once in the general circulation, a contaminant may be translocated throughout the body. In this process it may: *(1)* become bound to macromolecules; *(2)* undergo metabolic transformation (biotransformation) in specific organs; *(3)* be deposited for storage in depots, which may or may not be the sites of its toxic action; or *(4)* be excreted. Toxic effects may occur at any of several sites.

The biological action of a contaminant may be terminated by storage, metabolic transformation, or excretion, the latter being the most permanent form of removal.

Figure 6–2 provides a framework connecting pollutant sources, personal exposures, dose delivery to target organs and tissues, and health effects resulting from such exposures. Figure 6–3 shows various routes of absorption, distribution, and excretion of toxicants.

ENTRY OF ENVIRONMENTAL CHEMICALS INTO THE BODY

The portal of entry presents the first possible site of action of, and first line of defense against, environmental chemicals. Some environmental agents have multiple portals of entry, with the specific physicochemical properties in the exposure environment determining the significant entry path. The specific portal may be an important factor in determining the hazard from exposure.

Respiratory Tract

The respiratory tract is the prime portal of entry for airborne chemicals. It may be separated into two functional zones: the conducting airways and respiratory

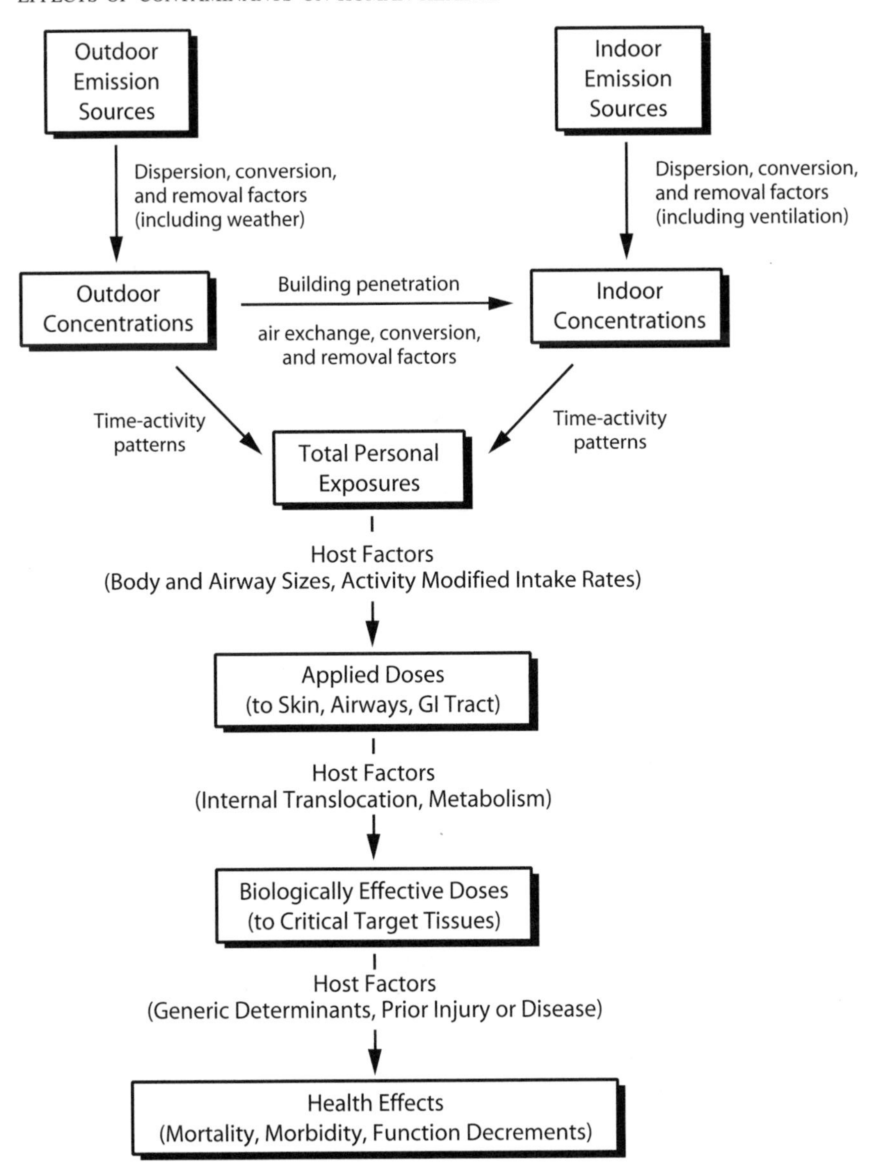

FIGURE 6–2. Framework for personal exposure assessment and exposure-response. (*Source*: Modified from NAS, 1985.)

airways (Fig. 6–4). The former extends from the upper respiratory tract (nasopharynx, pharynx, and larynx) through the terminal bronchioles, and serves as a conduit system for the transport of air into and out of the lungs. The latter zone, often called the alveolar, pulmonary, or gas-exchange region, consists of respiratory bronchioles, alveolar ducts, alveolar sacs, and alveoli, and is involved in the mutual gas exchange between air and the pulmonary circulation. The very

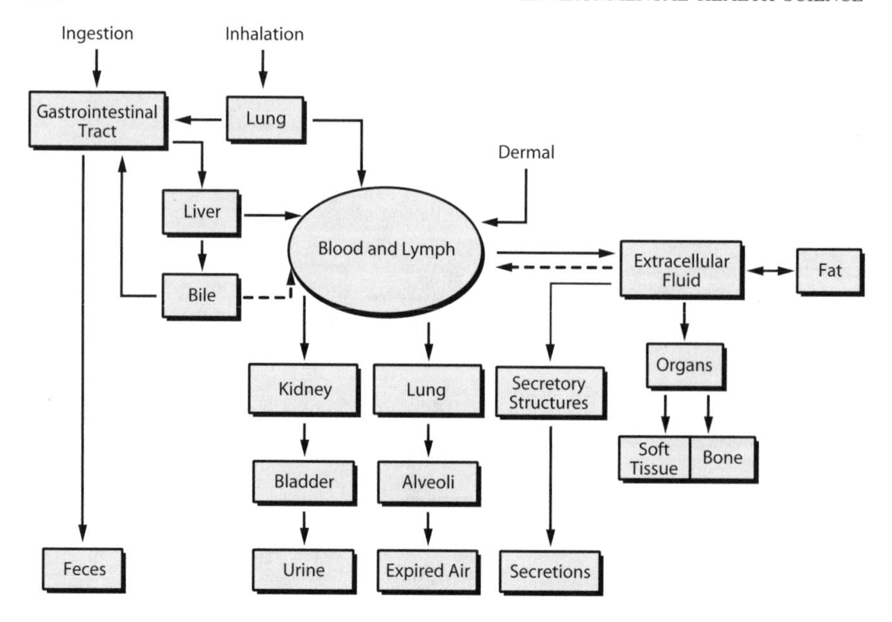

FIGURE 6–3. Routes of absorption, distribution, and excretion of toxicants in the body.

thin cellular layer between blood and air in the alveoli reduces the effectiveness of the lungs as a barrier to the systemic uptake of many inhaled chemicals.

The fate of a specific contaminant within the tract is dependent upon the form in which it exists, i.e., gaseous or particulate.

Particles

Deposition is a main factor in determining the fate of inhaled particles that are not subsequently exhaled. A variety of physical mechanisms act to remove suspended particles in various regions of the respiratory tract. The main processes affecting particle deposition are inertial impaction, sedimentation, Brownian diffusion, interception, and electrostatic attraction. The effectiveness of these various mechanisms depends upon airway geometry, breathing rate and pattern, and certain characteristics of the particle itself, such as size, shape, density, hygroscopicity, and charge. Particles with aerodynamic diameters greater than 10 μm are trapped in the nasal passages if breathed through the nose, or retained in the mouth, pharynx, and larynx if breathed through the mouth. Those from 2 to 10 μm are largely trapped in the nasal passages and/or bronchial tree, while those less than 2 μm penetrate extensively to the bronchioles and alveoli. Deposition

FIGURE 6–4. ICRP-1994 model for structure, function, epithelial cell types, and nomenclature of the human respiratory tract.

Functions	Cylology (Epithelium)	Histology (Walls)	Generation Number	Anatomy	Regions used in Model: New		Regions used in Model: Old*	Zones (Air)		Location		Airway Surface	Number of Airways
Air Conditioning; Temperature and Humidity, and Cleaning; Fast Particle Clearance; Air Conduction	Respiratory Epithelium with Goblet Cells: Cell Types: - Ciliated Cells - Nonciliated Cells: • Goblet Cells • Mucous (Secretory) Cells • Serous Cells • Brush Cells • Endocrine Cells • Basal Cells • Intermediate Cells	Mucous Membrane, Respiratory Epithelium (Pseudostratified, Ciliated, Mucous), Glands		Anterior Nasal Passages	ET_1		(N-P)	Conditioning	$0.175 \times 10^{-3} m^3$ (Anatomical Dead Space)	Extrathoracic	Extrapulmonary	$2 \times 10^{-3} m^2$	—
		Mucous Membrane, Respiratory or Stratified Epithelium, Glands		Nose, Mouth, Pharynx, Posterior, Larynx, Esophagus	ET_2	LN_{ET}						$4.5 \times 10^{-2} m^2$	—
		Mucous Membrane, Respiratory Epithelium, Cartilage Rings, Glands	0	Trachea	BB	LN_{TH} †	(T-B)			Thoracic		$3 \times 10^{-2} m^2$	511
			1	Main Bronchi									
		Mucous Membrane, Respiratory Epithelium, Cartilage plates, Smooth Muscle Layer, Glands	2 - 8	Bronchi							Pulmonary		
	Respiratory Epithelium with Clara Cells (No Goblet Cells) Cell Types: - Ciliated Cells - Nonciliated Cells • Clara (Secretory) Cells	Mucous Membrane, Respiratory Epithelium, No Cartilage, No Glands, Smooth Muscle Layer	9 - 14	Bronchioles	bb			Conduction				$2.6 \times 10^{-1} m^2$	6.5×10^4
		Mucous Membrane, Single-Layer Respiratory Epithelium, Less Ciliated, Smooth Muscle Layer	15	Terminal Bronchioles									
Air Conduction; Gas Exchange; Slow Particle Clearance	Respiratory Epithelium Consisting Mainly of Clara Cells (Secretory) and Few Ciliated Cells	Mucous Membrane, Single-Layer Respiratory Epithelium of Cuboidal Cells, Smooth Muscle Layers	16 - 18	Respiratory Bronchioles	AI		P	Gas-Exchange Transitory	$0.2 \times 10^{-3} m^3$			$7.5 m^2$	4.6×10^5
Gas Exchange; Very Slow Particle Clearance	Squamous Alveolar Epithelium Cells (Type I), Covering 93% of Alveolar Surface Area	Wall Consists of Alveolar Entrance Rings, Squamous Epithelial Layer, Surfactant	**	Alveolar Ducts					$4.5 \times 10^{-3} m^3$			$140 m^2$	4.5×10^7
	Cuboidal Alveolar Epithelial Cells (Type II. Surfactant-Producing), Covering 7% of Alveolar Surface Area	Interalveolar Septa Covered by Squamous Epithelium, Containing Capillaries, Surfactant	**	Alveolar Sacs									
	Alveolar Macrophages												
				Lymphatics			L						

* Previous ICRP Model

** Unnumbered because of imprecise information

† Lymph nodes are located only in BB region but drain the bronchial and alveolar interstitial regions as well as the bronchial region.

of particles in the nasal and/or oral airways and the bronchial tree is an important protective mechanism for those environmental agents that produce health effects only when they penetrate to and deposit in the gas-exchange region.

The conductive airways are lined with a ciliated epithelium, overlaid by a thin fluid layer composed largely of water and glycoproteins, and formed by secretions of specialized glands and individual cells (Fig. 6–4). This "mucous blanket" is propelled by the cilia towards the pharynx, where it may be swallowed or expectorated. A similar blanket in the nasal passages and sinuses also moves toward the pharynx. The rate of mucous transport varies in different regions of the tracheobronchial tree, and the composition and/or consistency of the fluid lining also differs in different regions.

Insoluble particles that deposit on the nasal passages and tracheobronchial tree may be cleared from the respiratory tract via this mucociliary system, with residence times ranging from minutes up to approximately 24–48 hours. Frequently, the rapidity and degree of clearance plays a major role in determining the risk from particulate matter exposure. Extended contact time between deposited toxic particles and the epithelium may lead to local damage or an increased degree of absorption and resultant systemic effects.

Soluble particles that deposit in conductive airways may dissolve in the mucus, moving with it out of the respiratory tract, or they may be absorbed through the epithelium into the circulatory and/or lymphatic system. The alveolar region of the lung does not contain cilia or mucus. Particles that reach and deposit within this zone are, however, also subject to clearance, but by different mechanisms, with half-times varying from days to years. Deposited particles may be taken up, via phagocytosis, by specialized cells known as alveolar macrophages, which are present on the alveolar surface. These cells may then follow a number of possible subsequent clearance routes. The macrophages, and also free particles, may penetrate the alveolar epithelium, entering the interstitial tissue where they may remain (parenchymal sequestration), or become absorbed into the lymphatic system. Macrophages carried in this system may be trapped in lymph nodes, which act as dust stores of the lung, or they may eventually drain with the lymphatic fluid into the systemic blood.

Another possible clearance mechanism is migration of the particle-laden macrophages to the level of the mucociliary blanket, and subsequent clearance via the mucociliary system. Free particles and macrophages may also move to the level of the mucociliary system by mechanisms that may involve respiratory motion of the alveolar walls, capillary action, tensile forces between alveolar fluid and mucus, the influence of ciliary beat in bronchioles, and the shearing effect of layers of mucus. Soluble particles depositing in the alveoli may be removed by direct translocation across the alveolar epithelium into the blood.

Other defense mechanisms of the respiratory system include sneezing, which serves to cleanse the upper respiratory tract, and coughing, which acts to clear the larger bronchial airways. Constriction of bronchi due to the contraction of surrounding smooth muscle following exposure to certain chemicals may act as a defense by decreasing further penetration to the deeper lung areas.

Gases and vapors

The site and extent of absorption of inhaled gases and vapors are, for the most part, determined by their solubility characteristics in water. Highly soluble gases, for example, SO_2, are largely absorbed in the upper respiratory tract, while those that are less water soluble, for example, NO_2 and O_3, reach the lower airways. Absorption is also dependent upon air flow rate and the partial pressure of the gas in the inspired air. Gases dissolved in the tracheobronchial tree may be cleared with the mucus.

Gastrointestinal Tract

Chemical contaminants that are waterborne or transported via food chains reach people via the gastrointestinal tract. Ingestion may also contribute to the uptake of chemicals that were initially inhaled, since material deposited on or dissolved in the bronchial mucous blanket is eventually swallowed.

The gastrointestinal (GI) tract may be considered to be a tube running through the body, but whose contents are actually external to the body (Fig. 6–5). Unless the ingested material affects the tract itself, any systemic response depends upon absorption through the mucosal cells lining the lumen. Although absorption may occur anywhere along the length of the GI tract, the main region for effective translocation is the small intestine. The enormous absorptive capacity of this region is due to the presence in the intestinal mucosa of projections, termed villi, each of which contains a network of capillaries; the villi result in a large effective total surface area for absorption.

Although passive diffusion is the main absorptive process, certain active transport systems allow essential lipid-insoluble nutrients and inorganic ions to cross the intestinal epithelium. These carrier systems may also be responsible for some contaminant uptake. For example, lead may be absorbed via the system that normally transports calcium ions.

Materials absorbed from the GI tract enter either the lymphatic system or the portal blood circulation; the latter carries material to the liver, from which it may be actively excreted into the bile, or diffuse into the bile from the blood. The bile is subsequently secreted into the intestines. Thus, a cycle of translocation of a chemical from the intestine to the liver to bile and back to the intestines, known as the enterohepatic circulation, may be established. Enterohepatic circulation usually involves contaminants that undergo metabolic degradation in the liver.

Various factors serve to modify absorption from the GI tract, enhancing or depressing its barrier function. A decrease in gastrointestinal mobility generally fa-

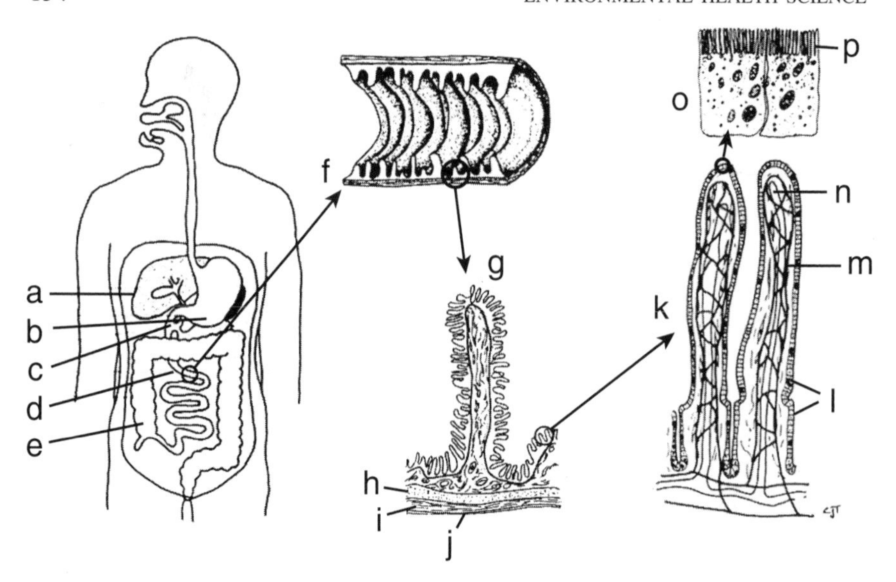

Figure 6–5. The mammalian gastrointestinal tract showing important features of the small intestine, the major site of absorption for orally administered compounds. *(a)* liver; *(b)* stomach; *(c)* duodenum; *(d)* ileum; *(e)* colon; *(f)* longitudinal section of the ileum showing folding that increases surface area; *(g)* detail of fold showing villi with circular and longitudinal muscles; *(h)* and *(i)* respectively, bounded by the serosal membrane; *(j)*; *(k)* detail of villi showing network of capillaries; *(m)* lacteals; *(n)* and epithelial cells; *(l)*; *(o)* detail of epithelial cells showing brush border or microvilli, *(p)*. The folding, vascularization and microvilli all facilitate absorption of substances from the lumen. (*Source*: Timbrell, J.A. Introduction to Toxicology, London: Taylor & Francis, 1989.)

vors increased absorption. Specific stomach contents and secretions may react with the contaminant, possibly changing it to a form with different physicochemical properties, for example, solubility, or they may absorb it, altering the available chemical and changing translocation rates. The size of ingested particles also affects absorption. Since the rate of dissolution is inversely proportional to particle size, larger particles are absorbed to a lesser degree, especially if they are of a fairly insoluble material in the first place. Certain chemicals, for example, ethylene diamine tetraacetic acid (EDTA), also cause a nonspecific increase in absorption of many materials.

As a defense, spastic contractions in the stomach and intestine may serve to eliminate noxious agents via vomiting or by acceleration of feces through the gastrointestinal tract, respectively.

Skin

The skin is generally a very effective barrier against the entry of environmental chemicals. In order to be absorbed via this route (percutaneous absorption), an agent must traverse a number of cellular layers before gaining access to the general circulation (Fig. 6–6). Skin consists of two structural regions, the epidermis and the dermis, which rest upon connective tissue. The epidermis consists of a number of layers of cells, and has varying thickness depending upon the region of the body; the outermost layer is composed of keratinized cells. The dermis contains blood vessels, hair follicles, sebaceous and sweat glands, and nerve endings. The epidermis represents the primary barrier to percutaneous absorption, the dermis being freely permeable to many materials. Passage through the epidermis occurs by passive diffusion.

The main factors that affect percutaneous absorption are degree of lipid solubility of the chemical, site on the body, local blood-flow, and skin temperature. Some environmental chemicals are readily absorbed through the skin, for example, phenols, carbon tetrachloride, tetraethyl lead, and organophosphate pesticides.

Certain chemicals, for example, dimethyl sulfoxide (DMSO) and formic acid, alter the integrity of skin and facilitate penetration of other materials by increasing skin permeability. Moderate changes in permeability may also result following topical applications of acetone, methyl achohol, and ethyl alcohol. In addition, cutaneous injury may enhance percutaneous absorption.

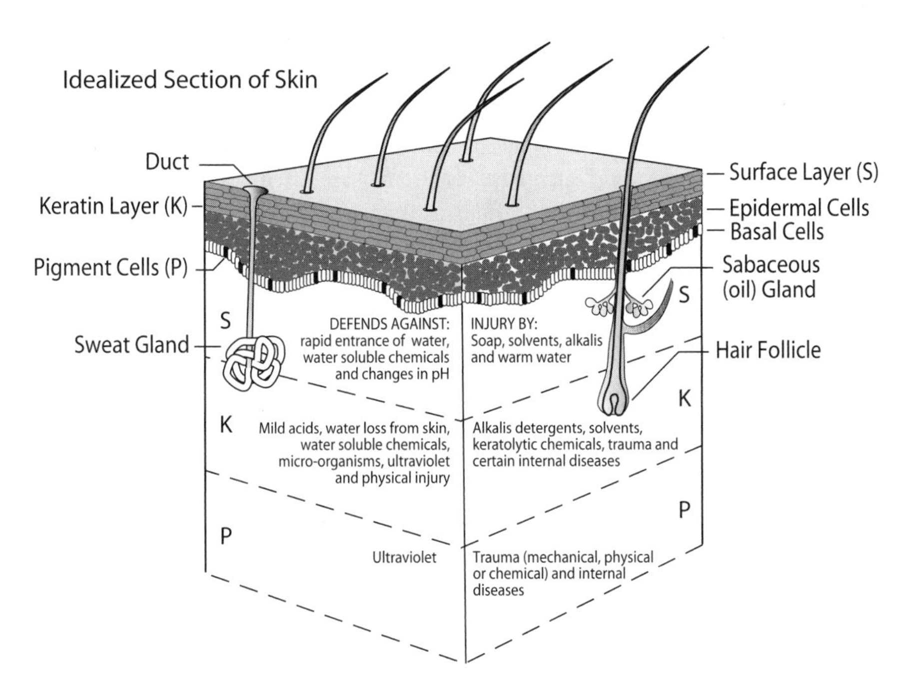

FIGURE 6–6. Idealized section of skin. (*Source*: Adapted from: Birmingham, D.J. Occupational Dermatoses: Their Recognition and Control. pp. 503–9 in The Industrial Environment—Its Evaluation and Control, U.S. H.E.W., Washington, DC, 1973.)

Interspecies differences in percutaneous absorption are responsible for the selective toxicity of many insecticides. For example, DDT is about equally hazardous to both insects and mammals if ingested, but is much less hazardous to mammals when applied to the skin. This is due to the poor absorption through mammalian skin, compared to its ready passage through the insect exoskeleton. Although the main route of percutaneous absorption is through the epidermal cells, some chemicals may follow an appendageal route, i.e., entering through hair follicles, sweat glands, or sebaceous glands.

FATE OF ENVIRONMENTAL CHEMICALS IN THE BODY

Once absorbed, chemicals may be translocated to storage sites, biotransformation sites, or sites of excretion. We shall consider each of these pathways before discussing specific biological responses to chemical exposures.

Metabolism of Chemicals: Biotransformation

Chemical contaminants that enter the body may undergo metabolic conversion in a process known as biotransformation. These chemical reactions are mediated by enzymes, and result either in alterations of the parent compound or formation of new product(s) via the combination of the parent with various endogenous substrates.

At one time, it was believed that all contaminants underwent biotransformation into less-toxic forms. Thus, these reactions were often referred to as detoxification mechanisms. However, certain of the reactions result in products that are more toxic than the parent (metabolic toxification). Contaminants having structures similar to certain normal substrates in the body may undergo biotransformation by enzymes that normally catalyze transformation of these substrates. For example, the enzyme monoamine oxidase catalyzes the metabolism of endogenous amines such as epinephrine; it is also involved in the reactions of foreign, short-chain amines, such as benzylamine.

The primary site of biotransformation is the liver. Liver cells, like most other cells, contain a system of internal, smooth- and rough-surfaced membranes, known as the endoplasmic reticulum. If these cells are homogenized and then subjected to ultracentrifugation, the smooth fraction of the endoplasmic reticulum separates into fragments termed microsomes. The enzymes involved in biotransformation reactions reside primarily in the microsomal fraction of the cells. Some of these enzymes are nonspecific, i.e., they act upon various substrates, and are capable of catalyzing a variety of biotransformation reactions. Some chemicals do, however, require specific enzymes for metabolic transformation. In addition, the enzymes generally do not act upon lipid insoluble material.

Most biotransformation mechanisms fall into two main classes of reactions: termed Phase 1 and Phase 2. Phase 1 reactions include hydrolysis, oxidation, and reduction. Phase 2 reactions, or conjugations, involve the production of a new product from the parent compound or a metabolite, and an endogenous substrate, generally a polar or ionic moiety. Conjugation includes numerous classes of reactions, for example, acetylation, alkylation, acylation, methylation, and esterification.

A number of biotransformation reactions have been found that do not fall into the above basic classes. These miscellaneous mechanisms include aromatic dehydroxylation, aliphatic dehydroxylation, nitrile hydrolysis, dehalogenation, cyclization, and ring scission.

More than one reaction type may be involved in the metabolism of a specific chemical. Sequential or parallel reactions, involving different mechanisms, often occur, and various metabolic products are formed from the parent compound. For example, Phase 1 reactions often produce metabolites that subsequently undergo conjugation reactions. The exact type of biotransformation reactions that an agent undergoes depends upon the particular structure of the chemical, and also upon its route of entry. Route of entry is important because liver cells are not the only sites for biotransformation mechanisms. Enzymes in blood plasma, kidneys, respiratory tract, gastrointestinal tract, and skin are capable of catalyzing metabolic transformation reactions. Certain components of the detoxification system and the extent of biotransformation activity do, however, differ in different tissues.

Various host and environmental factors serve to modify biotransformation mechanisms. The host factors include age (e.g., infants have incompletely developed enzyme systems), nutritional status, and genetic deficiencies (e.g., lack of certain enzymes or excess enzymatic activity). The environmental factors involve exposure to certain chemicals that result in induction or inhibition of microsomal enzymes.

A variety of chemicals can increase the amount and activity of enzymes. These include drugs, such as phenobarbital; organochlorine insecticides; certain herbicides, for example, Herban and Diuron; the food additive BHT; and various polycyclic aromatic hydrocarbons, for example, benzo(a)pyrene. If detoxification is the normal result of metabolism, induction would tend to be protective; if, however, metabolic toxification is the result, induction may increase harmful effects in the host. Other chemicals may nonspecifically inhibit microsomal enzymes. These include organophosphate insecticides, carbon tetrachloride, O_3, and CO. Enzyme inhibition would result in the persistence of a chemical that would normally be metabolized.

Induction and inhibition of biotransformation enzymes are important when one realizes that people are generally exposed to more than one chemical contaminant; thus, exposure to some may increase susceptibility to what alone would be relatively nontoxic levels of other contaminants due to modulation of microsomal enzymes.

Some contaminants may be altered by undergoing bacterially mediated and nonenzymatic reactions. For example, gastrointestinal flora may reduce aromatic nitro groups into potentially carcinogenic aromatic amines. Carcinogenic nitrosamines may be formed in the low pH environment of the stomach from secondary or tertiary amines, which naturally occur in a variety of foods, and nitrite, which is used as an additive in smoked meats. Another example is the development of a disease called methemoglobinemia in infants who ingest water and foods having high-nitrate contents. The condition, which results in a decrease in the oxygen-carrying capacity of blood, occurs due to differences in the pH and bacterial content of the gastrointestinal tract of infants compared to adults, resulting in greater conversion of nitrate to nitrite, the actual causative agent, in the former. Bacterially mediated reactions in the gastrointestinal tract may also result in the prolongation of action of certain chemicals via deconjugation, causing reabsorption of a chemical that had been previously conjugated in the liver and secreted with bile into the intestine.

Storage of Chemicals

Some contaminants tend to concentrate in specific tissues due to physicochemical properties, such as selective solubility, or to selective absorption onto, or combination with, macromolecules such as proteins. Storage of a chemical often occurs when the rate of exposure is greater than the rate of metabolism and/or excretion.

Storage or binding sites may not be the sites of toxic action. For example, CO produces its effect by binding with hemoglobin in red blood cells; on the other hand, inorganic lead is stored primarily in bone, but acts mainly on the soft tissues of the body.

If the storage site is not the site of toxic action, selective sequestration may be a protective mechanism, since only the freely circulating form of the contaminant produces harmful effects. Until the storage sites are saturated, a buildup of free chemical may be prevented. On the other hand, selective storage limits the amount of contaminant that is excreted. Since bound or stored toxicants are in equilibrium with their free form, as the contaminant is excreted or metabolized, it is released from the storage site.

Contaminants that are stored may remain in the body for years without effect, for example, organochlorine pesticides. On the other hand, accumulation may produce illnesses which develop slowly, as occurs in chronic cadmium poisoning. Table 6–1 lists the major storage sites, with examples of chemicals selectively stored there.

Excretion of Chemicals

The major role in elimination of toxicants is played by the kidneys. Extrarenal routes may be important in elimination of certain specific substances; these routes

TABLE 6–1. Main Storage Sites of Contaminants

STORAGE SITE	EXAMPLE OF CHEMICAL SELECTIVELY STORED	MECHANISM OF STORAGE
Fat	DDT, PCB	Dissolution
Bone	Inorganic Lead, ^{90}Sr	Substitutes for calcium in bone matrix
Kidney	Cadmium	Binds with intracellular protein

are the lungs, GI tract, skin, and elimination via body secretions, such as saliva and milk.

When the blood is filtered by the kidneys, contaminants are subject to the same removal mechanisms as are normal metabolic end products. As the filtrate travels through the renal tubules, an agent may be reabsorbed into the blood, or remain in the filtrate to be excreted in the urine. In general, lipid-insoluble substances are poorly reabsorbed, although reabsorption via active transport may occur regardless of solubility characteristics. Biotransformation is an important mechanism for the conversion of chemicals into metabolites that may then be more readily excreted by the kidneys than the parent compound. They may occur, for example, by conversion of a highly lipid-soluble agent into a less lipid-soluble metabolite. On the other hand, biotransformation reactions may also produce metabolites with increased lipid solubility.

Contaminants appear in the feces if they are not absorbed after ingestion, if they are excreted into bile, or are excreted along the GI tract. The GI tract is the primary route of excretion for many trace metals, for example, Cr, Mn, Pb, and certain large molecules, for example, many pesticides.

Since the circulation from the GI tract goes to the liver prior to entering the general circulation, the liver may serve to remove materials following GI absorption, preventing distribution to the systemic circulation. The contaminant or its metabolites may then be excreted into the bile, entering the small intestine. Generally, lipid-insoluble substances are more readily excreted into bile; once in the intestines, the agent may be reconverted into a more lipid-soluble form and be reabsorbed, or be excreted with the feces.

The lungs may serve as an organ of excretion for substances that exist in the gas phase at body temperature. Ingested volatile organic compounds, such as carbon tetrachloride (CCl_4), may be partially excreted from the lungs as vapors, via diffusion. In general, gases with low solubility in blood at body temperature will be more readily excreted through the lungs than will those with high solubility.

Although of minor importance, contaminants may be excreted in sweat, tears, saliva, and milk. Generally, lipid-soluble materials are passively diffused into these secretions. Contaminants in mother's milk may be passed along to the suckling infant. Excretion into saliva may result in reabsorption via the GI tract. Contaminants can also be eliminated by incorporation into hair and nails, which are periodically trimmed.

BIOLOGICAL RESPONSES TO CHEMICAL CONTAMINANTS

The action of chemical contaminants covers the entire range of effects, from a mere nuisance to extensive tissue necrosis and death, from generalized systemic effects to highly specific attacks on single tissues and even individual enzyme systems. Multiple sources and multiple insults via different environmental routes may increase the risk of disease from environmental chemicals. Biological effects may be the result of exposure to an individual agent, or be due to interaction between different agents. A specific chemical may produce more than one effect upon its target, while completely different agents may result in similar, or even identical, pathological manifestations.

A number of host and environmental factors serve to modify the effects of chemicals; the ultimate response is the result of the interaction between these factors. The main host factors are: *(1)* age, for example, older age groups tend to be more susceptible to morbidity and mortality during periods of increased air contamination. This is usually due to chronically reduced cardiovascular and respiratory function, resulting in the inability to cope with additional stresses. Newborns and infants are more sensitive to some toxicants than are adults, partly because of the inability to synthesize specific biotransformation enzymes and due to the high cell turnover rates that occur during maturation of organ systems; *(2)* state of health, for example, concurrent disease or dysfunction may result in enhanced toxicity following exposure, or may make an organ more susceptible to damage; *(3)* nutritional status; *(4)* immunological status; *(5)* gender, and other genetic factors, for example, enzyme-related differences in biotransformation mechanisms, such as deficient metabolic pathways, and inability to synthesize certain detoxification enzymes; *(6)* psychological state, for example, stress, anxiety; and *(7)* cultural factors, for example, cigarette smoking, which may affect normal defenses, or may potentiate the effect of other chemicals.

The environmental factors that affect biological response include the concentration, stability, and physicochemical properties of the agent in the exposure environment and the duration, frequency, and route of exposure. Acute and chronic exposures to a chemical may result in different pathological manifestations.

Any organ can only respond in a limited number of ways, although there are numerous diagnostic labels for the resultant diseases. Thus, similar responses may occur in different systems. The following sections discuss common, broad types of responses which may occur following exposure to environmental chemicals.

Irritant Response

A pattern of generalized, nonspecific tissue inflammation and destruction may result at the area of contaminant contact. This type of reaction is caused by a class of chemicals termed irritants. It is a portal of entry response, which occurs whether or not the agent is absorbed into the systemic circulation. A list of some common chemical irritants is presented in Table 6–2.

Some irritants produce no systemic effect because the irritant response is much greater than any systemic effect, for example, mustard gas in the respiratory tract, or the irritant response is significantly greater than any other potential toxicity, for example, sulfuric acid in the respiratory tract. Some irritants also have significant systemic effects following absorption, for example, H_2S absorbed via the lungs causing respiratory paralysis.

Exposure to irritants may result in death if critical organs are severely damaged. On the other hand, the damage may be reversible or it may result in permanent loss of some degree of function, such as impaired gas exchange capacity in the lungs or malabsorption of nutrients in the GI tract.

The respiratory tract is a common site of irritant exposure. Acute exposure results in a common inflammatory response in all affected regions: rhinitis, pharyngitis, and laryngitis in the upper respiratory tract, bronchitis in the bronchial tree, edema and pneumonia in the alveolar region. Longer-duration exposure may result in a chronic inflammation of small bronchi, and hyperplasia (an increase in size) and/or metaplasia (transformation of one cell type into another) of mucus-secreting glands and goblet cells. Other responses also include deposition of connective tissue (fibrosis), alteration in structural proteins, and loss of lung elasticity.

Changes in respiratory function without development of a specific disease state have been seen in response to exposure to many inhaled irritants, for example, SO_2, NO_2, and O_3. These changes are often due to constriction of bronchi caused by a reflex response, or by the release of endogenous chemicals, such as histamine. Another important effect of exposure to many pulmonary irritants is alteration of the normal functioning of the mucociliary and/or alveolar clear-

TABLE 6–2. Some Chemical Irritants

Sulfur dioxide	Ozone
Sulfuric acid and other strong acids	Peroxyacetylnitrates
Ammonia and other strong bases	Aromatic hydrocarbons, e.g., benzene, ether
Nitrogen dioxide	Particulate sulfates, e.g., zinc sulfate, ammonium sulfate
Hydrogen fluoride	Organic selenides
Formaldehyde	Numerous pesticides
Acrolein	
Chlorine	

ance systems. Those chemicals showing this effect include NO_2, SO_2, and H_2SO_4.

The skin is also a portal of entry frequently subject to environmental chemical irritation. However, most environmental skin disorders arise from occupational exposures to irritants. Most reactions to these are eczematous in nature, and include ulceration and granuloma formation.

Fibrotic Response

A number of environmental agents are etiological factors in the development of a group of chronic lung disorders termed pneumoconioses. This general term encompasses many fibrotic conditions of the lung, i.e., diseases characterized by scar formation in the interstitial tissue. Pneumoconioses are due to the inhalation and subsequent selective retention of certain dusts in the alveolar region, from which they are subject to interstitial sequestration.

Pneumoconioses are characterized by specific fibrotic lesions, which differ in type and pattern according to the dust involved. For example, silicosis, due to the deposition of crystalline free silica, is characterized by a nodular type of fibrosis, while a diffuse fibrosis is found in asbestosis due to asbestos-fiber exposure. Certain dusts, such as iron oxide, produce only altered radiology (siderosis) with no functional impairment, while the effects of others range from minimal disability to death. Some important dusts involved in fibrosis of the lung are listed in Table 6–3.

Table 6–3. Pulmonary Fibrotic Agents

MATERIAL	DISEASE DESIGNATION
Inorganic Fibers and Dusts	
Crystalline silica (quartz, cristobolite)	Silicosis
Asbestos	Asbestosis
Talc	Talcosis
Coal (mine dust)	Coal workers' pneumoconiosis
Kaolin	Kaolinosis
Graphite	Graphite lung
Organic Fibers and Dusts	
Cellulose	Bagassosis
Cotton	Byssinosis
Flax	Byssinosis
Hemp	Byssinosis
Metallic Fumes	
Tin oxide	Stannosis
Iron oxide	Siderosis
Beryllium oxide	Berylliosis

Dusts initially inhaled may be translocated to other parts of the body. For example, fibrotic nodules due to occupational exposure to asbestos can also be found in the spleen and peritoneum, possibly due to translocation by lymph or blood, or to swallowing of fibers carried to the larynx via the mucociliary system. The fate of inhaled fibers, and their potential effects in terms of producing lung fibrosis, lung cancer, and cancers of the plueral and peritoneal mesothelium are highly dependent on fiber length, fiber diameter, and their biopersistence (dissolution rate).

Asphyxiant Response

Some chemicals having the respiratory tract as a portal of entry can cause death by their action in preventing an adequate oxygen supply from reaching the tissues of the body. These chemicals are known as asphyxiants. Some "biologically inert" asphyxiants prevent tissues from receiving enough oxygen simply by displacing oxygen in the air. Examples of these are CO_2, and CH_4. Other asphyxiants prevent oxygen from being carried by the blood, for example, CO, or from being utilized by the tissues, for example, hydrogen cyanide. Chronic exposure to asphyxiants may result in systemic disorders due to a persistent impairment of the oxygen supply to vital organs.

Allergic Response

Allergic agents, termed allergens, generally affect the respiratory tract and skin, although they may also affect other organs such as the intestines (allergic colitis). Some chemical allergens are listed in Table 6–4.

Allergic responses involve the phenomenon known as sensitization. Initial exposure to an allergen results in the induction of antibody formation; subsequent exposure of the now "sensitized" individual results in an immune response, i.e., an antibody-antigen reaction (the antigen is the allergen in combination with an endogenous protein). This immune reaction may occur immediately following exposure to the allergen, or it may be a delayed response.

TABLE 6–4. Some Chemical Allergens

Organic Chemicals	Metals
Herbicides	Nickel
Organophosphate insecticides	Cobalt
Carbamate herbicides	Arsenic
Toluene diisocyanate	Chromium
Acrolein	Beryllium salts
Epoxy resins	

TABLE 6–5. Some Known or Suspected Chemical Mutagens

DDT	Sodium arsenate
2,4-D	Cadmium sulfate
2,4,5-T	Lead salts (some)
Benzene	Nitrite

The primary respiratory allergic reactions are bronchial asthma, reactions in the upper respiratory tract involving the release of histamine or histamine-like mediators following immune reactions in the mucosa, and a type of pneumonitis (lung inflammation) known as extrinsic allergic alveolitis. Skin reactions include urticaria (hives), atopic dermatitis, which is due to ingestion or inhalation of an allergen, and contact dermatitis, due to direct skin contact with an allergen. In addition to these local reactions, a systemic allergic reaction (anaphylactic shock) may follow exposure to some chemical allergens.

Mutagenic and Teratogenic Response

Mutagens are agents that produce mutations, or changes in genetic material, i.e., DNA. When the changes occur in the sperm and/or egg cells, the effects may be manifest in future generations. A variety of environmental chemicals have been found to be mutagenic, at least in test systems of cell cultures of mammalian and nonmammalian cells; these may, therefore, pose potential hazards to humans (Table 6–5).

A related effect is teratogenicity. A teratogen produces a generative change during early embryonic development, resulting in anatomical defects or other functional or biochemical developmental errors. Numerous chemicals, especially drugs, have been shown to be teratogenic in experimental animals (Table 6–6); and these, too, may be potential hazards to humans.

Carcinogenic Response

Cancer is a general term for a group of related diseases characterized by the uncontrolled growth of certain tissues. Its development is due to a complex process of interacting multiple factors in the host and the environment. It has been esti-

TABLE 6–6. Some Known or Suspected Chemical Teratogens

Dioxin	Cadmium sulfate
Organic mercury	Sodium arsenate
Phthalic acid esters	Phenylmercuric acetate

mated that up to 90% of all cancer in the human population in the United States is dependent upon either known or unknown dietary, lifestyle and other environmental factors. In some cases, specific-cancer causing chemicals (carcinogens) are involved, especially in occupational environments. In fact, the first documented cases of cancer produced by exposure to environmental chemicals, in this instance coal tar, were scrotal cancers in men and boys employed as chimney sweeps in eighteenth-century Britain.[2] However, there are numerous carcinogens present in the ambient environment.

One of the great difficulties in attempting to relate exposure to a specific chemical to cancer development in man is the generally long latent period, typically from 15 to 40 years, between onset of exposure and disease manifestation. Research studies of the carcinogenicity of chemicals, therefore, generally involve bioassay techniques in experimental animals. Although the ultimate relation of any positive results to humans is not always clear, evidence for carcinogenicity in such model systems generally results in the classification of the chemical as a potential human carcinogen.

Certain chemicals are carcinogenic as they exist in the environment; these are termed complete carcinogens. On the other hand, other environmental agents (termed procarcinogens) can become carcinogenic after they undergo conversion to some other form. Most of these procarcinogens are converted by biotransformation reactions, although some undergo nonenzymatic hydrolytic reactions to produce carcinogenic intermediates. It is not always clear whether a specific chemical is a complete or procarcinogen.

Some known and suspected human carcinogens are listed in Table 6–7. Many other environmental chemicals have been shown to produce cancer in laboratory animals and, thus, may be potential human carcinogens. These include N-mustards,

TABLE 6–7. Some Environmental Chemicals Carcinogenic in Humans

Organic Chemicals	Inorganic Chemicals
Benzidine	Arsenic (trivalent)
4-aminobiphenyl	Chromate
_-naphthylanine	Nickel carbonyl
_-naphthylamine	Beryllium
Benzene	Cadmium oxide
Vinyl chloride monomer	Asbestos
Bischloromethylether	
Soot, tar (probably due to polycyclic aromatic hydrocarbons)	**Radionuclides**
	Strontium-90
	Thorium dioxide
	Radium-226
	Radon and daughters

epoxides, small-ring lactones, urethane, thioamides, nitrosamine, and azo dyes. The list is quite long.

Current evidence suggests that most organic carcinogens belong to a limited number of chemical classes and, within each class, specific structures appear to be associated with carcinogenicity. However, it is not yet possible to predict from chemical structure whether a specific chemical is carcinogenic, since very slight differences in molecular structure and orientation result in wide variability of carcinogenic potential.

The site of development of malignant tumors may be at various areas of the body other than the initial portal of entry. Thus, for example, inhaled asbestos produces cancer at its portal of entry, the lung, but also in the peritoneum; azo dyes produce tumors in the liver, their site of biotransformation; radium produces bone cancer at its storage site; aromatic amines produce tumors in the bladder, their site of excretion.

Systemic Responses

Many environmental chemicals produce a generalized systemic disease due to their effects upon a number of target sites. Table 6–8 presents the main target sites for selected chemicals that may be classified as systemic toxicants. Some of the metals listed are essential to life at low levels, but quite toxic at high concentrations. In addition, the specific form in which a chemical exists in the exposure environment may affect its toxicity. For example, selenium as selenate and methylated forms of mercury are much more toxic than are other forms of these elements.

Finely dispersed particles (fumes) of several metal oxides are often associated with an acute systemic syndrome known as metal fume fever. This response is most often due to oxides of cadmium, manganese, and zinc.

INTERACTIONS OF CONTAMINANTS

Most people are generally exposed to more than one contaminant at any one time; thus, interactions of chemicals, as these may relate to health effects, are quite important. In one such interaction, the biological response following simultaneous exposure to a combination of two or more chemicals may be much greater than would be expected from the additive action of each individual agent. This potentiation of the combined effect is termed synergism. For example, while both carbon tetrachloride and ethanol are liver toxicants, when exposure occurs to both chemicals the extent of injury is greater than would be predicted by merely comparing the sum of the responses if exposure was to each alone.

TABLE 6–8. Main Target Sites of Selected Systemic Chemical Agents

CHEMICAL	RESPIRATORY TRACT	HEMATOPOIETIC SYSTEM	SKIN	GASTROINTESTINAL TRACT	LIVER	KIDNEY	BONES, TEETH	ENDOCRINE SYSTEM	NERVOUS SYSTEM (CENTRAL AND/OR PERIPHERAL)
Mercury	X	X		X	X	X			X
Lead		X		X		X			X
Cadmium	X	X		X		X	X	X	X
Arsenic	X	X	X	X	X	X		X	X
Fluoride		X		X			X		
Molybdenum		X			X				
Selenium			X	X	X	X	X		
Organophosphate pesticides		X	X						X
Organochlorine pesticides					X				X
Carbamate pesticides									X
Carbon tetrachloride					X	X			
Chlorinated biphenyls			X		X				X

The generally accepted view of synergism extends beyond simple potentiation to include other increases in toxic reactions, such as gas-particle interaction in the lungs. Gases adsorbed onto particulates may reach deeper lung areas than they normally would if inhaled in the gas phase. For example, the irritant potency of SO_2 was increased in guinea pigs undergoing simultaneous exposure to H_2SO_4 mist.[3]

An important area of concern is the synergistic effect of certain environmental chemicals in the pathogenesis of cancer. Some agents termed promoters, or cocarcinogens, potentiate the carcinogenic effect of other chemicals, although they are not carcinogenic themselves. In some classic examples, the combination of SO_2 with benzo(a)pyrene resulted in respiratory tract tumors in hamsters and rats, while no tumors were found following inhalation at similar concentrations of either agent alone or to SO_2 at any level.[4] Asbestos workers and uranium miners who smoked cigarettes were found to have a significantly greater risk of developing lung cancer than did their nonsmoking counterparts.[5,6]

In another type of interaction, an environmental chemical may act in an antagonistic manner with respect to another, i.e., there is a decrease in toxic effect below that expected by sole exposure to the latter. As opposed to synergism, exposure to both agents does not have to be simultaneous to produce antagonism.

A further type of interaction involves environmental chemicals and viable agents. A nonspecific response to certain chemicals, primarily irritants, is a depression of the immune response, making the host more susceptible to viable pathogenic agents. Increases in the susceptibility of experimental animals to respiratory tract infections, for example, bacterial pneumonia, have been observed following exposures to oxidant gases such as O_3 and NO_2.

A special type of interaction is termed tolerance. Tolerance is a phenomenon demonstrated in acute studies with experimental animals; tolerant individuals are not killed by levels of certain chemicals which are lethal to their nontolerant counterparts. Exposures of rodents to sublethal levels of O_3 afford protection against subsequent exposure to what would be lethal levels of O_3. Treatment with low concentrations of O_3 also confers protection against the acute effects of other chemicals, for example, NO_2. This phenomenon, termed cross-tolerance, also occurs between many other oxidants.

EPIDEMIOLOGICAL EVIDENCE FOR CONTAMINANT HEALTH EFFECTS

Epidemiology is the study of the distribution and frequency of a disease in a specific population. Epidemiologists seek associations between environmental factors, for example, levels of certain contaminants, and rates of morbidity and mortality in the exposed population. Effects of contaminants are generally expressed in terms of excess morbidity or mortality, with excess measured relative to the expected statistical mean for a reference population within a certain time period.

Epidemiologic analyses are beset with inherent problems, making it quite difficult to obtain a quantitative link between long-term exposure to contaminants and health effects. One major problem is separation of the effects of a specific contaminant from the possible mediating effects of other factors that affect health, such as concurrent disease, diet, living conditions, cultural factors, and occupational exposures. The isolation of the effect of only one factor upon health requires data from large populations that ideally differ only with respect to exposure to the contaminant in question. Because of the many unknown factors, assumptions are often made that these factors are identical for all groups, or vary randomly with respect to levels of the contaminant. Other problems in epidemiologic studies involve: *(1)* possible synergism, antagonism, and other interaction between individual contaminants, especially since most communities are exposed to combinations that often make isolation of any one contaminant as the primary culprit of observed effects quite difficult; *(2)* the accuracy of the classification and reliability of the records of symptoms during the period under study; and *(3)* reliability and accuracy of the measurements of ambient levels in the area under study and the relationship between these levels and actual personal exposures to the population(s) of concern.

In recent years, there have been numerous epidemiological studies of rates of daily mortality and hospital admissions for pulmonary and cardiovascular causes, as well as of total non-traumatic mortality, in large populations in relation to daily levels of ambient air pollution. These studies, known as time-series, are not significantly confounded by variations in smoking, diet, climate and lifestyle, since the same population is at risk each day. As discussed below, such studies have consistently indicated significant associations between daily, area-wide concentrations of fine particles and both daily mortality and hospital admission rates. However, similar associations can often be seen with other regularly measured ambient air pollutants, such as O_3, SO_2, NO_2, and CO, making it difficult to assign a causal role for the short-term health effects of any of the specific constituents within ambient particulate matter, or for co-pollutant gases.

For epidemiologic studies of the effects of chronic or cumulative exposures, it is usually necessary to rely on cross-sectional (intercommunity) differences in exposures and responses, or on prospective cohort studies based on individual risk-factor data for large numbers of subjects. The former are confounded by intercommunity differences in smoking and other influential factors, while the latter require large and long-term committments of resources that have seldom been available.

Thus, care must be taken in interpretation of epidemiological studies; the finding of an association between specific contaminants and a health effect does not necessarily prove a causal relationship. However, these studies sometimes provide the only data on the effects of long-term, chronic exposures of large populations to ambient levels of contaminants and, as such, are often used as the basis for policy decisions by governmental agencies.

Air Contaminants

Acute exposure

The severe effects of air contaminants upon health were initially brought to general attention following some acute air pollution crises known as episodes. Concentrations of some contaminants were reached that were clearly hazardous to human health, as indicated by abrupt increases in morbidity and mortality of the exposed population; there was left little doubt that air pollution was the cause of these effects.

Although some historic episodes were due to accidental industrial release of chemicals, most were associated with buildups of generally prevalent pollutants caused by abnormally poor ventilation conditions due, in large part, to characteristics of local topography. Most episodes involved a combination of aerosol and gaseous contaminants, since most occurred under conditions in which water droplets (e.g., fog) were present. The specific contaminant(s) that seemed to be responsible and reached greater than normal levels were almost always the reducing type, i.e., characterized by SO_2, related sulfur-containing species, and suspended particulate matter (such as smoke). However, no single agent has been irrevocably indicted as the cause for the excess mortality and morbidity, which occurred mainly among the elderly and people with preexisting pulmonary and/or cardiovascular disease. Table 6–9 presents some of the major historic air pollution episodes. Note that the concentration and often the nature of specific contaminants during the early episodes were unknown, and were generally estimated at a later date.

The acute episodes presented in Table 6–9 are by no means the only ones that have resulted in excess morbidity and mortality. The lethal fog in London in December 1952, which produced an official count of approximately 4000 excess deaths in the weeks following it, or 12,000 in a recent reanalysis,[7] was an extreme episode that led to a change in fuel to "smokeless fuel" over the next 10 years, markedly reducing the concentration of black smoke. When a similar atmospheric inversion occurred in December 1962, the peak smoke level was approximately 2 mg/m^3, but the peak SO_2 level, about 4 mg/m^3 was similar to that measured in December 1952. As shown in Figure 6–7, the clearly observable excess in deaths that followed the episode, cumulating to approximately 700, was much lower than the nominal 4000 seen in 1952, suggesting that black smoke, or its strong acid component, was a more important component than SO_2 in causing mortality.

Table 6–9. Major Historic Air Pollution Episodes Associated with Excess Mortality

LOCATION	DATE	TOPOGRAPHY, METEOROLOGICAL CONDITIONS	CHEMICAL AGENTS INVOLVED	MAIN SOURCES	MORTALITY/MORBIDITY
Meuse Valley, Belgium	Dec. 1–5, 1930	River valley; temperature inversion, weak winds, fog	Responsible agents not definitively known; those implicated include SO_2, fluorides, H_2SO_4. Estimated 9.6–38.4 ppm_v SO_2	Industry (steel mills, glass factories, Zn smelters, H_2SO_4 plants)	64 excess deaths; several hundred attributable illnesses; higher mortality in older age groups. Symptoms were respiratory tract irritation, coughing, chest pain, eye irritation
Donora, Pennsylvania	Oct. 26–31, 1948	River valley; temperature inversion, weak winds, fog	No conclusive proof for health effects from any single agent; combination of SO_2 and particulates implicated. Estimated 0.5–2.0 ppm_v SO_2, 4 mg/m^3 total particulates	Industry (steel mills, Zn smelter, H_2SO_4 plant)	20 excess deaths; 5000–7000 attributable illnesses; higher mortality in older age groups. Symptoms were respiratory tract irritation, eye irritation, cough, nausea
Poza Rica, Mexico	Nov. 24, 1950	Flat terrain; temperature inversion, weak winds, fog	Hydrogen sulfide (H_2S)	Single industrial plant accidental discharge	22 excess deaths; 320 attributable illnesses. Persons of all age groups affected. Symptoms: respiratory tract irritation and nervous system disorders
London, England	Dec. 5–9, 1952	River plain; temperature inversion, weak winds, fog	Health effects due to any single agent not proven; SO_2, H_2SO_4, particulate levels high; SO_2 maximum of 1.34 ppm_v, average 0.7 ppm_v; smoke particles above 5 mg/m^3	Space heating using coal in homes and factories	3500–12,000 excess deaths; excess morbidity, but no estimate of numbers made; higher mortality in older age groups. Symptoms: respiratory tract irritation, heart disease
New York City	Nov. 23–26, 1966	Temperature inversion, weak winds	Believed due to SO_2 and particulates. Maximum 24 hr average of hourly SO_2 concentration = 0.51 ppm_v; maximum hourly SO_2 = 1.02 ppm_v	General urban sources: household and industry	168 excess deaths; unknown number of attributable illnesses; higher mortality in older age groups

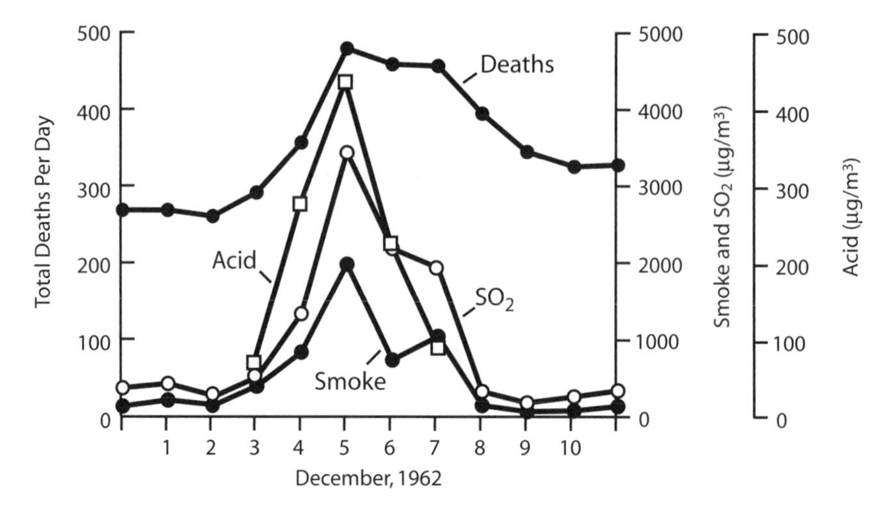

FIGURE 6–7. December 1962, London pollution episode.

While lesser peaks in smoke did not produce readily observable excess mortality, epidemiological analyses did demonstrate statistically significant exposure–response relationships during the period of generally high smoke pollution in London. One early time-series of daily mortality analysis is illustrated in Figure 6–8, which suggested that there was no threshold down to the then relatively "clean" days below 200 $\mu g/m^3$.

Recent time-series analyses in the U.S., where particulate matter concentrations are much lower, have shown significant excesses of daily total nonaccidential mortality associated with thoracic particulate matter less than 10 μm in aerodynamic diameter (PM_{10}) and/or fine particulate matter ($PM_{2.5}$). Figure 6–9 shows summary data for relative risk ($\pm$95% confidence intervals) for a change of 50 $\mu g/m^3$ of PM_{10} in various U.S. communities in relation to the concentrations of common gaseous air pollutants. This figure indicates that the association of daily total mortality with PM_{10} is not materially confounded by gaseous co-pollutants.

Figure 6–10 provides data that support a causal role for the PM association with total mortality. If total morbidity is increased, one would expect that mortality for respiratory causes would have a greater relative rise, with cardiovascular causes at an intermediate rate. One would also expect a larger increase in people needing acute medical attention, and that is also evident in Figure 6–10. Still higher rates of cough and respiratory symptoms would be expected, and the data in Figure 6–10 show such increased rates as well.

The relative risks indicated in Figures 6–9 and 6–10 are quite small, but since the entire population is at risk, the public health impacts can be substantial. While meteorological changes can produce similar effects, as suggested by Figure 6–11,

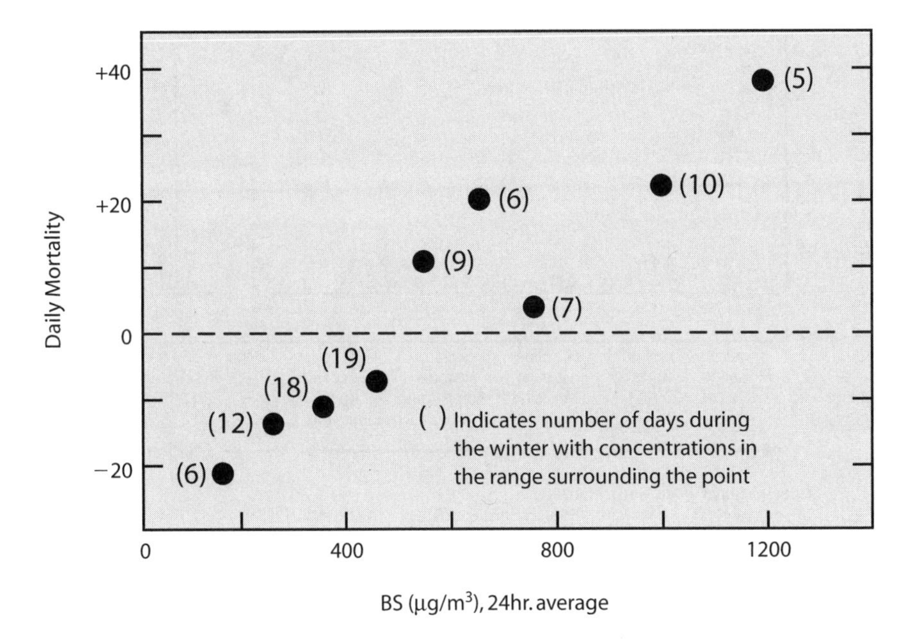

FIGURE 6–8. Martin and Bradley (1960) data for winter of 1958–1959 in London as summarized by Ware et al. (1981), showing average deviations of daily mortality from 15-day moving average by concentration of black smoke (BS).

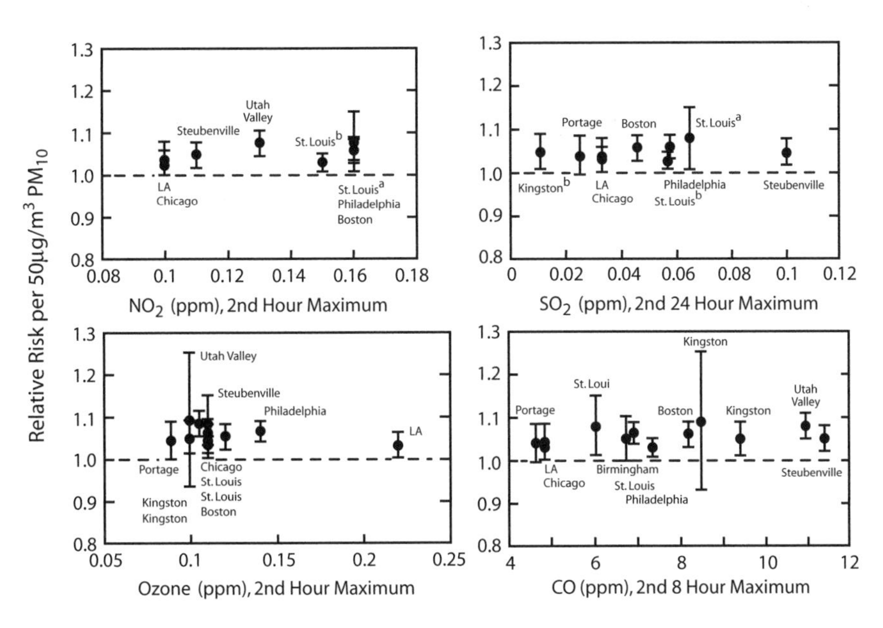

FIGURE 6–9. Relative risks of daily mortality in relation to a 50 $\mu g/m^3$ increment in PM_{10} for the indicated cities in relation to co-exposures to pollutant gases in those cities.

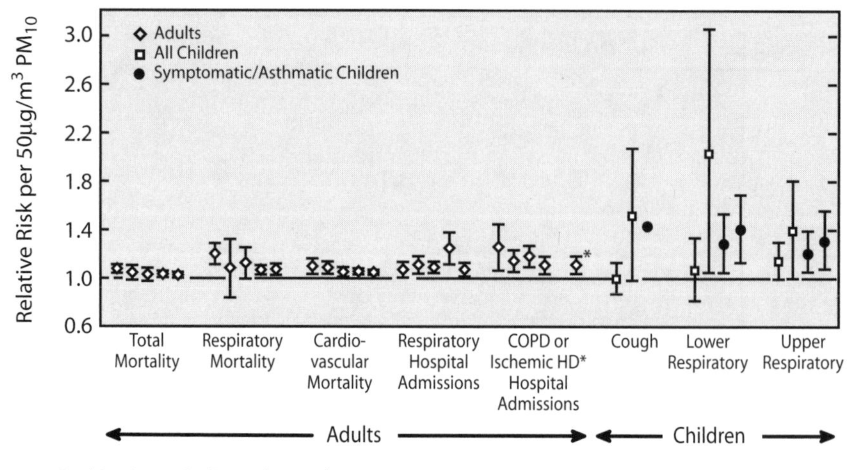

Total, Respiratory, Cardiovascular Mortality
1. Pope et al. (1992) 2. Schwartz (1993) 3. Styer et al. (1995) 4. Ostro et al. (1995a)
5. Ito and Thurston (1996)

Respiratory Hospital Admissions
1. Schwartz (1995) New Haven, CT 2. Schwartz (1995) Tacoma, WA 3. Schwartz (1996) Spokane, WA
4. Ito and Thurston (1994) Toronto, Canada

COPD or Ischemic HD* Hospital Admissions
1. Schwartz (1994f) Minneapolis, MN 2. Schwartz (1994c) Birmingham, AL
3. Schwartz (1996) Spokane, WA 4. Schwartz (1994d), Detroit, MI
*5. Schwartz & Morris (1995), Detroit, MI, Ischemic HD

Cough, Lower Respiratory, Upper Respiratory
1. Hoek and Brunekreef (1993) 2. Styer et al. (1994) 3. Pope & Dockery (1992), symptomatic children

FIGURE 6–10. Relative risks for various human health effects for ambient air PM_{10} concentration difference of 50 $\mu g/m^3$. (*Source*: U.S. Environmental Protection Agency.)

the effects of PM remain significant when weather variables are included in multipollutant regression analyses.

An unresolved issue in the role of PM, a complex mixture of particles from various sources, is the identification of one or more components that have the greatest impact on health. Figure 6–12 shows an analysis of data collected in six U.S. cities by investigators from the Harvard School of Public Health. These data indicate that thoracic particles (PM_{10}) are more closely associated with mortality risk than the coarser ambient particles, and that the fine fraction ($PM_{2.5}$) of PM_{10} is more closely associated with mortality than the fraction between 2.5 and 10 μm. However, the data did not provide any effective discrimination by chemical class, in that both the sulfate and non-sulfate fractions of $PM_{2.5}$ were both highly associated with mortality.

Chronic exposure

The acute episodes have established levels of contaminants that were associated with almost immediate adverse effects upon human health. Quantitative

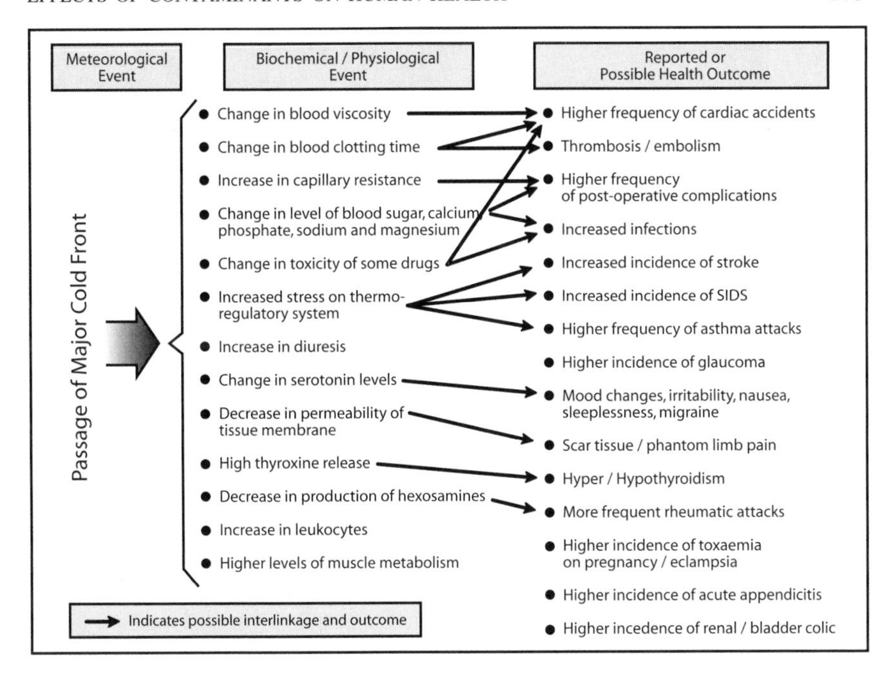

FIGURE 6–11. Health responses due to frontal passage. (*Source*: Curson, P. In: Climate Change: Developing Southern Hemisphere Perspectives. A. Henderson-Sellers and T. Giambelluca (Eds.) Chichester: John Wiley and Sons, 1996.)

analyses of effects of chronic effects occurring at lower levels of air contaminants are much more difficult to establish.

The available epidemiological evidence suggests that ambient air contaminant concentrations are contributors to the pathogenesis and/or exacerbation of certain chronic diseases in urban populations. Estimates of excess mortality due to air contamination range from 0.1% to 10%; the exact excess morbidity is not clear. The main diseases associated with general air contamination involve the respiratory tract—chronic bronchitis, pulmonary emphysema and, perhaps, lung cancer, and the cardiovascular system—coronary disease and stroke.

Chronic bronchitis is an inflammation of the bronchial tree, accompanied by excessive production of mucus and a persistent, productive cough. The main etiologic agent currently implicated in chonic bronchitis is cigarette smoke, a fact that complicates analysis of the effects of air contamination. Figure 6–13 presents the results of one historic study of British postal workers that examined the interaction of smoking and air contamination by comparing the incidence of chronic bronchitis for smokers and nonsmokers in areas of high and low smoke pollution.[8] Significantly higher levels of chronic bronchitis were observed in smokers in every age group above 35 years old who lived in the areas with greater

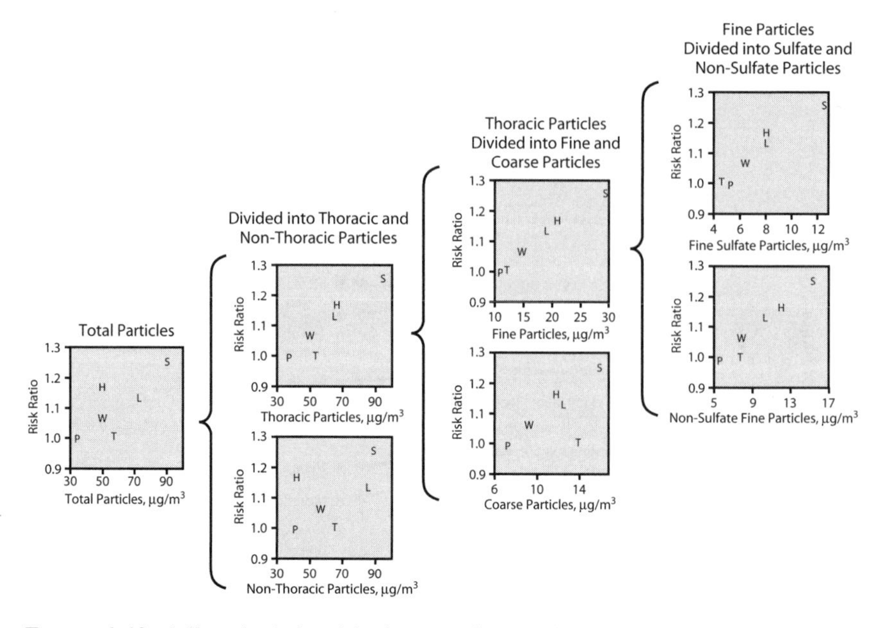

FIGURE 6–12. Adjusted relative risks for mortality are plotted against each of seven long term average particle indices in the Six City Study, from largest size range (total suspended particulate matter *lower left*, through sulfate and nonsulfate fine particle concentrations *upper right*). Note that a relatively strong linear relationship is seen for fine particles, and for its sulfate and non-sulfate components. Topeka, which has a substantial coarse particle component of thoracic particle mass, stands apart from the linear relationship between relative risk and thoracic particle concentration.

pollution levels. Thus, air pollution seemed to intensify the effects of smoking. As smoke pollution declined dramatically in the United Kingdom (UK) beginning in the late 1950s, annual mortality rates for respiratory tract diseases also dropped dramatically, as illustrated in Table 6–10.[9]

Recent cohort mortality studies in the U.S. have shown that annual mortality rates are significantly associated with fine particle concentrations ($PM_{2.5}$ and sulfates) at the much lower particle concentrations prevalent in the U.S. since the early 1970s. These studies accounted for personal risk factors such as smoking, diet, and occupational exposures to dusts and gases. They reported comparable risks for both fine particle pollution and environmental tobacco smoke for both lung cancer and for a category that combined other pulmonary and cardiovascular diseases.

Water Contaminants

Relatively little work has been done to analyze the effects of drinking water in relation to disease in the general population, even though a vast array of chem-

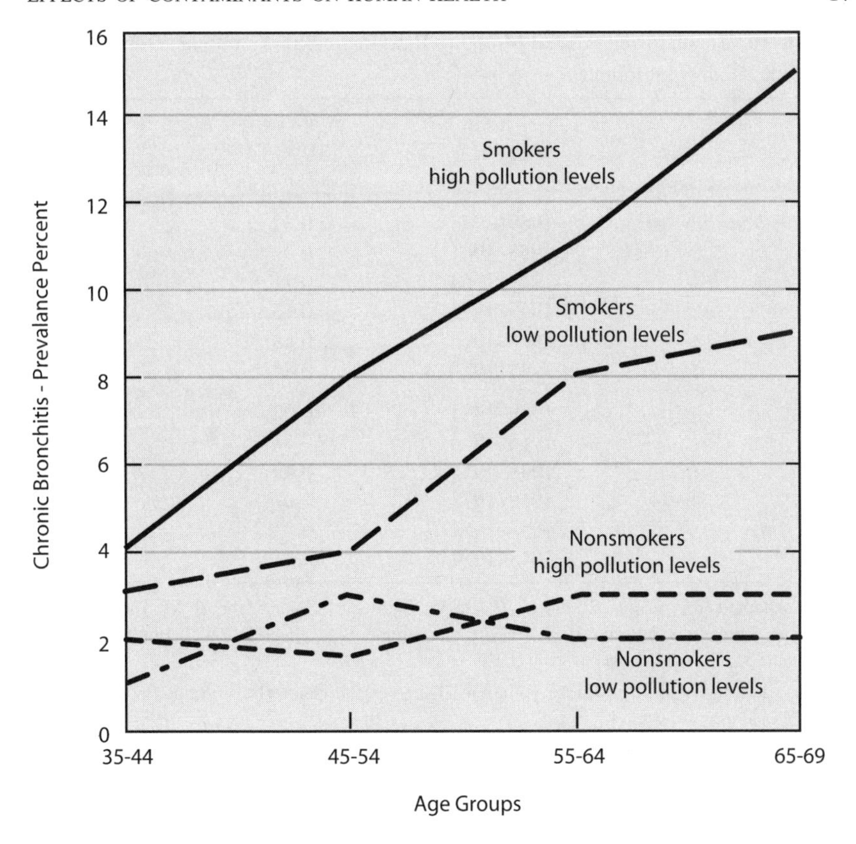

FIGURE 6–13. Prevalence of chronic bronchitis in smokers and nonsmokers in areas of high and low air pollution levels.

icals are found in drinking waters. Some studies suggest a statistical association between cancer mortality rates and water containing organic chemicals. Many epidemiological studies have been stimulated by the knowledge that disinfection of drinking water supplies using chlorine results in reactions with humic substances dissolved in the water, leading to the production of chloroform and other trihalomethanes that are known animal carcinogens. Bull[10] has summarized the findings of 17 case-contol and cohort studies of chlorinated drinking water, of which 16 indicated at least some small excess cancer risk in the colon, rectum, bladder, stomach, or pancreas. These risks must, of course, be balanced against the substantial risks of not using chlorine as a disinfectant, and the unknown risks of the by-products of other means of disinfection. A few epidemiological studies suggest a relation between certain inorganic contaminants, for example, asbestos[11] and arsenic[12] in drinking water and human cancer. However, definitive epidemiological studies have not been conducted, so very little is known of the

Table 6–10. Standardized Annual Mortality Rate Regression Coefficients on Smoke for 64 U.K. County Boroughs

SEX	AGE (YEARS)	MORTALITY IN	CANCER OF TRACHEA, BRONCHUS, LUNG	CHRONIC BRONCHITIS
Men	45–64	1969–1973	0.07	0.02
		1958–1964	0.53**	0.32*
		1948–1954	0.71***	0.48***
	65–74	1969–1973	0.15	−0.06
		1958–1964	0.68**	0.31
		1948–1954	0.87***	0.37*
Women	45–64	1969–1973	−0.02	−0.02
		1958–1964	−0.64**	0.33*
		1948–1954	0.49*	0.49**
	65–74	1969–1973	0.07	0.03
		1958–1964	0.25	0.40*
		1948–1954	0.61**	0.31

(*Source*: Adapted from Chinn, S., Florey, C., du V., Baldwin, I.G., and Gorgol, M. The relation of mortality in England and Wales 1969–1973 to measurements of air pollution. J. Epidemiol. Commun. Health 35:174–179, 1981.)

Note: Based on index of black smoke pollution 20 years before death (Daly: *Br. J. Prev. Soc. Med.* 13: 14–27, 1959).

*$p < 0.05$.

**$p < 0.01$.

***$p < 0.001$.

health effects of long-term exposure to ambient levels of most drinking water contaminants.

One exception involves nitrite and nitrate. Ingested nitrate per se has little toxicity. However, nitrate may be reduced to nitrite by bacteria in the gastrointestinal tract, resulting in the development of methemoglobinemia in infants. Nitrite in drinking water may also be involved in the formation of carcinogenic nitrosamines in the environment, or in the gut.

Some epidemiologic studies show an association between cardiovascular disease and soft water (water with a low-mineral content). Higher cardiovascular death rates were found in soft-water regions compared with areas having hard water; however, the specific etiologic agents responsible for the disease soft-water relationship are not known.

There have been incidences of chronic poisoning due to high levels of certain chemical contaminants in water. Two of the better-known ones involved cadmium and mercury. In the late 1950s, a large factory on the Jinzu River in Japan discharged cadmium into the water that was subsequently used to irrigate rice fields. A number of people developed cadmium poisoning, characterized by softening of bone and kidney failure. In the second episode, also in Japan, which occurred between 1953–1960, about 111 people were disabled and, of those, 43 died as a result of the industrial discharge of inorganic mercury waste into Minimata Bay. The mercury was methylated in the aquatic sediments and eventually reached the population via fish they ate.

In recent years, some studies have linked the consumption of drinking water meeting conventional modern standards for disinfection with the incidence of GI illness. Payment et al.[13] studied 600 Montreal households, half of which used a reverse osmosis unit to filter the tap water, and reported a 35% reduction in GI illness in comparison to those using regular tapwater. In a follow-up study of 1400 Montreal homes, there was a 14% to 19% excess of GI illness in families using tap water in comparison to those using bottled water as a control.[14] Furthermore, they estimated that the preventable fraction would have been closer to 50% if those using bottled water at home had also used it outside of the home. In an evaluation of population of Philadelphia in a time-series analysis, Schwartz et al.[15] used the variations in the turbidity of the tap water as a surrogate measure of the variability of pathogen contamination. They reported increases in admissions to hospital for GI illness for children over 2 years in age of up to 31% (CI: 10.8% to 55%), with a lag of ~6 days for a turbidity change over the interquartile range. For emergency department visits for GI illness, the corresponding increase with turbidity was about 7%.

The adequacy of current state-of-the-art water treatment has also come into question as a result of the outbreak of fatalities attributed to cryptosporidium contamination of the public water supply of Milwaukee, WI in 1998, as discussed previously in Chapter 1.

REFERENCES

1. Mehaffey, K.R., McKinney, J., and Reigart, J.R. Lead and Compounds, Chapter 14 in Environmental Toxicants: Human Exposures and Their Health Effects, 2nd Ed. (M. Lippmann, Ed.), New York: Wiley, Interscience, 2000, 481–521.
2. Pott, P. Chirurgical observations relative to the cancer of the scrotum, 1775. Reprinted in *Nat. Cancer Inst. Monogr.* 10:7–13, 1963.
3. Amdur, M.O. Physiological response of guinea pigs to atmospheric pollutants. *Int. J. Air Pollut.* 1:170–183, 1959.
4. Kuschner, M. The causes of lung cancer. *Am. Rev. Respir. Dis.* 98:573–590, 1968.
5. Selikoff, I.J., Hammond, E.C., and Chung, J. Asbestos exposure, smoking and neoplasia. *J. Am. Med. Assoc.* 204:106–112, 1968.
6. Archer, V.E. and Wagoner, J.K. Lung cancer among uranium miners in the United States. *Health Physics* 25:351–371, 1973.
7. Bell, M.L. and Davis, D.L. Reassessment of the lethal London Fog of 1952: Novel indicators of acute and chronic consequences of acute exposure to air pollution. *Environ. Health Perspect.* 109(Suppl. 3):389–394, 2001.

8. Holland, W.W. and Reid, D.D. The urban factor in chronic bronchitis. *Lancet* 1:445–448, 1965.
9. Chinn, S., Florey, C., du V., Baldwin, I.G., and Gorgol, M. The relation of mortality in England and Wales 1969–1973 to measurements of air pollution. *J. Epidemiol. Commun. Health* 35:174–179, 1981.
10. Bull, R.J. Drinking water disinfection, Chapter 9 in Environmental Toxicants: Human Exposures and Their Health Effects, 2nd Ed. (M. Lippmann, Ed.), 267–317, New York: Wiley, Interscience, 2000.
11. ATSDR. Toxicological Profile for Asbestos (update). Agency for Toxic Substances and Disease Registry, USHHS, Atlanta, GA 30333 (September 2001).
12. NRC. Arsenic in Drinking Water—2001 Update. National Research Council, National Academy Press, Washington, DC, 2001.
13. Payment, P., Richardson, L., Siemiatycki, J., Dewar, R., Edwards, M., and Franco, E.L. A randomized trial to evaluate the risk of gastrointestinal disease due to consumption of drinking water meeting current microbiological standards. *Am. J. Public Health* 81:703–708, 1991.
14. Payment, P., Siemiatycki, J., Richardson, L., Renaud, G., Franco, E., and Prevost, M. A prospective epidemiological study of gastrointestinal health effects due to the consumption of drinking water. *Int. J. Environ. Health Res.* 7:5–31, 1997.
15. Schwartz, J., Levin, R., and Hodge, K. Drinking water turbidity and pediatric hospital use for gastrointestinal illness in Philadelphia. *Epidemiology* 8:615–620, 1997.

7

Anthropogenic Impacts on Environmental Quality: Their Influence on Human Health and Welfare

Humans are not independent of their natural environment. We consume natural resources, and generate waste products. Moreover, the wastes are often discharged into systems that cannot handle them effectively, often upsetting the balance of nature that is essential to human well being.

Chemical contaminants may affect the environment in various ways; the result is often expressed in terms of changes in environmental quality. This term is hard to define, for environmental quality means different things to different people and is related to cultural and social attitudes. To some, a quality environment is a virgin forest, while to others it may be a thriving metropolis. Yet all would probably agree that no matter what specific environment is ideal, certain factors can reduce its quality. A quality environment may, thus, be defined as one that does not adversely affect the health or welfare of its human inhabitants or its ecological stability.

AIR CONTAMINANTS

Effects on Animals

Like humans, both domestic and wild animals are subject to the acute and chronic effects of air contaminants. During various acute air pollution episodes, many animal pets and livestock became ill, and some died from cardiopulmonary disorders. For example, in London, during the Killer Fogs of December 1883 and December 1952, prize cattle in the annual Smithfield Cattle Shows died of bronchitis and pneumonia. Incidences of severe pollution damage to animals have also occurred downwind[1,2] of some primary industries, such as smelters and fertilizer plants.

Chronic poisoning of animals is more common than is acute, and arises from inhalation exposure or feeding on forage upon which air contaminants have accumulated. Chronic poisoning of livestock due to arsenic from smelters, as well as arsenic poisoning of game animals and bees were reported as long ago as the early part of the twentieth century.[3,4] Airborne fluorides have caused more damage to domestic animals, on a worldwide basis, than any other air contaminant. One of the earliest descriptions of fluoride poisoning was provided in 1937, and involved livestock near an aluminum smelter in Italy.[5] Numerous insects have been victims of fluoride poisoning due to contaminant deposition on plant surfaces.[6]

Another air contaminant of historical importance in terms of damage to animals is lead. For example, in Germany in 1955, cattle and horses near a foundry developed symptoms of lead poisoning,[7] while cattle and horses grazing within 5 km of a smelter in Canada were found to have lead induced damage.[8] Captive animals in city zoos were also subject to poisoning; as they licked their fur, these animals ingested lead accumulated primarily from automobile exhaust emissions.[9] Table 7–1 describes the effects of selected air contaminants upon animals.

Effects on Vegetation

In the early history of air pollution, there were well-documented cases of the destruction of vegetation around certain industries. Today, the scope of the prob-

Table 7–1. Effects of Air Contaminants on Animals

CHEMICAL	SYMPTOMS
Arsenic	Colic, ulcers, hair loss, scleroderma (increase in thickness of upper layer of skin), bone malformation
Lead	Nervous system disorders, swollen joints, emaciation
Fluoride	Loss of appetite, weight loss, gastrointestinal disturbances, decreased milk production, lameness, worn teeth, bone disorders
Organic mercury	Nervous system disorders, listlessness, vomiting
Selenium	Loss of hair, abnormal hoof growth, systemic effects
Molybdenum	Gastrointestinal disturbances, limb stiffness, hematological disorders

lem has changed, with more widespread, but generally less severe, effects predominating. Although industrial sources do account for a certain amount of injury to vegetation, the larger problem is associated with more ubiquitous air contaminants, such as O_3 and SO_2, which are common to urban centers. For example, large natural forests in Southern California have been severely depleted by oxidant damage to pine trees. Pollution damage to vegetation is an increasing problem in the corridor extending from Washington, DC, to Boston.

Phytotoxic air contaminants may cause damage to natural plant communities, as well as to agricultural crops and ornamental vegetation. Different species of plants, different varieties of one species, and even different parts of one plant may vary widely in sensitivity to a specific chemical. In addition, some contaminants are associated with specific manifestations in particular plants; this often allows identification of the type and range of a specific agent. The sensitivity of any plant is affected by a number of factors, such as the age of the tissue, amount of moisture in the soil, air temperature, plant nutritional status, and intensity of light.

Contaminants may enter plants following wet or dry deposition on aerial structures (leaves, stems), or from the soil via the roots. Most gases enter via leaves, in the course of normal respiration, through the stomata, small openings between cells on the lower leaf surface. Particles are generally not injurious unless they are corrosive, or deposit in very heavy layers.

Injury to vegetation may be acute or chronic. Short-term exposure to relatively high concentrations of phytotoxicants produce necrotic patterns on leaves due to cell collapse, and perhaps eventually plant death. More commonly, however, plants are subject to long-term exposure to lower contaminant levels. Numerous types of chronic injury may occur. The most common are stunting of growth, destruction of leaf tissue, and chlorosis, a reduction and loss of chlorophyll. Other responses are premature aging, leaf abscission, small fruit, and flowering or fruiting abnormalities. Genetic and biochemical changes, such as alterations in activity of certain enzymes, may occur without any visible injury. Chronic exposures may also increase the susceptibility of plants to other environmental stresses, such as pests and disease.

Table 7–2 lists some of the more important phytotoxic air contaminants, and presents typical effects and some examples of the more sensitive plants. The list is not all-inclusive. Other contaminants, such as mercury vapor, ammonia, hydrogen sulfide, sulfuric acid and, of course, herbicides, may affect plant life. Furthermore, combinations of contaminants may produce synergistic effects in some plants. Plant activity may also be indirectly affected by specific classes of contaminants, such as the restriction of growth due to alterations in soil chemistry caused by acidic rain water.

Some plants may accumulate chemicals. For example, during the time in which leaded gas was used, high levels of lead were found in vegetation near highways.[10,11] In some cases a contaminant may be beneficial to vegetation; large

TABLE 7–2. Effects of Air Contaminants on Vegetation

CHEMICAL	SYMPTOM	SENSITIVE PLANTS[a]	EXAMPLES OF CONCENTRATION FOR SENSITIVITY
Chlorine	Bleaching, leaf-tip and margin necrosis, leaf abscission, spotting chlorosis	Radish, alfalfa, peach, buckwheat, corn, tobacco, oak, white pine	Radish, 1.3 ppm_v
Fluorides	Leaf-tip and margin necrosis, chlorosis, dwarfing, leaf abscission, decreased yield	Gladiolus, tulip, apricot, blueberry, corn, grape, blue spruce, white pine	Gladiolus, apricot, 0.1 ppb_v
Nitrogen oxides	Brown spots on leaf, suppression of growth	Azalea, sunflower, mustard, tobacco, pinto bean	Pinto beans, 3 ppm_v
Sulfur dioxide	Bleached spots on leaf, chlorosis, suppression of growth, early abscission, reduced yield	Barley, pumpkin, alfalfa, cotton, wheat, lettuce, apple, oats, aster, zinnia, birch, elm, white pine, ponderosa pine	Alfalfa, barley, cotton, 0.3 ppm_v
Ozone	Reddish brown flecks on upper surface of leaf, bleaching, suppression of growth, early abscission, premature aging	Alfalfa, barley, bean, oat, onion, corn, apple, grape, tobacco, tomato, spinach, aspen, maple, privet, white pine, ponderosa pine	Tomato, tobacco, 0.5 ppm_v
Oxidant gases, e.g., peroxyacetyl nitrate	Glazing, silvering or bronzing of lower surface of leaf	Pinto bean, mustard, oat, tomato, lettuce, petunia, blue grass	Petunia, lettuce, 0.2 ppm_v
Unsaturated hydrocarbons, e.g., ethylene	Leaf abscission, dropping of flowers, loss of flower buds, epinasty, chlorosis, suppression of growth	Orchid blossom, carnation blossom, azalea, tomato, cotton, cucumber, peach	Orchids, 0.005 ppm_v Tomatoes, 0.1 ppm_v

[a]Certain varieties of these plants are sensitive.

increases in atmospheric CO_2 may enhance photosynthetic activity in terrestrial forests, resulting in increased biomass.

Effects on Materials

There is significant damage to nonliving material by air contaminants in many areas. Material corrosion rates, for example, are significantly higher in contaminated urban and industrial atmospheres than in rural atmospheres. Damage may be the result of various mechanisms. These include abrasion destruction and the deposition of particulate matter on surfaces, resulting in the soiling of their appearance. The most important mechanism, however, is chemical attack. This may be direct, i.e., the contaminant reacts directly with the material, as in the tarnishing of silver and the blackening of lead-based paints by H_2S, or indirect, i.e., damage is due to a product of chemical conversion following absorption of the contaminant, as in the absorption of SO_2 by leather and conversion to sulfurous and sulfuric acid. The basic processes that lead to the deterioration of masonry surfaces are illustrated in Figure 7–1.

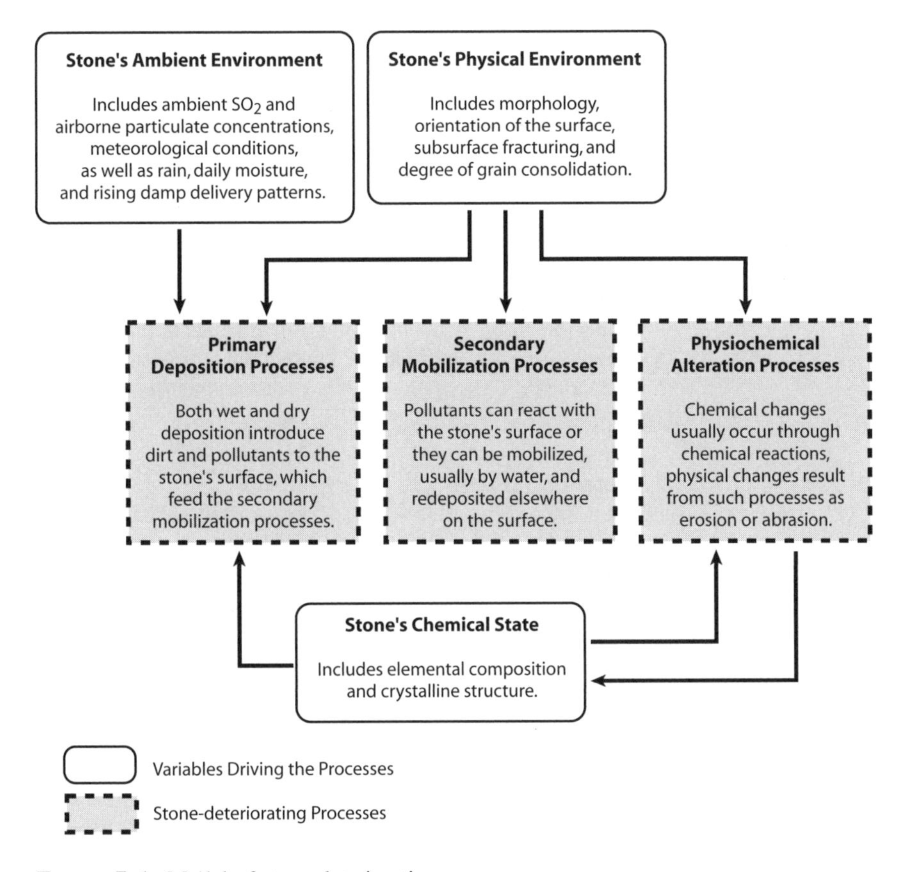

FIGURE 7–1. Model of stone deterioration processes.

A number of factors affect the extent of deterioration. Degree of moisture is one of the most important. Oxides of sulfur, carbon, and nitrogen in moist air may be converted into sulfuric, carbonic, and nitric acids, respectively, leading to corrosion of numerous materials. Acidic rainfall in certain regions of the world has resulted in enhanced corrosion. On the other hand, rain may decrease corrosion rates to the extent that corrosive contaminants are washed away.

Another mediating factor in material deterioration is temperature, which affects the rate of those chemical reactions responsible for deterioration, and also has an influence on the degree of moisture condensation on surfaces.

Other factors affecting deterioration include sunlight, which may promote photochemical reactions; air movement, which carries contaminants to surfaces; and position of the surface in space with respect to deposition or accessibility to a contaminant. Table 7–3 presents a survey of the types of damage to material caused by the major air contaminants.

TABLE 7–3. Effects of Air Contaminants on Materials

CHEMICAL	PRIMARY MATERIALS ATTACKED	TYPICAL DAMAGE
Carbon dioxide	Building stones, e.g., limestone	Deterioration
Sulfur oxides	Metals	
	Ferrous metals	Corrosion
	Copper	Corrosion to copper sulfate
	Aluminum	Corrosion to aluminum sulfate (white)
	Building materials (limestone, marble, slate, mortar)	Leaching, weakening
	Leather	Embrittlement, disintegration
	Paper	Embrittlement
	Textiles (natural and synthetic fabrics)	Reduced tensile strength, deterioration
Hydrogen sulfide	Metals	
	Silver	Tarnish
	Copper	Tarnish
	Paint	Leaded paint blackened due to formation of lead sulfide
Ozone	Rubber and elastomers	Cracking, weakening
	Textiles (natural and synthetic fabrics)	Weakening
	Dyes	Fading
Nitrogen oxides	Dyes	Fading
Hydrogen fluoride	Glass	Etches, opaques
Solid particulates (soot, tars)	Building materials	Soiling
	Painted surfaces	Soiling
	Textiles	Soiling

Air contaminants are responsible for damage to art treasures in many areas of the world. For example, the ancient Egyptian obelisk known as Cleopatra's Needle has undergone more deterioration since it was moved to New York City than in previous thousands of years in Egypt. In Athens, the Acropolis and other ancient temples in the Parthenon have been subject to cracking and decay due to the growth of nitrate, sulfate, and chloride salts penetrating into cracks in the building structure.

Effects on Climate

One of the most potentially devastating ways in which air contaminants may affect the environment is alteration of climate. As discussed in Chapter 2, the earth-atmosphere energy balance is maintained by minor atmospheric constituents, for example, CO_2; this suggests that small changes in their levels due to human activities could have major effects on this balance. There are essentially three ways in which this balance may be subject to perturbation: *(1)* increasing anthropogenic release of waste heat; *(2)* increasing levels of CO_2 and other greenhouse gases; and *(3)* increasing fine particle load and associated scattering of incident solar radiation. The potential effects of each of these are discussed in the following sections.

Elevation of regional ambient temperatures

Waste heat released into the atmosphere has the potential to alter local climate, primarily by causing an increase in the average surface temperature in urban areas. The primary sources of waste heat are electric power–generating plants and space heating, and changes in the surface heat capacity.

On a global scale, the rate of energy used and released as heat is small compared with the solar input to the earth's surface; net solar radiation is over 6000 times greater than the anthropogenic source strength. However, energy use is usually concentrated on a local or regional scale in highly populated areas; in these regions, the natural and anthropogenic source inputs may be on the same order of magnitude.

Urban heat release has affected the character of the local climate, producing what is known as the urban heat island. Average urban temperatures in many areas often exceed those in surrounding rural areas by 1°–2°C, with nighttime differences as great as 5°C. The thermal capacitance for solar input of buildings and streets in built-up areas is also a factor in formation of this heat island.

Local or regional heat islands could conceivably result in changes in atmospheric motions that would be global in scope; however, anthropogenic heat output would have to increase by approximately 50-fold before there would be climate changes comparable to the natural year-to-year variations on a global scale in general atmospheric circulation patterns. It is more likely that local heat islands would disturb the character of natural regional climates. One possibility is that very large concentrations of surface heating could, under appropriate environmental conditions, trigger convective instabilities that would lead to convective storms, for example, thunderstorms, hailstorms, and tornadoes. Thermal loading may also contribute to an increase in general cloudiness.

Particles

Particulate matter suspended in the troposphere may affect the radiative energy balance and, therefore, climate—either directly or indirectly. The direct effect involves the absorption and scattering of both incoming solar radiation and long-wave terrestrial radiation. The indirect effect involves influences in the formation and structure of clouds.

Tropospheric concentrations of suspended particles has increased in a belt that girds the Northern Hemisphere between 30° and 70° N latitude. A decrease in surface-incident radiation has been noted in many areas in this belt, with the most pronounced effect near urban areas. The possible climatic effects of the increasing tropospheric particulate load are quite conflicting. By absorbing and scattering the incoming solar radiation, particles tend to reduce the amount of this radiation reaching the ground, resulting in a reduction in heating both within and below the particulate layer. By absorption of the long-wave terrestrial radiation, particles would tend to increase the heating in the absorption layer, enhancing the greenhouse effect. The net effect is not clear, and depends upon a number of factors. These include optical characteristics of the aerosol, such as refractive indices at various wavelengths, concentration, aerosol-size distribution, and reflectivity of the underlying earth surface. For example, the size of the aerosol affects the relative proportion of radiation that is scattered in the forward versus the backward (towards space) direction, as well as the interaction with specific wavelengths of radiation (the greater the size, the greater is the potential to interact with longer wavelengths). While it seems logical that a global increase in aerosols would result in a net cooling of the surface of the earth, the situation is not entirely clear, since the actual effect is dependent upon the radiant energy absorption of the specific aerosols. In addition, increases in particulate load are mainly regional, rather than global, in extent.

In addition to any direct effect, particles may alter climate by influencing the type, structure, formation, location, or optical properties of clouds. This could affect the earth-atmospheric energy balance, since clouds are a contributory factor both to the amount of solar radiation that is reflected back to space, and to the greenhouse effect. Many anthropogenic aerosols can act as condensation nuclei for water vapor, increasing cloud droplet number and reflectivity to incoming solar radiation.

On the other hand, increased cloud cover would also absorb more outgoing terrestrial radiation. The net effect of increasing cloud cover is not clear. However, the increased particulate levels and effects on cloud formation may be a factor in the increased precipitation that occurs in, and downwind of, urban areas compared to upwind and remote rural areas.

Carbon dioxide and other greenhouse gases

The global background level of atmospheric CO_2 prior to the Industrial Revolution was estimated to have been 290–300 ppm_v, a level believed to have prevailed for about 10,000 years.[12] Currently, the level is approximately 360 ppm_v.[13] This increase in atmospheric CO_2 is due primarily to the combustion of fossil fuels. The annual rate of increase in CO_2 concentration jumped from 0.7 ppm_v/year in the late 1950s (when the first reliable measurements were made), to over 1.5 ppm_v/year at the end of the twentieth century. Numerous predictions of future trends of atmospheric CO_2 levels have been made; however, levels depend upon whether the current rate of increase in fossil-fuel consumption will continue, decline, or level off (see Chapter 15). Nevertheless, most predictions call for an increase in atmospheric CO_2 concentration to at least 400 ppm_v by the year 2010.

Even though it is a trace constituent of the atmosphere, CO_2 plays a major role in the energy balance. Because it absorbs terrestrial long-wave radiation and reradiates most of it back to earth, increases in atmospheric CO_2 increase the earth-surface temperature.

Numerous atmospheric models have been employed in attempts to ascertain the magnitude of any temperature change. They predict that an increase in CO_2 to 400 ppm_v could raise the average global surface temperature of the earth by about 0.5–1.0°C, while a doubling of current atmospheric levels could increase the average temperature by 2°–3°C.

Other gaseous contaminants, for example, fluorocarbons that were formerly used as refrigerants, CH_4, N_2O, and NH_3, have infrared absorption bands, and absorb in the spectral regions where H_2O vapor and CO_2 are poor absorbers, thus partially interfering with the atmospheric window that transmits most of the reradiated infrared radiation from the earth's surface and lower atmosphere to space. Thus, anthropogenic emissions of these gases may also affect climate by increasing the surface temperature of the earth. Some key data on the concentrations of these gases and their trends is shown in Table 7–4.

Overview of climatic effects

Over the course of the earth's history, the climate has changed numerous times. These changes have all been attributed to various natural processes, such as alterations in incident solar radiation or changes in the earth's orbit. However, since the Industrial Revolution anthropogenic activity has the potential to produce climatic changes that are global in extent.

Between approximately 1880 and 1940, the mean earth-surface temperature of the Northern Hemisphere increased approximately 0.6°C. From 1940 to 1970, a

TABLE 7–4. Summary of Key Greenhouse Gases[a]

	CO_2	CH_4	REFRIGERANT-11 CCl_3F	REFRIGERANT-12 CCl_2F_2	CH_3CCl_3	CCl_4	N_2O
Preindustrial atmospheric concentrations (1750–1800)	275–280 ppm	0.7–0.8 ppm	0	0	0	0	285–288 ppb
Approximate current atmospheric concentrations (1985–1990)[b]	345–353 ppm	1.72 ppm	220–280 ppt	380–484 ppt	130 ppt	120 ppt	304–310 ppb
Current rate of annual atmospheric accumulation	1.8 ppm (+0.46%–0.5%)	0.015 ppm (+0.9%–1.1%)	9.5 ppt (+4.0%–10.3%)	17 ppt (+4%–10.1%)	−(+15.5%)	−(+2.4%)	0.8 ppb (+0.25%–0.35%)
Projected atmospheric concentrations mid 21st century[c]	400–600 ppm	2.1–4.0 ppm	700–3000 ppt	2000–4800 ppt	—	—	350–450 ppb
Atmospheric lifetime[d]	50–200 yr	10 yr	65 yr	130 yr	—	—	150 yr

[a]% = percent by volume, ppm = parts per million by volume, ppb = parts per billion (10^9) by volume, ppt = parts per trillion (10^{12}) by volume.

[b]1990 concentrations are based on extrapolation of measurements reported for earlier years.

[c]Mid 21st century concentrations are based on current annual rate of atmospheric accumulation, and do not consider activities aimed at reducing emissions.

[d]Atmospheric lifetime is the ratio of atmospheric content to the total rate of removal. CO_2 lifetime is a rough indication of the time necessary for CO_2 concentrations to adjust to changes in emissions.

[*Source*: Linak, W.P. and Kramlich, J.C. A review of nitrous oxide behavior in the atmosphere, and in combustion and industrial systems. In: Schneider, T., (Ed.) Air Pollution in the 21st Century. Amsterdam: Elsevier, 1998, pp. 265–313.]

cooling of 0.2°–0.3°C occurred. However, it is still not entirely clear to what extent, these warming and cooling trends were due to anthropogenic activity. Furthermore, the mid-century cooling at high northern latitudes was accompanied by a warming at high southern latitudes. Evidence for a secular increase in mean atmospheric temperature has become much stronger since the mid-1980s, as illustrated in Figure 7–2. An indication of the warming trend at the end of the twentieth century was the observation that there was open ocean at the North Pole during the winter of 1999–2000 for the first time in recorded history. Despite these unusual observations, any theory of climatic change is difficult to prove, especially when fluctuations are within the range of normal variability. In addition, many factors control the energy systems that determine climate, and much uncertainty exists in our knowledge of climate cause-and-effect links.

The effects upon overall climate of any isolated contaminant is hard to predict, since possible synergism and numerous feedback mechanisms in the real

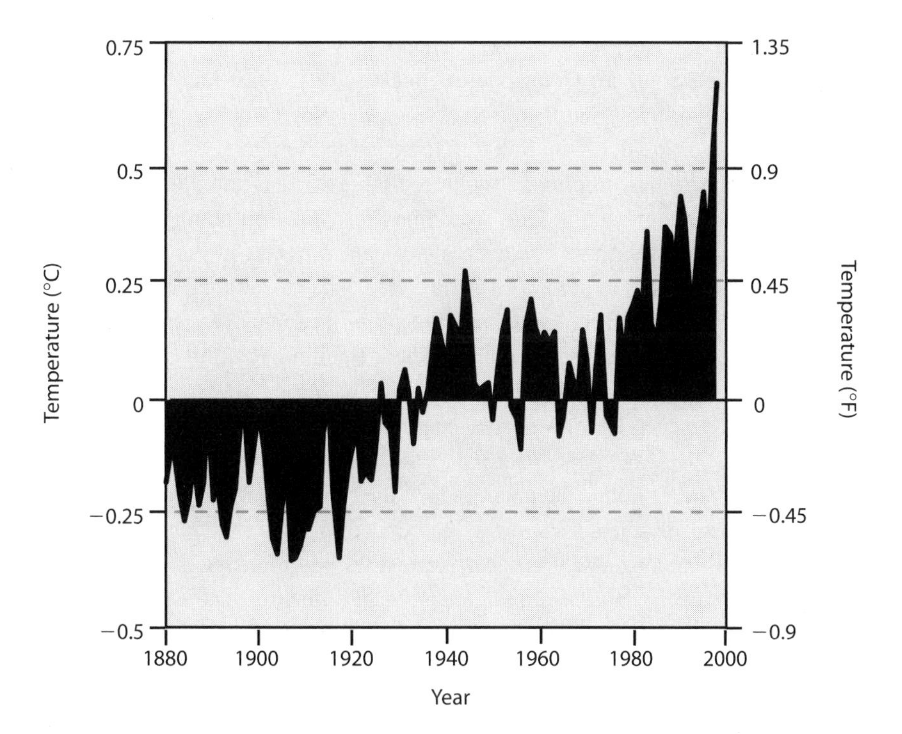

FIGURE 7–2. Average global land and ocean temperature anomalies (deviations from average); 1880–1998. "Zero degrees" represents the overall average during that time period. Seven of the ten warmest years have occurred in the 1990's. (*Source*: National Climate Data Center/NESDIS/NOAA.)

climatic system are largely unknown or hard to model. Some of the possible mitigating feedback mechanisms are outlined below:

1. An increase in earth-surface temperature due to high CO_2 levels would probably be accompanied by an increase in cloudiness. This increased cloudiness, by acting to decrease incoming solar radiation, could counteract any warming trend. On the other hand, CO_2 is less soluble in water at higher temperatures, so that increases in sea-surface temperature due to increasing atmospheric CO_2 levels could result in a decrease in ocean uptake, enhancing the warming trend by upsetting the ocean-atmospheric CO_2 balance.
2. If earth-surface temperatures increase, snow and ice cover may melt to some extent. This would decrease surface albedo, increase absorption of solar radiation, and thus enhance any warming effect. On the other hand, cooling of the surface could increase ice cover, increasing the albedo, decreasing absorption and enhancing the cooling effect.
3. Differential heating of the earth sets up heat gradients, which drive wind and ocean currents. Altered gradients due to temperature changes could feed back on winds, etc., to change many other aspects of climate.

Different mixing rates of CO_2 and particles may affect climate differently in the Northern and Southern Hemispheres. Because of the fast latitudinal mixing of CO_2 in the two hemispheres, differences in CO_2 levels between them would be small; however, particles are unlikely to be completely mixed globally. Thus, any effects of particles on climate would be intensified in the Northern Hemisphere, whereas effects due to CO_2 would be more equal in both regions.

Over recent decades, there has been significant progress in the development of mathematical models to predict climatic changes due to air contaminants. Nevertheless, inadequacies of the models still result in inconclusive results. Our current knowledge of climate theory is insufficient to eliminate fully even the most pessimistic of the present estimates of climatic change.

The generally accepted view is that continued release of heat, CO_2, and particulate matter into the atmosphere has the potential to produce significant changes in climate, although the magnitude of the change is not accurately known. The current state of scientific knowledge concerning anthropogenic influences on global heat exchange with our extraterrestrial environment is illustrated in Figure 7–3. However, in dense urban areas, local climatic changes have already occurred, and as urban areas are extended and energy production increases, the scale of influences upon climate may increase from this local urban scale to larger regional areas. Furthermore, most advanced climate models predict that wider fluctuations in weather (e.g., more severe storms) will precede dramatic changes in average temperature (see Table 7–5).

The most potentially devastating climatic effect of air contaminants is a significant alteration of the earth-surface temperature. In terms of relative signifi-

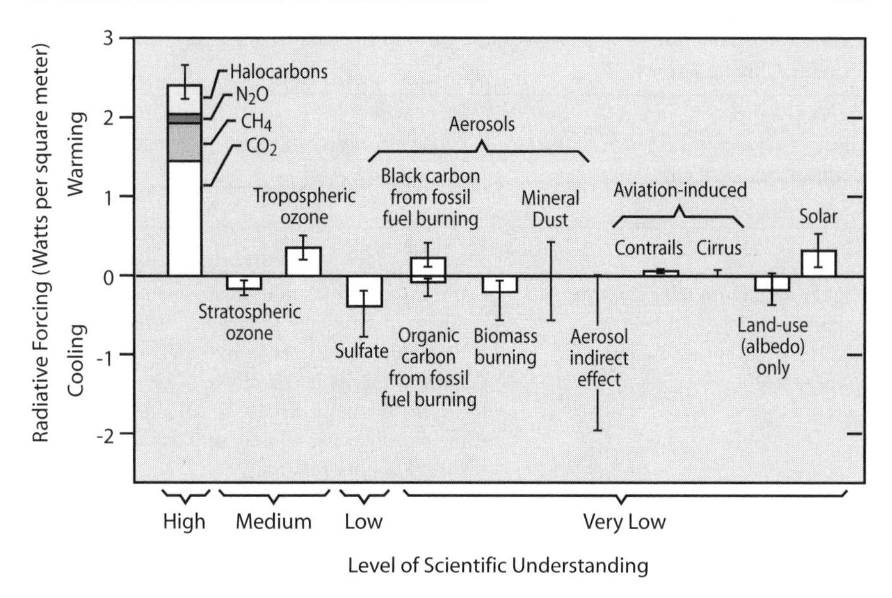

FIGURE 7–3. Estimated global mean radiative forcing exerted by gas and various particle phase species for the year 2000, relative to 1750.

cance, a difference of 6°C distinguished the glacial from the interglacial conditions during the Pleistocene Ice Age. Smaller surface temperature changes, perhaps as low as 2°C, could result in an advance or retreat of the polar ice caps, depending upon the direction in which the temperature was altered. Changes in levels of the oceans would result from changes in the size of the ice caps. Temperature changes may also affect the evaporation–condensation pathway of the hydrologic cycle, with possible significant alterations in the amount and global distribution of precipitation. The widespread effects of the El Niño and La Niña patterns of water flow and temperature in the eastern Pacific Ocean at the end of the twentieth century produced such changes.

A slight but persistent change in temperature could have serious ecological consequences. It could tip the balance in favor of certain organisms that may have been held in check by previous climatic conditions. Changes in patterns of winds and currents may also disrupt previously adapted organisms. Finally, any increase in the instability of global weather patterns is a definite threat to world food production.

Effects on the Stratosphere

Most of the potential effects of air contaminants upon climate involve the troposphere. However, certain alterations of the stratosphere may also affect climate.

Table 7–5. Examples of Impacts Resulting from Projected Changes in Extreme Climate Events

Projected changes during the twenty-first century in extreme climate phenomena and their likelihood[a]	Representative examples of projected impacts[b] (*all high confidence of occurrence in some* areas)[c]
Simplex extremes	
Higher maximum temperatures; more hot days and heat waves[d] over nearly all land areas (*very likely*)	• Increased incidence of death and serious illness in older age groups and urban poor • Increased heat stress in livestock and wildlife • Shift in tourist destinations • Increased risk of damage to a number of crops • Increased electric cooling demand and reduced energy supply reliability
Higher (increasing) minimum temperatures; fewer cold days, frost days, and cold waves[d] over nearly all land areas (*very likely*)[a]	• Decreased cold-related human morbidity and mortality • Decreased risk of damage to a number of crops, and increased risk to others • Extended range and activity of some pest and disease vectors • Reduced heating energy demand
More intense precipitation events (*very likely*[a] over many years)	• Increased flood, landslide, avalance, and mudslide damage • Increased soil erosion • Increased flood runoff could increase recharge of some floodplain aquifers • Increased pressure on government and private flood insurance systems and disaster relief
Complex extremes	
Increased summer drying over most mid-latitude continental interiors and associated risk of drought (*likely*)[a]	• Decreased crop yields • Increased damage to building foundations caused by ground shrinkage • Decreased water resource quantity and quality • Increased risk of forest fire
Increase in tropical cyclone peak wind intensities, mean and peak precipitation intensities (*likely*[a] over some areas)[c]	• Increased risk to human life, risk of infections, disease epidemics, and many other risks • Increased coastal erosion and damage to coastal buildings and infrastructure • Increased damage to coastal ecosystems such as coral reefs and mangroves
Intensified droughts and floods associated with El Niño events in many different regions (*likely*)[a] (see also under droughts and intense precipitation events)	• Decreased agricultural and rangeland productivity in drought- and flood-prone regions • Decreased hydro-power potential in drought-prone regions

(*continued*)

TABLE 7–5. (*continued*)

PROJECTED CHANGES DURING THE TWENTY-FIRST CENTURY IN EXTREME CLIMATE PHENOMENA AND THEIR LIKELIHOOD[a]	REPRESENTATIVE EXAMPLES OF PROJECTED IMPACTS[b] (*ALL HIGH CONFIDENCE OF OCCURRENCE IN SOME* AREAS)[c]
COMPLEX EXTREMES	
Increased Asian summer monsoon precipitation variability (*likely*)[a]	• Increased flood and drought magnitude and damages in temperate and tropical Asia
Increased intensity of mid-latitude storms (little agreement between current models)[d]	• Increased risks to human life and health • Increased property and infrastructure losses • Increased damage to coastal ecosystems

[a]Likelihood refers to judgmental estimates of confidence used by TAR WGI: *very likely* (90%–99% chance); *likely* (66%–90% chance). Unless otherwise stated, information on climate phenomena is taken from the Summary for Policymakers, TAR WGI. TAR WGI = Third Assessment Report of Working Group 1.[21]

[b]These impacts can be lessened by appropriate response measures.

[c]High confidence refers to probabilities between 67% and 95%.

[d]Information from TAR WGI, Technical Summary.

[e]Changes in regional distribution of tropical cyclones are possible but have not been established.

(*Source*: Intergovernmental Panel on Climate Change (IPCC). Climate change 2001: Impacts, adaptation, and vulnerability. Contribution of working group II to the third assessment report of the IPCC. Cambridge: Cambridge University Press, 2001.)

Jet plane flight in the stratosphere, on a large-scale basis, increases the cloudiness of the upper atmosphere, via formation of contrails, i.e., trails of water vapor. Increasing stratospheric moisture content could intensify the atmospheric greenhouse effect.

Solid particles injected into the stratosphere, because of their longer residence time than those in the troposphere, may also have an effect upon climate. To date, however, the main stratospheric aerosols are volcanic dust. Although these dusts warm the stratosphere as a result of absorption, surface air may be cooled due to a reduction in radiation reaching the earth's surface.

One stratospheric effect that has generated a great amount of interest and international action is the depletion of the ozone (O_3) layer due to releases of certain halogenated air contaminants. About 90% of the O_3 present in the Earth's atmosphere can be found in the stratosphere. This stratospheric O_3 is considered to be beneficial because of its ability to screen out potentially harmful solar radiation. Much of this O_3 is created over the equator (where the sun's rays are most direct) and is transported by global air currents toward the poles.

The stratospheric O_3 has quite different health and environmental implications than the tropospheric O_3. In the boundary layer of the troposphere, which we share with vegetation and other animals, O_3 is an important component of community air pollution, as discussed in Chapter 6.

Ozone concentration is a balance of processes that produce ozone and those processes and reactions that remove ozone. Natural formation of stratospheric O_3 involves two steps: *(1)* the sun's rays split apart oxygen molecules (O_2) into single oxygen atoms (O); *(2)* these single atoms are very unstable, and will react readily with nearby atoms or molecules to become more stable. When O atoms combine with nearby O_2 molecules, O_3 is formed.

Stratospheric O_3 levels fluctuate periodically. Under some circumstances, the fluctuations are extreme. For instance, atmospheric conditions can at times isolate a portion of the stratosphere, effectively keeping it from mixing with surrounding O_3-rich and warmer pockets of air. Should there be a high concentration of O_3 depleting substances in the isolated pocket, O_3 destruction can out-pace O_3 replacement and result in a sharp decrease in O_3 concentration and consequently, less screening out of the sun's ultraviolet-B (UV-B) rays.

This extreme depletion occurs during the southern spring (September through November) creating the Antarctic "ozone hole." Atmospheric conditions there clearly favor the annual phenomenon (extremely cold winter temperatures support the formation of a "polar vortex"—an impenetrable core in the atmosphere) where O_3 depleting substances accumulated throughout the winter can be activated by springtime solar radiation to break down O_3. Additionally, ice crystals present in this region of the stratosphere act as reaction "platforms" for enhanced O_3 breakdown. This process is illustrated in Figure 7–4.

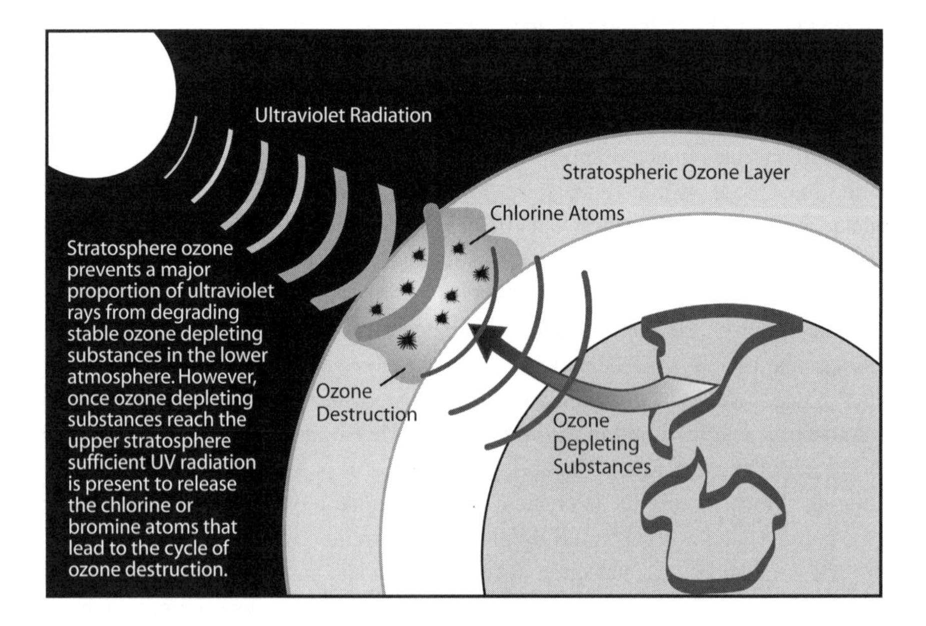

FIGURE 7–4. Basic processes affecting stratosphere ozone depletion.

The stable O_3 depleting substances don't just destroy one O_3 molecule; a chain reaction occurs. Using chlorofluorocarbons (CFCs) as an example, solar radiation breaks down the CFCs, which in turn releases chlorine atoms. A series of reactions take place, with chlorine acting as a catalyst, that result in destruction of O_3 and the formation of diatomic oxygen O_2. The chlorine from the CFCs is available to begin the O_3 destruction cycle again. The bases for concern about stratospheric O_3 depletion are illustrated in Figure 7–5.

A discussed in Chapter 10, energy is transferred from the sun to the earth in the form of electromagnetic energy. Photons that transfer energy have both a wavelength and energy level. The electromagnetic spectrum is divided into ultraviolet, visible, and infrared regions. The ultraviolet (UV) region is composed of UV-C, UV-B, and UV-A. Ozone differentially removes wavelengths of UV-B between 295 and 320 nm; UV-A in wavelengths above 350 nm is not removed, nor is visible light (400–900 nm). Ozone removes all UV-C. Wavelengths between 295 and 300 nm are generally more biologically effective (i.e., able to cause damage) than other wavelengths in UV-B and even more so than UV-A radiation.

The adverse effects of increased UV-B radiation at the earth's surface range from a greater frequency in eye and skin disease in humans and animals, in-

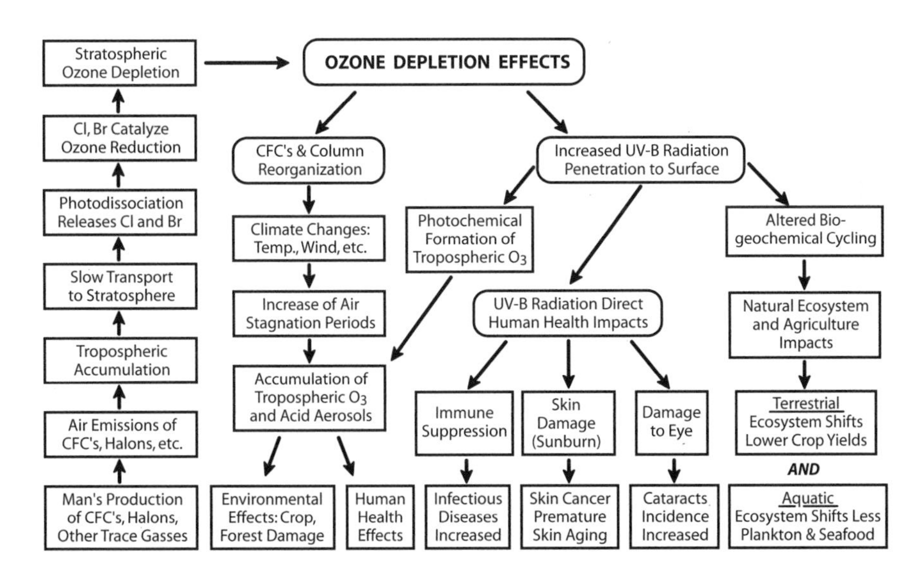

FIGURE 7–5. Processes involved in stratospheric ozone depletion because of anthropogenic production of CFCs, halons, and other trace gases are shown to the left. The types of effects caused by stratospheric ozone depletion and consequent increased UV-B penetration to the Earth's surface are hypothesized to include both direct effects on human health (e.g., increased cancer rates, immune suppression, etc.) and other terrestrial and aquatic ecological effects resulting from increased alterations of biogeochemical cycles.

cluding skin cancer and cataracts, to taxing the food chain in the natural environment, especially in the polar environments where the ozone layer is most severely depleted. The first countries to be affected by O_3 depletion over Antarctica were Argentina, Chile, South Africa, and New Zealand. By September and October of 1991, the Antarctic ozone hole was, for the first time, large enough to allow a large human population in the southern tip of South America to be exposed to increased levels of UV-B. The affected location with the greatest population density was the city of Punta Arenas in southern Chile (110,000 inhabitants).

In terms of the sensitive ecosystems in the Antarctic Ocean, plants and animals have adapted to the harsh environmental conditions. These species are greatly dependent upon one another for survival. Adverse effects to one species in a food web may cause harmful effects to other species and the ecosystem as a whole. A major concern is that UV-B may cause a major decline in plankton, which serve as a primary source of nutrients for the Antarctic marine food chain, which is illustrated in Figure 7–6.

Though injurious UV-B effects have been documented on some individual species within marine ecosystems, the nature and extent of ecosystem responses to UV stress are not well understood. Is the structure and function of the total marine ecosystem more or less sensitive than its components? Will negative effects (e.g., increased UV-B) on the base of the food web cascade through the system and reduce fish production?

At this point, such questions remain unresolved. It is possible that differences in UV-B tolerances between species will be great enough to create a competitive advantage for one particular species over another. What if animals dependent upon a certain species of phytoplankton for food cannot readily adapt to feeding on other species? Will more and more species in the food web also decline? How will decreased or different, more UV-tolerant phytoplankton populations affect the carbon cycle and global climate change?

While the connection between stratospheric O_3 depletion and global climate change remains speculative, we do know that carbon dioxide (CO_2) is a key heat-absorbing compound in the atmosphere and is used up by plants and phytoplankton during photosynthesis. Significant reductions in plant and phytoplankton populations due to increased levels of UV-B radiation can be expected to exacerbate the global warming phenomenon.

The direct effects of UV-B radiation on long-term growth and metabolism in representative phytoplankton species are being studied in order to develop models to predict the effects of increased UV-B radiation on the structure and function of marine phytoplankton communities. Growth rings in the shells of long-lived Antarctic bivalves (e.g., clams) can be examined, much like the rings in cross-sections of trees. Fluctuations in growth ring sizes of these filter feeders (i.e., they filter phytoplankton out of water for food) to determine if they corre-

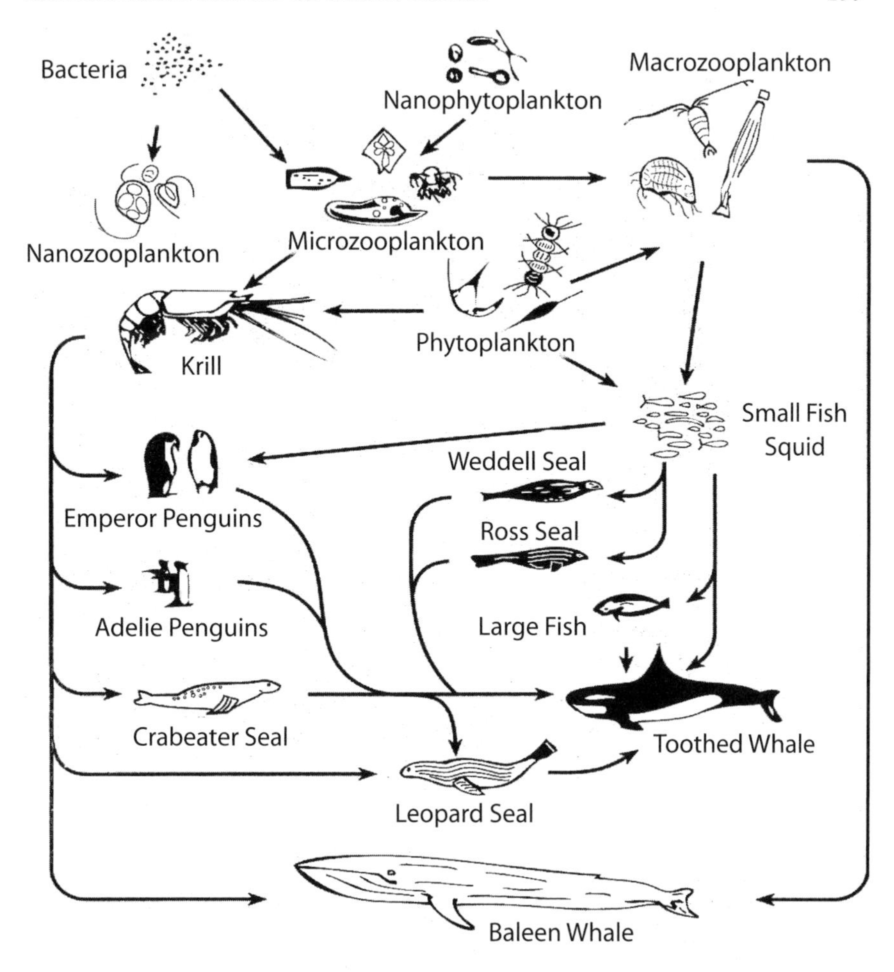

FIGURE 7–6. Antarctic marine food chain. (*Source*: Adapted from EPA/640/K-95/004.)

late well with the annual Antarctic ozone hole (first documented in 1979). If so, bivalve growth rings could be used as indicators of phytoplankton population reductions resulting from stratospheric ozone depletion.

O_3 depletion is also occurring, albeit to a lesser extent, in the Arctic. Kerr and McElroy[14] demonstrated that UV-B exposures at the Earth's surface increased seasonally between 1989 and 1993 (more so in winter than in summer months) linking increased levels of ground-based UV-B energy (at a wavelength of 300 nanometers) to stratospheric O_3 depletion.

In view of the long lead times for ground based emissions of stratospheric O_3 depleting chemicals to reach the stratosphere, and the expectation that there will be serious consequences of stratospheric O_3 depletion over a very long period of time, 26 of the major nations of the world adopted, in September of 1987, the Montreal Protocol on Substances that Deplete the Ozone Layer, a landmark international treaty dealing with a worldwide problem in a coordinated way.

However, given the stability of the O_3 depleting substances already in the atmosphere, the continued (albeit decreased) release of these substances, and the anticipated emissions of temporary alternatives (that deplete O_3 to a lesser extent), most scientists believe that the lowest levels of worldwide stratospheric O_3 (and the greatest potential effects of UV radiation exposure) are yet to come.

Acidification of Surface Waters and Terrestrial Soils

Ordinary rain should have an average pH of approximately 5.7, based upon atmospheric CO_2 in equilibrium with the precipitation. However, large regions of eastern North America (northeastern United States and southeastern Canada) and southern Scandinavia have received highly acidic precipitation, having a weighted average pH of 4.0–4.4, and a range extending as low as 2.8. The acidity is due primarily to atmospheric formation of H_2SO_4 and, to some extent, HNO_3 from SO_2 and NO_x, respectively. Acid precipitation occurs especially in areas downwind (up to thousands of kilometers) of dense urban and industrial complexes. For example, changes in pH have occurred in some lakes of the Adirondack Mountains of New York State, and many of these lakes no longer support fish populations.

The pH of an aquatic environment reflects both the acidity of the precipitation and the ability to neutralize incoming acid via chemical weathering and ion exchange processes in the watershed. Numerous lakes and rivers, especially those with naturally poorly buffered waters, i.e., having low mineral content, have shown the most dramatic increase in acidity, often having a pH less than 5. With continued acid precipitation, however, even those waters with better buffering capacity may show changes.

Acidification of waters affects all aspects of the aquatic environment. Extensive depletion of fish populations in acidified lakes and streams took place in many of the areas receiving acid rain. The causes were usually direct toxic action of acid waters on eggs and/or larval fish stages, reduction in the number of eggs due to interference with reproductive physiology, and changes in food supply due to the effects of acidity upon other aquatic biota. If the waters are very acidic, a direct toxic action to adult fishes results via interference with ion exchange across the gill membranes.

Like waters, soils having high buffering capacity are not as susceptible to increased acidification. However, many areas do show increased soil acidity. This results in the alteration of some properties of the soil, with an increase in the leaching of certain ions. The ecological effects include a decrease in the growth rate of forests and changes in nutrient cycling.

The concerns about acidic deposition led to a major U.S. federally sponsored effect to determine the extent and significance of the environmental impacts, as well as federally mandated controls on emissions of SO_2 and NO_x. Table 7–6 summarizes findings, as of 1996, that were reported to Congress by the National Acid Precipitation Assessment Program (NAPAP) in 1998.[15]

Aesthetics

It is often the changes in aesthetics caused by the clearly visible effects of air contaminants that spur the public to demand the control of the sources of contamination. Some aesthetic effects of air contaminants have already been mentioned, such as the soiling of buildings and damage to ornamental plants. Two others of importance, decreased visibility and odors, are discussed in the next sections.

Visibility

One of the most obvious effects of air contamination is the deterioration of visibility, which is not only an aesthetic problem, but also a safety hazard. Airline pilots have reported increases in ground haze and air pollution domes over cities since the 1950s and 1960s; cities previously visible from aerial distance of about 30–60 km are now often not visible for more than 16 km or even less during pollution episodes.

Visibility may be defined in meteorologic terms as the greatest distance in a given direction at which it is just possible to see and identify, with the unaided eye: *(1)* in the daytime, a prominent dark object against the sky at the horizon; and *(2)* at night, a known, preferably unfocused, moderately intense light source. After visibilities are determined around the entire horizon, they are resolved for reporting purposes into a single value of prevailing visibility.

The reduction of visibility is due both to the absorption and scattering of visible light by gas molecules and particles in the atmosphere, although scattering is the primary mechanism responsible.

Scattering is the deflection of the direction of travel of light by airborne matter. Particles in the size range of 0.4–0.7 μm are most effective in scattering, because their size is close to the wavelength of visible light. In addition to size, the degree of scattering is also influenced by particle shape, surface roughness, and refractive index.

The coloration of some contaminated atmospheres is due to the selective absorption of specific wavelengths of light by various atmospheric contaminants.

Odors

Malodors due to air contaminants are mainly a problem of aesthetics, although property values may be adversely affected in areas where odors are common.

TABLE 7–6. Selected Policy-Relevant Developments Since 1990[a]

WHAT'S NEW SINCE 1990	SIGNIFICANCE
SULFUR CONCENTRATION IN PRECIPITATION	
Sulfur concentration levels in wet deposition decreased 10%–25% over large areas of the eastern United States in 1995, with the largest decreases in and downwind of the Ohio River Valley. Similar decreases were found in sulfur concentrations in dry deposition.	The significant drop in acid deposition (and emissions) in 1995 provides a unique scientific (and economic) opportunity to validate atmospheric deposition models and dose-response relationships.
AQUATIC EFFECTS FROM NITROGEN	
Nitrogen is now recognized as playing a greater role in watershed acidification.	There may be limited recovery in some sensitive systems because NO_x reductions under Title IV may not be sufficient enough to result in measurable improvements in chemical or biological changes.
SURFACE WATER TRENDS	
Concentrations of sulfate in lake and stream waters have decreased in many areas, with evidence of recovery from acidification in New England. However, the majority of Adirondack lakes have remained fairly constant, while the sensitive Adirondack lakes continue to acidify.	Reductions in sulfur deposition to date may be insufficient in some areas to improve the acid-base status of acidified surface waters.
HIGH-ELEVATION SPRUCE-FIR DIEBACK	
Strong linkage was confirmed between acid deposition and damage to high-elevation spruce-fir forest ecosystems.	There is a higher likelihood of some short-term benefits from controls of acid deposition precursors.
CULTURAL RESOURCES	
Dry deposition of SO_2 and aerosols is now thought to be more damaging to stone than wet deposition.	The role of dry deposition and its relative impact on benefits to cultural resources must be reviewed.
VALUATION OF ECONOMIC BENEFITS	
Expected benefits are greater than previously thought, especially in the areas of human health and visibility.	The magnitude of valued benefits in these areas exceeds the costs of Title IV, independent of benefit estimates for other areas.

[a]This information represents the significant developments since the NAPAP 1990 Integrated Assessment Report.

Some odorants are merely a nuisance, while others will also produce systemic effects, such as nausea and appetite loss. In addition, odors may interact synergistically or antagonistically.

The olfactory system is quite sensitive. Even when gases are present in the ppb_v range, odors may still be so annoying as to affect personal comfort. However, people do differ widely in their sensitivity to odorants. In addition, the sense of smell is often rapidly fatigued, i.e., continued exposure results in loss of smell of the odorant.

Many natural sources of odor exist; these are all primarily due to sulfur compounds formed during microbial decomposition of plants and animals, largely in stagnant and insufficiently aerated waters, such as swamps and sewers.

Anthropogenic odorants are the result primarily of industrial operations, although mobile combustion sources, such as gasoline and diesel engines, are also contributors in certain areas. The principal industries responsible for odorant release are petroleum refineries, natural gas plants, chemical plants, food processing plants, smelters, paper mills, and tanneries. Table 7–7 lists some common chemical odorants.

WATER CONTAMINANTS

The hydrosphere has long been considered an infinite sink for the disposal of all kinds of wastes. It was assumed that running waters were always able to "purify" themselves, and the vastness of the oceans was such that they were able to assimilate any and all of the chemicals and flotable wastes we cared to dump into them. Although water does have certain self-purification capabilities, very

TABLE 7–7. Selected Odorants

CHEMICAL	CHARACTER OF ODOR	ODOR THRESHOLD[a]
Acetic acid	Sour	1.0
Ammonia	Sharp, pungent	47
Chlorine	Pungent, irritating, bleach	0.3
Ethyl mercaptan	Decayed cabbage, sulfidelike	0.001
Hydrogen sulfide	Rotten eggs, nauseating	0.0005
Isocyanates	Sweet, repulsive	[b]
Ozone	Slightly pungent, electric sparks	0.05
Selenium compounds	Putrid, garliclike	[b]
Sulfur dioxide	Pungent, mustiness	0.5
Tars	Rancid, skunklike	[b]

[a]This represents odor recognition thresholds for a panel of four trained observers. The concentrations are in ppm_v and are those at which all panelists recognized the odor.

[b]Not tested.

often these are simply overwhelmed by contaminant discharge. Today, all aquatic environments are threatened, some to a greater degree than others. These include coastal regions near cities, as well as remote lakes and ocean waters thousands of miles from land areas. The extent of contemporary water quality impairment by source, by pollutant, and by type of water body is illustrated in Figure 7–7.

Water quality is a value judgment, since water which is unfit for one use may be fine for another, or water unfit for one species may be quite suitable for another. Even natural waters are never 100% pure. Therefore, an aquatic environment may be considered as polluted if the water becomes unsuitable for its intended use, or changes occur due to human activities that disrupt the natural ecological balance.

Contaminants may alter aquatic environments in various ways. The type and degree of effect depends upon the type and amount of contaminant and characteristics of the receiving waters, such as temperature, pH, flow rate, degree of dilution and mixing, and the presence of other contaminants that may interact with each other.

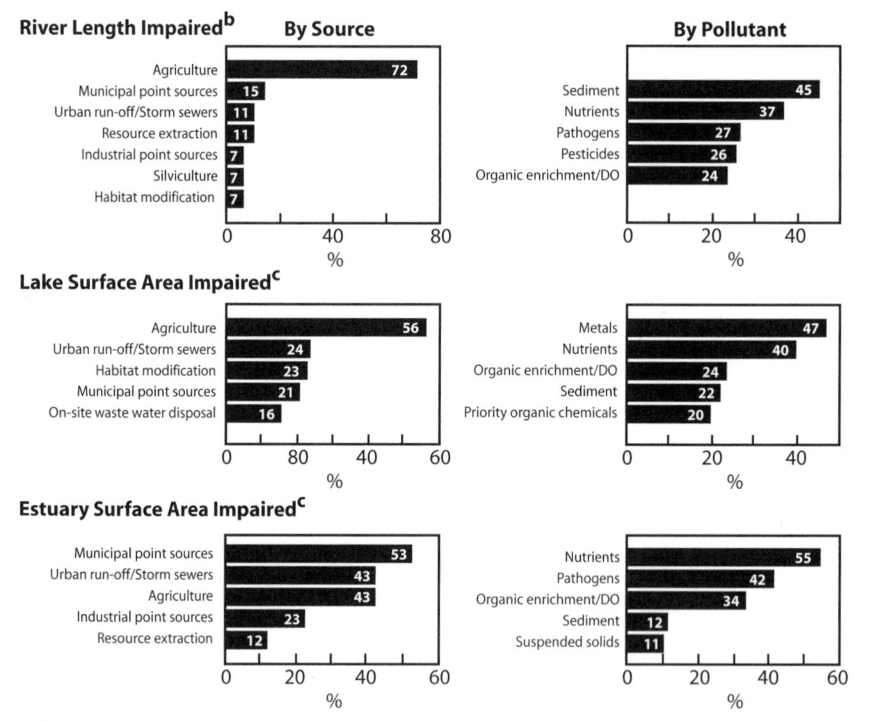

FIGURE 7–7. Sources and causes of water quality impairment, early 1990s.

The effects of water contaminants upon aquatic life may be divided into two broad types: direct and indirect. An agent is said to exert direct action if it affects characteristics of the organism itself, for example, growth, reproduction, and physiology. Indirect effects involve alterations of the organism's environment, either abiotic or biotic, so as to make the habitat unsuitable for continued existence or reproduction, for example, affecting food resources, changing turbidity, or DO content. Indirect effects may be just as critical to species survival as are the direct effects.

Contaminants may be quite selective in their action, or they may affect many types of organisms. Often, only certain tolerant species survive, resulting in a change in the population balance. As food sources are destroyed, animals on higher trophic levels die or move out. In addition, stressed individuals are often more susceptible to disease and parasites, further reducing the reproductive potential of the population. Certain chemicals act as repellents to aquatic life, so that, for example, fish are driven out of an area, making the entire region biologically unproductive. Other types of contaminants may result in extreme overproduction and overenrichment of a body of water. The end result of any disturbance is an alteration, often slow and subtle, of the character of the waterway over a certain period of time.

All contaminants do not adversely affect aquatic life. Some may affect the aesthetics of the water, such as color, or the ability to use it for specific purposes, such as drinking or recreation, without affecting the natural biotic communities.

In the following sections, water contaminants will be discussed by broad classes. Effects upon the physicochemical properties of the aquatic system are presented together with discussions of the effects upon aquatic life.

As with air contaminants, the aesthetic effects of water contaminants contain components of the entire range of environmental problems. People enjoy waterways of high quality used for recreational purposes, or which may add a degree of natural beauty to some area. No one likes a beach blackened by floating oil, or a lake that smells of rotting sewage.

Waste Heat

Waste heat is released into receiving waters by electric power–generating stations, and by the many industrial processes that require cooling waters. Although cooling towers are often used in attempts to dissipate the heat before the water is discharged into the environment, the water is still released warmer than when it was taken up.

Certain other human activities may affect water temperatures. Removal of forest canopies, removal of brush and shade trees along streams, impounding of river waters, reduction of stream flows, and return of irrigation waters often lead to increases in temperature in the nearby waterways. The temperature of water naturally varies from season to season, year to year, and even between night and day. Human activities have often served to extend this normal range of variability, sometimes beyond the limits to which the native biota are adapted.

Except for birds and mammals, other aquatic organisms are poikilotherms ("cold blooded"); their body temperature is at or near the temperature of their environment, and is subject to change as the environmental temperature changes. Within a certain range of tolerance, however, aquatic organisms can adjust and survive. Problems may arise when the temperature exceeds this limited range.

The chemical processes of life are, like all chemical reactions, very sensitive to the temperature of the environment in which they occur. As environmental temperature changes, so does the rate of metabolic reactions, which increase with rising temperature. As the metabolic rate increases, so does the demand for oxygen. However, with rising water temperature, the solubility of oxygen in the water decreases; thus, just as increased demand occurs, less oxygen is available, and levels of DO may fall below the critical value. Of course, if temperatures are high enough, complete enzyme inactivation and cellular disruption may occur.

Aside from affecting metabolic reactions, temperature influences all facets of life, such as hormonal and nervous control, digestion, respiration, osmoregulation, and behavior. Behavioral changes may be just as detrimental as physiologic changes, for example, attempts to spawn too early in the season or premature migration triggered by changes in temperature.

Many nuisance species of plants and animals thrive at higher temperatures than do more desirable species. For example, blue-green algae survive quite well at around 24°–34°C, while certain more desirable plankton have their optimal range at about 14°–24°C. As the water temperature increases, the algae have a selective competitive advantage, and their numbers increase, fouling the stream, and further reducing DO upon their death and decomposition. In extreme conditions, i.e., above 60°C, only a few bacterial species are able to survive.

The effects of waste heat also depend, to some extent, upon the season and weather conditions, tending to be more harmful in hot climates than in cold areas. Rapid changes in temperature and intermittent or nondependable fluctuations, such as those due to intermittent discharges, are often more harmful to biota that could otherwise have been able to adapt to slower, more constant changes of temperature greater than their optimal level. Waste heat is also a greater problem in small streams and rivers than in larger waterways having better circulation and mixing.

In addition to direct biological effects, waste heat may affect the action of other contaminants in the water. Temperature affects the susceptibility to some chemicals, resulting in increased hazard from these agents. Some examples are the synergistic effects of heat and methyl mercury, PCB, and a number of insecticides.

Suspended Solids

Solids may produce effects on aquatic environments while carried in suspension or after settling to the bottom of the waterway.

Suspended solids increase the turbidity of the water, thus decreasing the penetration of light by absorption and scattering of the sun's rays. This directly affects the photosynthetic activity in the waterway, which ultimately appears as a reduction in biological productivity. Extreme turbidity can result in almost complete cessation of photosynthesis. Increased turbidity may also interfere with the vision of animals, possibly preventing them from sighting their prey and thus reducing the efficiency of food use.

If the concentration of suspended particulates is high enough, they may interfere with the feeding of filter-feeding organisms; in addition, physical injury to delicate eye and gill membranes may occur by abrasion.

Once solids settle to the bottom, the benthic environment may be disturbed, for example, by actually burying bottom habitats. Destruction of bottom dwellers and fish larvae, essential parts of certain food chains, could disrupt entire biological communities.

Plant Nutrients: Organic

As described in Chapter 5, organic material introduced into receiving waters undergoes a normal process of decomposition by microbial action, which depends primarily on the oxygen dissolved in the water. If sufficient amounts of organic matter are introduced, the rate of oxidative decomposition could exceed the rate of oxygen replenishment, and the DO concentration in the receiving waters will decline. The exact rate and extent of this decline depends upon the differential between the rates of oxidation and replenishment.

Most healthy streams and rivers have DO levels of 5–7 mg/L. Values consistently less than 4 mg/L tend to indicate organic overloading. Except for the purest of natural waters, all waters have a measurable BOD, which may be as high as 5 mg/L. Many domestic and industrial wastes have BODs of several hundred mg/L which, if inadequately diluted in receiving waters, will produce severe oxygen depletion.

Organic wastes released into waters are, of course, sources of nutrients and food for the microbial decomposer organisms. These wastes may encourage their growth, and the resultant increased production may result in other problems, such as health risks and malodors. Suspended microorganisms may increase turbidity and result in discoloration of the water. Organic waste discharges often lead to the growth of bacteria and other microorganisms in the stream bottom, producing what is known as sewage fungus. Not only is this an aesthetic problem, but it may clog water supply inlets or the nets of fishermen, and may change the benthic environment to make it unsuitable for its natural inhabitants.

Organic waste discharge and resultant oxygen depletion may have both direct and indirect effects upon all aspects of aquatic life. It can result in fish kills due to oxygen depletion, or make an area unsuitable for desirable species. In lakes, as DO levels decrease in deep waters, certain species may disappear, while those better able to tolerate reduced oxygen tension may increase in number. In rivers and streams, the typical example of effects on aquatic life is the succession of communities downstream from a sewage outfall, a process discussed in Chapter 5.

The classic scheme for describing the biological effects of organic waste discharge was introduced by Kolkwitz and Marsson.[16,17] This is known as the saprobic system of zones of organic enrichment, which classifies aquatic biota according to areas in which these species are found. Later systems have been patterned after this one, with differences in nomenclature and in delineation of specific zones. Although there are difficulties in attempting to present a rigid and arbitrary classification of an environment as dynamic as a river, the zonation system is of value in ordering, to some extent, interrelationships in rivers receiving organic wastes. The zonal regions proposed by Kolkwitz and Marsson are presented in Table 7–8 in simplified form. It should be kept in mind that in nature there are no clear boundaries between classes, and both the extent and location of any zone within river reaches may vary with time, with flow conditions, and with the seasons of the year.

Table 7–8. The Zonation of Contaminated Streams

Zone	Level of Contamination	DO	Predominant Biota	Bacterial Count (per mL H_2O)
I (polysaprobic)	Heavy	Zero to very low	Bacteria, sludge worms, maggots, some algae	$> 10^6$
II[a] (mesosaprobic)	Strong, but diminishing	Low to fully saturated	Bacteria, protozoa, worms, rotifers, midge larvae, diatoms, algae, carp	10^4–10^5
III (oligosaprobic)	Low or none	Fully saturated	Diverse plants and animals including game fish	$< 10^3$

[a]This zone is actually separated into a heavily contaminated subdivision which adjoins Zone I, and a less contaminated region which adjoins Zone III.

DO: dissolved oxygen.

Plant Nutrients: Inorganic

The primary inorganic nutrients are nitrates and phosphates, one or both of which are generally the limiting factors to plant growth. The main effect of either of these is the "fertilization" of water, resulting in accelerated eutrophication.

Eutrophication is the term generally applied to the process of natural evolution of a lake. It involves the slow change with time from a biologically unproductive, nutrient-deficient lake having a sparse biotic community (oligotrophic lake), to one which is highly productive, nutrient-rich, and supports diverse biota (eutrophic lake). The gradual addition and buildup of nutrients in the lake from natural sources in the surrounding watershed and internal mineral fixation leads to this enrichment and biological development. The rate of normal eutrophication in a lake depends upon such factors as soil type, type of vegetation in the drainage basin, and local geology.

At some point in this process, a stable condition results where the rate of biological productivity approximately equals the rate of decomposition. This results in a fairly constant, homeostatic chemical and biologic aquatic environment where small disturbances may cause rates of productivity and decomposition to vary, but in balance. By introducing excessive amounts of inorganic plant nutrients, humans are responsible for accelerated eutrophication in many aquatic environments, as these homeostatic mechanisms are overwhelmed.

There are predilective sites for accelerated eutrophication. The prime ones are impounded (naturally or artificially) bodies of water, such as small lakes and dammed reservoirs. In these, added nutrients may recycle for many years, since there is little removal via water exchange of any introduced chemicals. Semi-enclosed bodies of water such as estuaries and coastal regions of large lakes, especially in those areas downstream to waste discharge sites or runoff from non-point agricultural sources, are also prone to accelerated eutrophication. The rate of accelerated eutrophication is dependent upon the size of the body of water, the rate of nutrient input, and the homeostatic condition that existed prior to any disturbance.

Nutrient input initially results in the increased growth of some plankton species, primarily blue-green algae, and certain rooted aquatic weeds. The previously dominant phytoplankton disappear, decreasing the variety of food for herbivores and reducing total plant species diversity. An overview of the major sources of nutrient overload is illustrated in Figure 7–8.

Upon algal death, oxidative decomposition in the sediments increases the BOD of the water, decreasing the level of DO. Deep stratified lakes that are eutrophic have little or no DO in the hypolimnion. As the deeper waters are robbed of oxygen, those fish species which require deep, well-oxygenated waters, for example, trout and herring, disappear, being replaced by other species, for example,

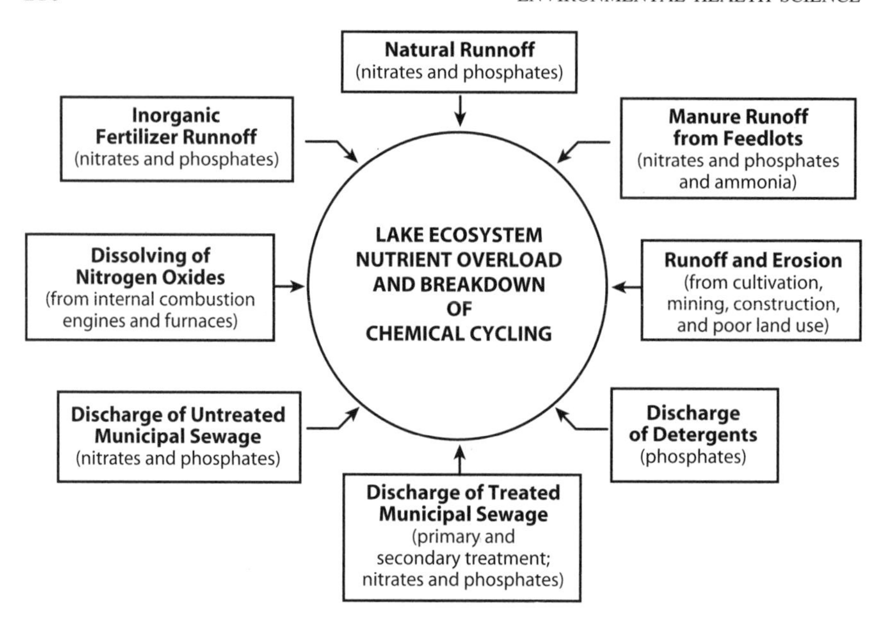

FIGURE 7–8. Major sources of nutrient overload in slow moving lakes.

sunfish and carp, which require less oxygen and are supported on shorter food chains. In addition, upon algal death and decomposition, the nitrogen and phosphorus bound in the algae are released back into the water. The spring overturn carries these nutrients to surface layers, where they may promote new blooms. Thus, as mentioned, added nutrients may continually recycle in lakes.

With increasing algal growth, the water becomes more turbid, a condition that restricts the penetration of light to deeper water layers, further depressing photosynthesis below the surface layer. At its worst, the lake becomes stagnant, supporting only anaerobic organisms involved in decay food chains; the decay results in the gradual filling of what is now an odorous (NH_3, H_2S, amines), discolored, and generally unsightly body of water. Thus, the biotic and chemical composition of the lake has changed, making it unsuitable for domestic, industrial, or recreational uses, or even for other wildlife.

The most important example of accelerated eutrophication in the United States is Lake Erie. Effects in this lake occurred mostly between 1910 and 1965, due to the large increase in population within its drainage basin. The main source of water into Lake Erie is Lake Huron, via a river system that services industrial Detroit. Lake Erie also receives additional water from rivers that drain agricultural lands and flow through industrial cities such as Toledo and Cleveland. Over the past 100 years there have been major changes in the chemical composition of the lake and severe oxygen depletion in the central basin. The accelerating deterioration of the lake led to a joint United States–Canadian effort to reverse the trend, and significant progress was made since the mid-1960s in controlling the discharge of nutrients into Lake Erie; this has resulted in greatly improved water quality.

That control and elimination of nutrient sources to a lake can sometimes prevent algal blooms is also evidenced by the reversal of accelerated eutrophication in Lake Washington due to the elimination of phosphate input by the diverting of sewage effluents.[18]

Although the term eutrophication is generally not directly applied to rapidly running waters such as rivers and streams, a response similar to those in lakes does occur following enrichment, with increased algal and bottom growth (Chapter 5). This response usually abates if effluent discharge is ended.

Dissolved Solids and Minerals

The total content of dissolved minerals is referred to as salinity. Excessive mineral content may affect the taste of drinking water and be harmful to people who have specific illnesses. "Hard water," i.e., with excess minerals, primarily calcium and magnesium ions, affects use of the water for domestic, irrigation, and many industrial purposes.

Freshwater fauna are adapted to low salt levels, and discharges that produce excess salt in freshwater environments may be lethal.

Excess minerals may affect certain aspects of water chemistry. The addition of chloride and sulfate, primarily as sodium salts, affects the solubility equilibrium of waters, primarily via absorption of the sodium onto clay particles. This produces a decrease in the pH, especially if the sodium is exchanged with a less alkaline cation. These changes will affect carbonate dissociation and buffering capacity of the water.

The discharge of inert brines of, for example, Na_2SO_4 or NaCl, may promote eutrophication. This occurs because phosphate tends to be released from bottom sediments formed under a region of low total dissolved salt but bathed by waters having higher ionic strength.

Some dissolved chemicals may color the water, with a possible decrease in light penetration and, therefore, photosynthetic activity.

Industrial Chemicals

Multitudes of industrial wastes are discharged into aquatic environments. These may be derived from specific factory point sources via direct discharge or accidental release, or be general watershed runoff.

Many waters contain certain levels of natural toxic chemicals leached from surrounding rocks and soils, for example, mercury, or produced during the decomposition of plants and animals, for example, H_2S. Depending upon the specific mechanism that has evolved to handle it, an aquatic organism will most likely tolerate a certain amount of these natural toxicants. However, human activities have often resulted in increasing the levels of many natural toxic chemicals above the tolerable levels, and have also resulted in the introduction of other chemicals for which the organisms have no defense.

The effects due to discharge of large amounts of toxic chemicals are quite different from those due to sewage discharge described above. While certain species may become severely depressed by sewage release, others become quite abundant. On the other hand, most toxic chemicals do not benefit aquatic organisms, and are probably deleterious to most, except for a few types of microorganisms that may be able to use specific chemicals as a source of energy. Thus, large increases in populations of particular aquatic species are usually not found after toxic chemical release.

High concentrations of toxic materials have obvious deleterious effects. The most dramatic of these are fish kills, which are due primarily to acute effects of chemical poisons. More often, levels of chemicals that are released are not high enough to produce fish kills but, rather, result in other effects that may or may not be clear cut. These may be, for example, tumors, fungal diseases, systemic pathology, abnormal larval growth, and decreased reproductive potential. Behavioral changes involving migratory, territorial, feeding, and social behavior may also be induced. All of these effects may ultimately result in decreased population size and biologic productivity of the waterway.

Certain chemicals may accumulate in bottom sediments and in food chains. In 1971, the FDA temporarily banned the sale of swordfish because a large number of samples tested had excessive levels of mercury. High levels of other chemicals often result in the temporary banning of commercial fishing in many areas of the United States.

Numerous chemicals, when present in low, sublethal levels may impart unpleasant tastes to fish and shellfish used as food by man. Only trace amounts are sometimes enough to produce a noticeable effect, without changing the distribution or abundance of biota. For example, unpleasant tastes in fish will occur when chlorophenol is present at levels of 0.0001 mg/L. Other chemicals that impart tastes at low levels are benzene, oil, and 2,4-D. This action affects recreational and commercial fishing, and may also make the water undrinkable.

No aquatic environment has an unlimited ability to accommodate contaminants. Even open ocean areas thousands of miles from any population center show evidence of chemical contaminants. For example, waste oil and associated debris have been found in the central Atlantic Ocean, and a decline in plankton primary production since the 1950s has occurred in the North Atlantic. Table 7–9 presents some important industrial chemical contaminants found in aquatic environments, and describes their biological effects. The list is by no means inclusive; it would take a whole volume to present the industrial chemicals found in aquatic systems. Bear in mind that environmental conditions, such as water

TABLE 7–9. Effects of Selected Industrial Chemical Contaminants in Aquatic Environments

CONTAMINANT	EFFECT UPON AQUATIC ENVIRONMENT
Petroleum	Contains many water-soluble compounds that are toxic to plant and animal species; coats benthic environment when it sinks; oil films decrease light penetration and oxygen absorption; coats body surfaces of aquatic birds and destroys waterproofing; some products may impart unpleasant flavors to fish and shellfish; may act to concentrate other fat-soluble toxic chemicals in the water; interferes with recreational use and is aesthetically unpleasing; oil-laden sediments may move with bottom currents to other areas
Organochlorine pesticides (e.g., DDT)	Reduction in thickness of eggshells in birds which feed upon fish containing residues; decreased survival of fish fry; inhibits phytoplankton photosynthesis; acutely toxic to some aquatic fauna via food chain accumulation
Polychlorinated biphenyls	Similar to DDT; eggshell thinning in aquatic birds
Heavy metals	Toxic to many forms of aquatic life; some may be carcinogenic to fish and shellfish

pH and temperature, and the presence of other chemicals, may modify the hazard from each of these contaminants.

Acidity

Aside from acid rainfall, a major source of acidity, especially in streams, is acid mine drainage, primarily from coal mines. When exposed to air during mining operations, iron sulfide ores (pyrite) become oxidized, resulting in numerous products, including sulfates. Water draining through the mines dissolves these products, and the resulting acidic solution (H_2SO_4) runs off into surface waters and may percolate to groundwater. These acidic waters often contain several kinds of metals, whose solubility in water is increased at the lower pH. The effects of acidity upon aquatic life have been described previously, in the discussion of acid rain.

CHEMICAL CONTAMINANTS AND THE DISRUPTION OF NATURAL ECOSYSTEMS

Natural ecosystems, upon which humans ultimately depend, are complete functional units, which create and maintain patterns of energy flow, nutrient cycles, growth, sanitation and, within limits, self-regulation and self-restoration. If these limits are exceeded, however, disruption and degradation may occur. It may only require imbalance in a few components to upset the entire ecosystem.

Disruption of Biogeochemical Cycles

Biogeochemical cycles are integral components of the ecosystem, serving to maintain steady-state levels of various chemical elements via equilibrium in a number of continuing processes.

Disruption of biogeochemical cycles is one of the greatest problems caused by human activity. Many contaminants enter natural cycles, becoming redistributed and/or concentrated at some stage as the cycle strives to regain an equilibrium. What results is too little here, and too much there; this redistribution of cycle intermediates may result in an effect on human health and welfare. Local and, in some cases, even global disruptions of cycles are already in evidence.

The carbon cycle shows evidence of a global disruption. Exchange of CO_2 between the hydrosphere and atmosphere had resulted in a balanced, relatively constant CO_2 concentration in the latter until about the time of the Industrial Revolution. Since then, the ever-increasing combustion of fossil fuels is returning to circulation carbon that had been fixed into biota, and then subsequently trapped as coal and petroleum millions of years ago. This has resulted in an upsetting of the dynamic equilibrium between the atmosphere and hydrosphere.

Although the total amount of CO_2 injected into the atmosphere is small when compared to the total amount of CO_2 in global circulation, the atmospheric reservoir is also small. CO_2 cannot be absorbed into the much larger hydrospheric reservoir as fast as it is being generated. The result of this, as discussed previously, is a gradual increase in atmospheric levels of CO_2.

The nitrogen cycle shows evidence of imbalances on a more local scale. For example, runoff of nitrates from fertilized land areas into lakes and streams may result in overenrichment of these waters. Balanced nutrient cycles would have maintained optimal levels of plant nutrients in these waterways.

Organic nitrogen from farm wastes and untreated or inadequately treated domestic sewage may ultimately be oxidized to nitrate, again resulting in accelerated eutrophication.

Plants that are grown in soils containing high levels of nitrogen fertilizers may assimilate nitrate faster than it is fixed into organic molecules, resulting in an accumulation of nitrate within the plant. These high nitrate levels may adversely affect livestock and people feeding on these plants.

Imbalances, especially excesses, at certain stages of the cycle may have other implications in terms of human health. For example, high levels of nitrate in potable water may cause methemoglobinemia in infants.

Prior to the Industrial Revolution, the amount of N_2 removed from the atmosphere via biological fixation was essentially balanced by the amounts returned by denitrification processes. However, the rate of nitrogen fixation in the biosphere is now increasing very rapidly due to the large amount of fixation by various industrial processes, such as fertilizer manufacture and various combustion processes, and the increased agricultural cultivation of legumes that fix nitrogen through symbiosis with certain bacteria. This accelerated rate of fixation may overwhelm the ability of natural denitrification processes to keep pace, or result in increases in denitrification products, producing an imbalance in the nitrogen cycle. If sustained for continued periods of time, this imbalance could result in overall global consequences of which we are not as yet aware.

As with nitrogen, steady-state levels of certain sulfur-cycle intermediates normally maintained in undisturbed ecosystems may be upset by human activities. For example, bacterial reduction of sulfate to H_2S under anaerobic conditions is part of the normal sulfur cycle. However, release of sulfate-rich effluents from, for example, paper mills may be responsible for fish kills in waterways, as secondarily derived H_2S reaches lethal levels.

Various naturally occurring toxic chemicals have, due to ecological processes controlling their synthesis and degradation, tended to maintain a global distribution that remains fairly constant. As humans produce many of these materials and release them into the environment, an imbalance between degradation and synthesis may occur. A classic example is mercury.

Mercury occurs naturally in the environment, but generally only in trace amounts. The biogeochemical mercury cycle is shown in Figure 7–9. Under partial to total aerobic conditions in aquatic sediments, microorganisms convert inorganic and phenyl compounds to methyl and, to some extent, dimethyl mercury. These alkyl compounds are the most toxic forms. They are quite stable and, in addition, if taken up by biota, are only very slowly excreted; thus, they tend to become concentrated in biological organisms and may be long-term environmental hazards.

As with other cycles, interconversions of various mercury compounds result in a homeostatic system and, under undisturbed conditions, a steady-state concentration of highly toxic methyl mercury in the aquatic sediments. Humans have often upset this balance.

A number of other elements besides mercury may be methylated by microbes in aquatic sediments and terrestrial soils. These include gold, palladium, platinum, tin, thallium, selenium, and tellurium. Like methyl mercury, most of these alkyl metals are quite stable in the aquatic environment. The use of palladium and platinum catalysts in automobile emission control systems and heavy metal alkyls in gasoline additives instead of lead alkyls may thus pose a potential environmental problem.

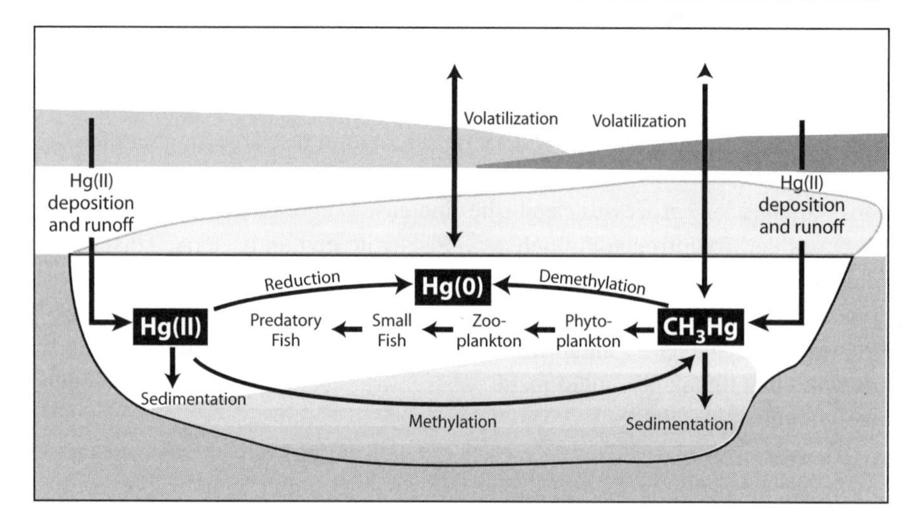

FIGURE 7–9. Mercury entering lakes—by direct surface deposition or terrestrial runoff—typically includes elemental mercury, Hg(O); oxidized mercury, Hg(II); and extremely small amounts of methylmercury, CH_3Hg. Most lake methylmercury, however, is produced when anaerobic bacteria in the water and sediments methylate oxidized mercury through a metabolic process. Methylmercury is bioaccumulated by plankton and other organisms and then passed up the food chain to fish, where it also concentrates. While this diagram represents major processes in the aquatic mercury cycle, the overall cycle is complex and cannot be generalized for all lakes.

Disruption of Ecosystem Structure

The introduction of chemical contaminants into the environment often leads to complex changes in overall ecosystem structure and function. Details of the pattern of alteration have been demonstrated clearly in only a few instances. Although the effects of some contaminants may be more conspicuous than others, the effects of all were found to be parallel; the resultant changes followed similar and broadly predictable patterns for both terrestrial and aquatic ecosystems.

A mature, undisturbed ecosystem is a dynamic unit that maintains some degree of stability. An ecosystem reaches this stage via an orderly development with time, if not disturbed by humans or by natural catastrophes; this evolutionary process is termed ecological succession. Succession involves the interplay between the biotic and abiotic components of the environment, leading towards development of stable communities, with maximum biomass and diversity of organisms in relation to the physical constraints of the environment. Succession proceeds through a sequence of biological community types until a climax community is reached; this is the final and most stable stage. The climax is self-perpetuating if not disturbed, and its complexity results in resistance to perturbances of the physical environment. The biogeochemical cycles are "conservative," i.e., only very small amounts of nutrients are lost, as, for example, via drainage water from terrestrial ecosystems.

A classic broad outline of the pattern of ecosystem alteration due to environmental contaminants has been described by Woodwell,[19] and is presented below.

The disturbance of any ecosystem is accompanied by a reduction in biotic community structure, with a resultant trend toward simplification and monotony of total ecosystem structure. A diversity of specialized species of plants and animals is shifted towards a monotony of a larger number of only a few species of plants or animals which are smaller and have a more rapid reproduction rate. For example, hardy shrubs replace trees in a forest, and algae replace the diverse phytoplankton of a lake. Food chains become shortened. Any disruption of community structure poses the greatest risk to those consumers at the apex of the trophic pyramid, for example, humans.

As a result of the reduction in community structure, a change in cycling of nutrients occurs. Terrestrial communities tend to become "leaky," with nutrient depletion, while nearby aquatic communities become overburdened due to accelerated nutrient input.

The ultimate result of disturbance is that a balanced, stable ecosystem becomes unbalanced and unstable. Often, short-lived disturbances may be "repaired" by the natural successional processes of the ecosystem. However, cumulative and chronic effects may produce more severe changes, with long time intervals necessary for recovery, if corrective measures are taken in time.

While much is still unknown about physicochemical and biological processes in the environment, a summary of the linkage among ecosystem goods and services can now be made in broad terms, as illustrated in Figure 7–10. However, accurate predictions of effects are not always possible, and long-term changes are difficult to assess. This is especially true since individual ecosystems are not discrete entities but are all interconnected with each other in some fashion, especially via food webs.

CONTAMINATION AND EVOLUTION

The diverse forms of life in the biosphere are the products of evolution, the mechanism of which is natural selection as proposed by Charles Darwin in 1838. Natural selection is the power of the environment to select characteristics of the next generation of a population, leading to organisms which are better adapted to their surroundings.

Chemical contamination is an environmental change that produces new selection pressures. Given the presence of heritable variation in the population, these new pressures may cause a change in gene frequency and, therefore, a change in the genetic makeup of the population involved. Thus, environmental contamina-

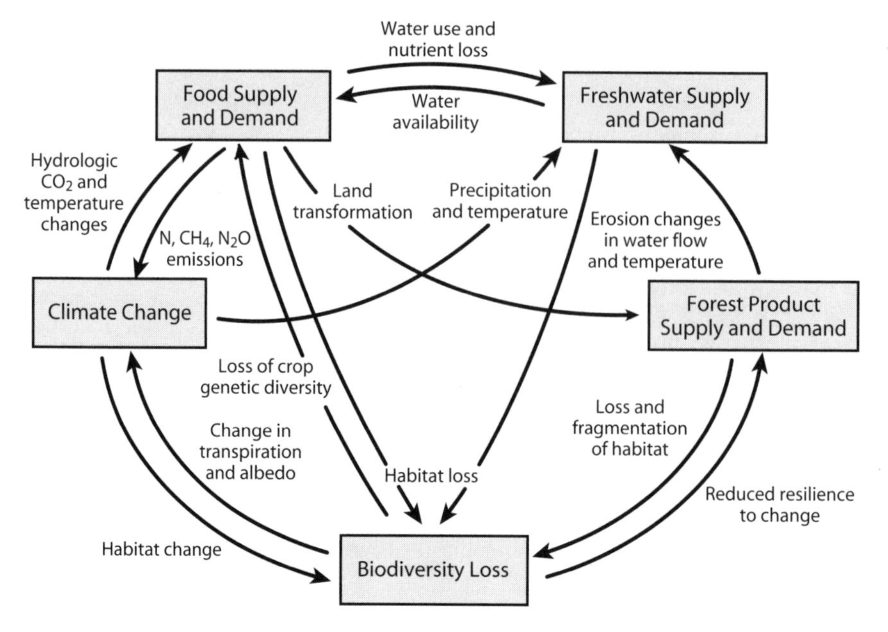

FIGURE 7–10. Linkages among various ecosystem goods and services (food, water, biodiversity, forest products) and other driving forces (climate change).

tion may be expected to cause evolutionary changes in exposed populations of plants and animals. The evolution of populations resistant to the destructive effects of specific chemicals, or otherwise adapted to life in contaminated areas, enables continued existence of the species under conditions that might otherwise have resulted in their extinction.

Contaminant-related evolution is widespread among many plant and animal species, and in response to many different chemicals. For example, there is evidence of populations of plants that are specifically adapted to many known chemical contaminants.[20]

Most evolutionary processes are slow. The rapidity, often in one or two generations, of some evolution is evidenced by the presence of plants adapted to life under conditions of contamination that have been in existence for only a short time.

Thus, changes in population characteristics may be one of the effects of exposure to chemical contaminants, and some of these changes have direct implications for human health and welfare, such as pesticide-resistant insects.

REFERENCES

1. Anon. The effects of the fog on cattle in London. The Veterinarian XLVII (No. 553), (Fourth Series, No. 229) (Jan. 1874) pp. 1–4, 32, 33.

2. Ministry of Health, Mortality and Morbidity During The London Fog of December 1952. London: Her Majesty's Stationary Office, 1954.
3. Harkins, W.D. and Swain, R.E. The chronic arsenical poisoning of herbivorous animals. *J. Am. Chem. Soc.* 30:928–946, 1908.
4. Prell, H. Die Schadigung der Tierwelt durch die Fernwirkungen von Industrieabgasen. *Arch. Gewerbepathol.–Gewerbehyg.* 7:656–670, 1937.
5. Bardelli, P. and Menzani, C. La fluorosi (fluorosis), part 2. *Atti Ist. Veneto Sci.* 97:623–674, 1937.
6. Lillie, R.J. Air Pollutants Affecting the Performance of Domestic Animals: A Literature Review. Agriculture Handbook No. 380, Washington, DC: U.S. Dept. of Agriculture, 1970.
7. Hupka, E. Uber Flugstaubvergiftungen in der Umgebung von Metallhutten. *Wiener. Tierarztl.* 42:763, 1955.
8. Schmitt, N., Brown, G., Devlin, E.L., Larsen, A.A., McCausland, E.D., and Savillo, J.M. Lead poisoning in horses. *Arch. Environ. Health* 23:185–197, 1971.
9. Bazell, R.J. Lead poisoning: Zoo animals may be the first victims. *Science* 173:130–131, 1971.
10. Cannon, H.L. and Bowles, J.M. Contamination of vegetation by tetraethyl lead. *Science* 137:765–766, 1962.
11. Chow, T.J. Lead accumulation in roadside soil and grass. *Nature* 225:295–296, 1970.
12. Barrie, L.A., Whelpdale, D.M., and Munn, R.E. Effects of anthropogenic emissions on climate: A review of selected topics. *Ambio.* 5:209–212, 1976.
13. Manahan, S.E. Environmental Chemistry. Boca Raton, FL: Lewis, 2000.
14. Kerr, J.B. and McElroy, C.T. Evidence for large upward trends of ultraviolet-B radiation linked to ozone depletion. *Science* 262:1032–1034, 1993.
15. NAPAP, Biennial Report to Congress: An Integrated Assessment. Silver Spring, MD: U.S. National Acid Precipitation Program, 1998.
16. Kolkwitz, R. and Marsson, M. Ökologie der pflanzlichen Saprobien. Berichte der Deutschen Botanischen Gesellschaft 26a:505–519, 1908. Translated: Ecology of plant saprobia. In Biology of Water Pollution, L.E. Keup, W.M. Ingram, and K.M. Mackenthun, (eds.), Federal Water Pollution Control Administration, U.S. Dept. of the Interior, 1967, pp. 47–52.
17. Kolkwitz, R. and Marsson, M. Ökologie der tierischen Saprobien. Beitrage zur Lehre von der biologischen Gewasserbeurteilung. Inter. Revue der Gesamten Hydrobiologie und Hydrogeographie. 2:126–152, 1909. Translated: Ecology of animal saprobia. In Biology of Water Pollution Control, L.E., Keup, W.M. Ingram, and K.M. Mackenthun (eds.), Federal Water Pollution control Administration, U.S. Department of the Interior, 1967, pp. 85–95.
18. Edmondson, W.T. Phosphorus, nitrogen and algae in Lake Washington after diversion of sewage. *Science* 169:690–691, 1970.
19. Woodwell, G.M. Effects of pollution on the structure and physiology of ecosystems. *Science* 168:429–433, 1970.
20. Bradshaw, A.D. Pollution and evolution. In Effects of Air Pollutants on Plants, T.A. Mansfield (ed.), Cambridge: Cambridge University Press, 1976, pp. 135–159.
21. Intergovernmental Panel on Climate Change (IPCC). Climate change 2001: The scientific basis. Contribution of working group I to the third assessment report of the IPCC. Cambridge: Cambridge University Press, 2001.
22. Intergovernmental Panel on Climate Change (IPCC). Climate change 2001: Impacts, adaptation, and vulnerability. Contribution of working group II to the third assessment report of the IPCC. Cambridge: Cambridge University Press, 2001.

8

Human Exposure Assessment

As discussed further in Chapters 9, 10, and 11, exposure assessment is a key element in risk assessment and risk management. There are a number of pathways for making quantitative exposure assessments (Fig. 8–1). Some, such as personal monitoring of concentrations in the breathing zone of selected individuals, can provide relatively precise information on those individuals, but only point estimates for a population at risk. Measurements of concentrations in environmental media (air, drinking water, food) can also be precise for the samples that are collected and analyzed, but of somewhat limited relevance for individuals in the population. Population distributions of exposure are often estimated using mathematical models with varying degrees of validation. This chapter focusses initially on techniques for direct measurements of exposures and concentrations in environmental media, and ends with a discussion of the limitations of the measurement data and models for exposure assessments in populations.

TECHNIQUES FOR DIRECT MEASUREMENTS OF ENVIRONMENTAL CONCENTRATIONS AND EXPOSURES

Accurate and reliable qualitative identifications and quantitative determinations of chemical contaminants in the environment are essential for: *(1)* the quantita-

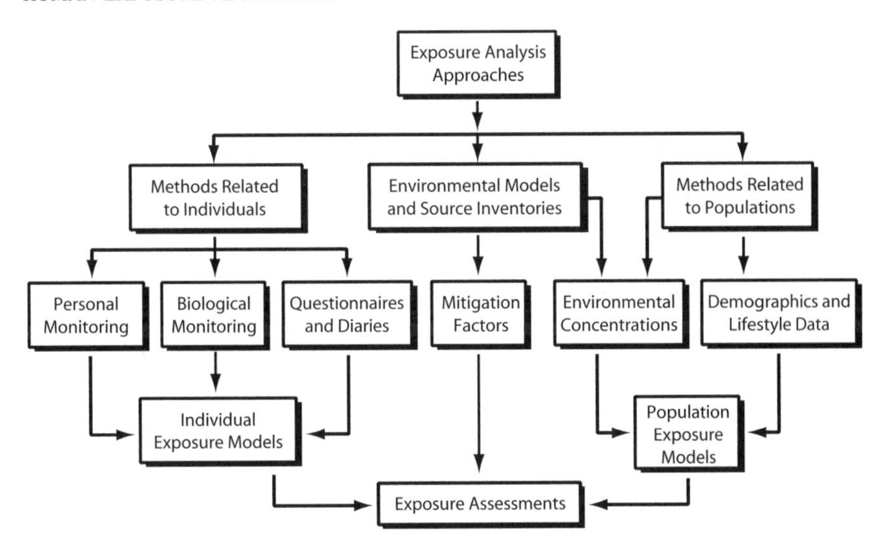

FIGURE 8–1. Possible approaches for analysis of contaminant exposures.

tive evaluation of potential hazards to human health and welfare; *(2)* for identifying and evaluating sources; and *(3)* for monitoring changes in environmental levels resulting from changes in source characteristics. Unfortunately, the level of available technology and the skills of the analysts have often been inadequate in relation to the needs. On the other hand, there has been substantial progress in recent decades in instrument capabilities, and in the adoption of guidelines and procedures for quality control, and the certification of analytical laboratories.

In practice, a large proportion of the problems in evaluating environmental contaminant levels are not related to the accuracy of laboratory evaluations but, rather, to biases resulting from the selection of nonrepresentative locations and times for sampling environments, and/or to errors introduced in the process of sample collection and field evaluations. Considerations of sampling location, sampling frequency, duration and volume, the performance characteristics of sampling instruments and collection substrates all influence the results obtained, and poor choices can bias the results. The exposure assessor generally needs both extensive technical training and professional experience in order to make optimal and appropriate choices. Some of the important considerations in environmental sampling and measurements are discussed in this chapter.

Factors Affecting Sampling Schedules and Locations

Concentrations of contaminants in the environment may be expected to vary continuously and considerably for many reasons. The rates of anthropogenic contaminant release depend upon the level of human activity and the degree of effort expended in limiting discharges. The source strengths of natural contaminants will vary with time, since they depend upon variable biological, geochemical, and meteorological factors. Ambient concentrations will also depend on the degree of dilution that takes place between the source and the sampling site, which in turn depends upon the volume of dilution fluid and its mixing characteristics.

Temporal variations

Temporal variations can have several different time constants. There may be rapid fluctuations due to fluid turbulence, which are superimposed on diurnal cycles associated with variations in sources, strengths, and dilution rates. For example, atmospheric dilution depends upon wind pattern and lapse, which, in the boundary layer, varies with solar flux and radiation from the ground surface. Dilution in aquatic environments depends upon surface-water flow, which varies greatly with rainfall.

Seasonal variations in contaminant concentrations depend on changes in source strength and mixing characteristics. Because of annual growth cycles, source strength is the dominant factor for natural contaminants, such as terpenes from coniferous forests, or pollens from plants. The contaminant releases associated with space heating also have an annual surge associated with cold weather. On the other hand, the release of the chemical raw materials involved in photochemical smog formation has little seasonal variability, and the large observed seasonal patterns in oxidant levels are attributable to the differences in solar radiation and atmospheric ventilation at various times of the year.

Spatial variations

Concentrations of contaminants vary spatially as well as temporally. Thus, it is often necessary to analyze samples drawn from many different locations in order to adequately characterize the average level in, for example, a given airshed, work environment, stream, or food source.

In practice, the choice of sampling sites may be limited by such factors as isolation from local sources and flow disturbances, accessibility for sample changing and sampler maintenance, assurance of sample integrity in relation to tampering, theft, or vandalism, and the need for utilities and/or environmental controls for proper sampler performance. These considerations, and the cost of multiple sampling sites, may lead to dependence on a sampling location not fully representative of the whole. Further evaluations may, therefore, be needed to establish the correspondence, if any, between contaminant levels measured at a fixed site and those in the larger environment it is supposed to represent.

Selection of Materials and Methods

Materials sampled

Environmental samples are generally categorized as air samples, water samples, food samples, soil samples, sediment samples, biota samples (plants and animals), and biological samples (tissues, blood, excreta, etc.).

Most air and some water sampling is done by extractive techniques, whereby the sampled fluid is passed through a collector that extracts the contaminant onto a suitable substrate and passes the fluid. The resulting contaminant samples are much less bulky, and, therefore, are generally easier to package and transport than samples that include the fluid medium as well as the contaminant. Filters are widely used for extractive sampling of suspended particles in both air and water.

Another technique used in both air and water sampling is adsorptive extraction of organics on granular beds of activated carbon or another solid sorbent. Extractions of ions from water samples can also be performed with ion exchange resins, which exchange and bind ions from the aquatic medium. Other extractive techniques that are primarily limited to air sampling include thermal and electrostatic precipitation and inertial impaction for airborne particles, and scrubbing with liquids for both particles and soluble gases.

In occupational health hazard evaluations, most of the samples collected will be on sampling substrates. Biomarker samples can also be used to evaluate the degree of chemical exposures or their effects, and are also frequently collected. They may include blood, urine, exhaled air, and occasionally other materials, such as hair, fingernails, and feces.

In ambient air evaluations, most of the samples would, of course, be extracted from the sampled air. Other samples that may occasionally be useful are sediment, either as dust fall in a collector or as constituents of surface soil, and biota. Plants can be analyzed for their uptake of contaminant or for pathological features attributable to exposure.

In water contaminant evaluations, bulk samples of water are most widely collected, and the samples for analysis are extracted in the laboratory rather than in the field. Sediment samples and biota, including rooted plants, shellfish, and finned fish, are also frequently collected. The biota may be analyzed for contaminant burdens, for pathology, or for changes in population density associated with level of contaminant.

Sample handling and preservation

Certain precautions are necessary in the handling of samples in order to ensure that the characteristics of the sample to be analyzed are not altered. Some important considerations are: *(1)* to minimize the time interval between sample collection and analysis; and *(2)* to tag or label the sample properly, and to collect supporting data to indicate the purpose of the sampling, the exact identification or location of the sampling point, the date and time(s) of sampling, the results of any measurements of ambient conditions at the sampling site, the identity of the individual who collected the sample, and the nature and extent of human activities going on in the vicinity of the sampler that could influence the air concentration being measured.

If the contaminant of interest is produced or affected by biological action, or if the material sampled is chemically or thermally unstable, or can be adsorbed on the container surface, the samples will require special handling to prevent changes in composition between sample collection and analysis.

Since available preservation techniques may not be sufficient in all cases, some analyses are usually performed only at the sampling site, for example, pH and DO measurements in aquatic environments.

Types of samples

There are many kinds of samples that can provide information useful to contaminant evaluations, and it is important not to confuse or misinterpret the contaminant levels found in specific samples. The basic types of samples are: *(1)* source; *(2)* ambient; *(3)* personal; and *(4)* process.

Source samples include stack samples for airborne effluents and discharge-pipe or channel samples for liquid effluents. They can provide essential information on source strengths, but are of very limited value in evaluating exposures to populations.

Ambient samples provide information on environmental contaminant levels in representative locations within airsheds and waterways. They can be used to indicate whether established standards are being exceeded, and to monitor trends in contaminant levels. The samples are of limited value in identifying or locating specific sources, or for estimating exposure levels for individuals within the population.

Personal samples are used to determine air contaminant exposure levels within the immediate environment of specific individuals. The samplers need to be light in weight and self-contained, so as not to limit the mobility or normal activity of the wearer. They are most widely used to evaluate inhalation exposures of workers, and are also used in some community epidemiological studies where indoor exposures are of special interest.

Process samples are samples collected within process equipment and transfer lines, which are taken to characterize mass flowrates or stream composition. Samples up- and downstream of a pollution-control device belong in this category. The concentrations measured may be very high, but may bear little relation to quantities discharged to the environment, and even less to ambient environmental levels.

Sampling efficiency

It is generally desirable to select the sample collector and its operating conditions so that the fraction of the contaminant of interest that penetrates the collector will be negligible. However, the analyses can be just as reliable when the collection efficiency is much lower, provided that it is known and constant. In this case, a correction factor can be applied. The collection of gases and vapors in air, and dissolved chemicals in water, can generally meet this criterion (provided that the ambient temperature is constant), since each molecule of a particular contaminant is essentially equivalent to every other in terms of capture probability. However, the same consideration does not apply to contaminants present as particles, since an additional variable affecting collection efficiency, i.e., particle size, is involved. Particle samplers should have essentially complete collection to avoid any sampling bias.

Sample size and analytical sensitivity

Every analytical procedure has a lower detection limit at which the accuracy of measurement falls below an acceptable level. If the results of the analysis are to be useful, the amount of the specific contaminant in the sample must be as large as, and preferably many times greater than, this limit. Therefore, for a contaminant of interest, the quantity to be sampled depends on two factors: *(1)* its estimated environmental concentration; and *(2)* the size of the sample to be analyzed.

In extractive sampling, the amount sampled depends on: *(1)* the rate of sample flow; and *(2)* the duration of the sampling interval. Sample size can be increased either by increasing the time interval or the sampling rate. However, freedom to change the rate may be limited in some cases, since sampling efficiency may be rate-dependent. Sampling rates may also be limited by the size, power requirements, or suction capacity of the sampling equipment.

The selection of an appropriate sample size in a given situation must also involve a consideration of the basic reason for collecting the sample. If the purpose is to compare an ambient level to an established standard or specified action level, the sample should be large enough to permit the determination of a specified fraction of that standard or level. The fraction used is generally 1/10, although equipment limitations may dictate acceptance of a fraction as high as 1/2.

Time of sampling

In the measurement of contaminant levels, it is important to characterize both the total time and specific time intervals of sampling. In deciding when and how long to sample, the kind and degree of temporal variability likely to occur must be considered, as well as whether it is more important to determine peak levels or average levels. In other words, the individual specifying the sampling frequency and duration should appreciate and anticipate the uses to be made of the resulting data.

Samples that are collected within a brief period are called "grab" samples. Samples collected at a constant rate over a longer period of time are known as integrated samples. While there is no precise demarcation between grab and integrated samples, the former are generally collected in less than a few minutes.

In most cases, grab sampling involves filling a container of a known volume with the fluid being sampled. Examples include filling a 1 liter bottle with water from an effluent discharge or stream, or filling a plastic bag with exhaled air for breath analysis. By contrast, integrated samples are usually of the extractive type.

Sampling substrate

In extractive sampling, the contaminant of interest is deposited onto or into materials that will retain it effectively throughout the balance of the sample collection process, and through any subsequent transport and storage prior to analysis. The material that retains the extracted substance is known as the sampling substrate. A good substrate must not only efficiently retain the sampled material prior to analysis, it must also permit it to be analyzed efficiently in the laboratory. It must either be possible to separate the sampled material from the substrate quantitatively, or it must be possible to perform the analysis in the presence of the substrate. A given substrate may be ideal for some analyses and entirely unsuitable for others where, for example, its presence may preclude the analysis of choice, or where it may contain constituents that would interfere with the analysis.

Specificity and interferences

One of the most difficult aspects of the analytical chemistry of environmental contaminants is that one is generally applying trace microanalytical techniques to samples of mixed composition. The presence of cocontaminants of unknown composition and concentration may either enhance or depress the response characteristic of the material being analyzed. When the potential for interferences is known, it is generally desirable to achieve greater analytical specificity by performing chemical separations prior to the analyses.

Legal requirements

When sampling is performed to demonstrate conformance with legal codes or standards, it may be necessary to use certain specified sampling and analytical procedures rather than, or in addition to, those best suited to scientific investigation.

Sample collection vs. direct measurements

In this discussion, sample collection refers to the collection of a defined weight or volume of sampled material for a subsequent laboratory analysis or series of analyses. The analyses are performed at a later time, and the results are not generally available until long after the sampling has been completed. In other words, there is no possibility of feedback to guide further sampling or to initiate immediate reduction of exposure.

In direct measurements, on the other hand, the sampling and analysis are performed in the same instrument. This technique allows feedback during the sampling period at the sampling site, so that the site and/or frequency of sampling may be modified so as to permit a more thorough evaluation of exposure and its determinants or to justify a prompt shutdown or evacuation when exposures are acutely hazardous.

Some direct reading instruments are known as continuous analyzers. In these, an intrinsic property of the contaminant is measured as the sampling stream passes through a sensing zone. There may be no sample collection, and an uninterrupted output response is a direct function of the concentration of the contaminant of interest. The output can be recorded, and can also be integrated to yield average concentrations over specified time intervals.

Other types of direct measurements are based upon extractive sample collection and immediate analysis of the sample. These instruments perform collection and analysis within the same housing, and are known as semicontinuous analyzers. A representative fraction of the contaminant is obtained and analyzed, and the process then repeats itself. The measurement phase is generally performed on a liquid, after controlled dosage of a reagent chemical, using electrochemical or colorimetric techniques. In air sampling, the contaminant is first extracted by a collecting liquid in a gas washer or scrubber. Ideally, the analyzing period is sufficiently short so that no significant chemical changes occur before another sample is measured. However, because of the finite time lag (on the order of a few minutes) between the sampling and measurement steps, and as a result of the mixing and diffusion within the liquid stream, a monitor of this type has a slower response than does a continuous gas-phase analyzer.

In using direct-reading instrumentation, accurate calibration is essential to the correct interpretation of instrument response. Calibration, which may be defined as the determination of the true values of the scale readings of the instrument, generally involves a comparison of instrument response to that of a reference instrument or to a standardized atmosphere or solution.

There are a number of advantages to direct measurements. These include: both peak and average concentrations can be determined; results are immediately available, permitting one to track down sources and initiate corrective actions as appropriate; continuous and unattended operation is possible under some circumstances, continuous recordings of concentrations may be useful in retrospective data evaluations and, in industry, as legal documentation of employee exposures for compliance with established standards.

On the other hand, there are many distinct advantages in sample collection with subsequent laboratory evaluations. For example, sample collection is a much simpler operation than is quantitative chemical analysis, and the hardware needed for collection is less expensive, smaller, and less sensitive to mechanical and thermal stresses. Being smaller and more portable in most cases, the sampling equipment is easier to transport and operate in the field, and can be set up in locations not suitable for continuous monitors. The analyses performed in the laboratory on field-collected samples can be more sensitive, accurate, and reliable. The samples can be analyzed by highly specialized equipment units that cannot be incorporated into field monitors. A series of different analyses can be performed on each sample, and the effects of cocontaminants can be eliminated by preliminary chemical separations.

Measurements of Fluid Flow

Characterization of chemical contamination in air or water generally requires data on fluid flow as well as quantitative chemical analyses. For example, when extractive sampling techniques are used, the determination of concentration requires measurement of both the sampled volume as well as the amount of chemical contaminant in the sample. Furthermore, the concentration at the sampling location may be different from that at other locations, and the determination of contaminant transport in a surface stream or airborne plume may require measurements of flow and concentration at many points.

Flowmeters can be divided into three basic groups on the basis of the type of measurement made; there are integral-volume meters, flowrate meters, and velocity meters. In volume meters and flowrate meters, the whole fluid stream passes through the instrument. In this respect, they differ from velocity meters, which measure the velocity at a particular point of the flow cross section. Since the flow profile is rarely uniform, the measured velocity will almost always differ from the average velocity, and it may be necessary to make a large number of measurements in order to determine the average value. However, when the flow field is very large, velocity sensors may be the only indicators than can be used.

Integral-volume meters

Some integral-volume meters are used exclusively for measurements in air; these include the wet-test meter and dry-gas meter. Others, which operate by positive displacement, are available for both air and liquid flow metering.

A wet-test meter (Fig. 8–2) consists of a partitioned drum half submerged in a liquid (usually water), with openings at the center and periphery of each radial chamber. Air or gas enters at the center and flows into an individual compartment causing it to rise, thereby producing rotation. This rotation is indicated by a dial on the face of the instrument. The volume measured will be dependent on the fluid level in the meter, since the liquid is displaced by air.

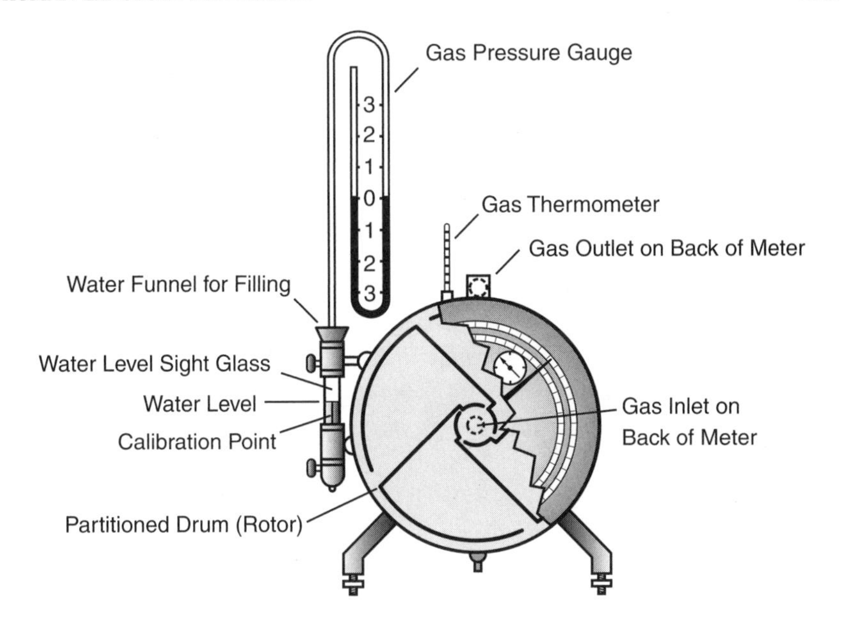

FIGURE 8–2. Schematic diagram of a wet-test meter.

The dry-gas meter shown in Figure 8–3 is very similar to the domestic gas meter. It consists of two bags interconnected by mechanical valves and a cycle-counting device. The air or gas fills one bag while the other bag empties. When the cycle is completed, the valves are switched and the second bag fills while the first one empties. The alternate filling of two chambers as the basis for volume measurements is also used in twin-cylinder piston meters. Such piston meters can also be classified as positive displacement devices.

Positive-displacement meters consist of a tight-fitting moving element with individual volume compartments that fill at an inlet and discharge at an outlet. Another type of multicompartment continuous rotary meter uses interlocking gears.

Volumetric flowrate meters

The integral-volume meters discussed above are all based upon the principle of conservation of mass; specifically, the transfer of a fluid volume from one location to another. On the other hand, the flowrate meters described in this section operate upon the principle of the conservation of energy; they are based upon Bernoulli's theorem for the exchange of potential energy for kinetic energy and/or frictional heat. Each consists of a flow restriction within a closed conduit. The restriction causes an increase in the fluid velocity and, therefore, an increase in kinetic energy, which requires a corresponding decrease in potential energy, i.e., static pressure. The flowrate can be calculated from a knowledge of the pressure drop, the flow cross section at the constriction, the density of the fluid, and the

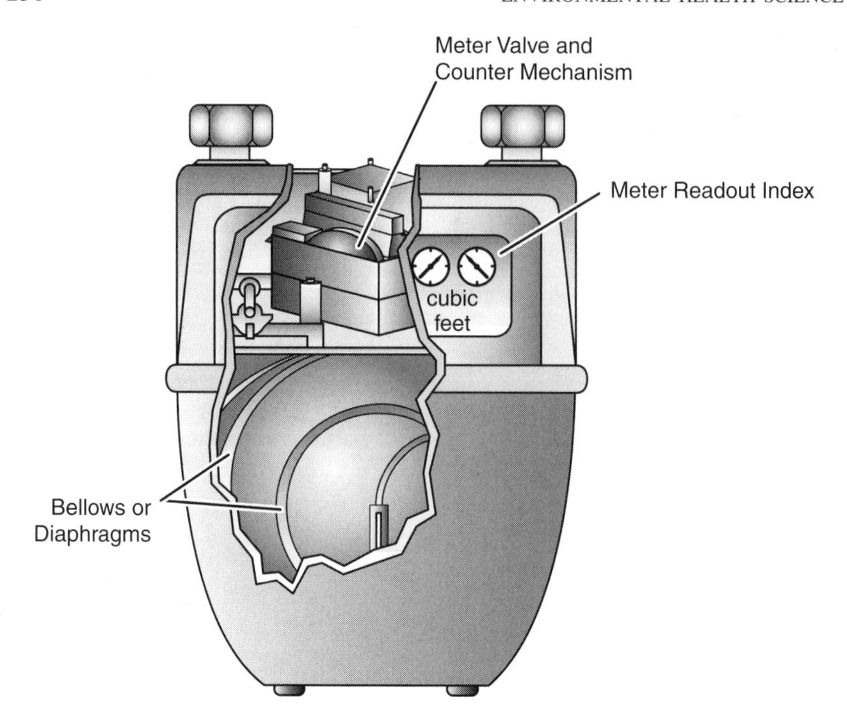

FIGURE 8–3. Schematic diagram of a dry-gas meter.

coefficient of discharge, which is the ratio of actual flow to theoretical flow (and makes allowance for stream contraction and frictional effects).

Flowmeters that operate upon the conservation of energy principle can be divided into two groups. One group, which includes orifice meters, venturi meters, and flow nozzles, consists of devices that have a fixed restriction; these instruments are known as variable-head meters, because the differential pressure head varies with flow. A special subclass of this group includes weirs and flumes specifically used to measure flowrates of water. In these, the flow channel is only partially filled with water, and the height of the water column in the restriction varies, providing an indication of the flowrate. The other, smaller, group, which includes rotameters, are known as variable-area meters, because a constant pressure differential is maintained by varying the flow cross section.

A rotameter (Fig. 8–4a) contains a "float," which is free to move up and down within a vertical tapered tube that is larger at the top than the bottom. The fluid flows upward, causing the float to rise until the pressure drop across the annular area between the float and the tube wall is just sufficient to support the float. The tapered tube is usually made of glass or clear plastic, and has a flowrate scale etched directly on it. The height of the float indicates the flowrate. Floats of various configurations are used, as indicated in Figure 8–4b. The term ro-

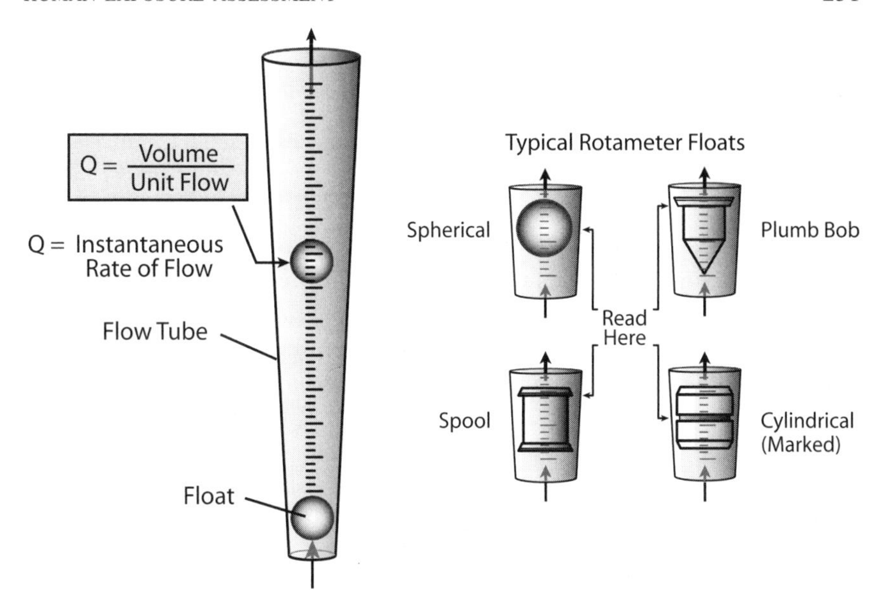

FIGURE 8–4. Typical rotameter.

tameter was first used to describe variable-area meters with spinning floats, but now is generally used for all types of tapered metering tubes.

The simplest form of variable-head meter is the square-edged, or sharp-edged, orifice illustrated in Figure 8–5. It is also the most widely used, because of its ease of installation and low cost. While the square-edged orifice can provide

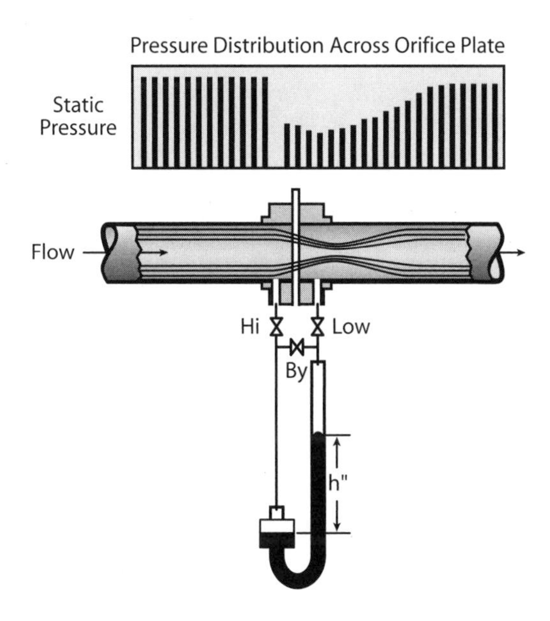

FIGURE 8–5. Pipe-line orifice.

accurate flow measurements at low cost, it is inefficient with respect to energy loss. The permanent pressure loss for an orifice meter due to turbulence will often exceed 80%.

Venturi meters have converging and diverging angles of about 25° and 7°, respectively. They have high pressure recoveries, i.e., the potential energy, which is converted to kinetic energy at the throat, is reconverted to potential energy at the discharge, with an overall permanent loss of only about 10%. The characteristics of various other types of variable head flowmeters, for example, flow nozzles (Fig. 8–6), centrifugal flow elements, etc., are similar in most respects to those of either the orifice meter, venturi meter, or both.

For water flow in open channels, the most common flow measurement techniques utilize weirs or flumes. A weir is essentially a dam or obstruction placed in the stream. It generally consists of a vertical plate with a sharp crest; the top of the plate is either straight, notched, or rectangular shaped (Fig. 8–7). The water level at a given distance upstream from the weir is proportional to the flow rate.

There are a number of different types of flumes. The Parshall flume (Fig. 8–8) is a device that is similar to a venturi meter in that it consists of a converging section, a throat, and a diverging section. The level of the floor in the converging section is higher than the floor in the throat and diverging section. The head of the water surface in the converging section is a measure of the velocity through the flume and, therefore, of flowrate.

The flowrate in a pipe or tube may be strongly dependent on the flow resistance, and flowmeters with a very low resistance may be bulky and/or expensive. A metering element used in such cases is the bypass rotameter, which actually meters only a small fraction of the total flow; however, this fraction is proportional to the total flow. As shown schematically in Figure 8–9, a bypass flowmeter contains both a variable-head element and a variable area element. The pressure drop across the fixed orifice or flow restrictor creates a proportionate flow through the parallel path containing the small rotameter. The scale on the rotameter indicates the total flow.

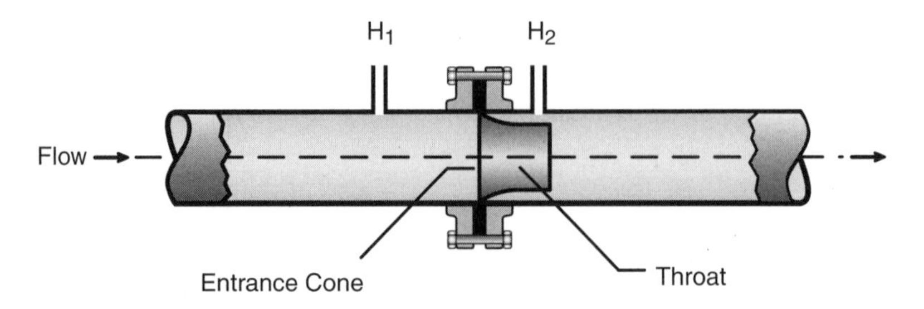

FIGURE 8–6. Flow nozzle (in a pipe).

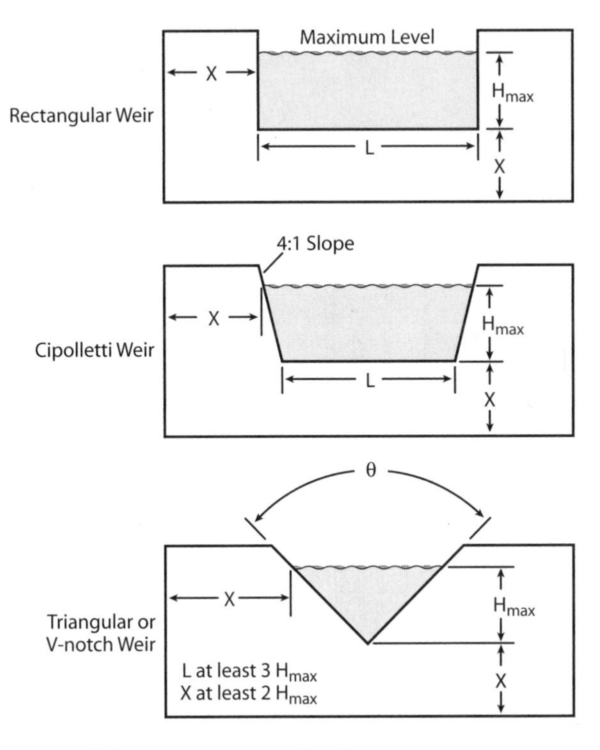

FIGURE 8–7. Common types of weirs.

Flowrates of aqueous discharges from pipes can also be estimated by measuring the distance the flow is projected from the end of an open pipe, as illustrated in Figure 8–10.

For small volumetric flows of water, where the stream can be diverted into a vessel of known volume, the rate of flow can be determined by measuring the

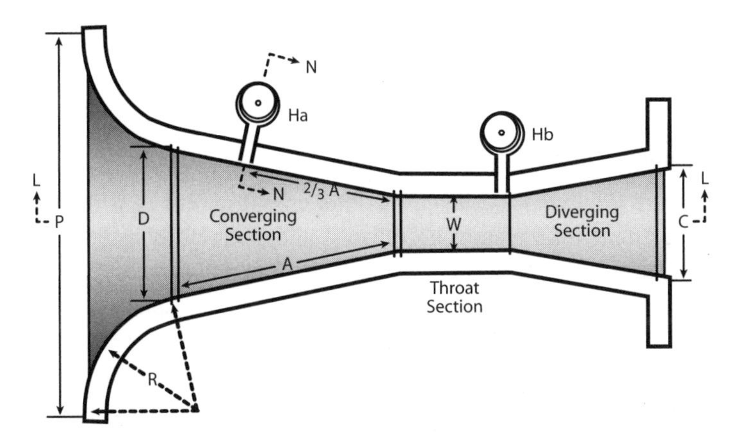

FIGURE 8–8. Parshall flume.

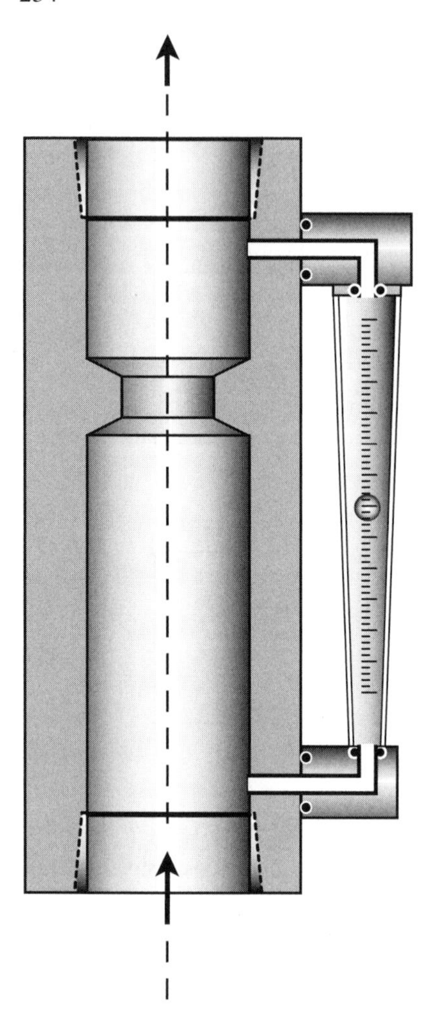

FIGURE 8–9. Schematic of a bypass flowmeter.

time required to fill the vessel. This is known as the bucket and-stopwatch technique.

Flow velocity meters

One type of flow velocity meter, the Pitot tube (Fig. 8–11), is often used as a reference instrument for measuring velocity, and, if carefully made, will need no calibration. It consists of an impact tube whose opening faces axially into the flow, and a concentric static pressure tube with eight holes spaced equally around it in a plane that is eight diameters from the impact opening. The difference between the static and impact pressures is the velocity pressure. Bernoulli's theorem applied to a Pitot tube in a stream simplifies to the dimensionless formula:

$$V = \sqrt{2gP_v} \tag{8–1}$$

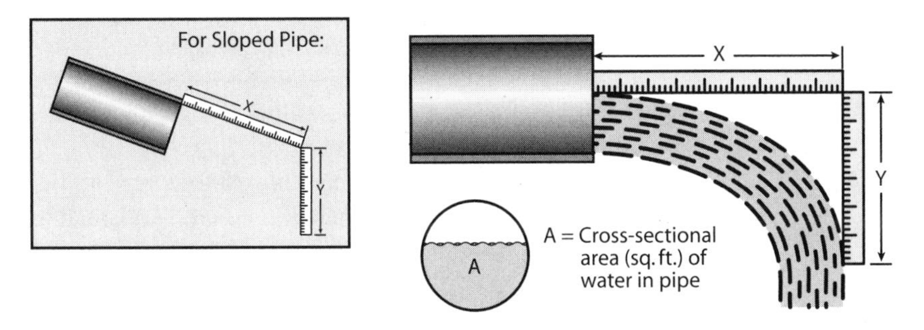

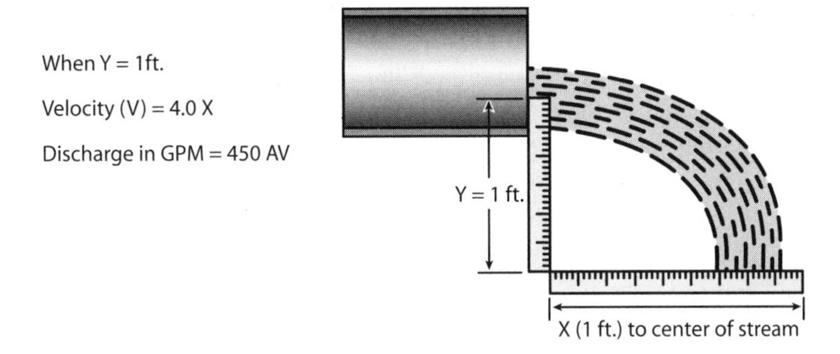

FIGURE 8–10. Flowrate measurements based upon the distance a stream is projected from the end of an open pipe.

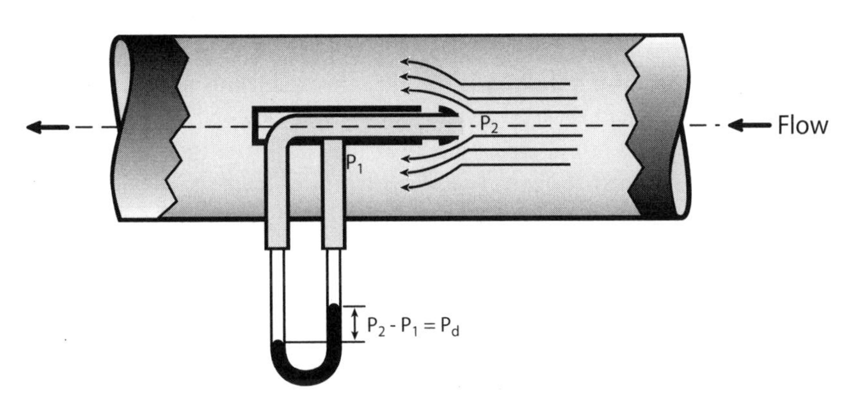

FIGURE 8–11. Pitot tube.

where:

V = linear velocity

g = gravitational constant

P_v = pressure head of flowing fluid (velocity pressure)

There are several other ways beside the Pitot tube to utilize the kinetic energy of a flowing fluid to measure velocity. One technique is to align a jeweled-bearing turbine wheel axially in the stream and count the number of rotations per unit time. Such devices are known as rotating-vane flowmeters. Some are very small and are used as velocity probes. Others are sized to fit the whole duct and become indicators of total flowrate; these latter devices are sometimes called turbine flowmeters.

Mass flow and tracer techniques

A thermal meter measures mass flowrate with negligible pressure loss. It consists of a heating element in a pipe or duct section between two points at which the temperature of the stream is measured. The temperature difference between the two points is dependent on the mass rate of flow and the heat input.

The principle of mixture metering is similar to that of thermal metering. However, instead of adding heat and measuring temperature difference, a tracer is added and its increase in concentration is measured, or clean fluid is added and the reduction in concentration is measured. The measuring device may react to some physical property, such as thermal conductivity or vapor pressure.

Mass flow may also be obtained using an ion-flow meter. In this device, ions are generated from a central disc and flow radially toward a collector surface. Airflow through the cylinder causes an axial displacement of the ion stream in direct proportion to the mass flow.

An instrument specifically used for measuring water flow is the magnetic flowmeter (Fig. 8–12). This apparatus operates according to Faraday's Law of Induction, i.e., the voltage induced by a conductor moving at right angles through a magnetic field will be proportional to the velocity of movement of the conductor through the field. In this device, the water is the conductor and a set of electromagnetic coils in the meter produces the field. The induced voltage is measured to obtain the flowrate.

Factors affecting the selection of flow-metering devices for aqueous streams are rated in Table 8–1.

The surface velocity of water may be measured by placing floating objects (e.g., wood, cork, etc.) in the stream and measuring the time required for the object to traverse a measured distance between two points. The velocity within a given length of channel may also be obtained by the use of dyes.

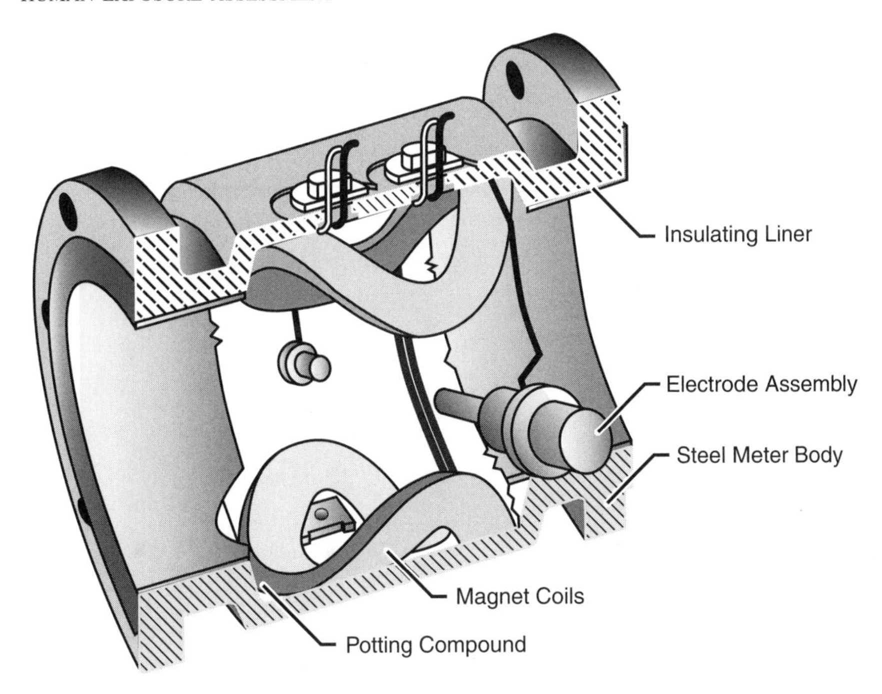

FIGURE 8–12. Magnetic flowmeter.

Air Sampling

Instrumentation

A description of available instrumentation for air sampling can easily occupy a large reference volume. Therefore, for a more comprehensive review, the reader is referred to other sources, such as Air Sampling Instruments[1] or to the appropriate chapters in the multivolume reference works of Patty.[2] The discussion to follow will be limited to the more fundamental considerations in the selection of instruments and sampling techniques for air contaminant evaluations.

Elements of an air-sampling train

There are a number of essential elements that comprise a sampling system, known as a sampling train. These may all be incorporated into a single compact housing or portable instrument, or they may be separate elements.

A sampling probe is needed when sampling in a moving stream, such as in a duct or stack, and, when used, is the first element in the train. It is not needed when sampling from relatively still air in the ambient atmosphere or at the breathing zone of a worker. In such cases, it should not be used, since it would present some opportunity for sample losses without any corresponding benefit.

TABLE 8–1. Selection Chart for Water Flow Measuring Devices

	ORIFICE							
	CONCENTRIC	SEGMENTAL OR ECCENTRIC	VENTURI	NOZZLE	PITOT	ELBOW	LO-LOSS TUBE	MAGNETIC FLOW METER[a]
Accuracy, and amount of empirical data	E	F	G	G	*	P	G	E
Differential for given flow and size	E	E	G	G	F	P	E	None
Pressure recovery	P	P	G	P	E	E	E	E
Use on dirty service	P	F	E	G	VP	P	G	E
For liquids containing vapors	E[b]	E	E	G	F	F	G	E
For vapors containing condensate	E[c]	E	E	G	P	F	G	None
For viscous flows	F	U	G	G	†	U	F	E
First cost small size	E	G	P	F	G	E	P	P
First cost large size	E	G	P	F	G	E	P	P
Ease of changing capacity	E	G	P	F	VP	VP	P	E
Convenience of installation	G	G	F[d]	F	E	E	F[d]	F[e]

All ratings are relative: E, excellent; G, good; F, fair; P, poor; VP, very poor; U, unknown.

*For measuring velocity at one point in conduit, the well-designed pitot tube is reliable. For measuring total flow, accuracy depends on velocity traverse.

†Requires a velocity traverse.

[a]Restricted to conducting liquids.

[b]Excellent in vertical line if flow is upward.

[c]Excellent in vertical line if flow is downward.

[d]Both flange type and insert type available.

[e]Requires pipe reducers if meter size is different from pipe size.

(*Source*: U.S. Environmental Protection Agency.)

In sampling quiescent air, the inlet configuration of the sampler is a significant element of the train, and one whose influence is not always recognized, especially when sampling for particulate matter. The inlet size and configuration, in conjunction with the sampling flowrate, establish an actual upper size cutoff for particle acceptance; particles larger than this size will not be aspirated into the inlet.

The next element in the train is the sample collector. It should precede other elements, such as flow-measuring devices and pumps, which could remove or add contaminants to the sample stream. The selection of the type of sample collector depends on the nature of the sample to be collected and is discussed in the next section.

A pressure sensor should be located downstream of the sample collector, preceding the inlet to the flow-metering element. There will usually be a significant pressure drop between the inlet to the probe or sample collector and the inlet to the flowmeter, due to the flow resistance of the sample collector and the flow path itself. Most flowmeters are calibrated for atmospheric pressure inlets and, therefore, require a correction when used with a reduced inlet pressure. The necessity for, and magnitude of, the correction can be determined by a static pressure measurement at this point.

The accuracy of the concentration measurement is equally dependent on the sampled volume as on the mass of the collected sample. The sampled volume can either be determined directly by an integrating flowmeter, or from the product of the flowrate and the sampling interval. Flowrate measurements are made more frequently than integrated volume measurements, because the meters are generally smaller, lighter, and less expensive. The precision of many flowmeters used in air sampling is, unfortunately, frequently poor, and may act to limit the overall reliability of the concentration determination. Care should be taken to avoid leakage between the inlet of the sampler and the inlet of the flowmeter, so that the volume measured represents only sampled air. Leakage downstream of the flowmeter can reduce the sampling rate, but would not affect the accuracy of the measurement. The most commonly used flowrate meters in air samplers are rotameters and orifice meters.

The final element of the train is the air mover or suction source. It can be an air pump, a blower or fan, or an ejector. An ejector is a device that uses a stream of high-pressure fluid flowing through a jet to create a secondary stream of sampled air. The fluid can be compressed air, steam, or water. The selection of air-mover type and size is dependent on the choice of sampling rate and the pressure drop to be overcome in maintaining the desired flow.

The sequence of the train elements is important, but not sacred. Circumstances sometimes lead to the selection of a different configuration, and this is acceptable when it can be demonstrated that excessive losses or errors are not introduced. Some typical sampling-train elements and their normal sequence are illustrated in Figure 8–13.

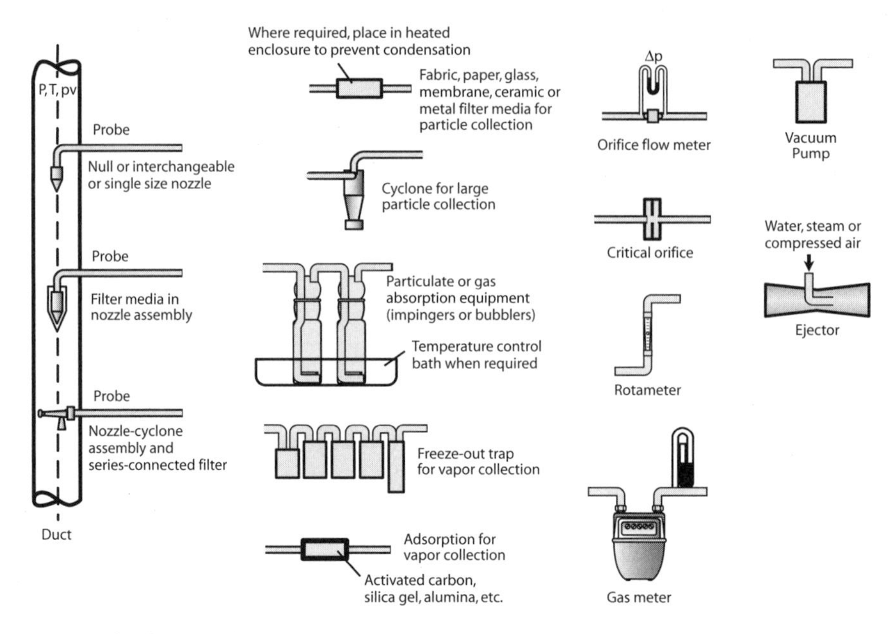

FIGURE 8–13. Sampling system components.

Sample collectors for gases and vapors

Gases and vapors can be extracted from an airstream by absorption, adsorption, or condensation. The most common absorption technique involves intimate contact between gas bubbles and an absorbing liquid. Gas washers in various configurations are illustrated in Figure 8–14. Table 8–2 presents examples of some gases commonly collected in liquid sorbents.

The airstream may be broken down into bubbles by a submerged jet, as in impingers (Fig. 8–14, gas washer *A*) and simple bubblers (Fig. 8–14, gas washer *B*). Finer bubbles, and, hence, greater gas-liquid contact and removal efficiency, can be obtained by passing the air through a porous plug or frit rather than a single orifice jet. Such a device, known as a fritted bubbler, is illustrated in Fig. 8–14, gas washer *D*.

Absorption can also take place into a liquid film on a solid support. The support can be a screen or filter that has been coated with a reagent chemical. The airstream can be drawn through the screen or filter, or these devices can be used as passive samplers. In the latter, the gas or vapor molecules to be trapped reach the collection surface by molecular diffusion. The NO_2 sampler[3] illustrated in Figure 8–15 utilizes an orifice as a diffusion barrier of known characteristics in order to eliminate the effects of bulk fluid motion on the transport rate of NO_2 from the ambient source to the collection surface at the screen.

Gases and vapors can also be captured by adsorption onto surfaces. The most commonly used adsorption collectors are cylinders filled with granules of an ef-

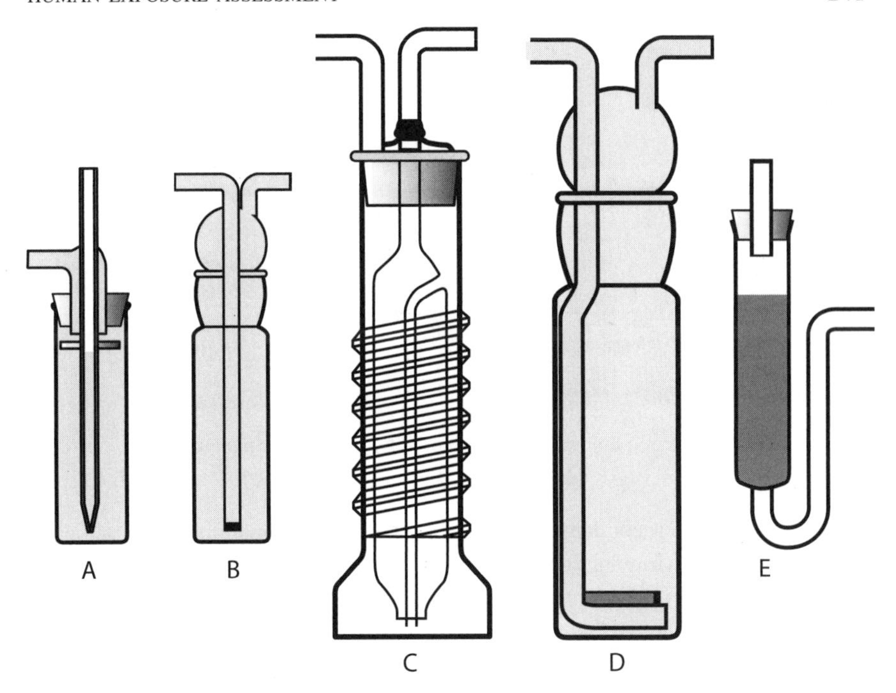

FIGURE 8–14. Various gas washers: (A) Midget impinger; (B) simple gas washer; (C) spiral absorber; (D) fritted bubbler; (E) glass-bead column.

ficient adsorbent, such as activated charcoal or silica gel. As a gas stream is drawn through such a bed, the molecules reach the surfaces of the granules by molecular diffusion. The O_2, N_2, and Ar molecules are not retained, but molecules of the contaminant of interest can be adsorbed by granules of suitable composition. Solid sorbents are generally used for the collection of organic gases and vapors.

TABLE 8–2. Some Gases and Vapors Collected in Liquid Sorbents

CHEMICAL	SAMPLE COLLECTOR	SORPTION MEDIUM
Ammonia	Impinger	Sulfuric acid
Carbon dioxide	Fritted bubbler	Barium hydroxide
Formaldehyde	Fritted bubbler	Sodium bisulfite
Hydrogen sulfide	Impinger	Cadmium sulfate
Methyl mercury	Impinger	Iodine monochloride in hydrochloric acid
Ozone	Impinger	Potassium iodide in potassium hydroxide
Sulfur dioxide	Impinger	Sodium tetrachloromercurate

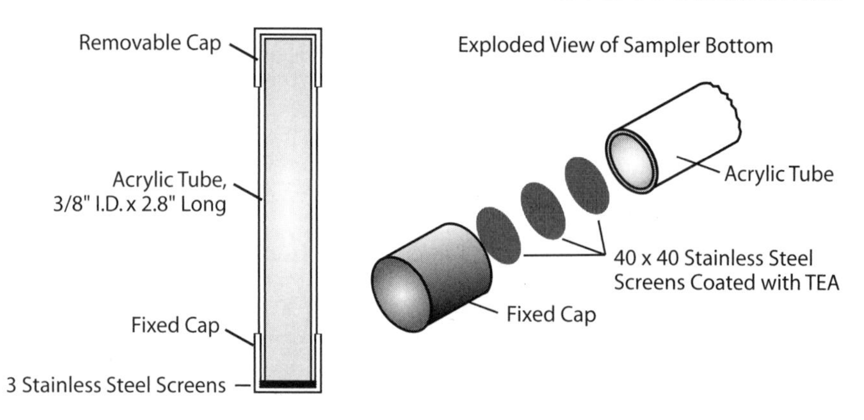

FIGURE 8–15. Schematic diagram of personal NO_2 sampler (Palmes tube).

Contaminants that condense into liquids or solids below ambient temperature can be removed by drawing them past cooled collection surfaces, which are sometimes called "cold traps." One complication is that the condensate will generally include a large volume of water unless the water vapor in the atmosphere can be removed before the cold trap.

Sample collectors for aerosols

While useful for gas sampling, the impinger, shown in Figure 8–14a, was actually designed to sample mineral dusts. The airstream is accelerated as it passes through the orifice nozzle, and particles larger than about 0.75 μm are efficiently collected when they strike the submerged plate and are wetted. The standard formerly used for silica-bearing dusts was based on the particle concentration measured in the suspension within the flask.

In more recent years, almost all particle sampling has been performed using dry-collection techniques. These include other inertial samplers, such as impactors, cyclones, and centrifuges, as well as filtration, electrostatic precipitation, and thermal precipitation.

Inertial Collectors. An impactor is very similar to an impinger, but does not use a trapping liquid. The airstream is accelerated through a nozzle and directed at a collection surface. Particles larger than a certain size (known as the cut-size) strike the surface and may be retained; smaller particles, having less momentum, are carried away with the carrier flow. The cut-size depends on the velocity in the jet. At ambient pressures, the smallest cut-size readily attainable is about 0.5 μm diameter; lower cut-sizes can be attained by operating the sampler within a vacuum chamber. If the particles and the collection surface are both dry, the particles are more likely to bounce and escape rather than be retained. Impactors can only be used successfully for such applications when the collection plate is coated with an adhesive layer. However, even with the use of an adhesive, collection must be limited to avoid particle bounce. The adhesive can rapidly become saturated, and particles striking those already collected are poorly retained.

In a series or cascade impactor (Fig. 8–16), the same volumetric flow is passed through a series of impaction jets, with each successive stage having a smaller jet cross section and particle cut-size. It, therefore, sorts the aerosol into a series of fractions on the basis of aerodynamic particle size. Knowing the proportions of the sample mass on each stage, and the stage constants (i.e., the cut-sizes of each stage), the overall size distribution of the sampled aerosol may be estimated.

Another widely used type of inertial sampler is the cyclone. In the cyclone configuration illustrated in Figure 8–17, the sampled air is drawn into a tangential inlet. The flow follows a spiral path downward along the outer wall and then forms a tighter spiral as it flows up the axial exit pipe. Particles larger than the cut-size strike the outer wall and either remain there or migrate slowly down the wall into the conical section at the bottom. The major application of cyclones as samplers is as the first stage of a two-stage collector. They can also be used for aerodynamic size distribution evaluations in a multicyclone array, with each cy-

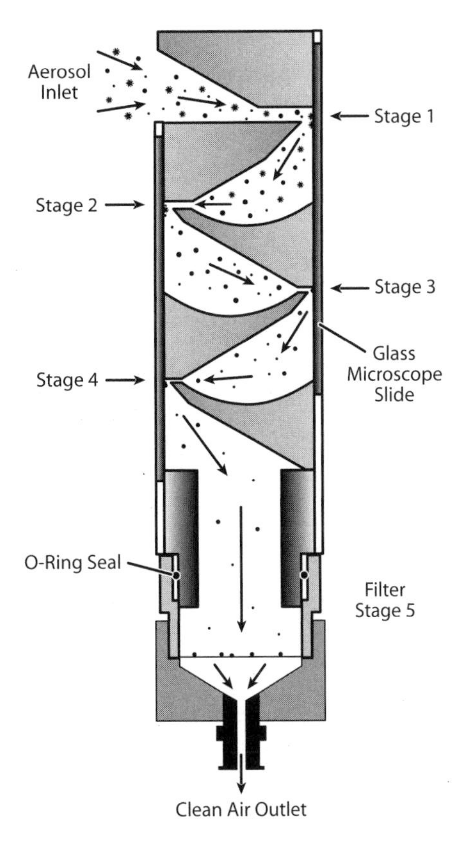

FIGURE 8–16. Diagrammatic cross-sectional view of a cascade impactor while sampling. The particle size is exaggerated.

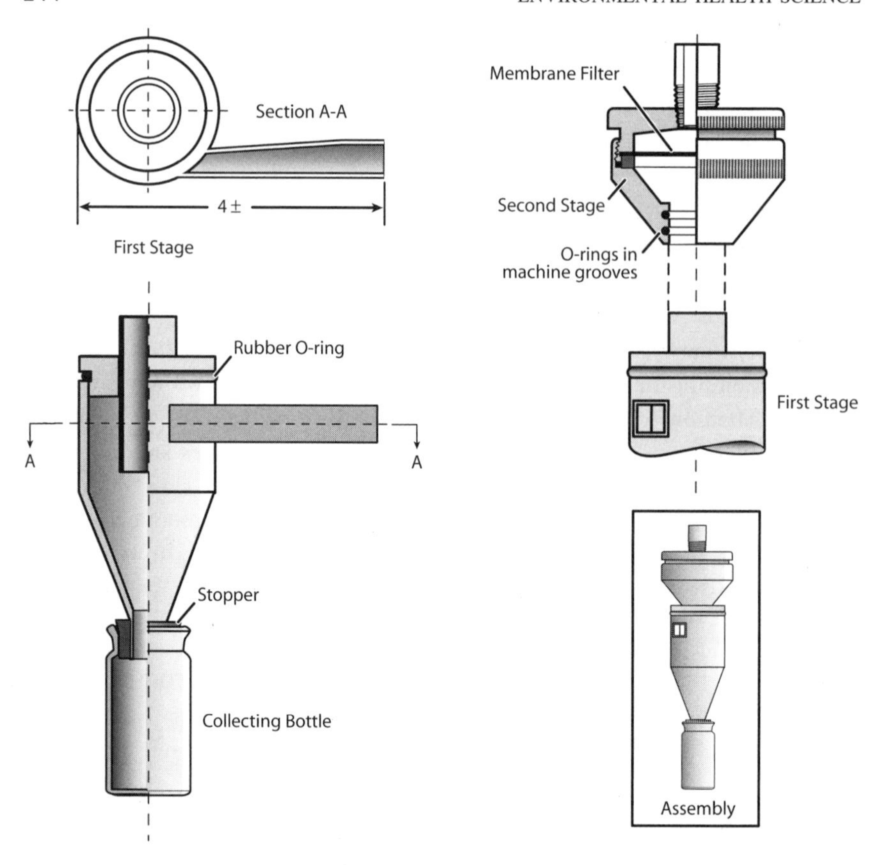

FIGURE 8–17. A miniature cyclone-filter unit for two-stage sampling of aerosols.

clone having a different cut-size. Their advantage over cascade impactors for such applications lies in the much larger sample masses that can be collected without artifacts due to particle bounce.

More precise separations and collection capabilities for smaller particles can be achieved using aerosol centrifuges. The particles enter at one side of a laminar flow channel and are deposited gently along a collection foil according to their aerodynamic diameter. However, the aerosol centrifuges are basically laboratory instruments, their sampling flowrates are very low, and they are relatively large and expensive.

Filtration. Filters are currently the most widely used type of aerosol sampler. While no single type of filter is suitable for all applications, filters are available in a wide variety of types, ratings, and sizes, so that there is generally one or more that are well suited for each particular application. Thus, one can generally take full advantage of their inherent advantages: minimal equipment, low cost, and convenience with respect to sample handling.

There are four basic types of filters: *(1)* fibrous filters, consisting of a mat of randomly oriented fibers of cellulose, glass, asbestos, polystyrene, etc.; *(2)* membrane filters, consisting of a plastic material with a gel structure having interconnecting pores; *(3)* polycarbonate pore filters, which are a solid sheet with uniform parallel holes; and *(4)* granular beds. The basic structures of polycarbonate pore and fiber filters are illustrated schematically in Figure 8–18.

In selecting a filter for a given task, the following factors should be considered: *(1)* physical size, composition, and structure of the filter, and whether these would limit the analyses to be performed; *(2)* collection efficiency and flow resistance, and how they may be expected to change during the sampling interval (e.g., with loading); and *(3)* the characteristics of the available sampling pumps, and whether they can provide the desired suction capacity and sampling rate throughout the sampling interval.

While filters may appear to be very simple devices, the mechanisms by which they capture airborne particles are frequently misunderstood. The most common misconception is that they function like the sieves or screen collectors used to separate large particles from liquid streams, and that particles smaller than the pore or void size will penetrate. This is generally not the case in air filtration, where particles much smaller than the void size can be collected with very high efficiency.

The major mechanisms of particle collection operative in air filters are inertial impaction, Brownian diffusion, and interception. In some cases, where the particles or the filter material have high levels of electrical charges, electrostatic precipitation may contribute significantly to the overall collection efficiency.

While the flow path through polycarbonate pore filters is relatively simple, the flow through all other types is quite complex. The air undergoes accelerations, decelerations, and numerous branchings and directional changes in negotiating

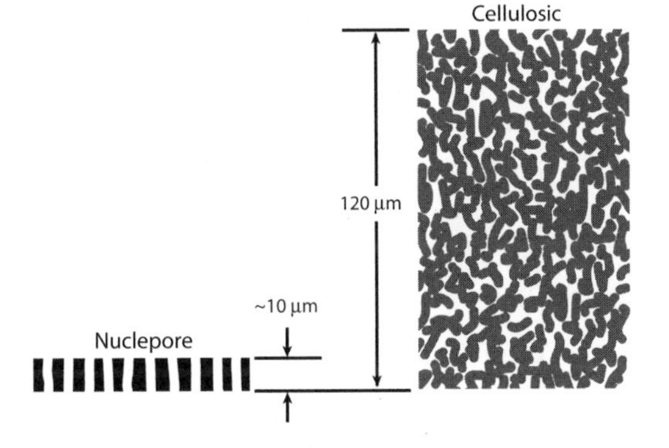

FIGURE 8–18. Cross-sectional comparisons of Nuclepore and cellulose-fiber filter thicknesses.

its way through the complex web of pores or voids. As the aerodynamic particle size and flow velocity increase, the probability of particle retention by impaction increases; with decreasing particle size and flow velocity, the particles' Brownian displacement and retention time within the filter structure increase, increasing the percentage of retention by this mechanism.

The particles most likely to penetrate the sampling filter are those that have both minimal Brownian displacement and minimal momentum. Under most conditions, maximum penetration occurs for particle diameters of about 0.3–0.5 μm. For some widely used sampling filters, such as most membrane filters with pore sizes below 3 μm and most glassfiber filters, the maximum penetration will be less than 1%. On the other hand, some commonly used cellulose fiber filters may have particle penetrations as high as 70%, and polycarbonate pore filters may have even greater penetrations. These considerations are illustrated in Figure 8–19. It can be seen that the collection efficiency of filters having characteristic penetration minima can be greatly improved when they are operated at face velocities (the velocity normal to the filter face) that are greater or lower than those at which the minima occur.

In fibrous and granular filters, there is defense in depth, i.e., the particles are collected by impaction on and diffusion to the granular or fiber surfaces throughout the depth of the filter. In order to analyze the material collected, one must either extract it from the filter or analyze it on the filter itself. On the other hand, in membrane and polycarbonate pore filters, which are much thinner, the particles are collected on or close to the upstream surface. This makes it possible to

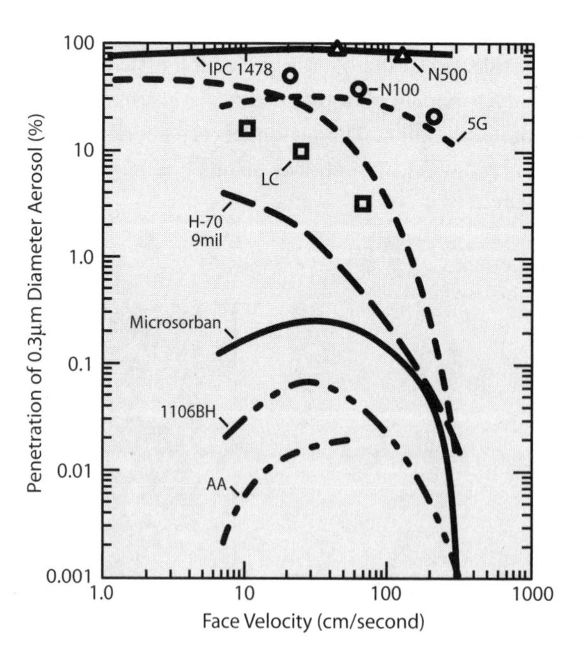

Figure 8–19. Penetration characteristics for various filters: AA-cellulose membrane, 0.8 μm pores; 1106BH-glass fiber; Microsorban-polystyrene fiber; H-70-cellulose-asbestos mixed fiber; W-41-Cellulose fiber; LC-teflon membrane, 10 μm pores; 5G-thin glass fiber; IPC 1478-thin cellulose-fiber mat; N100-Nuclepore, 1 μm pores; N500-Nuclepore, 5 μm pores.

perform some kinds of analyses without removing the sample from the surface. These include electron or optical microscopic examinations of the particles, counting of α-particle emissions without excessive α-particle absorption within the filters, and X-ray fluorescence analysis of elements with low-energy X-ray emissions.

Thermal Precipitation. Particles can be extracted from a sample stream by thermophoresis in a device known as a thermal precipitator. Prior to the mid-1950s, these were widely used in Europe to collect particles for microscopic determinations of particle number concentration and size distribution. A heated wire causes an unequal bombardment of particles by gas molecules, creating a net migration of the particles away from the wire and, in effect, a dust-free zone around the wire. When the temperature is high enough and the sampling flow-rate is low enough, the diameter of the dust-free zone can be larger than the width of the flow channel. In this situation, essentially all of the particles are collected on a linear trace, as illustrated in Figure 8–20.

Electrostatic Precipitation. When an airstream containing particles carrying electrical charges passes through a flow channel having a potential gradient normal to the flow, the charged particles will be deflected toward the electrode closer to ground potential. The efficiency of collection increases with the number of

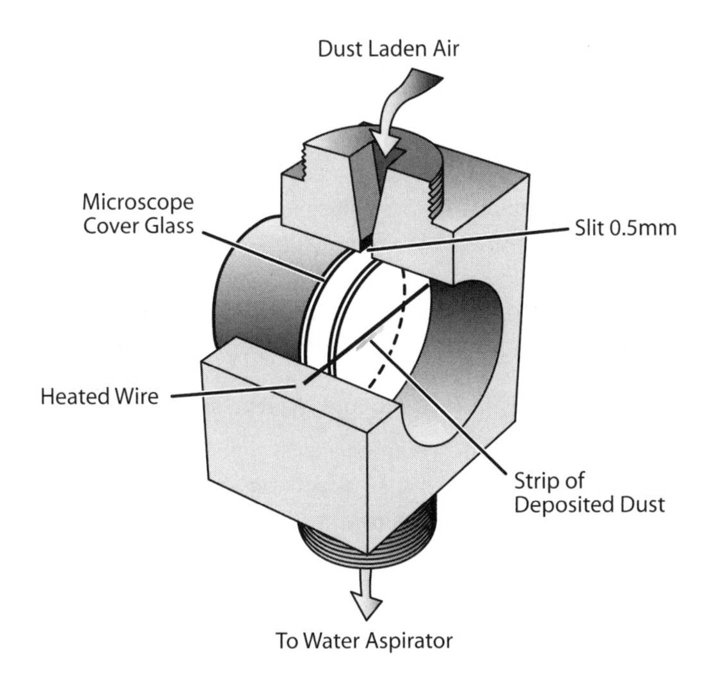

FIGURE 8–20. Sampling head of a thermal precipitator.

charges on the particle and the potential gradient. Very high collection efficiencies can be achieved in electrostatic precipitator samplers.

Electrostatic-precipitator samplers were widely used for particle sampling in the 1930s and 1940s because of their high collection efficiency and their low and constant flow resistance. Their use was limited by the precautions needed to avoid unintended high-voltage discharges. Also, they could not be used in atmospheres containing combustible vapors. With the development of improved filters for air sampling, which were simpler to use and much less expensive, electrostatic precipitation has since become limited to special sampling applications.

Special considerations in ambient air sampling

Ambient air concentrations of chemical contaminants are greatly influenced by meteorological factors, and their interpretation is, therefore, facilitated by knowledge of wind speed and direction, mixing layer depth, temperature profile, humidity, etc. It is generally desirable to have appropriate weather instrumentation that can represent ambient conditions at the sampling site.

As indicated previously, the selection of sampling sites requires a compromise between an ideal of a relatively large number of sites at strategically located positions and practical limitations imposed by fiscal constraints, availability of sites secure from malicious mischief, accessibility for sample changing and maintenance, and availability of power.

There are some special considerations in the selection of instrumentation for ambient air sampling. For airborne gases and vapors, the trend in recent years has been to use direct-reading continuous instruments having rapid-response gas-phase sensing, with each instrument being specific for a particular contaminant. Direct-reading instruments have also been favored for measurement of particle size distributions. For aerosol composition determinations, the trend has been toward sample collection in discrete aerodynamic size fractions. A size cut is made at about 2.5 μm in aerodynamic diameter, when sampling for fine particles that derive primarily from gaseous precursors. The larger particles, which derive from mechanical processes and were emitted as discrete particles below 10 μm in aerodynamic diameter, represent coarse particles that deposit in the thorax ($PM_{10\text{-}2.5}$).

Special considerations in occupational hygiene sampling

Air sampling in occupational environments is generally much more highly focused than ambient air sampling. It is usually designed to determine exposure levels for specific individuals or groups of individuals engaged in a common activity. It is also concerned with only one or, at most, a limited number of specific air contaminants at each work site.

There are two basic approaches available for determining an individual's average exposure. The more traditional one involves breaking up the workday into a number of specific subfractions during which the air concentration is reasonably constant or reproducible. Samples are then collected in sufficient numbers in each activity interval to permit a reliable characterization of the exposure in that activity. The product of the exposure concentration at a given activity and the time devoted to that activity during each workday represents the contribution of that activity toward the overall exposure. The time-weighted average exposure is the sum of all the products of concentration and time, divided by the total daily work time. A representative determination of a time-weighted average occupational exposure is illustrated in Table 8–3.

An alternate approach to the determination of average daily exposure became available in the 1960s, with the development of lightweight, self-contained samplers and battery-powered pumps that could be worn by individual workers with-

TABLE 8–3. Sample Determination of a Time-Weighted Average Occupational Exposure

Given: Workers perform three different operations which involve potential exposure to airborne lead (Pb) during each workday. Breathing zone (BZ) air samples were collected at each of the operations, and general air (GA) samples were collected that represent the workers' exposure during the balance of the workday.

Sampling rate for all samplers: 15 L/min
Sampling interval for BZ samples: 10 min
Sampling interval for GA samples: 60 min
Sample collections: Operation #1: 20.6, 24.3, and 18.2 μg
Operation #2: 35.2, 33.5, and 39.1 μg
Operation #3: 6.5, 9.7, and 7.8 μg
General air: 3.7, 1.9, and 5.1 μg
Working time/day: Operation #1: 60 min
Operation #2: 90 min
Operation #3: 90 min
General air: 4 hr (240 min)

CALCULATION

OPERATION	AV. SAMPLE (μg Pb)	SAMPLED VOLUME (LITERS)	Pb CONCENTRATION (C) (μg/m^3)	EXPOSURE TIME (t) (MIN)	$C \times T$ (μg-MIN/m^3)
1	21.0	150	140.2	60	8,413
2	35.9	150	239.6	90	21,560
3	8.0	150	53.3	90	4,800
GA	3.6	900	4.0	240	951
			Totals	480	35,724

Time-weighted average exposure = 35,724/480 = 74.4 μg/m^3

Note: Threshold limit value (for 2000) = 50 μg/m^3, so the workers in this case are overexposed. Operation #2 accounts for 60% of the daily exposure. If, by application of engineering controls, the concentration at Operation #2 was reduced to 25 μg/m^3, the time-weighted average would drop to 34.2 μg/m^3.

out restricting their mobility. The sampling rates are low, but the sampled volume accumulated over a workday is usually large enough to permit an accurate determination of the average exposure for the day. Although there are fewer samples to analyze using this approach, it provides no information on the peak levels of exposure, or which of the activities during the day may have accounted for the bulk of the overall exposure.

The trend in recent years has been toward a greater reliance on personal samplers for routine monitoring of exposures. In sampling airborne particles, there has been a growing utilization of size-selective samplers, where the particles are aerodynamically separated into sample fractions on the basis of their presumed fate in the respiratory tract. The largest application of these is for dusts that produce pneumoconioses following deposition in the alveolar region of the lungs. The dust that penetrates to this region is simulated by the second stage of a two-stage sampler having a first-stage collector removing that fraction expected to be deposited in the head and tracheobronchial tree, and a second stage which collects all of the particles penetrating the first stage.

Special considerations in source sampling

The air flowing in discharge ducts and stacks generally has much higher concentrations of contaminants than does the ambient air or workroom air. As a result, it is important to use sampling substrates that: can retain relatively large sample masses without losses due to resuspension in the sample stream, and that do not exhibit changes in sampling rate due to clogging.

When the flow channel is large and/or where there are branch entries or elbows near the sampling port, the flow pattern and contaminant concentration across the channel are likely to be far from uniform. Thus, in order to determine

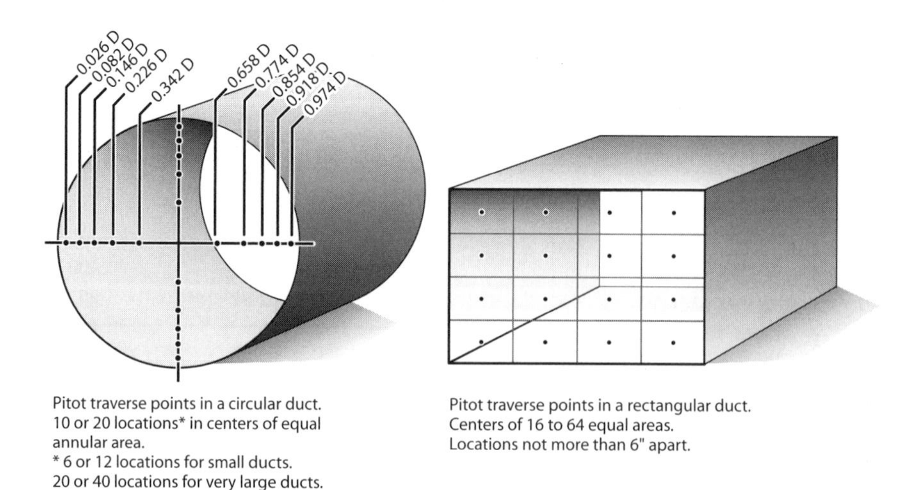

FIGURE 8–21. Traverse points for flow measurements in ducts.

the average concentration or total mass discharge rate, it is necessary to measure both the flowrate and concentration at numerous points across the channel. Such a series of measurements is known as a traverse; standardized traverse locations for circular and rectangular cross sections are available, and are shown in Figure 8–21.

It is important that the stream drawn into the sampler probe at each traverse point be representative of the stream at that point. No special precautions are needed when sampling most gases, or particles with diameters smaller than approximately 2 μm. However, for larger particles moving in high velocity airstreams, the particle momentum may lead to a biased sample. The bias may be either for or against the larger particles, depending on the velocity and orientation of the sampling probe with respect to the stream flow. Representative samples of aerosols containing larger particles can only be taken using the technique of isokinetic sampling, where the probe inlet faces into the airstream, and the velocity in the probe is equivalent to that of the stream flowing past it. Isokinetic sampling is illustrated in Figure 8–22.

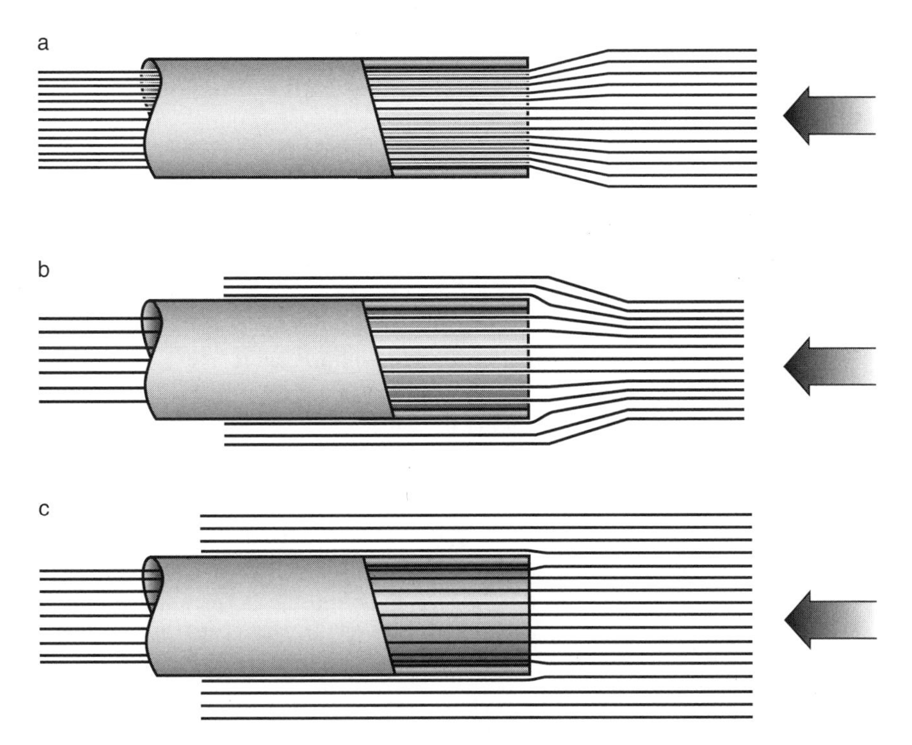

FIGURE 8–22. Various cases of aerosol sampling. (a) Isokinetic sampling; (b) Flowrate less than isokinetic rate. Flow streamlines diverge outward near the edge of the probe, causing larger particles to diverge into probe, and smaller particles to follow streamlines; thus, sample has too many large particles. (c) Flowrate greater than isokinetic rate. Streamlines diverge inward; sample has too few large particles.

In some stacks, such as vents for hot industrial processes or furnace discharges, the discharge stream may be much warmer than ambient temperature, and may also be high in moisture content. When hot, moist air passes through a tube whose wall temperature is lower than the dew point, the moisture will condense on the inside walls of the tube. If such condensation takes place before the stream reaches the sample collector, some or all of the sample can be lost. Insulated or heated sampling lines may be needed to avoid such complications.

When the stream is hot, it may also be difficult to obtain an accurate measurement of the sampling rate or sampled volume because of the change in air density with temperature and humidity. Elevated temperatures may also enhance chemical reactions between gas-phase constituents and the walls of the sampling line, resulting in line losses.

Water Sampling

The evaluation of water-quality parameters requires characterization of both the quantity of flow in the waterway as well as its contaminant load. Since water generally is confined to pipes, channels, and defined streams, it is possible to establish mass flowrates at critical sampling points. Total waste load is then obtained by multiplying mass flowrate and the concentration of contaminant. This knowledge should help to identify both source locations and strengths for contaminants, and also the effectiveness of installed controls.

Grab sampling

A grab sample of water is usually obtained with a very simple instrument, such as an empty jar or a bottle with a tight-fitting removable cap. The sample of water containing the contaminants of interest has a volume equal to the internal volume of the bottle, and the sample is collected within a short time interval. The sample may be obtained at the surface, or at various depths by use of weighted bottles which are opened and closed at the selected collection depth.

Intermittent sampling

The temporal pattern of contaminant levels can be determined by analyzing a series of manually collected grab samples. However, since it is usually less expensive to automate such a simple task, it is more common to use devices which collect samples periodically according to a preselected schedule. A series of individual samples can be collected, or a composite sample may be preferred, representing a mixture of equal-volume increments collected throughout a day or duty-cycle.

Continuous sampling

Intermittent sampling at fixed time intervals can miss surges in contaminant discharge, and, therefore, it may be desirable to draw the sample continuously.

Continuous samplers are generally operated at a very low flowrate to avoid processing larger volumes than those needed for the laboratory analyses.

Proportional sampling

Samples of constant volume collected on a fixed time schedule and samples collected continuously at a constant sampling rate can be used to determine the flux of contaminant directly only when the stream being sampled moves at a constant rate. When the stream flow varies, both the flowrate and the concentration must be determined in order to obtain the average or total mass flux of contaminant. Alternatively, the samples can be collected at variable rates that are proportional to the flow.

There are two basic types of proportional samplers. One type collects a definite volume at irregular time intervals; the other collects a variable volume at equally spaced time intervals. Both are flow dependent: in one, flow dictates the time interval; in the other, flow regulates the sample volume. In most of these, the pressure differential needed to extract the sample is provided by the moving stream itself, ensuring the required proportionality. A schematic diagram of a proportional-sampler control system is presented in Figure 8–23.

A variety of approaches have been used in flow proportional sampling. In some, a constant sampling flow is pumped through a pipe. After a predetermined volume has passed through the flowmeter, a diverter is activated and a sample is taken. An air-lift automatic sampler can be used to obtain samples when a pump cannot be used. When the compressed air supply is shut off (the air-control valve is connected to a timing relay from the flow-measuring device), a spring in the sampler raises a

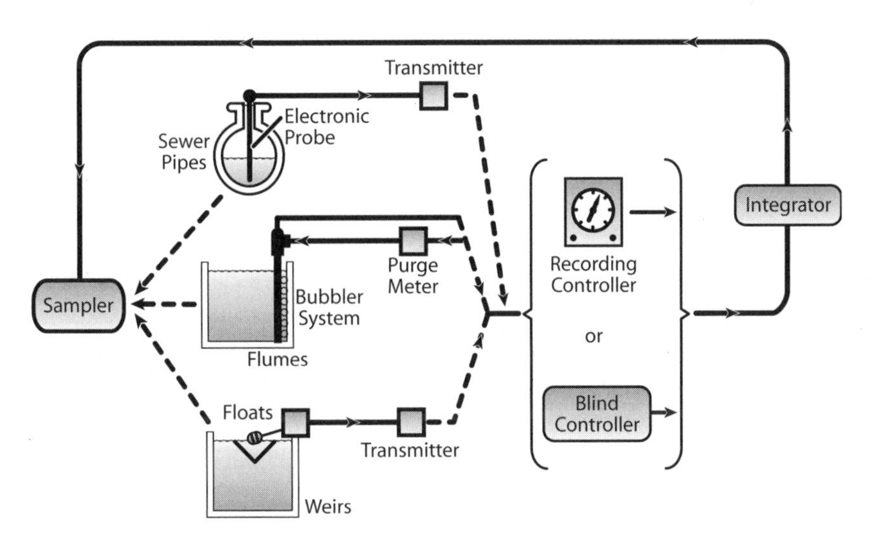

FIGURE 8–23. "Flow-proportional" sample-control systems.

piston (normally kept closed by the air) which opens an inlet so that water enters the sampler and goes to the sample container. The air valve is then opened and the piston is forced down, closing the inlet. The air passes through the air-escape port into the main chamber of the sampler and forces the liquid up the sample line into the collecting container. The cycle is then repeated.

In a vacuum-type sampler, which is very often used in water with high suspended-solids content or corrosive properties, a signal from a flowmeter activates the vacuum system, which lifts liquid through a suction line into the sample chamber. When the chamber is filled, the vacuum line is automatically closed. The pump then turns off, and the sample is drawn into the sample container. A float check prevents any liquid from reaching the pump.

Another type of automatic sampler consists of a cup or dipper on a chain. When activated by a signal, the cup is carried down through the stream and returns filled with a sample, which is emptied into a container.

In theory, most automatic-type samplers may be connected to flow-measuring devices in order to obtain proportionate samples.

Extractive sampling

Extractive techniques have many advantages for water sampling, corresponding to those previously discussed for air sampling. The samplers are much lighter, more compact, and are easier to preserve and ship, and they allow the concentration of contaminants from large volumes of water in a practical manner. Unfortunately, effective and reliable extractive techniques have not been developed for a large number of water contaminants of interest, including many of the soluble gases and salts, and most colloidal solids.

Effective extractive techniques are available for suspended solids, many organics, and some of the toxic metallic ions. Membrane and glass-fiber filters are widely used for collecting suspended solids. In liquid filtration, sieving is an important mechanism of collection, and a major fraction of the particles smaller than the void or pore size can penetrate the filter. Membrane filters are available with pore sizes as small as 0.01 μm, but the smaller-pore-size filters have large pressure drops and, therefore, have very low flow capacity, limiting the sample size that can be drawn through them.

Adsorption is the most widely used extractive sampling technique for the collection of water-soluble organic material. Activated carbon and various organic resins (e.g., XAD, Tenax) are commonly used in pipes or columns of varying capacities and configurations through which the water percolates.

Ion exchange is a widely used technique for extractive sampling of contaminants in ionic form; it is applicable to both organic and inorganic contaminants. This technique involves the reversible transfer of ions between the water solution and a solid material capable of binding the ions. The resins used in ion exchange are graded powders or beads of porous compounds, packed into columns.

A number of materials have ion-exchange properties. Among the solid inorganic materials commonly used are natural aluminum silicate minerals (zeolites); hydrous TiO_2 or ZrO_2; metal phosphates, for example, zirconium phosphate, microcrystalline ammonium molybdophosphate; oxides of A1(III), Si(IV), Fe(III), and Mn(IV). The solid organic resins include cellulose, lignin, cation-exchange resins such as natural clay, chelating resins (with amine carboxylates as functional groups), and anion resins (usually in OH^- or Cl^- forms). The selectivity for specific ions depends largely upon the chemical structure of the resin and its physical configuration (e.g., degree of cross-linking).

Special considerations in stream sampling

It is especially difficult to collect representative samples of water in a free-flowing stream or river. The velocity profile in a stream is very variable, depending as it does on the cross section for flow, the volumetric rate of flow, the disturbances introduced upstream by bends in the stream, tributary streams, surface winds, stream bed obstructions, etc. The stream flow varies in the short term with the recent history of precipitation, and in the longer term with seasonal variations in runoff. Variations in flow affect both the levels of contaminants attributable to surface runoff and the resuspension of contaminants from the stream sediments.

Since no one point in the stream cross section can be considered representative of the overall stream, it follows that contaminant flux can only be determined accurately from an analysis of samples collected at a series of representative locations across the flow cross section. Unfortunately, the appropriate traverse locations are not as easily defined as those for the circular and rectangular cross sections of Figure 8–21; it may be necessary to sample at only one or a few points and to accept the uncertainties introduced by the circumstances. Although, ideally, the sample should be taken from mid-stream where the velocity is greatest and the possibility that any solids have settled is minimal, in practice most samples are collected at the edge of the stream and near the upper surface. One potential error introduced by such a practice is illustrated in Figure 8–24.

Special considerations in effluent sampling

The collection of representative samples of effluent waste waters is relatively simple in comparison with sampling of process lines or free-flowing streams. In most cases, the number of outfalls of discharge points will be limited, their volumetric rate of flow will generally be known, or at least definable, and the flow will be relatively well mixed. The major variables will usually be in the temporal aspects of the waste discharges. Industrial wastes may be expected to vary greatly in both composition and volume with time, reflecting the batch nature of many production operations, the periodicity of routine cleanup and maintenance operations, and the consequences of accidental, unanticipated releases.

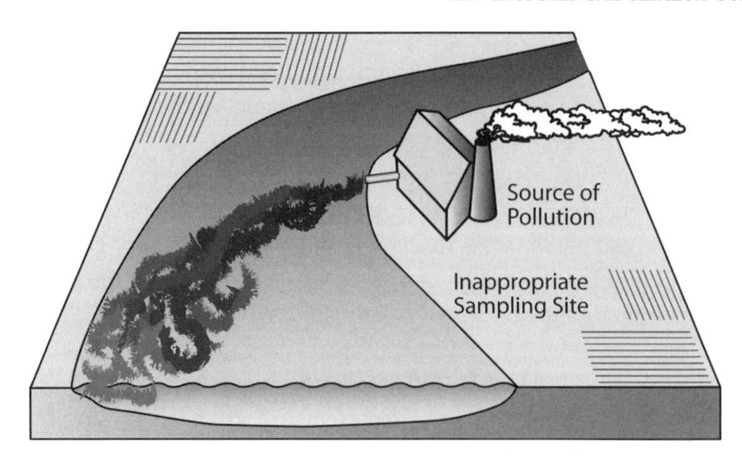

FIGURE 8–24. An illustration of a potential problem encountered by sampling near the edge of a stream.

The first step in designing an effluent sampling program is to define all of the significant discharge points. The next step is to determine their likely variability in discharge, and to select the best means of characterizing the discharges from each. If the total amounts discharged are of primary concern, it may be satisfactory to continuously collect an integral sample whose volume is proportional to the overall flow. On the other hand, if the objectives include identifying the contributions of the component sources to the overall discharge, it may be necessary to collect a series of effluent samples at appropriate times throughout the production or other cycle. Some of these considerations are illustrated in Figure 8–25.

Special considerations in sample handling and preservation

Some special precautions are necessary in the handling of water samples. Water that is contaminated with chemicals is often contaminated with microorganisms as well. Since the metabolism of these microorganisms may add or subtract materials of interest between the time of collection and the subsequent laboratory analyses, water samples are often refrigerated to minimize such complicating effects.

Many other time-dependent changes may occur in water samples after their collection. These may include changes in pH, loss of some dissolved gases and absorption of others from the atmosphere, change in valence state of metal ions via oxidation-reduction reactions, and precipitation of metal cations due to chemical reactions. Procedures for sample preservation for the analysis of various contaminants are discussed in detail in elsewhere.[4] It is important that the procedures used to stabilize one contaminant of interest do not affect the determination of another.

Some precautions which may be needed in a water-sampling train to preserve contaminants of interest are illustrated in Figure 8–26.

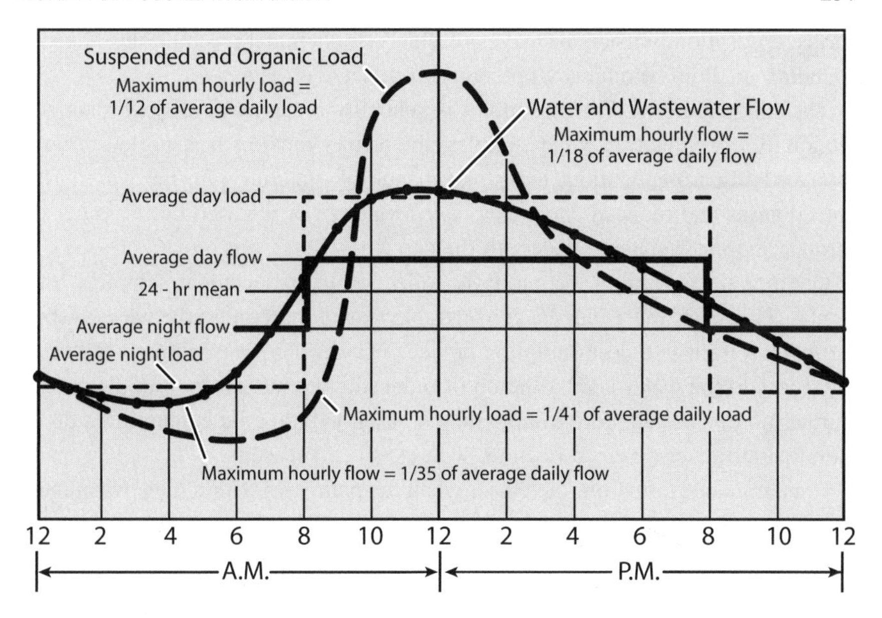

FIGURE 8–25. Flow variations of water and waste water and variation in the strength of waste water.

Sampling of Biota, Sediments, and Soil

A complete evaluation of the extent and significance of environmental contamination by a given material will frequently require the analysis of soil and aquatic sediments and biota, since they can act as temporary or permanent sinks for the material. As long as the contaminant is available for ingestion by mobile life

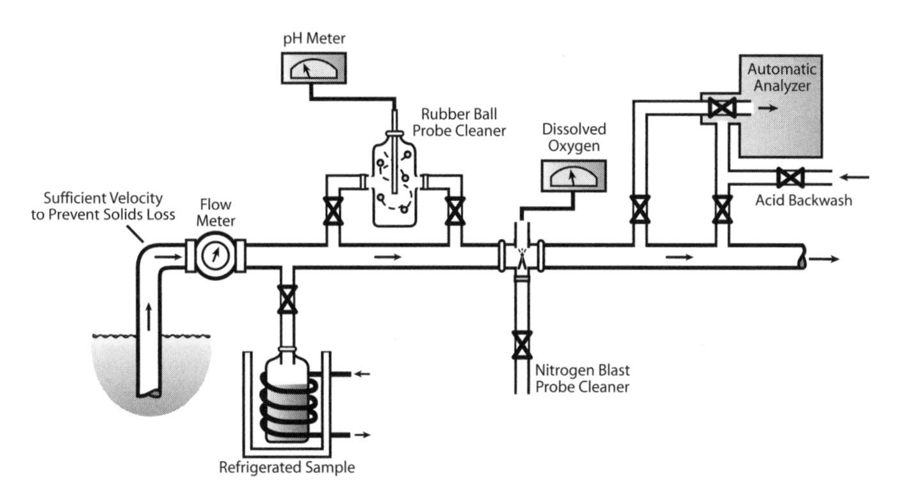

FIGURE 8–26. Examples of possible precautions needed in a sampling train to prevent changes in composition in the water sample.

forms, absorption by roots or leaves of plants or chemical leaching into the surrounding medium, it retains a potential for adverse effects.

The collection of sediment samples is generally much more difficult than collection of representative water samples; the former must be transported through the overlying water without loss or exchange of material with the water. Dissolved gases and reduced chemicals may be altered or released during transport through more oxygenated waters to the surface.

One popular sampling technique is collection of a flocculent sample with a dredge. However, there may be considerable loss of material to the water. A better method utilizes a core-sampling device. This technique minimizes both material loss to the water and oxidation of reduced materials during sample ascent. Furthermore, an intact core sample may be used to study the contaminant deposition pattern over a period of time, such as several seasons.

Contaminant evaluations are easier when the pathways within the environment are well established. In such cases, a sample from an established indicator organism may provide a sufficient index of the extent of the contamination. When less is known about contaminant behavior, a larger range of materials and a greater number of samples will be required.

An indicator organism is a plant, animal, or microbe that provides an index of environmental conditions by its presence, absence, or specific characteristics. The narrower the tolerance of the indicator organism for a specific condition, the greater is the accuracy in describing ecologic conditions. For example, presence of an aquatic organism that can only survive in a pH from 7.0 to 8.0 is an accurate field monitor of mild alkalinity in the waterway.

Indicator plants may be used in evaluating the extent of chemical contamination of the ambient air by characteristic pathological changes. For example, intercoastal markings on the leaves of violets indicate high SO_2 levels; banding on snowstorm petunia leaves indicate aldehydes; white flecks on tobacco leaves indicate high O_3 levels. Other plants may accumulate chemicals, and are thus serve to provide an index of ambient levels. For example, samples of Spanish Moss growing in the southeastern U.S. on trees downwind of highways were collected in order to determine their Pb content, on the basis that this content was proportional to traffic density.

Some of the best biological indicators of chemical contamination can be found in the aquatic environment. Some filter-feeding crustacea extract organic contaminants and metallic ions very efficiently from the water. Aquatic plants may also greatly concentrate some of the trace metals that accumulate in the bottom sediment of streams and lakes. Certain algae, such as the green and blue-green types, are indicators of high-nutrient content in waterways. Samples of aquatic biota may be obtained with nets, dredges, or an artificial substrate, such as glass slides for microorganisms.

Certain plants on land are associated with the presence of particular chemicals in the soil. For example, the growth of Eastern Colombine in the eastern United

States is indicative of high soil calcium carbonate content, and plants of the genus Astragalus in the western United States grow in association with selenium in soil.

Food Sampling

Concern about the extent of chemical contamination of food may lead to several kinds of sampling programs. One involves identification of specific batches of contaminated, adulterated, or spoiled food products that may reach the market. The random- and spot-sampling programs of the FDA and various state agencies fall into this category. When the samples indicate that the quality of the food is substandard, the batch of food product represented by the sample will be destroyed or diverted to another usage where its quality would be acceptable.

A second type of program focuses on the definition of pathways and accumulation rates for materials of interest that do not present immediate hazards, but may be worthy of concern and continued observation. One example was the worldwide food-sampling program and analysis for ^{90}Sr content during and after the period of atmospheric testing of thermonuclear weapons in the 1950s and 1960s. Another is the continuing monitoring of pesticides in foods.

In much of this large-scale food sampling, the extent of the problem is determined from a relatively limited number of composite samples rather than from large numbers of analyses of individual foods. The approach is generally known as market-basket sampling. In it, a representative diet is selected and the food products needed to prepare this diet are purchased from regular retail outlets. The foods are prepared for cooking as they would be in the home, i.e., wrappings, bones, trimmings, etc., are discarded. The parts that would be consumed are then analyzed for their content of the contaminant(s) of interest.

Market-basket sampling has several important advantages for routine monitoring of overall contaminant levels and their trends. These are: *(1)* fewer samples need to be analyzed; *(2)* the samples are relatively large, avoiding problems of too limited analytic sensitivity; and *(3)* the results are directly relatable to an average population exposure. On the other hand, there are important limitations: *(1)* there is no information on the major sources within the overall diet; and *(2)* there is no information on maximum levels of exposure within the population attributable to unusual dietary patterns.

Biological Media Sampling—Biomarkers of Exposure

The sampling and analysis of ambient air, drinking water, and foods can indicate the contaminants to which people are exposed. However, environmental data cannot define the fractions retained after, for example, inhalation or ingestion either initially or at later times. For most toxicants, the amount retained is very variable among individuals, and with time in a given individual. Furthermore, the basic metabolic pathways are poorly defined for many contaminants. For these reasons, it is usually a good practice to use biological samples as supplements to environmental samples in evaluating the health significance of exposures to environmental contaminants.

Biological samples have, in the past, been most widely used in occupational health evaluations, as discussed in Chapter 12, and Biological Exposure Indices have been suggested for various chemicals, their metabolites, or the alterations they produce in biological constituents or physiological functions. The kinds and sizes of the samples needed for such analyses depend on the contaminant and its metabolism, and the sensitivity of the assay.

The easiest kinds of samples to collect are urine and exhaled air. Hair and fingernails may also be useful and can also be collected fairly readily in many cases. It is usually more difficult to obtain the cooperation needed for the collection of blood or fecal samples, but they frequently are needed and can be successfully collected. Table 8–4 lists some biological indices of contaminant exposure.

An ever-present problem in the collection and handling of all of these types of samples is contamination, and extreme caution must be exercised in the selection and handling of the sample container. The material to be analyzed must not be extractable from the container itself, and anyone handling the sample must be aware of all the possible means of introducing artificial material, and must avoid them. For example, industrial workers usually have much more of the chemical of interest on their hands than in their urine and, if they haven't first washed thoroughly, can easily contaminate a urine bottle while filling it.

TABLE 8–4. Some Biological Samples Used as Exposure Indices

CONTAMINANT	SPECIMEN FOR EVALUATION	CHEMICAL INDICATOR
Arsenic	Urine, blood, hair	Arsenic
Benzene	Urine	Phenol
	Blood, exhaled breath	Benzene
Cadmium	Hair, nails	Cadmium
Carbon monoxide	Blood	Carboxyhemoglobin
Cyanide	Blood	Cyanmethemoglobin
Fluoride	Urine, hair	Fluoride
Hydrogen sulfide	Blood	Sulfhemoglobin
Lead	Hair, blood	Lead
	Urine	Lead, delta amino-levulinic acid
Nitrite	Blood	Methemoglobin
Organic mercury	Urine, hair	Mercury
Parathion	Urine	P-nitrophenol
Polycyclic aromatic hydrocarbons	Urine	Analysis for parent compound
Vinyl chloride	Exhaled breath	Vinyl chloride

Another problem is the collection of a representative sample. Most biological samples are short-interval (grab) samples containing a material of interest whose body concentration varies considerably with time. Proper interpretation may depend on the availability of supplementary information, such as the times of exposure relative to the times of sampling, and the characteristic metabolic time constants.

For some contaminants, especially radioactive materials, the overall retention in the body and within various organs can sometimes be determined by noninvasive, external measurements of emitted radiation. Estimates of individual and population burdens of contaminants can also be made by analysis of tissues taken at autopsy from accident victims. However, the great difficulties associated with obtaining adequately sized samples of this type generally precludes the acquisition of a significant body of data through this approach.

MEASUREMENT OF CONTAMINANT CONCENTRATIONS

Concentrations of contaminants may be measured by sample collection and subsequent laboratory analysis, or by use of direct-reading instrumentation in the field. Many of the instruments used in the field are merely more compact and/or rugged versions of those used in the laboratory.

Laboratory Analysis of Environmental Samples

All of the samples of air contaminants, water, soil, biota, food, and biological materials brought to the analytical facility can be analyzed by similar techniques. While they may differ considerably in their nature, such samples generally have a number of common characteristics. These include: the likely presence of a variety of cocontaminants at concentrations equal to or greater than the contaminant of interest, and the presence of a collection substrate or matrix from which the contaminant must be extracted prior to analysis. Thus, the first task in a laboratory evaluation is generally to separate the contaminant of interest from its co-contaminants and matrix, so that it can be further analyzed unambiguously.

Separation is often combined with preconcentration procedures. Preconcentration improves the sensitivity of the analytical method and increases the precision and accuracy of analysis. The necessity to concentrate prior to analysis is dependent upon the specific analytical method that is to be used and the lower limit of detection of the procedure. For example, organic constituents of water are sufficiently numerous and usually present at such low concentrations that they require preconcentration and separation. Many inorganics are present at concentrations above the sensitivity limits of analytical methods; however, numerous interferences can arise from other agents that should be removed prior to analysis. Many of the current analytical methods are subject to well-characterized interferences, which are noted in standardized procedures for contaminant analysis.[4,5]

Contaminants collected by extractive sampling techniques generally need to be separated from the collection matrix. Following adsorption on activated carbon, the organic chemicals are extracted from the carbon using a chloroform wash, sometimes followed by methanol. Following evaporation of the solvent, the weights of the organic extract residues are expressed in units of μg/L as carbon chloroform–extract (CCE) and carbon alcohol–extract (CAE). These extracts may be further separated into groups, for example, bases, weak acids, strong acids, etc., via differential solubility techniques.

Recovery of contaminants from ion-exchange resins is performed by elution with a solvent appropriate for the particular material being analyzed. Ion exchange is a particularly useful separation technique for selective removal of ions that may interfere with the analysis of other ions.

A number of specific separation techniques are used in contaminant analyses. These are presented in Table 8–5. Often, more than one procedure is required prior to final analysis. Many of these separation techniques can also be used for the preconcentration of contaminants.

ANALYTICAL INSTRUMENTATION

The full range of analytical instrumentation that can be used for the qualitative and quantitative analyses of environmental samples could not be adequately described in a whole volume, let alone a small part of this chapter. Thus, the reader is referred to several of the more concise descriptions in a number of the standard references in the Bibliography. An overview of some of the more commonly used techniques and their typical applications are presented in Table 8–6.

The selection of the best analytical techniques in a specific situation is often quite difficult. Factors to consider in any choice are: *(1)* any sample preprocessing required; *(2)* specificity with regard to the chemical being analyzed; *(3)* influence of the matrix; *(4)* amounts needed for determination of the chemical; *(5)* accuracy for the concentration ranges expected; and *(6)* time and cost.

Direct Measurement of Environmental Concentrations

As mentioned earlier, many instruments may be used for direct measurements of contaminants in the field. This discussion of equipment for the direct determination of air and water concentrations will be brief. It will be limited to an illustration of some of the more common or innovative approaches to the general

TABLE 8–5. Some Common Chemical Separation Techniques

TECHNIQUE	PRINCIPLE	TYPICAL SEPARATION APPLICATIONS
Coprecipitation	Removal of an ion from solution via adsorption on a carrier precipitate	Trace metals
Liquid-liquid extraction (solvent extraction)	Physical separation based upon the selective distribution of a substance in two immiscible solvents (e.g., water and a water-immiscible organic solvent)	Many organic and inorganic compounds, especially water-immiscible organics and metal ions
Freeze concentration	Water in sample is frozen, yielding pure ice crystals and leaving water-soluble impurities in a liquid phase with a reduced volume	Wide range of inorganic and organic solutes
Adsorptive bubble separation	Passage of gas bubbles through a solution or suspension in a vertical column; material of interest may be adsorbed at bubble-solution interface or onto bubble surface	Surface active agents; colloids and some other particles
Distillation, evaporation, sublimation	Separation from water via removal of a component as a gas or vapor	Organic compounds; dissolved inorganic gases
Centrifugation	Decrease time required for particles to sediment by increasing the gravitational forces affecting them	Macromolecules; suspended and colloidal particles

(*continued*)

Table 8–5. Some Common Chemical Separation Techniques (*continued*)

TECHNIQUE	PRINCIPLE	TYPICAL SEPARATION APPLICATIONS
Chromatography	Based upon the differential migration of substrates due to their selective retention in a fixed phase while subjected to movement by a flowing bulk phase (gas or liquid)	Wide applicability; generally used for organics
Gel filtration	Lodging of colloidal particles and high-molecular-weight organic compounds in pores of a cross- linked gel packed in columns	Colloids; organics
Chelation separation	Complexing of metals by certain reagents	Metals
Liquid-anion exchange (ion-pair formation)	Separation of metal complexes by formation of an ion pair with an onium cation (e.g., trialkyl ammonium) formed by use of a strongly basic solvent	Metals
Dry ashing	Combustion of material (e.g., filter, biological tissues) and recovery of contaminants of interest in unburned residue or in gaseous emissions	Metals
Wet ashing	Oxidation of material in acid to separate contaminant of interest from an organic matrix	Metals

TABLE 8–6. Some Common Methods of Contaminant Analysis

METHOD	PRINCIPLE OF OPERATION	INSTRUMENTATION	SAMPLE[a]	SPECIFICITY[b]	SENSITIVITY[c]	TYPICAL APPLICATIONS
1. Gravimetric	Isolation of component of interest in the form of one of its compounds which shows insolubility under test conditions and has a known chemical composition; weigh the product	Conventional lab equipment	SLG	Good	1–10 μg	Numerous analyses for inorganic and organic materials
2. Titrimetric (e.g., acid-base; oxidation-reduction; precipitation)	Reaction of material in predictable manner with a standard solution of known concentration	Conventional lab equipment	L	Good	10^{-6}–10^{-7} M in solution	Numerous analyses, e.g., acidity, alkalinity, water hardness (Ca^{-2}, Mg^{-2}), Cl^-, S^{-2}, transition metals, DO
3. Absorption spectrophotometry						
a. Visible	Measure of selective absorption or transmission of visible light, usually following reaction with a reagent	Colorimeter; spectrophotometer	SLG	Fair	0.005 ppm	Metals (e.g., Fe, Cu); nutrients (NO_2^-, NO_3^-, PO_4^{-3}), NH_3, phenol SO_2, NO_x, oxidant gases (O_3), COD, TOC
b. Ultraviolet	Absorption of UV light	UV spectrophotometer	SLG	Fair	0.005 ppm	Organic compounds, some inorganic gases, e.g., SO_2, O_3, NO_2

(continued)

TABLE 8–6. Some Common Methods of Contaminant Analysis (*continued*)

METHOD	PRINCIPLE OF OPERATION	INSTRUMENTATION	SAMPLE[a]	SPECIFICITY[b]	SENSITIVITY[c]	TYPICAL APPLICATIONS
c. Infrared	Absorption of IR (from heated filament)	IR spectrophotometric	SLG	Fair	1 ppm	Organic compounds, some inorganic gases, e.g., CO, CO_2, SO_2, NO_x, NH_3, O_3, TOC
4. Emission spectroscopy						
a. Flame photometry	Spectral-emission analysis following excitation by flame (arcs or sparks are also used)	Flame photometer; spectrograph (arc)	SL	Good Excellent	0.001–0.1 ppm	Metals, halogens, phosphorus, sulfur (depending on specific method)
b. X-ray fluorescence spectrometry	Spectral-emission analysis following X-ray excitation	XRF spectrometer	SL	Good	10 ppm	All elements having atomic numbers above 11
c. Spectrofluorimetry	Reemission of radiation absorbed by dissolved molecules	Recording spectrofluorimeter	SL	Good	0.001 ppm	Organic compounds; some inorganic constituents
d. Chemiluminescence	Emission of spectral radiation resulting from a chemical reaction	Chemilumi--nescence analyzer	G	Excellent	ppb	O_3, NO_x
5. Atomic absorption spectrophotometry	Absorption of radiation by free atoms in a vapor state	AA spectrometer	SL	Excellent	0.001 ppm	Most metals

6. Chromatography (gas; liquid; thin-layer)	Differential migration of agents due to selective retention in a fixed phase while subjected to movement by a flowing bulk phase	Gas chromatograph, liquid chromatograph	LG (gas chr) SL (liquid chr) SL (thin-layer)	Excellent (gas) Good (liquid)	ppb–ppm (TLC)	Organic compounds, trace metals, anions
7. Electrochemical						
a. Conductivity	Measurement of electrical conductivity following absorption of an agent through a solution	Conductivity meter	LG	Poor	0.01 ppm	Any gas which forms electrolytes in aqueous solution, e.g., SO_2, NO_2, Cl_2, H_2S, NH_3
b. Anodic stripping voltammetry	Electrolysis of solution and electrodeposition followed by stripping at various potentials	DC-pulse polarograph	L	Good	0.001 ppm	Some metals, e.g., Cd, Cu, Fe, Pb, Zn
c. Coulometry	Quantitative electrochemical conversion from one oxidation state to another	Coulometer	L	Good	1 ppm	SO_2, NO_2, O_3, H_2S, olefins, F^-, mercaptans
d. Polarography	Electrolysis of solution and measurement of current-voltage relation	Polarograph	L	Good	0.1 ppm	Some organic compounds and some metals, e.g., Sb, As, Cd, Cr, Ni, Zn
8. X-ray diffraction	Recording of scattered X-rays from sample subject to X-ray beam	X-ray diffractometer	S	Good	—	Solids of crystalline structure, e.g., asbestos, quartz
9. Microscopy (polarizing; fluorescence)	Optical analysis of enlarged images	Various types of microscopes	S	Excellent	—	Nature and size of particles, e.g., fibers, dusts

(*continued*)

TABLE 8–6. Some Common Methods of Contaminant Analysis (*continued*)

METHOD	PRINCIPLE OF OPERATION	INSTRUMENTATION	SAMPLE[a]	SPECIFICITY[b]	SENSITIVITY[c]	TYPICAL APPLICATIONS
10. Mass spectrometry	Determination of material by creation of ionic current via electrostatic or electromagnetic field and separation of the ions according to their mass. Generally used in conjunction with gas chromatographs	Mass spectrometer	SLG	Excellent	ppb	Organic compounds
11. Neutron activation analysis	Measurement of emitted ionizing radiation following production of radionuclides by neutron bombardment	—	SL	Excellent	ppb to ppm	Hg, As, Pb, Fe, and about 66 other elements which can become radioactive when bombarded with neutrons

[a]Sample: Most usual form of sample suited to the specific method; S = solid; L = liquid; G = gas.

[b]Specificity: This is an indication of the general ability of the method to measure the material in the presence of matrix interferences. The classification are very broad and use of preconcentration or separation methods may increase specificity.

[c]Sensitivity: Typical lower limits of detection are presented; these may differ depending upon the specific chemicals analyzed and the background concentrations present.

DO, dissolved oxygen; UV, ultraviolet; IR, infrared radiation; TOC, total organic carbon; XRF, X-ray fluorescence; AA, atomic absorption; TLC, thin-layer chromatography; DC, direct current.

task. For a more comprehensive description, the reader is once again referred to the references provided in the Bibliography.

Bear in mind that similar instrumentation may be used for both water and air sampling. The determining factor is the specific state in which the sample must be introduced to the instrument.

Direct-reading instrumentation for airborne contaminants

Gases and Vapors. Any characteristic physical property of a chemical can be utilized in its detection and measurement. A variety of instrumental principles can be employed to maximize sensitivity, specificity, and precision. A widely used instrument for monitoring airborne carbon monoxide (CO) is based on the capacity of CO to absorb specific wavelengths of infrared radiation (IR). Thus, CO molecules in the path between an IR source and an IR sensor will reduce the incident flux at the sensor. A higher concentration or longer path length will increase the attenuation. Other gases and vapors present in relatively high concentrations in the air, including methane and water vapor, will also absorb IR. However, they do not absorb at the same wavelength as does the CO and, by using an IR beam of an appropriate wavelength, the instrument response can be limited to CO. It also follows that the same basic instrument can be used to make specific measurements of the concentration of other airborne molecules by using appropriate wavelengths.

A schematic diagram of an IR instrument is shown in Figure 8–27. It uses both a sensing cell and a sealed reference cell, and the signal is proportional to the difference in the heat absorbed by the two detectors which, in turn, varies with

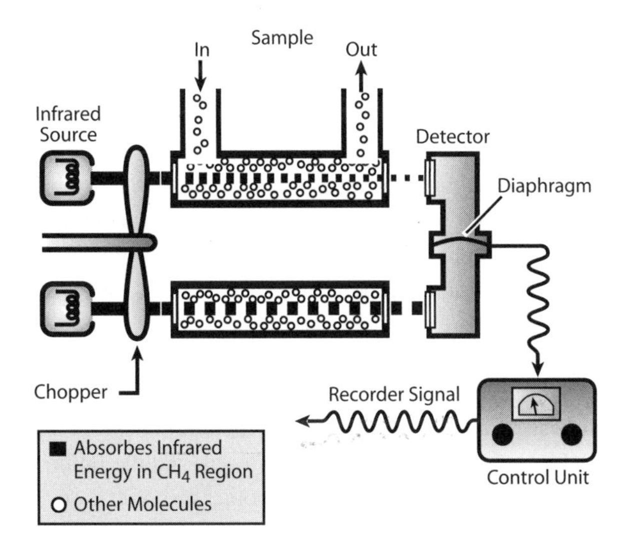

FIGURE 8–27. Schematic of an infrared analyzer.

the CO content of the sample cell. In this configuration, small variations in IR output by the source affect both detectors equally, and do not significantly affect the output signal.

Instruments have also been developed for airborne contaminants, such as mercury vapor and benzene, which strongly absorb ultraviolet light. More recently, instruments have become available that detect molecules that fluoresce upon excitation by a radiant source. In this case, the detector is tuned to the fluorescence frequency, rather than the source frequency. Instruments of this type are currently being used for carbon monoxide and sulfur dioxide analysis.

Of still greater complexity are some relatively new instrument designs that analyze patterns in the radiant spectra of excited molecules rather than just total absorption over a given wavelength band. These second derivative spectrometers can be used to monitor a wide variety of gases and vapors, including SO_2, NH_3, NO_2, and benzene.

Another approach to continuous measurement of gas and vapor contaminants is to react them with other chemicals in the stream, or at surfaces in contact with the stream, and to measure the rate of reaction or the presence of reaction products. One of the earliest applications of this approach, and one still widely used, is the combustible gas indicator. A gas stream is passed over a catalytic filament at which combustible vapors burn. The heat of combustion raises the temperature of the filament, reducing its electrical resistance. The change in resistance provides an indication of the concentration of combustible material. A schematic diagram of this type of instrument, in which the catalytic filament is one leg of a Wheatstone bridge, is shown in Figure 8–28.

A slightly more sophisticated approach, which has also been used for many years, is utilized in the halide meter. It employs the "Beilstein" reaction, in which halogen atoms in contact with a copper element at high temperature emit an intense green light. In the halide meter, halogen containing hydrocarbons are burned in a copper arc, and the intensity of the spectral emission indicates the concentration of the vapor.

Neither the combustible gas meter nor the halide meter can provide accurate or specific determinations when there are mixtures of air contaminants. The former responds to all combustible vapors, and its response depends on the heat of combustion. The halide meter responds only to halogens, but has a different degree of response for different halogen compounds.

Some of the newer instruments utilizing gas-phase conversions achieve specificity by employing highly individual chemical reactions. For example, the ozone monitor illustrated in Figure 8–29 utilizes the chemiluminescent reaction between ozone and ethylene. An excess of ethylene is used, and the luminescence is limited by the ozone concentration. None of the other airborne gases react with ethylene, so there are no significant interferences.

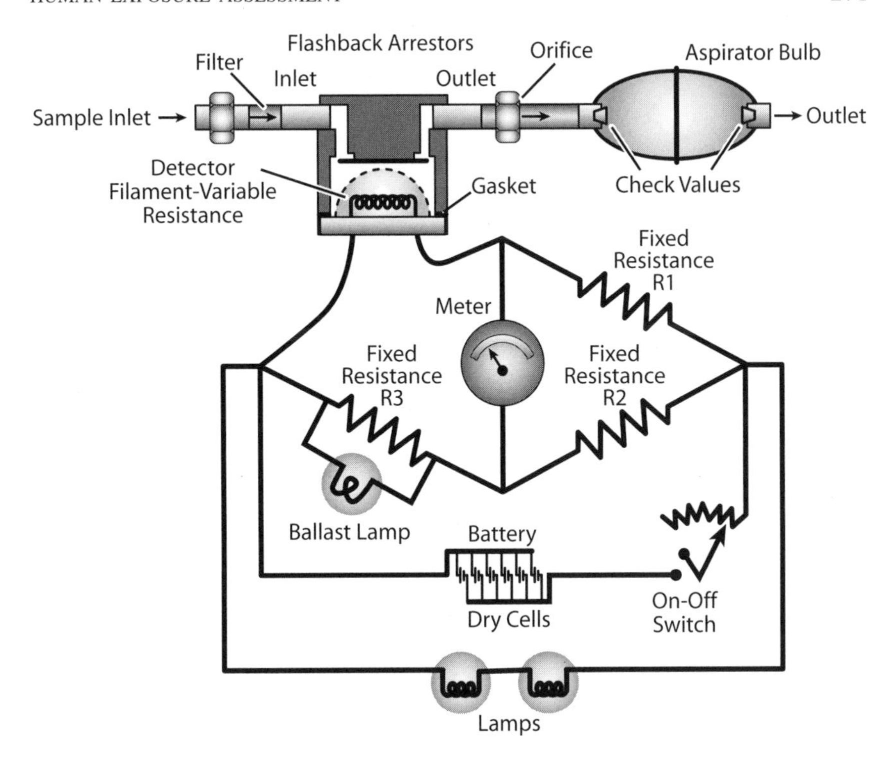

FIGURE 8–28. Schematic of a combustible-gas indicator flow system with circuit diagram.

Particles. There are very few methods for measuring particle concentrations in airstreams without sample collection, and almost all of these utilize the light-scattering properties of the particles. Some measure the integral scatter of an aerosol. Since the amount of light scattered by each particle varies greatly with particle size, these instruments have little value unless the size distribution is known and constant. Other instruments measure the scattered light from individual particles as they pass through the sensing zone, and sort the pulses by size. Thus, they can accumulate number concentrations within defined size intervals for particles larger than about 0.3 μm diameter. They are calibrated for reflective spherical particles and, therefore, may not be accurate for size analyses of particles with other shapes and optical properties.

Sample collection with on-line measurements

In on-line systems, the analysis instrumentation is combined with the sampling instrumentation. A sample is collected as a grab, composite, or continuous sample, and then analyzed by a direct-reading instrument. Most sample-collecting instruments with direct-measurement capabilities combine one of the extractive-

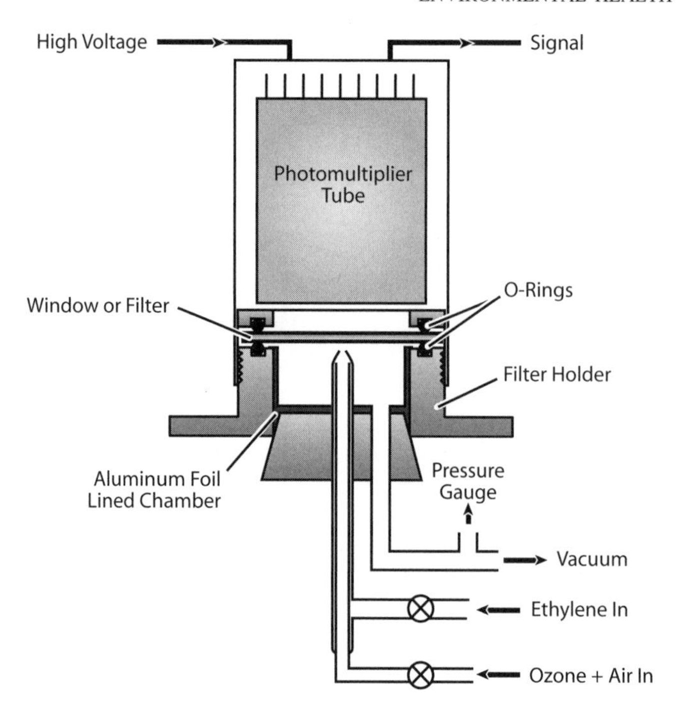

FIGURE 8–29. Schematic of ozone monitor utilizing ozone-ethylene chemiluminescent reaction and photometric detection.

sampling techniques previously described with a simplified version of a laboratory-type analytical instrument.

Many of the older on-line instruments used wet chemical techniques following extraction of the air contaminant by a bubbler or gas washer. A once widely used SO_2 instrument passed the scrubbing solution through an electrical conductivity cell. However, it was not specific for SO_2, since other ionizable contaminants in the air would also contribute to the conductivity. Other two-stage instruments used colorimetric reagents to collect the contaminants, and could give more specific analyses, provided that co-contaminants in the air did not produce or quench color changes at the wavelengths used in the built-in colorimeter.

Most of the newer instruments use dry collection techniques. For example, the gas chromatographic flame photometric analyzer illustrated in Figure 8–30 collects various sulfur gases simultaneously on a chromatographic column. When the sampled gases are eluted from the column into the flame photometric detector, they each give essentially the same signal per mole of sulfur. However, since each compound has a different retention time on the column, they give distinct peaks, and the quantity of each can thus be determined.

Perhaps the simplest example of sample collection with a rapid readout of concentration is that provided by detector tubes. Glass tubes of the type illustrated

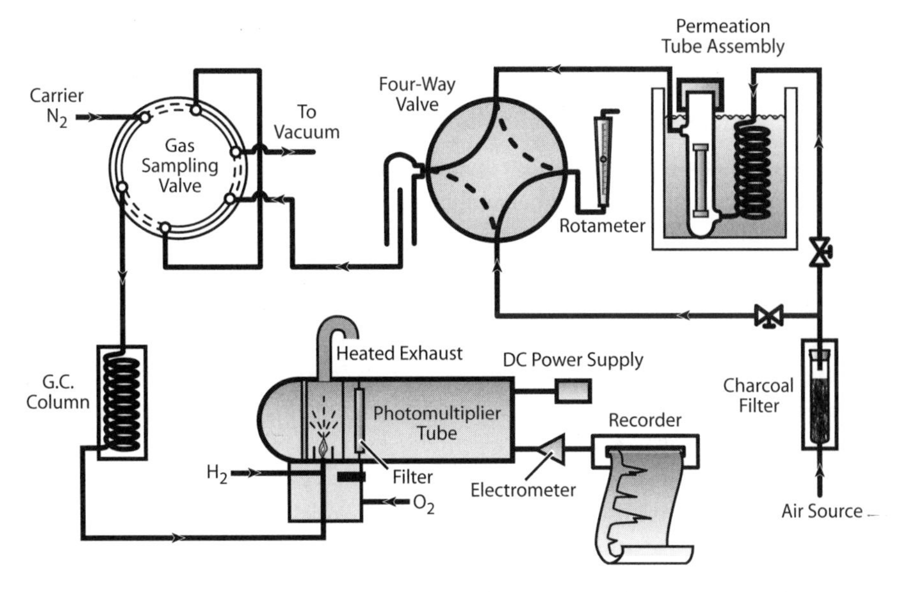

FIGURE 8–30. Schematic of an automated gas chromatograph/flame photometric detector system for analysis of SO_2 and other sulfur compounds.

in Figure 8–31 are filled with adsorbing granules coated with a colorimetric chemical reagent that changes its color after reacting with a specific gas or compound class.

A specific small volume of air, typically 100 cm^3, is drawn through the tube from one end toward the other, usually with a hand-powered pump; the contaminant of interest reacts with the adsorbed chemical, changing its color. The capacity of the granules to take up the chemical is limited, so that the penetration of contaminant into the tube before its molecules are captured is dependent on concentration. The length of color change is, therefore, an index of the concentration. Detector tubes were developed for occupational health and safety evaluations, and are currently available for about 200 gases and vapors. However, their accuracy is generally not very good; only 39 tube types for 14 gases have been demonstrated to have accuracies equal to or better than +25%, according to tests conducted by the NIOSH. Some detector tubes have been calibrated for long-period sampling using mechanical sampling pumps and can, therefore, be used to determine lower airborne concentrations in industrial and community environments.

FIGURE 8–31. A detector tube.

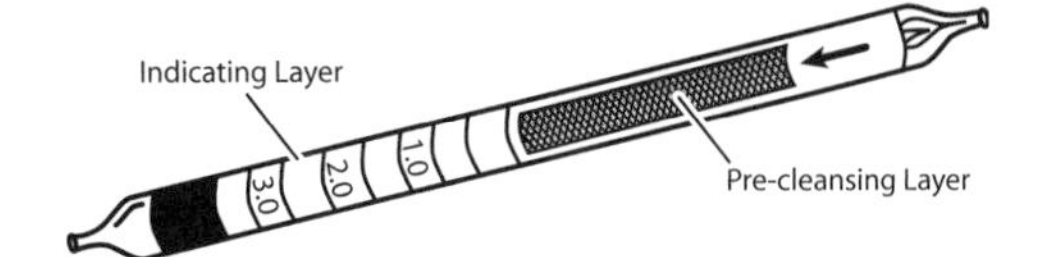

While there are many direct-reading instruments that are specific for gases and vapors, there are virtually none for airborne particles.

Direct-reading instrumentation for waterborne contaminants

Direct-reading instruments are commonly used for the measurement of water-quality parameters other than contaminant concentrations, such as temperature, pH, and dissolved oxygen. Examples of these instruments are presented in Table 8–7.

One of the more commonly used methods for the direct measurement of dissolved contaminants is the ion-selective electrode. A variety of electrodes are available that respond rather selectively to specific ions; their response depends upon the potential of a measuring electrode vs. a reference electrode. Among the contaminants for which selective electrodes exist are NH_4^+, CN^-, SO_4^{-2}, F^-, Na^+, and Ag^+. Spectrophotometric methods utilizing the IR- or UV-absorption characteristics of specific contaminants are also widely used. Some of their applications are for measurement of total organic carbon and certain dissolved in-

Table 8–7. Direct Measurements for Some Nonspecific Water-Quality Parameters

PARAMETER MEASURED	TYPICAL INSTRUMENTATION	PRINCIPLE OF OPERATION
pH	pH meter	Voltage difference between a measuring electrode (a glass tube having a special membrane which responds to H^+ at one end) and a reference electrode
DO	DO electrode or DO probe (gas membrane electrode)	Gas dissolved in the water diffuses through a semipermeable membrane into an electrochemical cell compartment, which is comprised of a sensing electrode, reference electrode, and supporting electrolyte. DO reacts at sensing electrode to produce a current flow
Turbidity	1. Turbidimeter	1. Measures amount of light passing directly through the water
	2. Nephelometer (low turbidity ranges)	2. Measures light-scatter in water
Temperature	1. Thermometer	1. Expansion and contraction of a liquid
	2. Thermocouple	2. Measures voltage generated at junction of two wires made of different metals
	3. Thermistor	3. Electrical resistance varies with temperature in special resistors

DO, dissolved oxygen.

organic gases. Electrochemical methods, such as coulometry, potentiometry, and polarography, are used for the measurement of a wide range of metals in water.

Sample collection with on-line measurements

The water-quality instrumentation that measures a rate or product of reaction between a contaminant and a reagent is essentially the same as that described earlier for air contaminants, except that a reactor vessel replaces the scrubber, and the sampled stream contributes water as well as contaminant to the mixture in the reactor.

Quality Assurance

The accurate determination of the concentrations of trace contaminants in environmental media is no small or simple task, as should be evident from the preceding discussion. It should, therefore, not be surprising that many of the data in the literature are at least partially suspect. One unfortunate result is that there is a great deal of confusion and controversy about the status and significance of many chemicals in the environment.

Fortunately, there has been a much greater awareness of the problems of quality assurance of environmental data in recent years, and significant progress is being made in the availability of standard reference materials and calibration instrumentation and techniques for analysis of specific contaminants. There are an increasing variety of laboratory certification programs, and programs for interlaboratory evaluation of analytical methods. Some of these important activities are summarized in Table 8–8. More complete discussions of standardization and calibrations are presented in a variety of standard reference works in the Bibliography.

EXPOSURE DATA RESOURCES AND DATA MANAGEMENT

There are multiple needs for exposure data throughout the risk assessment and risk management continuum. Exposure data are needed to: *(1)* establish baseline exposure levels for populations and to observe trends in those levels as a measure of the success or failure of risk management efforts (e.g., regulations); *(2)* perform surveillance functions, i.e., using data to identify high exposure/high risk groups where public health interventions might be appropriate and effective before harmful effects occur; *(3)* investigate exposure-response relationships for environmental health hazards (e.g., epidemiologic research); and *(4)* better inform regulatory decisions by supporting population exposure assessments, cost estimates, and other aspects of regulatory analyses.

The ultimate goal of these applications is the protection of public health. Each requires direct measures of exposure or the monitoring of environmental factors

Table 8–8. Organizations Publishing Recommended or Standard Methods and/or Test Protocols Applicable to Air Sampling Instrument Calibration

ABBREVIATION	FULL NAME AND ADDRESS
ANSI	American National Standards Institute, Inc. 11 W. 42nd Street, 13 Floor New York, NY 10036
ASTM	American Society for Testing and Materials D-22 Committee on Sampling and Analysis of Atmospheres and E-34 Committee on Occupational Health and Safety 100 Barr Harbor Drive West Conshohocken, PA 19428
AWMA	Air and Waste Management Association 1 Gateway Center, Third Floor Pittsburgh, PA 15222
EPA/NERL	U.S. Environmental Protection Agency National Exposure Research Laboratory Quality Assurance Division Research Triangle Park, NC 27711
NIOSH	National Institute of Occupational Safety and Health Editor, *NIOSH Manual of Analytical Methods* (NMAM®) Division of Physical Sciences and Engineering 4676 Columbia Parkway Cincinnati, OH 45226

that will permit an estimation of those exposures. To be useful, repositories of exposure data should contain not only measurements of contaminant concentrations in relevant media, but also information about the circumstances that give rise to the concentrations and to potential exposures to those media, i.e., simultaneous measurements of the activities of populations of interest. This section discusses some salient aspects of current exposure databases and the manner in which current assumptions and practices in exposure monitoring affect the nature and usefulness of such data.

The last two decades have seen a change in the availability of methods for sampling and analysis of environmental exposures, as well as in the means to store and manipulate data through ever cheaper and more efficient computers. Coupled with the regulatory legislation of the same period, these changes have triggered an explosion in the volume of quasi exposure-related data collected and stored. Substantial financial, human and technological resources are devoted to this task throughout the nation. However, the quality, availability, and usefulness of the resulting data resources leave much to be desired for their application to long-term assessment of exposure and changes in exposure. Present data collection approaches are neither comprehensive nor cost effective, and the collected data have not been optimally used.

Government agencies, particularly the EPA and the FDA, are the major collectors of human exposure data, with the notable exception of the occupational environment, where the OSHA, NIOSH and the Mine Safety and Health Administration (MSHA) have primary domain. EPA typically monitors contaminants in source emissions (i.e., industrial stacks or discharge pipes), in the environment (i.e., air and drinking water) and, much less frequently, in human tissue or blood (i.e., the former National Human Adipose Tissue Survey). The data, however, are frequently inadequate for estimating exposure in various exposure assessment applications. The monitoring is largely driven by regulatory or legal mandates related to compliance with source emission or environmental standards. Environmental monitoring focused on measuring contaminants in the air, water, food, and soil does not provide actual measures of human exposure. Furthermore, as a result of the current regulatory structure, the measurement of environmental contaminants is highly compartmentalized among and within various government agencies (OSHA, EPA, FDA, etc.). This compartmentalization frequently results in artificial barriers that limit the ability of any one agency or industry to assess total human exposure and develop effective mitigation strategies.

Assessing exposures to air contaminants provides a good example of the problems posed by the current regulatory structure. The EPA has regulatory responsibility for monitoring community air quality, and OSHA and the regulated industry have responsibilities for monitoring air in the work place. Indoor residential sources, despite their importance (particularly for the susceptible segments of the population), are not assessed on any routine basis by any agency and are not considered in establishing exposure standards. The ability to foresee and effectively address emerging environmental issues will require such regulatory barriers to be removed, minimized, or adapted in ways that promote multiple uses of that data.

Regulatory efforts frequently separate contaminants by whether they are found in these different media, whether they are ingested, inhaled or absorbed through the skin, and by the environment in which the exposure occurs (e.g., work place, home). Contaminants in multi-environmental media and multi-human exposure pathways, such as pesticides, automotive fuels, polycyclic aromatic hydrocarbons, and heavy metals, are not monitored in a systematic way, so that the media and pathway of exposures can be assessed or actual exposures quantified.

A primary justification for human exposure assessment is to support actions that protect public health and welfare. Seldom, however, are environmental exposure data gathered in combination with measures of dose or effects. The National Health and Nutrition Examination Surveys (NHANES) of the National Center for Health Statistics (NCHS) are some of the few national health surveys that have gathered biomarker indicators of exposure in combination with health outcome data. These studies, however, have relied mostly on questionnaires to assess exposures, with some use of environmental monitoring data that were collected independently. Exposure monitoring needs to be linked to indicators of dose (i.e., biomarkers) and health or comfort outcomes, as well as to information about the sources and circumstances that gave risk to the exposures. In many ways the recently completed National Human Exposure Assessment Survey (NHEXAS) was being developed in a fashion that parallels, and significantly improves on, the limited exposure metrics that could reasonably be employed in the first four NHANES.

Since environmental contaminants, whether found in the air, water, food or soil, are generally found as part of a complex mix, current efforts to monitor environmental contaminants that focus on single compounds (specific pesticides, individual air contaminants, specific heavy metals, etc.) may not reflect the complex nature of the mix or the toxicity from interactions among the components. If monitoring efforts are to be tied to effects they must take into account the complex nature of contaminant mixtures.

Environmental monitoring networks are designed to assess environmental concentrations of regulated contaminants in areas of suspected high concentrations and media where the potential for large scale exposure exists (i.e., ambient air, soil, and water quality monitoring networks). While these monitoring networks may meet the mandated regulatory needs, they usually do not provide data for the direct measurement of human exposure or data necessary to estimate human exposure, characterize exposure distributions, or identify high-risk groups. Monitoring locations are rarely selected to be statistically representative of populations or geographic areas. Population time-activity patterns are not measured or considered in site selections, or in the interpretation of data.

When applying data in a risk assessment for a population, the distribution of the exposures needs to be described. Figure 8–32 outlines EPA's current recommendations for describing such a distribution.

Each database has associated with it potential sources of bias, error, and inconsistencies resulting from all aspects of the data gathering effort (site selection, frequency of sampling, sampling and analytical methods used, etc.). Quality control and quality assurance procedures vary greatly among these databases. Seldom are the documentation for the data presented and the limitations and inconsistencies identified. No standardized procedures exist for collecting or reporting environmental data. The lack of such procedures introduces considerable difficulties in combining existing monitoring data for the estimation of human exposures. Furthermore, much of the available environmental data are maintained in formats that are not easily accessible. The systems through which these data are stored, retrieved, analyzed, and reported are not designed to be easily accessible and usable by government or nongovernment groups interested in assessing human exposures. Those databases that are more easily accessible frequently do not contain the necessary documentation.

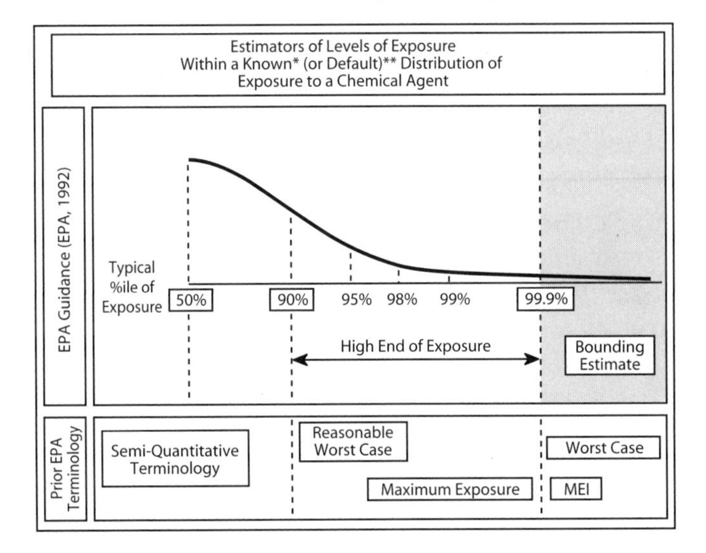

FIGURE 8–32. EPA Science Advisory Board recommendation on exposure terminology.

MODELLING OF EXPOSURES

Distributions of direct measurements of exposures based on actual measurements are seldom available for risk assessments of populations of interest. Therefore risk assessors generally rely on exposure models. They often begin with source characterization (See Chapter 3), extend through dispersion modelling in environmental media (Chapter 4), assume standard patterns of ventilation, ingestion, and activity sites and levels, and they correct, to the extent possible, for population distributions of age, sex, and socioeconomic variables. The use of such data is illustrated schematically in Figure 8–1.

Since there are numerous data gaps that confront the risk assessor when using exposure models, conservative assumptions (default values) are generally built into the exposure models to provide some assurance that exposures will not be underestimated in terms of either median levels or upper bound exposures. For general population distributions of exposures, the latest EPA Guidelines for Exposure Assessment provide a good description of a series of fairly detailed procedures.[6]

Constraints in Current Exposure Modelling Practices

To a large extent, exposure assessment for application in risks assessments is still performed under a number of assumptions that have been proven incorrect, or are not supported by common experience and systematic verification by direct observation. These assumptions and their shortcomings are summarized below.

Time-activity patterns

Consideration of the time spent by individuals in different locations and their activities have been incorporated to a very limited extent in exposure assessments conducted for risk assessment purposes. Current practice is generally based on the following questionable assumptions:

- time-activity patterns are invariant during an individual's lifetime,
- there are no significant differences in time-activity patterns of the population as a function of age, gender, socioeconomic status, or ethnic origin that may affect exposures, and
- there are no significant differences in time-activity patterns of the population in relation to regional variability, as well as urban, suburban, or rural place of residence.

Time-activity patterns at any given age can also change significantly over time due to societal trends. For example, children used to remain at home until school age. With more women working outside the home, however, more infants and preschoolers spend most of their day in child care settings. There is also a trend towards lengthening the school year, which could result in children spending less time in the home or outdoors, or in changed times of the year for school vacations. Children and adolescents are also increasingly involved in structured, competitive sports activities, either indoors or outdoors, for significant amounts of time. The duration and place where these activities are undertaken could impact children's exposures and their inhalation doses associated with elevated ventilation rates. The trend towards telecommuting and the increased number of home-based businesses increases the amount of time spent at home, as compared to a separate work place, for at least some fraction of the adult population. A large segment of the adult population also engages in sports or exercise activities, both indoors and outdoors, during significant amounts of time, for health maintenance or cosmetic reasons. As such adults age and have more free time, they are likely to engage in less strenuous, longer duration exercise and leisure activities (e.g., daily walks, golf) performed outdoors, resulting in less time spent indoors. Consideration of these societal trends means that activity patterns cannot be considered fixed in time.

Although time location budgets in the U.S. and abroad are rather consistent (i.e., approximately 90% of the time is spent indoors), there has been inadequate consideration of time-activity pattern variability as a function of socioeconomic status, gender, ethnic origin, or location of residence. For example, population subgroups in lower socioeconomic strata with significant levels of unemployment would be expected to have very different time-activity patterns than those in the middle or upper socioeconomic strata. They are also less likely to engage in the health maintenance and leisure activities previously described. The type of employment also can influence the outdoors vs. indoors time budget (e.g., construction, lawn maintenance). Gender also affects individual time-activity patterns. Even when over half the women with school-age children work away from the home, a significant number still remain within the home environment most of the day. There is also limited information on differences in activity patterns that may affect exposures as a function of the region of the country or urban vs. suburban vs. rural populations due, at least in part, to the lack of activity in behavioral science research. This is a critical gap in exposure analysis.

Exposure pathways

Although exposure assessments, as applied to risk assessment, have incorporated the consideration that certain exposure sources and pathways may be more important for some population subgroups (e.g., ingestion of contaminated soil by children), current practice is, by and large, based on the following assumptions:

- source emissions and concentrations of contaminants in media, foodstuffs, and consumer products to which an individual may be exposed are invariant during an average lifetime of 70 years.
- the relative importance of different exposure pathways does not change over an individual's lifetime (exception: soil ingestion by children).
- there are no significant differences in relevant exposure pathways as a function of gender, socioeconomic status, or ethnic origin.

Reformulation of consumer products, for example, cosmetics, cleansing agents, personal care products, occurs continuously, both in terms of the types and relative concentrations of the chemical constituents of such products. Emissions from mobile sources in particular, but those from industrial point sources as well, have shown a consistent trend of reductions during the last four decades, largely as a result of improvements in technology and regulatory pressures. The types of emissions have also changed in many cases. For example, benzene and other aromatic compounds have replaced tetraethyl lead as engine antiknock additives, with the consequent changes in airborne lead and benzene concentrations, as well as the exposures associated with mobile sources. Changes in the types and relative consumption of different fuels as well as improvements in combustion technology have also resulted in reductions of airborne concentrations of some pollutants such as sulfur oxides and particulate matter. As a result, exposures have changed both qualitatively and quantitatively well within the generally assumed 70-year life span, and current models do not account for increasing life expectancy.

The types and relative proportions of different foodstuffs in the diet and, consequently, food consumption-related exposures are generally assumed to be constant over a lifetime after infancy. However, food preferences can vary significantly with the age of the individual, as well as with societal trends. Young children may consume proportionally larger amounts of fruits and milk in their diet as compared to adults. Adolescents may consume significantly larger amounts of "fast" or "junk" foods. As adults, they may become more aware of the importance of a healthy diet and reduce their intakes of such foods, fat, and meat, and revert to an increased consumption of fruits and vegetables. Advice regarding what constitutes a healthy diet also changes over time, therefore affecting exposures as well. In addition, a significant fraction of the population at any given time may be on special diets (e.g., weight reduction diets).

Dietary sources of exposure also vary over time as a result of changes in agriculture and food production practices. For example, pesticides, herbicides, and other chemicals used in the production, preservation, and processing of foods vary as a result of regulatory and market pressures. New food products are introduced into the market place constantly, affecting dietary exposures. The levels of contaminants present in locally grown foods may not be a good indicator of dietary exposures for a particular population. Foods grown in one area of the country are distributed nationally; food imports have also increased significantly as a result of increased trade. The types and relative amounts of foods consumed also vary according to socioeconomic status, ethnic origin, and gender.

Lifestyle and other personal factors

Current EPA practice in exposure assessment assumes that in general, lifestyle and/or other personal factors do not impact exposures significantly and lifestyle and/or other personal factors that might impact exposures do not vary significantly throughout an individual's lifetime or across the population.

Lifestyle factors will significantly affect exposures. The most notorious behavioral factor with a strong influence on exposures to a wide range of contaminants is smoking. But other lifestyle factors are also potentially important. Dietary intakes of, for example, benzo(a)pyrene may not only be strongly affected by food preferences, but can also be strongly affected by the method used to cook the food.

Residential mobility

The typical current assumption by EPA is that individuals reside in the same location throughout their lifetime. The reality is, however, that the U.S. population is highly mobile, with the average family changing residences every 5 to 7 years on average. There may also be differences in mobility associated with socioeconomic status.

Reliability of predictive models based on sources and transport

Current EPA practice in exposure assessment is based on the assumption that exposures can be adequately assessed by using source emissions or concentrations of contaminants in media and environmental transport models, and a limited number of exposure situations (i.e., scenarios).

The sophistication and complexity of models used for exposure assessment have increased notably and has also led to the development of new models that attempt to link exposure to the internal dose of a chemical at a critical target site. However, there is a significant lack of validation of such models with actual data. All models are based on explicit and implicit assumptions about how contaminants move into, through, and across environmental compartments, as well as on some conceptual framework about the most significant routes of exposure. The weakness of this approach is that, frequently, neither the assumptions nor the model results are validated with actual exposure data. The results of EPA's total exposure assessment methodology (TEAM) studies are an excellent example in which measurements of volatile organic compounds in outdoor, indoor, and personal air demonstrated that the long-held assumption that populations living near industrial sources experience higher exposures to these compounds than those living in less industrialized areas was incorrect. They study showed, in fact, that indoor sources dominate exposures to many volatile organic compounds, and that exposures to the study populations were similar and not dominated by the presence of nearby sources. Another example is the assumption that ingestion is the dominant route of exposure for chemicals in potable water. In many cases, major contributions to internal dose derive from dermal contact via bathing or inhalation of vapors and aerosols released in showers and sprays.

Temporal variability at specific locations

Although EPA occasionally includes consideration of long-term accumulation of contaminants in environmental compartments, the Agency often assumes that the concentration of contaminants in media remains constant over time.

As a result of this very assumption, exposures associated with those contaminants and compartments are also assumed to be invariant over time. To a large extent, this assumption is related to the heavy reliance on environmental transport and fate models that are generally based on steady-state condition assumptions. Concentrations of contaminants in media can either increase or decrease over time due to changes in environmental conditions or human activities that may result in either enhancing or diminishing the release and bioavailability of the contaminant in specific compartments.

Independence of exposures to multiple individual agents and sources

Current EPA practice is based on the assumption that exposures can be assessed on a chemical-by-chemical basis, or, conversely, that there are no significant interactions between simultaneous exposures to more than one agent. There is, however, significant evidence that suggests that this assumption is not appropriate, since effects from a combination of agents may be more or less than additive.

Infiltration of outdoor air into indoor spaces

Although there has been some recognition that indoor environments are more significant contributors to solvent and NO_2 exposures than outdoor air, current

EPA exposure assessment practice is still largely based on the following assumptions: buildings do not significantly affect exposures to outdoor airborne pollutants, and that buildings are static and indoor concentrations of airborne contaminants can be modeled using steady state assumptions.

As noted, most of the population spends about 90% of their time indoors. As a result, indoor environments are typically more important in determining exposures to some airborne contaminants than ambient air. Indoor exposures to airborne pollutants are the sum of the fraction of the outdoor concentration that penetrates into a building plus the contribution from indoor sources. The extent of infiltration of outdoor air and contaminants into a structure depends on a number of variables related to the building itself (e.g., construction, ventilation system), environmental conditions (e.g., season temperature differences between outdoors and indoors), the type of contaminant (e.g., reactive or nonreactive, small or large particles), and human factors (e.g., opening of windows, obstruction of air intakes to maintain higher temperatures indoors, use of the space for purposes other than the original design).

Population distributions of exposure

Inherent in current EPA practice on exposure assessment are the assumptions that the population exposure to any contaminant can be described by one of the well characterized statistical distributions (e.g., log-normal), and that the distribution of exposures in the population is not affected by factors such as socioeconomic status, gender, ethnicity, and lifestyle factors.

The EPA generally assumes that population exposure distributions behave similarly because concentrations of contaminants in media generally approach one of the simpler statistical distributions (i.e., typically a unimodal, log-normal distribution). The idea that, for risk assessment purposes, an acceptable exposure can be established at a certain percentile in the upper tail of such distribution is also based on the assumption of a "well behaved" statistical distribution of exposures.

Figure 8–32 from EPA's Guidelines for Exposure Assessment (FR 57[104] 5/29/94, 22888–22938) shows the current terminology for describing exposures at the upper end of the population distribution. This guidance replaced "armchair" and uninterpretable terminology, such as maximally exposed individual. When total exposures occur via multiple media, and especially when indirect exposures to contaminants emitted into and transported through the atmosphere are involved, the situation can become quite complex. While data on population exposures and their distributions are very limited, there is some evidence that population exposure distributions are often skewed, i.e., they may be multimodal because the overall distribution of population exposures is a juxtaposition of different population subgroups' exposures.

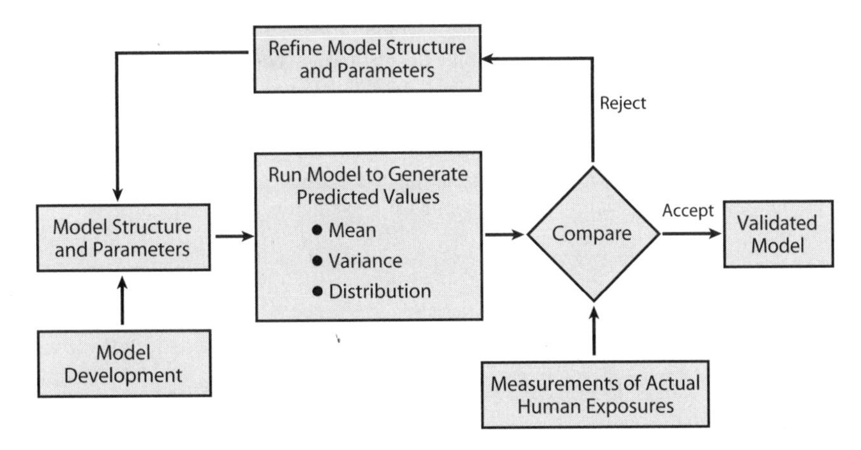

FIGURE 8–33. Diagram showing the importance of human exposure measurements for validating exposure models. (*Source*: Adapted from EPA materials.)

Currently Available Models

Current models for human exposure assessment provide estimates of chemical concentrations in environmental media, as well as mass flux from sources, through environmental compartments, to human receptor target organs, tissues, or cells. Most of the modeling effort has been focussed on the solution of chemical fate and transport equations for the prediction of concentrations in air, food, water, and soil. Common pathways of concern include drinking water, incidental ingestion of soil, inhalation of vapors and particulate matter, and ingestion of fish and garden vegetables.

Many of the current exposure models are undergoing in-depth evaluations and refinement. The basic approach to model validation is illustrated in Figure 8–33. There will need to be a long-term and serious committment to this model validation program before the quantitative risk assessments based on exposure model predictions became reasonably credible.

REFERENCES

1. ACGIH. Air Sampling Instruments—9th Edition. American Conference of Governmental Industrial Hygienists. Cincinnati, Ohio, 2000.
2. Patty, F., Clayton, G., and Clayton, F. Industrial Hygiene and Toxicology—5th Ed., Vol. 1. New York: Wiley, 2000.
3. Palmes, E.D., Gunnison, A.F., DiMattio, J., and Tomczyk, C. Personal Samplers for Nitrogen Dioxide. *Am. Industr. Hyg. Assoc. J.* 37:570–577, 1976.

4. APHA, AWWA, and WPCF. Standard Methods for the Examination of Water and Waste water—19th Ed. American Public Health Assoc., Washington, DC, 1995.
5. ASTM. Annual Book of ASTM Standards-Part 31, Water, and Part 26, Atmospheric Analysis. American Society for Testing and Materials, West Gonshohocken, PA, 1997.
6. U.S. EPA. Guidelines for Exposure Assessment. EPA/600/Z-92/001. Risk Assessment Forum. Office of Research and Development. Washington. DC, May 29, 1992.

9

Environmental Noise

Noise contamination can be defined quite simply as unwanted sound. At high sound pressure levels it can cause temporary and/or permanent losses in our capacity to hear and/or understand speech and in our ability to hear and enjoy music. At lower sound pressure levels it can still be a significant environmental sensory stress. In order to understand how environmental acoustic noise can damage auditory capacity and interfere with human comfort and performance, we need to understand the nature of sound in our environment, as well as our capacity and limitations in sensing and interpreting auditory signals.

SOUND AND HEARING

Sounds are generated by mechanical vibrations that propagate through a fluid medium, such as air or water. The discussions in this chapter will be limited to airborne sound. The vibrations displace air molecules and set up patterns of elastic molecular collisions moving outward from the source. A point source vibrating at a fixed frequency generates a pure tone, and the propagating wave form is sinusoidal. The speed of sound varies inversely with the square root of the fluid density, but is constant at a given barometric pressure for all frequencies. In air, at sea level and 20°C, it is 344 m/s. The speed of sound is the product of the frequency of the mechanical disturbance, and the wavelength, i.e.,

$$C = f\lambda \tag{9–1}$$

where:

f = frequency, generally expressed in cycles per second, also known as hertz (Hz)
λ = wavelength, generally expressed in meters (m)
c = speed of sound, generally expressed in m/s.

Figure 9–1 illustrates the relationship between wavelength and frequency in air.

The intensity of a sound varies with the energy producing the mechanical vibrations, and the total acoustic output of a source is called the sound power. However, it is more convenient to express intensity in terms of a more readily measured parameter, i.e., sound pressure level (SPL). Sound pressure level is related to the variations in air pressure caused by the sound. In a free field sound travels outward from a source, so that the power is distributed uniformly over a spherical surface. The dispersion of sound is, however, also influenced by other real world factors, such as absorption of energy and reflection of sound waves at environmental surfaces, surface curvatures, distortion of sound waves by convective processes such as ambient winds, and temperature gradients (lapse rates) in boundary level air. With the resulting interactions of the original wave forms and their harmonics, the sound field at the receptor (human ear or microphone of a sound level meter) is inevitably more complex than produced by a single source. Furthermore, there are almost always multiple sound sources in every human environment, and they generally produce multiple sound frequencies.

The Decibel Scale

Measuring pressure on a linear scale gives rise to certain problems when related to the performance of the human ear. The quietest SPL at 1000 Hz that can be

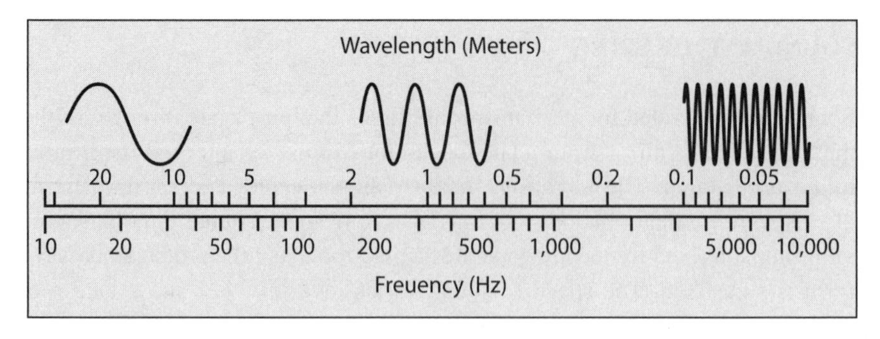

FIGURE 9–1. Wavelength in air versus frequency under normal conditions.

heard by an average person is about 20 μPascals, and this value has been standardized as the nominal hearing threshold for the purpose of sound level measurements. At the other end of the scale the threshold of pain occurs at a sound pressure of approximately 100 Pascals, a ratio of more than 5 million to 1. The direct application of linear scales to the measurement of sound pressure would therefore lead to the use of large and unwieldy numbers.

Additionally, the ear does not respond linearly, but rather logarithmically, to stimuli. For these reasons it is more practical to express acoustic parameters as a logarithmic ratio of the measured value to a standard value. This reduces the numbers to manageable proportions. The resulting unit, called the Bel (after Alexander Graham Bell), is defined as the logarithm to the base ten of the ratio of two acoustical intensities. This unit was found, in practice, to be too large, and a unit of one tenth of a Bel, the decibel (dB), is in general use. As the acoustic intensity, i.e., the power passing through a unit area in space, is proportional in the far field to the square of the sound pressure, a convenient scale for acoustic measurements can be defined as:

$$\text{Sound Pressure Level } (Lp) = 10 \log_{10} \left(\frac{p}{\mathrm{p_o}}\right)^2 = 20 \log_{10} \frac{p}{\mathrm{p_o}} \qquad (9\text{–}2)$$

where: p is the sound pressure being measured, $\mathrm{p_o}$ is the reference sound pressure, usually 20μPa, and the word level is added to sound pressure as an indication that the quantity has a certain level above some predefined reference value.

Any measurement may be expressed in dBs, as long as the absolute reference value for the unit used in the logarithmic ratio is quoted. Use of the dB scale thus reduces a dynamic range of sound pressures of a million to 1 to a more manageable range of SPLs of only 0 to 120, zero indicating the reference minimum threshold and 120 the approximate threshold of pain. This is far more convenient and easier to deal with, as the values lie within a more limited range; one unit, i.e., 1 dB, is about the smallest value of significance. In terms of perception, a change of 3 dB is barely perceptible, a change of 5 dB is clearly perceptible, and a change of 10 dB is generally considered to be twice as loud.

Because of the logarithmic nature of decibels, two identical sound sources, each producing 80 dB alone, will, when both operating, produce an SPL of 83 dB. For four 80 dB sources, the overall SPL would be 86 dB. For the addition of unequal sources, the total noise level can be obtained from a summary figure, such as Figure 9–2, by taking the difference between the dB level for the two sources and adding the value read from the y axis of the figure to the louder noise level.

Hearing

Hearing is necessary for communication, the enjoyment of music, and to locate sound sources, as well as the means of receiving undesirable noise. The recep-

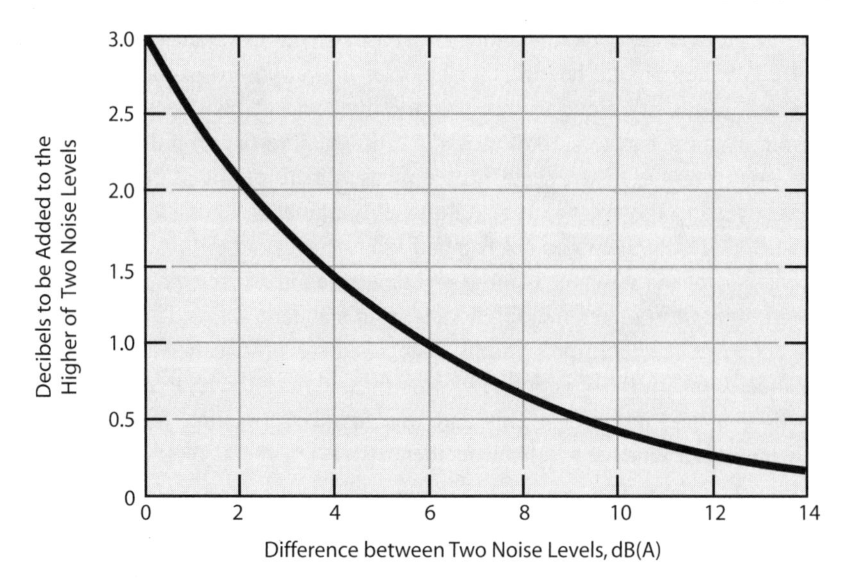

FIGURE 9–2. Noise level addition chart.

tion and analysis of sound is a complicated process that is not completely understood. The ear is a complex instrument capable of excellent discrimination over a wide range of frequencies and sound intensities.

The human ear consists of three main parts, as shown in Figure 9–3; an outer and middle ear collect the airborne sound waves and pass them to the liquid-filled inner ear, which acts as a transducer, converting mechanical vibration signals into neural impulses that transfer the acoustic information to the brain. The outer ear, consisting of the pinna and the ear canal, collects the airborne sound waves and channels them through the auditory canal, finally setting the eardrum into vibration. The middle ear has three small bones operating as a set of levers. These transfer the vibration of the eardrum to the inner ear.

The final link occurs in the inner ear, which consists of two separate systems, the semicircular canals, which are concerned primarily with balance, and the cochlea, which is concerned with hearing. The liquid-filled cavity of the cochlea is divided into two longitudinal canals by the basilar membrane, which extends along the cochlea's entire length, except for a small gap called the helicotrema at the far end. Figure 9–4 shows a longitudinal section of the unfurled cochlea and a section across it. When the stirrup, responding to an acoustic stimulus, moves the oval window, the resultant fluid disturbance passes along the upper canal, past the helicotrema, into the lower canal, and ultimately the round window deflects to accommodate it. During its passage through the canals the disturbance distorts the basilar membrane, on whose upper surface there are thousands of extremely sensitive hair cells. They register this distortion and transform

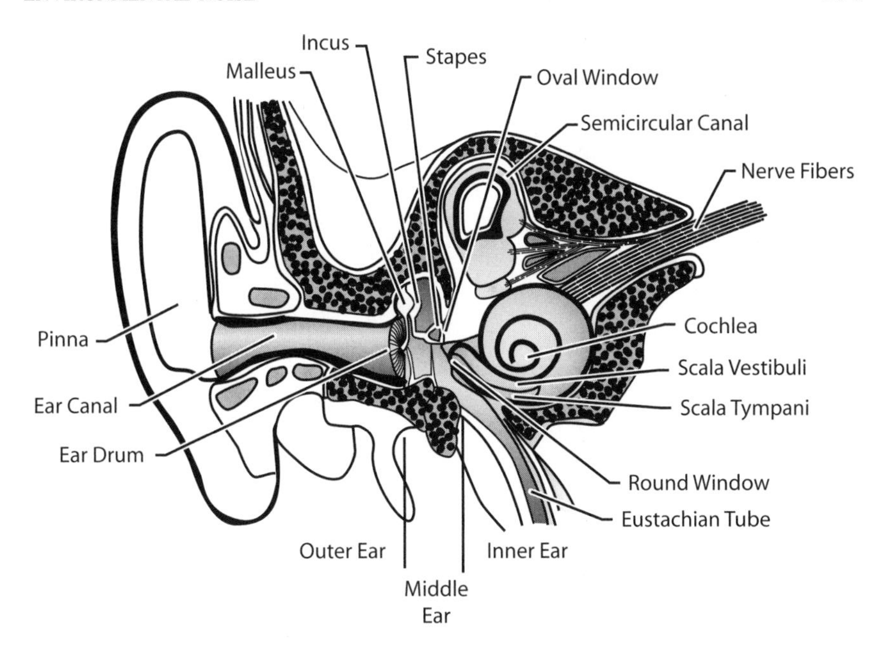

FIGURE 9–3. The main parts of the ear.

it into the nerve impulses that are transmitted to the brain. The frequency sensitivity varies with distance along the basilar membrane, the maximum response at high frequencies occurs near the oval window and that at low frequencies near the helicotrema. By this system of canals, levers, membranes, and hair cells, the ear is able to detect sounds over enormous ranges of frequency and intensity.

The ear is a remarkably sensitive organ. At certain frequencies, healthy human ears can hear sound that moves the tympanic membrane a distance equivalent to only 10% of the diameter of the hydrogen atom. Since this displacement approaches the threshold of thermal energy, any greater sensitivity would imply detection of Brownian motion. At the other extreme, the ear can sense sound pressures, such as those generated by jet engines, that are 15 orders of magnitude above the threshold of hearing. Such large SPLs can cause physical pain and, with prolonged exposure, losses in hearing acuity. The range of environmental SPLs and frequencies are illustrated in Figure 9–5, in terms of decibels. It can be seen that sensory perception varies with both frequency and intensity. It also varies with age, and we gradually lose hearing acuity, especially at the higher frequencies, as we get older. This condition is known as presbycusis.

There is not a simple relationship between the measured physical SPL and the human perception of the same sound. The loudness of a pure tone of constant sound level, perhaps the simplest acoustic signal of all, varies with its frequency,

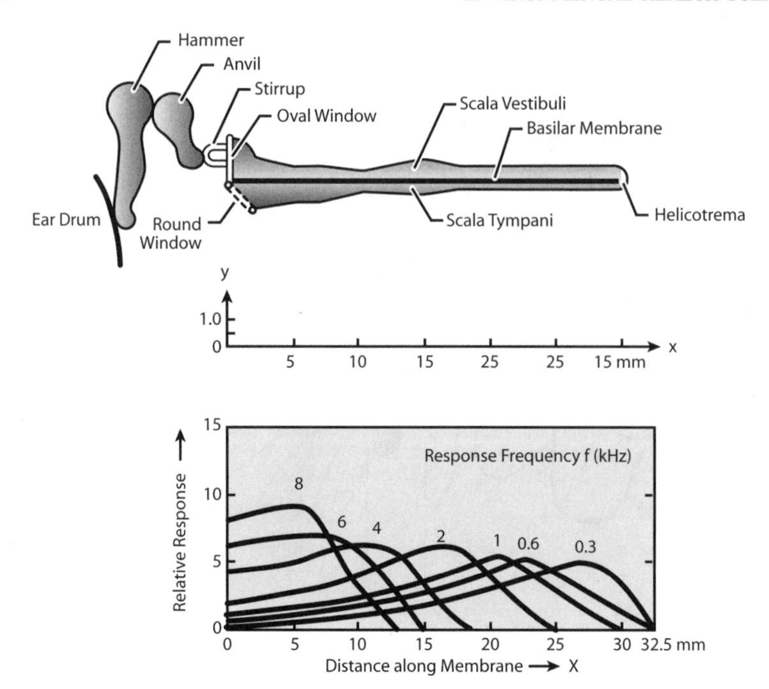

FIGURE 9–4. Longitudinal section of the cochlea showing the positions of response maxima.

and that of a short pulse will vary with its duration as well. The treatment of acoustic noise and its effects is a complicated problem, which must take a wide variety of parameters into account to achieve good correlation between measurements and the resultant human perception or reaction.

A pure tone at 1000 Hz will become very obnoxious or even painful at levels between 120 and 140 dB. As the frequency of a sound becomes greater or smaller than 1000 Hz, the auditory threshold becomes greater. For instance, the mean threshold of audibility for 10 Hz is 80 dB and for 16 kHz it is 44 dB. At the low infrasonic frequencies, sounds lose their tonal characteristics and are perceived more like rumbles. As the frequency of the sound becomes lower yet, a person is more likely to sense the vibration of the eardrum (or tympanic membrane), as well as a pressure buildup behind the eardrum. At very low frequencies, discomfort or pain may not occur until the SPLs exceed 180 to 190 dB. At 190 dB, the threshold of eardrum rupture is reached.

Actual hearing sensitivity is evaluated using a pure tone audiometer. This produces tones at 500, 1000, 2000, 3000, 4000, and 6000 Hz. Many audiometers include a tone at 8000 Hz and some also include tones at 125 Hz and 250 Hz. The intensity output from the audiometer can vary from 0 dB to about 110 dB and is often marked "hearing loss" or "hearing level" on the audiometer.

FIGURE 9–5. Envelope of human hearing and sensation.

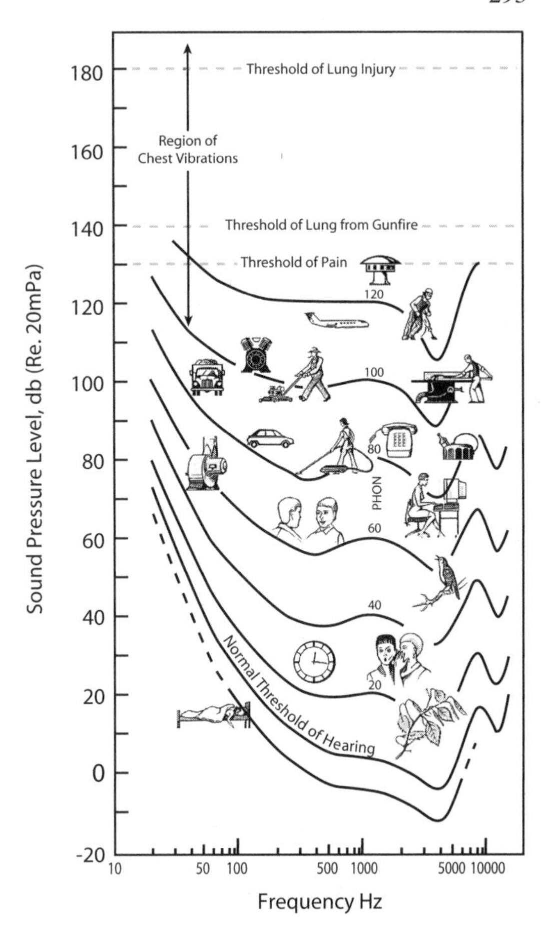

The zero reference on the audiometer ("0 dB hearing level") is the average level for normal hearing for different pure tones. Reference levels have been obtained by testing the hearing sensitivity of young healthy adults and averaging the sound level at specific frequencies at which the tones were just perceptible. If a person has a 40 dB hearing loss at 4000 Hz it means that the intensity of a tone at 4000 Hz must be raised 40 dB above the "standard" to be perceived by that person. Since the threshold of hearing is different for different frequencies, the sound pressure level required to produce 0 dB hearing level will also be different for different frequencies.

The audiogram serves to record the results of the hearing tests. The level of the faintest sound audible is plotted for each test frequency. Noise-induced hearing loss often is considered a "dip" at 4000 Hz, but for older individuals this dip might not show due to presbycusis effects at higher frequencies.

Loudness and Its Determination

The human perception of loudness of pure tones and other noise types has been exhaustively investigated and various sets of equal loudness level contours proposed. These curves are the result of a large number of different psycho-acoustical experiments, and each is, therefore, valid only for the particular experimental conditions of the test itself. The sound source may, for example, be a pure tone or a frequency band of various width; the subject may be in a free or reverberent field; a stimulus may be applied to one or both ears by means of sound sources in the room, or directly by earphones. The curves obtained are usually the result of smoothing and averaging the statistical properties over large groups of people with normal hearing in the age group 18 to 25 years. Figure 9–6 shows the loudness level contours which have been internationally standardized for pure tones heard under standard conditions, and demonstrates how the subjective loudness of a pure tone of given physical SPL varies with frequency. Tests are carried out by presenting the tone to be judged to the subject, who has adjusted a 1000 Hz reference tone until it appeared to have the same loudness. 1000 Hz is thus the reference for all loudness measurements, and all contours of equal loudness level,

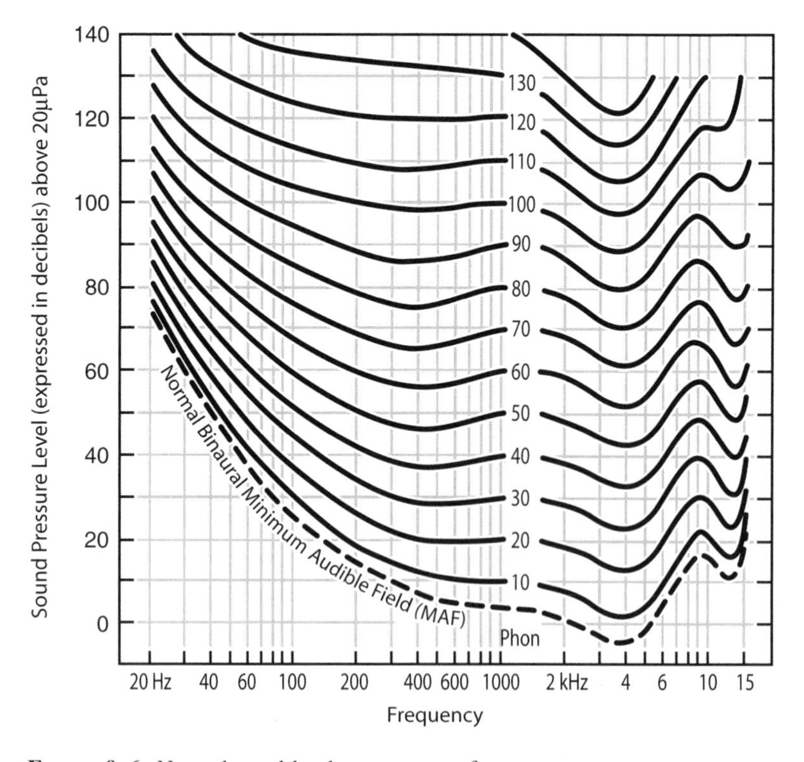

FIGURE 9–6. Normal equal loudness contours for pure tones.

expressed in Phons, have the same numerical value as the SPL at 1000 Hz. A 50 dB tone at 1 kHz thus has the same loudness level, 50 phons, as a 73 dB tone at 50 Hz or a 42 dB tone at 4000 Hz, the ear's most sensitive frequency. Generally, then, it can be seen that the loudness level of a pure tone at a given SPL falls off at low frequencies and at very high frequencies, and is a maximum at approximately 4 kHz. In addition, at very high SPL, tones of all frequencies tend to have similar loudness. The ear's assessment of loudness is, therefore, very nonlinear in relation to both frequency and absolute SPL but for a given noise, a rise of 10 dB in SPL corresponds approximately to a doubling of subjective loudness.

While it is useful to understand that there are sounds outside the range of normal hearing that may cause environmental problems, such problems are caused by sound with frequencies well inside the frequency range of 20 Hz to 20 kHz. Even with these sounds, there is a strong effect of frequency, and the common way of dealing with this is to use an A-weighting frequency network.[1] A-weighting deemphasizes both low and high frequencies, as shown in Figure 9–7. A-weighting is derived from an equal loudness curve, in which the sound pressure level is about 40 dB (more specially, the 40 phon curve shown in Fig. 9–5). The C-weighting network is derived from an equal loudness curve in which the SPL is ~100 dB. A-weighting has been found to be a good indicator for the evaluation of the effects of noise-induced hearing loss (NIHL), speech interference, and community noise in general. Therefore, A-weighting has become almost universally accepted as the unifying approach for the frequency content of noise. However, noise control engineers may use a more precise approach for

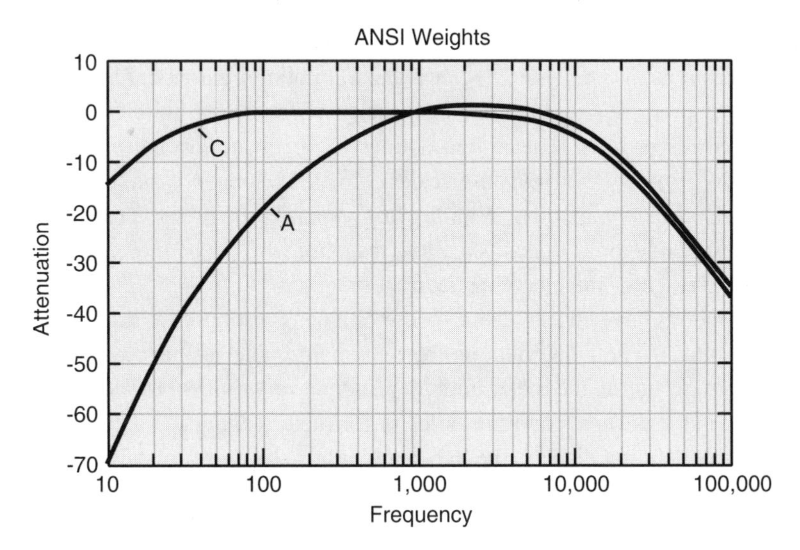

FIGURE 9–7. A-weighting and C-weighting curves.

frequency weighting when attempting to reduce the noise of a certain product or environment. For instance, aircraft certification uses a loudness descriptor, i.e., perceived noise decibel (PNdB).[2] While a precise description of the effect of noise on speech would use the speech interference level (SIL).[3]

Another necessary factor in dealing with environmental noise is the variability of the sound level with time. The commonly accepted method is to use an energy average. For community noise, a 24-hour day is broken up into day and night average sound level, with the abbreviations DL and NL. The daytime measure is the time-average sound level between 0700 and 2200 hours. The nighttime measure is the time-average sound level between 2200 and 0700 hours. Ten decibels are then added to the nighttime measure. The combined values of DL and NL are called the day–night average sound level abbreviation DNL. The approach of using logarithms for averaging sounds is well accepted and has proven to be a practical expedient in evaluating the overall impact of noise.

MEASUREMENT OF ENVIRONMENTAL NOISE

In order to properly evaluate environmental noise, it needs to be measured. The basic instrument for investigating noise levels is the sound level meter (SLM). The SLM consists of a microphone, a preamplifier, an amplifier with an adjustable and calibrated gain, frequency weighting filters, meter response circuits, and an analog meter or digital readout. Also, most meters have an output jack where the signal can be connected to a tape recorder or a graphic level recorder. There are three levels of precision available, classified by the American National Standards Institute (ANSI) as Types 0, 1, and 2. Type 0 is a laboratory standard; Type 1 is for precision measurements in the field; and Type 2 is for general purpose measurements. A Type 2 meter is the minimum requirement by OSHA for sound measurement equipment and is usually sufficient for noise surveys.

Most SLMs provide at least two options for frequency weighting: A and C. Some also provide other response scales. Most SLMs have two meter response characteristics: slow and fast. With the fast response, the meter very closely follows the sound level as it changes. Slow response tends to be more sluggish and gives an average of the changing sound level.

Some meters have an impulse response or a peak response for transient or impulsive sounds. The peak value is the maximum value of the waveform. With the impulse response, the meter initially responds very quickly to sounds of short duration, but it decays slowly in order to facilitate reading the value. On some meters with a digital display, the indicated impulse level can remain at the value until the user resets the meter.

Specifications of SPL meters and guidance on their use are provided by ANSI Specifications for Sound Level Meters.[1,4] These meters are available from many manufacturers, so the user needs only to verify that the manufacturer assures that the appropriate standards are met. The use of such meters requires field calibration. For community noise specifically, there are four standards that are appropriate.[5–8]

HEALTH EFFECTS OF ENVIRONMENTAL NOISE

Noise-Induced Hearing Loss

For the purposes of NIHL, the term noise is used to denote both wanted sound and unwanted sound, since both can damage hearing. NIHL has undoubtedly occurred throughout human history. With the advent of gunpowder and modern industrial processes, NIHL began to be recognized. However, before 1950, reliable dose-effect data were not available.

Currently American, European, and international standards relating to noise measurement and hearing acuity measurements are in reasonable agreement. An international standard[9] provides the method for predicting NIHL from noise exposure. A complete description of NIHL for various exposure levels and times can be calculated. An example of the data in this standard is provided in Table 9–1 which lists the noise induced permanent threshold shift (NIPTS) at various SPLs for several occupational exposure durations.

The main types of hearing loss are conductive hearing loss, sensorineural hearing loss, or a combination thereof.

Conductive hearing loss is any condition that interferes with the transmission of sound to the cochlea. Pure conductive losses do not damage the organ of Corti or the neural pathways. A conductive loss can be due to wax in the external au-

TABLE 9–1. Noise-Induced Permanent Threshold Shift in dB Averaged Across Audiometric Test Frequencies 0.5, 1, 2, and 3 kHz[a]

	NIPTS, DB											
	EXPOSURE TIME, YEARS											
	10			20			30			40		
	FRACTILES											
L_{AB}	0.9	0.5	0.1	0.9	0.5	0.1	0.9	0.5	0.1	0.9	0.5	0.1
85	0.5	1.0	1.5	1.0	1.3	2.0	1.0	1.3	2.3	1.0	1.8	2.3
90	1.0	2.5	4.8	2.3	3.5	6.0	2.8	4.0	6.8	3.3	4.5	7.3
95	2.3	5.8	10.8	5.0	7.8	13.5	6.3	9.5	15.0	7.3	10.3	16.5
100	4.5	11.0	21.0	9.5	15.5	26.5	12.5	18.0	29.8	14.5	20.0	32.3

[a]The average of noise-induced permanent threshold shift values from Tables F1 to F4 of ANSI S3.44-1996

ditory canal, a large perforation in the eardrum, blockage of the eustachian tube, interruption of the ossicular chain due to trauma or disease, fluid in the middle ear secondary to infection, or otosclerosis (i.e., fixation of the stapedial footplate). A significant number of conductive hearing losses are amenable to medical or surgical treatment.

A sensorineural hearing loss is almost always irreversible. The sensory component of the loss involves the organ of Corti, and the neural component implies degeneration of the neural elements of the auditory nerve. Damage to the hair cells is of critical importance in the pathophysiology of noise-induced hearing loss. Invariably, degeneration of the nerve fibers accompany severe injury to the hair cells. Sensorineural hearing loss may be attributed to various causes, including presbycusis, viruses (e.g., mumps), some congenital defects (e.g., heredity), and drug toxicity (e.g., aminoglycosides).

Excessive noise exposure to the ear can cause a noise-induced temporary threshold shift (NITTS), a noise-induced permanent threshold shift (NIPTS), tinnitus, and/or acoustic trauma.

Noise-induced temporary threshold shift

Noise-induced temporary threshold shift refers to a temporary loss in hearing sensitivity. This loss can be a result of the acoustic reflex, short-term exposure to noise, or simply neural fatigue in the inner ear. With NITTS, hearing sensitivity will return to the pre-exposure level in a matter of hours or days (without continued excessive exposure).

Noise-induced permanent threshold shift

Noise-induced permanent threshold shift refers to a permanent loss in hearing sensitivity due to the destruction of sensory cells in the inner ear. This damage can be caused by long-term exposure to noise or by acoustic trauma as defined below.

Tinnitus

The term tinnitus is used to describe the condition in which people complain of a sound in the ears. The sound is often described as a hum, buzz, roar, ring, or whistle. This sound is produced by the inner ear or neural system. Tinnitus can be caused by nonacoustic events, such as a blow to the head or prolonged use of aspirin. However, the predominant cause is long-term exposure to high sound levels, although it can be caused by short-term exposure to very high sound levels, such as firecrackers or gunshots. Many people experience tinnitus during their lives. Often the sensation is only temporary, although it can be permanent and debilitating. Diagnosis and treatment of tinnitus can be difficult because tinnitus is subjective and cannot be measured independent of the subject.

Acoustic trauma

Acoustic trauma refers to temporary or permanent hearing loss due to a sudden intense acoustic event, such as an explosion. The results of acoustic trauma can be a conductive or sensorineural hearing loss. An example of a conductive loss is when the event causes a perforated eardrum or destruction of the middle ear ossicles. An example of a sensorineural loss due to acoustic trauma is when the event causes temporary or permanent damage to the hair cells of the cochlea.

ACCEPTABILITY CRITERIA

The acceptability of noise can be judged by whether the level of the noise and exposure to the noise can cause hearing loss, annoy people, or interfere with speech communication, hearing or emergency warning signals.

Hearing Loss Criteria

Noise-induced permanent threshold shift affects 10–20 million workers in the U.S. Employees exposed to high noise levels each workday for a working lifetime without adequate hearing protection can develop permanent, irreversible hearing loss.

Table 9–1 provides the statistical differences in hearing levels between a population not exposed to occupational noise and a population exposed to a measurable occupational noise at the level indicated for each group. The table shows the difference for the better hearing 10% of the population at the 90th percentile, at the median, and at the poorer hearing 10th percentile, due to noise exposure. The values of Table 9–1 can be used to predict a statistical distribution of hearing levels for a community based population. There are several observations that can be made.

First, the part of the population distribution starting with the worst hearing changes the most. In other words, the 10th percentile point of a noise-exposed population changes more from noise exposure than the better hearing median. This is the result of adding a distribution of noise-induced hearing loss to a normal distribution of hearing. It does not mean that individuals with poorer hearing are more susceptible to more loss.

Second, as an amplification of the preceding thought, the predictions of NIHL (also called noise-induced permanent threshold shift, or NIPTS) in Table 9–1 are for populations, not individuals. For an individual with a hearing loss, there is no certain method for separating the noise component from the aging component.

Third, as the combined effects of noise and aging approach approximately 70 to 80 dB, a limit as to the amount of noise-induced hearing loss that can occur seems to be reached.

Finally, Table 9–1 is for sounds that are generally broadband (contain many frequencies) and are not greatly fluctuating in intensity. A noise with one or two tones could be more hazardous, and the L_{Aeq}, or time averaged sound level, values might need to be adjusted 5 dB downward. On the other hand, an intermittent noise with many quiet periods (periods below 75 dB) might well be 5 dB less hazardous.

For the most part, the major threat to hearing comes from occupational and recreational noise exposure. Attending rock concerts and race tracks and using firearms, chainsaws, fireworks, and the like, without hearing protection, are a few examples of potentially harmful non-occupational noise.

Generally, environmental noises are not a problem with respect to hearing loss. For example, even around a very busy airport, aircraft flyovers are broadband, are interrupted, and just do not have the energy necessary to significantly harm the auditory system. Annoyance, of course, is another problem.

Nonauditory Stress

A commonly held view is that noise exposure can adversely affect physical and mental health. Noise exposure not only interferes with various activities such as speech and sleep, which causes stress, but noise may directly affect psychological and physiological processes. However, at this time, there is no clear causal link between nonauditory disease and noise. While there are many cases in which workers exposed to noise have higher blood pressure levels than normal, these same workers are also exposed to the stresses of a typical industrial setting, such as dust, vibration, time constraints, and safety hazards. For this reason the U.S. EPA concluded that "If noise control sufficient to protect persons from ear damage and hearing loss were instituted, then it is highly unlikely that the noises of lower level and duration resulting from this effect could directly induce nonauditory disease." For this reason, noise-induced hearing loss was considered the controlling effect.

Sound-Induced Vibration

The resonance of the chest to low frequency is in the range of 50 to 60 Hz, although the resonance of a very large person may be somewhat lower and the resonance of a very small person may be higher. While many discotheques and other types of musical entertainment clubs use this effect as part of the musical experience, the imposition of such effects on an unwilling population is generally completely unacceptable.

Vibration effects first occur at low frequency sound levels above 105 dB. The American Conference of Governmental Industrial Hygienists (ACGIH)[10] threshold limit values (TLV) document states that any nonimpulsive level from 1 to 100 Hz is unacceptable if above 145 dB, even if such exposure is desired. For unwanted exposure to such low frequency sounds, a sound that can be sensed will probably be a problem and efforts should be made to control the exposure at the source.

COMMUNITY NOISE

In 1974, the EPA published the *Levels Document*.[11] This document, required by the Noise Control Act of 1972, provided information to protect the public health and welfare with an adequate margin of safety. In this document, the concept of the day–night sound level was promoted. Two major methods for assessing noise exposure were also put forth. The first was the annoyance or complaint frequency demonstrated by the exposed population. The second was the activity interference, such as speech or sleep interference, caused by noise. These two methods frame the next two sections of this chapter.

Annoyance—Community Response

The day–night average sound level is useful for predicting the annoyance of a community as a result of noise from a variety of sources, including railroads, highways, aircraft, and industrial sites. An overall annoyance response description is shown in Figure 9–8. From such data the EPA suggested that a DNL of

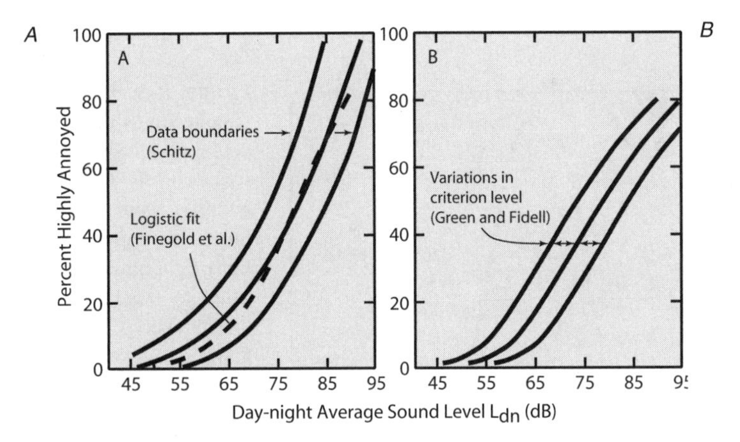

FIGURE 9–8. Various presentations of the relationship between "percent highly annoyed" and day–night average sound level L_{dn}. Boundaries in *Panel A* encompass 90% of the 161 data points from 12 "clustering survey" data sets. The solid centerline shows the fitted curve. The broken line in *Panel A* shows logistic fit to 400 data points from 28 survey data sets. *Panel B* indicates typical variations in the "annoyance criterion level," based on data from 34 survey data sets (453 data points). The central curve in *Panel B* is positioned to fit their average criterion level.

55 dB be identified as the maximum sound level for residential noise, as measured outside the home, if the public health and welfare are to be maintained with an adequate margin of safety. Unfortunately, traffic noise will cause this level to be exceeded in most urban areas. It was estimated for residential noise exposure that over 100 million people are exposed to more than 55 dB, 33 million to more than 65 dB, and 3 million to more than 75 dB. A distribution of the number of people exposed to various average day–night levels in the U.S. is shown in Figure 9–9. Note the dominance of road traffic noise. The Department of Housing and Urban Development (HUD) came up with guidelines on new developments that were intended to cover residential noise exposure. Basically, they only supported developments in which the exposure was 65 dB or lower. Such actions are a step in the right direction, but they will not solve the problem until quieter transportation vehicles (cars, trucks, aircraft, etc.) are produced.

Other guidelines for compatibility of land use are available from ANSI. Such guidelines are best used with master planning by local activities such that present or future land use can be evaluated. Figure 9–10 provides some of their guidance. Note that residential single family, which assumes outdoor use, has the most restrictive requirements. As outdoor use becomes less important, the yearly day–night average sound level (DNL) will be greater. Where there is no outdoor use, noise control by sound insulation becomes a viable option. This is why hotel, motels and transient lodging may be compatible with higher DNL's. Of course, one should always be aware of exceptions. For instance, a resort hotel based on outside activity should be treated like a single family residence.

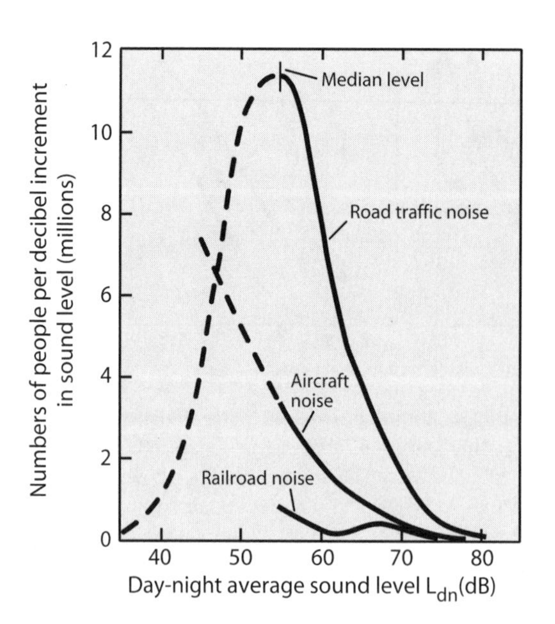

FIGURE 9–9. Population of the United States distributed by the day–night average outdoor sound levels to which various numbers were exposed in 1980 (nominal population: 20 million). Smooth curves have been fitted to tabulated estimates of the numbers of people exposed at various levels to noise from: air carrier aircraft noise, traffic on urban and rural roads and railroads, rail rapid transit systems, and rail yards. Broken lines are hypothetical extrapolations.

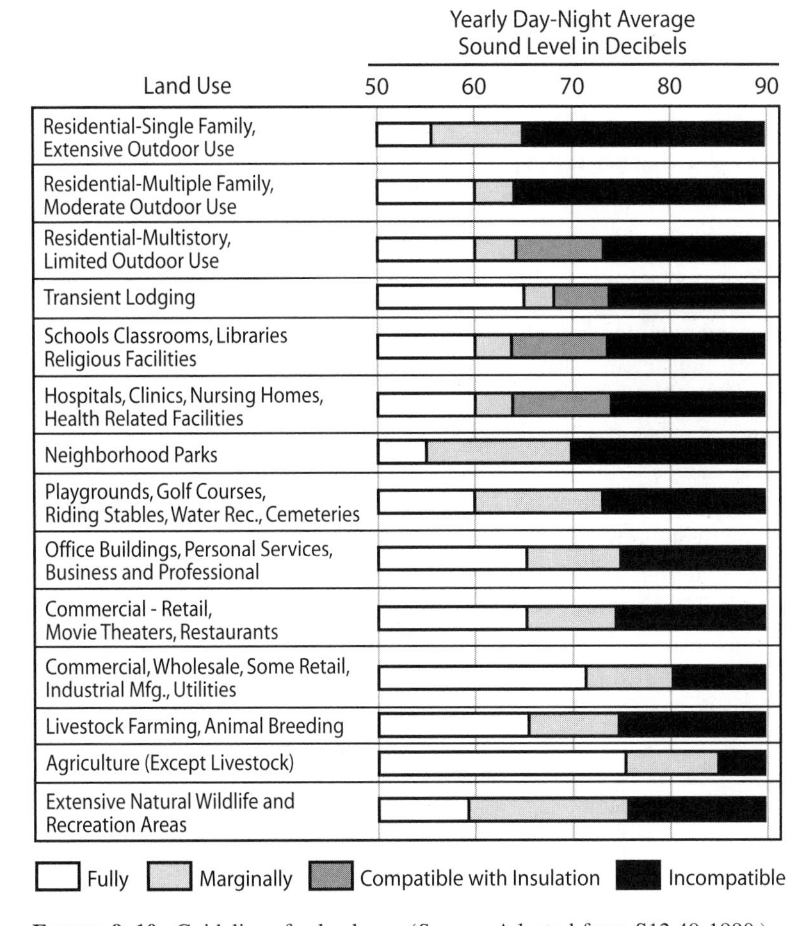

FIGURE 9–10. Guidelines for land use. (*Source*: Adapted from S12.40-1990.)

While the yearly DNL is a practical and useful measure for environmental noise, specific noise exposures might require additional analysis and review, for example, seasonal variations in land use, seasonal variations in sound exposure, interaction between noise occurrences, etc.[8] In addition, a recent standard provides adjustments for certain types of environmental noise. These special noise categories are impulsive noises (subdivided into regular impulsive, highly impulsive, and high-energy impulsive), noises with rapid onset rate, tonal noise, and noise with strong low-frequency content.[8]

The amount of correction for such special noise on the yearly DNL may be as much as 12 dB. The need for such special adjustments would most likely occur for residential areas near outdoor firing ranges, quarries, military bases with training missions requiring explosives, military operating areas with sonic booms or low level military overflights, and wind power production devices.

The yearly DNL can be measured or predicted through computer modeling. Contours of equal yearly DNL can be drawn around a noise source such as an airport, and the total number of highly annoyed residents can be predicted using the demographics of the area and a relationship shown in Figure 9–9. The impact of noise changes then can be presented in the overall change in total number expected to be highly annoyed.

Activity Interference

The second environmental impact of noise is the interference of activities such as speech, music, and sleep. The advantage of viewing noise by activity interference, in addition to annoyance, is that such interference occurs regardless of the exposed person's attitude about the noise or sound. For instance, participants in a discotheque will find it difficult to communicate regardless what their feelings are about the music. Sound insulation, such as could be placed around classrooms, is likely to be effective in reducing speech and sleep interference.

Speech interference is the effect that is easiest to quantify. Figure 9–11 shows the effect of a noise background on the distance at which two persons can carry on a conversation. The curves are adjusted such that as the background noise rises, the voice effort is also increased. Nevertheless, at some point it becomes

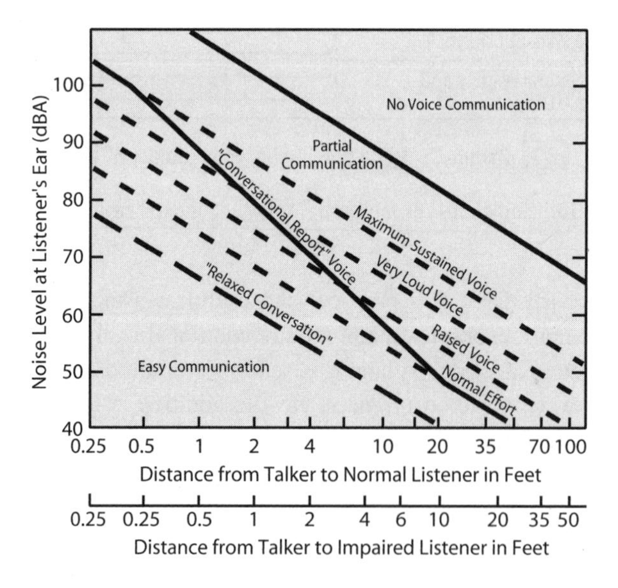

FIGURE 9–11. Maximum distances outdoors over which conversation is considered to be satisfactorily intelligible in steady noise. With one or both of the conversationalists with noise-induced hearing loss in which the signal to noise must be 6 dB or greater, the distance between the conversationalist needs to be halved. (*Source*: EPA levels document, 1974.)

impossible to communicate. Also shown on this figure, is the predicted effect on a mildly impaired person with a high-frequency noise hearing loss, such as occurs at 3 kHz and 4 kHz from noise exposure. The speech level must be as much as 6 dB greater for such persons for the same noise level. Using 6 dB as a nominal value, a legend for mildly hearing-impaired persons is also presented in Figure 9–11. This figure is one way to show the additional problems individuals with noise-induced hearing loss have with a noise exposure. Note that for the same degree of speech intelligibility, people engaged in conversation either have to talk louder or get closer when one of them has noise-induced hearing loss.

Sleep interference is a more difficult problem to analyze because individuals do adapt to sleep-interrupting noise. This is why laboratory studies will often show completely different results from field studies. This is best illustrated by some published relationships between noise exposure and sleep interference. Figure 9–8 gives the relationship proposed by some members of the Federal Interagency Committee on Noise (FICON) based on laboratory studies.[12]

The American National Standards Institute (ANSI) has set up a working group to review this issue, and they expect to propose the use of field studies. The proposed curve will, most likely, be like the Pearson's curve shown in Figure 9–12.[13] While the curve of the field studies shows less effect, it demonstrates an important problem in that not all individuals of an exposed population will adapt.

CONTROL OF ENVIRONMENTAL NOISE

Noise can be controlled in a variety of ways. Laws, voluntary standards, proper design of the sources, proper community planning, and public awareness are just some of the approaches. The more important approaches to control noise is discussed below.

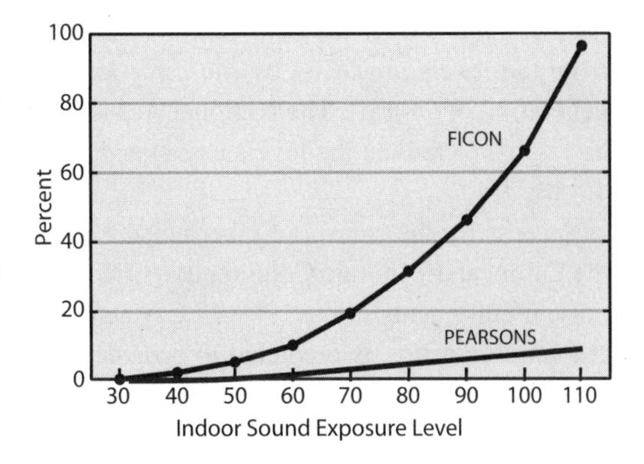

FIGURE 9–12. Dose–response curve adopted by FICON (1992) compared to curves considered by ANSI working group S12–37. Sleep disturbance is in a home environment and the event occurs within 5 minutes of awakening, which is defined by the sleeper pushing a button upon awakening.

Public Awareness

Awareness that noise is a problem and can sometimes be avoided is an important step in controlling noise. The inner ear can be protected by either avoiding excessive noise or by wearing hearing protection when participating in noisy events. For example there are plugs that are designed to attenuate rather evenly across frequencies in order to not unduly interfere with the enjoyment of music. Unfortunately, these are not universally accepted and one is likely to see only a few participants at a noisy recreational event wearing them. At shooting ranges, however, the wearing of hearing protection is more common. This is a step in the right direction, as nonoccupational noise exposures are at least as important as occupational noise exposures. In the workplace, the individual needs to follow the guidance from management. If such guidance appears to be inadequate, a complaint to the proper government authority is in order.

For nonhearing loss concerns, the aware individuals can do much. First, they can avoid living in areas with noise problems. They will avoid living next to an airport or busy highway. If a noise source tries to move next to them, they will be active in preventing such a move, requiring the noise source to reduce the noise impact to acceptable levels or providing compensation. They will also support their local government zoning activities. They will also try to buy quieter products. Aware teachers will ensure that their classrooms are quiet enough for all their students. Aware listeners will not accept not understanding what is said.

In summary, noise is best controlled by an aware society that wants it controlled.

Noise Control at the Source

The best and most efficient method for controlling noise is at the source. The most efficient action has undoubtedly been the various programs of government and the aircraft industry to reduce jet engine noise. Significant progress has been made over the years, as shown in Figure 9–13. Note the 20-dB drop from the levels produced by the early jet aircraft versus those by the current generation of aircraft. The National Aeronautics and Space Administration still has a goal to reduce the levels associated with the 1992 technology by another 10 dB.[14]

Success for the control of other noise sources has not been as good. However, the European Economic Community (EEC) has taken the lead by mandating low-noise requirements in the 1989 EEC Machinery Safety Directive.[15] In the world market, this action is predicted to provide an incentive for all manufacturers to try to reduce the noise from their products, although it is expected European manufacturers will take the lead.

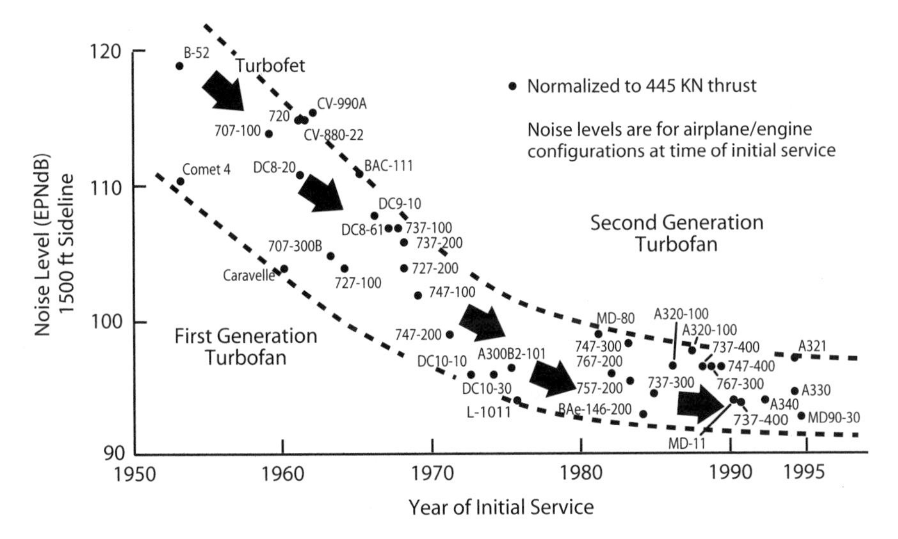

FIGURE 9–13. Progress in noise reduction. (*Source*: Stephens and Crazier, 1996.)

Voluntary Standards

Standards serve to harmonize the way noise is measured and its effects assessed throughout the world. While these standards do not set limits on noise exposure, they serve as the framework for setting limits. They also serve to provide reliable methods for evaluating how well noise control efforts are progressing. This effort is increasing. In the International Standards Organization (ISO), the number of work efforts was 17 in 1970 as compared to over 80 in 1994. These are too many to list, but a sample of the broad range of topics are as follows: hearing protector; earth moving machinery; determination of sound power levels of multisource industrial plants for evaluation of sound pressure levels in the environment.

Government Regulations

Ultimately, it is necessary for some public authority to decide how much noise is too much. For noise-induced hearing loss, most developed countries now have statutory regulations for work related exposures. These vary from the typical 85 dBA 8-hr Leq, where Leq is an equivalent frequency-weighted continuous noise level, based on a 3-dB trading relation to the more lenient 90 dBA 8-hr Leq based on the 5-dB trading relation adopted by the OSHA in the U.S.

For community noise, the lead has come from the more industrialized countries. Especially noteworthy is the effort of the EEC countries. By setting noise standards on many products, domestic U.S. manufacturers now have a goal if they expect to compete in the world market.[15]

In the U.S., one of the most important agencies in terms of noise control is Federal Aviation Administration (FAA). Initially applicable to aircraft manufactured after 1973, the FAA set noise standards for the certification of new aircraft. The standards, which are dependent on the weight of the aircraft, have become more restrictive over time and have led to categories of stage 1, stage 2, stage 3, and stage 4. Other countries have followed the U.S. lead to restrict the earlier aircraft from landing at their airports. Thus, this program has helped control aircraft noise worldwide.

New Technology

The ability to control noise can be enhanced by technological breakthroughs. Perhaps the most important achievement recently has been noise cancellation. The advent of the microchip has allowed development of feasible active noise–control devices in which the noise is measured and a canceling signal produced. These devices work best for noise signals below 1000 Hz, and they have proved effective for various low-frequency noise sources such as exhaust systems. Where the active noise–control device cannot directly reduce the noise, such as rotor noise from a helicopter, the device can be placed in a hearing protector. Noise canceling earmuffs have indeed proved effective for helicopter crews, as well as for anyone else in noise that is dominated by low frequency sound.

Another recent development is the recognition and increased use of "sound quality." Engineers are recognizing that just reducing the intensity of product noise is not as effective as making the noise both more pleasing and less intense. The concept of making noise more acceptable by use of listener panels or other techniques cannot but help to improve our acoustic environment.

In summary, the battle against environmental noise will probably never be completely won, but progress has been and will continue to be made. The need for some governmental group to provide leadership will remain necessary. In addition, the general public must increase their awareness that noise can be and should be controlled.

REFERENCES

1. ANSI (American National Standards Institute). 1994. *American National Standard Specification for Acoustical Calibrators. ANSI S1.40-1984 (R 1994).* New York: ANSI.
2. ANSI (American National Standards Institute). 1992. *American National Standard Procedure for the Computation of Loudness of Noise. ANSI S3.4-1980 (R 1992).* New York: ANSI.
3. ANSI (American National Standards Institute). 1986. *American National Standard for Rating Noise with Respect to Speech Interference. ANSI S3.14-1977 (R 1986).* New York: ANSI.

4. ANSI (American National Standards Institute). 1995. *American National Standard Measurement of Sound Pressure Levels in Air. ANSI S1.40-1984 (R 1994).* New York: ANSI.
5. ANSI (American National Standards Institute). 1992. *American National Standard Quantities and Procedures for Description and Measurement of Environmental Sound, Part 1: Measurement of Long-Term, Wide-Area Sound. ANSI S12.9-1992/Part 2.* New York: ANSI.
6. ANSI (American National Standards Institute). 1993. *American National Standad Quantities and Procedures for Description and Measurement of Environmental Sound, Part 1. ANSI S12.9-1988/Part 1 (R 1993).* New York: ANSI.
7. ANSI (American National Standards Institute). 1993. *American National Standard Quantities and Procedures for Description and Measurement of Environmental Sound, Part 3: Short-Term Measurements with an Observer Present. ANSII S12.9-1993/Part 3.* New York: ANSI.
8. ANSI (American National Standards Institute). 1996. *American National Standard Quantities and Procedures for Description and Measurement of Environmental Sound, Part 4: Noise Assessment and Prediction of Long-Term Community Response.* New York: ANSI.
9. ISO (International Organization for Standardization). 1990. *Acoustics: Determination of Occupational Noise Exposure and Estimate of Noise-Induced Hearing Impariment. ISO.* Geneva, Switzerland.
10. ACGIH (American Conference of Governmental Industrial Hygienists). 1999. TLVs and BEIs. Cincinnati, Ohio.
11. EPA (U. S. Environmental Protection Agency). Information on levels of environmental noise requisite to protect the public health and welfare with an adequate margin of safety. EPA 550/9-74-004. Washington, D.C., 1974.
12. FICON (Federal Interagency Committee on Noise). 1992. *Final Report: Airport Noise Assessment Methodologies and Metrics.* Washington, D.C.
13. Pearsons, K. I. 1996. Recent field studies in the United States involving the disturbance of sleep from aircraft noise. *Proceedings of Internoise 96, Liverpool, Eng. Inst. Of Noise Control Eng.*, pp. 2271–2275.
14. Stephens, D. G. and F. W. Cazier, Jr. 1996. NASA noise reduction program for advanced subsonic transports. *Noise Control Eng. J.* 44(3).
15. Brooks, B. M., T. J. DuBois, G. C. Maling, and L. C. Sutherland. 1996. A global vision for the noise control market place. *Noise Control Eng. J.* 44(3).

10

Nonionizing Electromagnetic Radiation

Electromagnetic radiation is emitted from sources in space and from anthropogenic sources on earth. It travels at a constant speed, i.e., the speed of light. The overall electromagnetic spectrum is illustrated in Figure 10–1. Energy is transmitted as a sinusoidal wave form, by time varying electric and magnetic fields. The transmission velocity, c, is described by the formula:

$$c = f\lambda \qquad (10\text{–}1)$$

where:

c = speed of light (generally expressed in meters/sec)
f = frequency (generally expressed in Hertz [cycles/sec])
λ = wavelength (generally expressed in meters)

The health effects of exposures to the various components of the electromagnetic spectrum vary greatly with frequency, and the discussion that follows outlines the sources, as well as the nature and extent of the effects that they produce. There are separate discussions on component bands within the overall spectrum, i.e., ionizing radiation, UV, visible, IR, and radio frequency (RF). The electric and magnetic fields induced by these radiations can also produce biological responses, and these responses will also be reviewed.

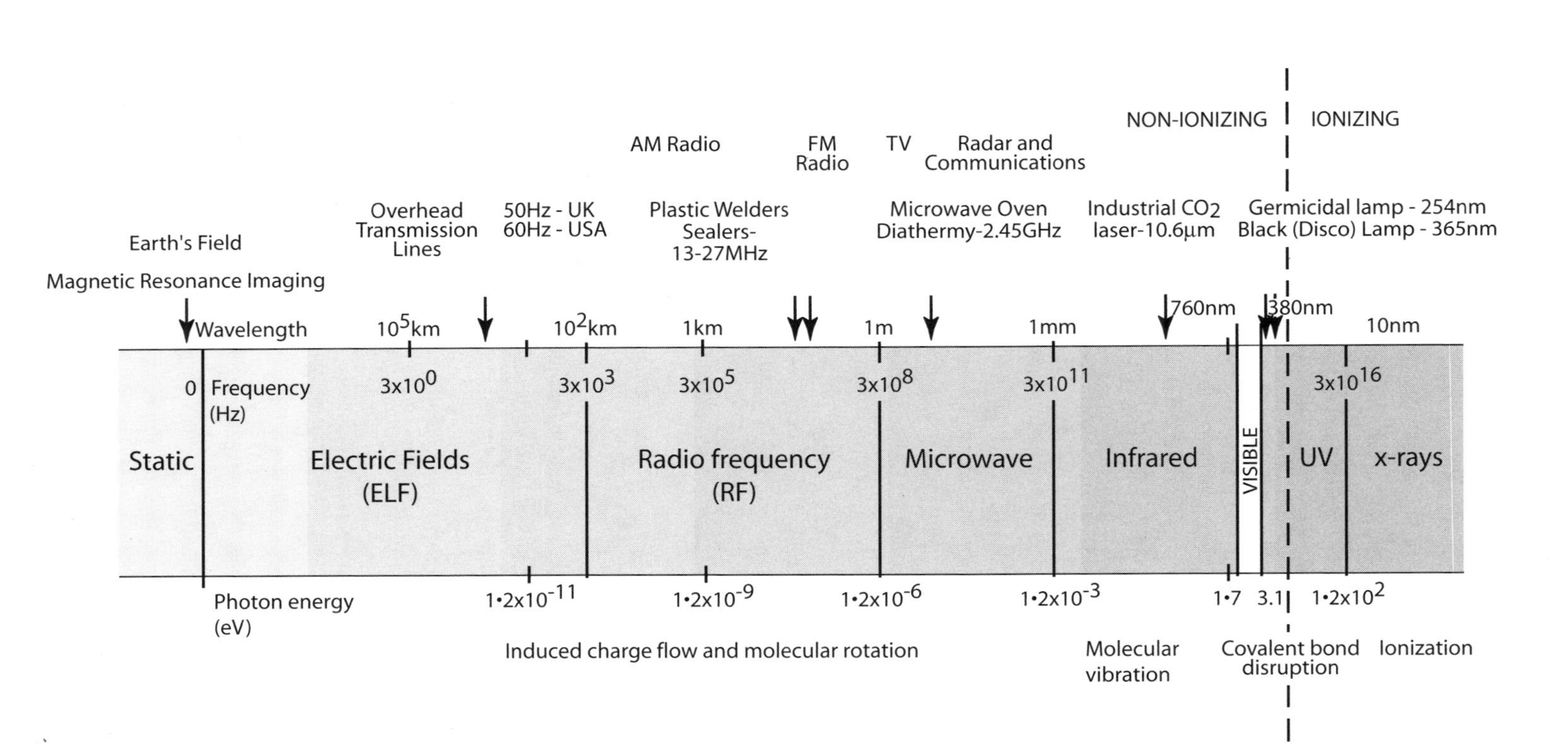

Figure 10–1. The electromagnetic spectrum.

While the energy travels in wave form, it consists of individual particles known as photons, whose energy can be expressed in terms of electron volts (eV). The photon energies decrease with increasing wavelength. Those with energies above 12.4 eV can ionize matter in their path, and are known as ionizing radiation. The ionizing radiation bands include cosmic radiation from distant stars, gamma (γ) radiation from radionuclide decay, and X-rays from anthropogenic sources. Ionizing radiation is discussed in Chapter 11. The balance of this chapter is devoted to the non-ionizing electromagnetic radiation.

Electric fields results from static charge differentials, while magnetic fields result from moving charges. The fields influence the flow of charges and their interactions with tissues through which they pass.

The discussion of human exposures and health-related responses to electromagnetic radiation begins with the radiation bands that can be analyzed in terms of conventional optics, i.e., the UV, visible, and IR bands. Ultraviolet and visible radiation are generated by electronic transitions in excited atomic systems. Infrared radiation is produced by changes in the vibrational, rotational, or translational energy states in molecules. The discussion of optical radiation is followed by a discussion of radio frequency radiation, which includes microwaves.

The optical radiation has been divided into component bands that differ in terms of their usage and biological effects, as indicated in Table 10–1. While these bands can be identified by either wavelength or frequency, they are generally described by their wavelength.

ULTRAVIOLET RADIATION

Interactions of UV radiation with matter include transmission, propagation, absorption, reflection, and refraction. Ultraviolet radiation incident on a surface may be reflected or transmitted into the material. Refraction is a change in the direction of propagation, and occurs at an interface between two transmitting media with different refractive indices.

TABLE 10–1. Spectral Bands for Optical Radiation

REGION	BAND	WAVELENGTH
Ultraviolet	C	100–280 nm
	B	280–315 nm
	A	315–400 nm
Visible		400–770 nm
Infrared	A	770–1400 nm
	B	1.4–3.0 μm
	C	3.0 μm–1 mm

Ultraviolet radiation is divided into three wavelength bands according to the effects they produce. These wavelength bands are defined in Table 10–1. Biological or hazard weighting factors are obtained from UV action spectra. An action spectrum is a graph of the reciprocal of the radiant exposure required to produce the given effect at each wavelength. All the data in such curves are normalized to the datum at the most efficacious wavelength(s).

Sources

The main environmental UV source is the sun, which has two components: the sun's beam and sky radiation. Sky radiation is diffuse, and is caused by scattering in the atmosphere. Global UV-A is a stable component of global radiation. Solar UV-B wavelengths less than about 290 nm are attenuated by stratospheric ozone. However, with the continuing depletion of stratospheric ozone, surface level UV radiation will continue to increase for several decades. In any case, individual habits in terms of exposures to sunlight greatly influence the risks associated with solar UV. Ultraviolet from artificial sources can also contribute significantly to exposure. Sources include sunbeds used for cosmetic tanning, radiant devices used for clinical therapy, and occupational sources, such as welding arcs.

Ultraviolet-B transmission is sensitive to the angle of the sun, and the time of year, and is greatest when the sun is overhead. The greatest sunlight exposures are received by horizontal surfaces, such as the tops of the feet, shoulders and ears. Although the UV irradiance is often sufficient to produce skin and eye effects for relatively brief exposure times, ocular effects generally do not develop because of shielding of the eye by the orbit, eyebrows, eyelashes, and squinting.

A number of outdoor occupational groups have been evaluated for UV exposure. These include fishermen, construction workers, landscape workers, outdoor athletes, etc. Of the man-made sources, welding and various lamps and lasers are the major sources of occupational exposure. Lamps that may emit relatively high levels of UV include metal halide, high-pressure xenon, mercury vapor, and other high-intensity discharge (HID) lamps. The spectral output of mercury vapor lamps varies with the gas pressure. Low pressure lamps emit line spectra characteristic of mercury (mostly 253.7 nm) and are used primarily for germicidal applications. Medium to high-pressure lamps are used for product curing and area lighting, such as in gymnasiums and parking lots. These lamps produce a bluish light and may be hazardous when viewed at close distances. Mercury lamps used for area lighting have two envelopes. The inner envelope is quartz (transparent to UV), while the outer envelope is made of materials that are largely opaque to UV. The output may produce hazardous exposures some distance from the lamp when the outer envelope is broken and the lamp continues to operate, which can occur in lamps that are not self-extinguishing. Ultraviolet-A, -B, -C are emitted by fluorescent lamps used in open fixtures, but UV-B and UV-C are filtered out when an acrylic diffuser is used with the fixture. High UV-B and UV-C irradiances are associated with high–output (HO) and super high–output (SHO) lamps.

Medical UV devices include phototherapy, photochemotherapy, tanning, and disinfection and sterilization. Dentists may use UV and blue-light-curable materials. Generally, handheld applicators that are properly designed, maintained, and used will minimize exposure to the dentist. However, improper use or excessive leaks may result in mouth burns to the patient.

The penetration of the body by UV radiation is effectively limited to the skin and the eye. Since the bony ridge above the eyes provides protection from sunlight overhead, many UV-induced ocular conditions are mainly related to high levels of reflected solar radiation. Damage to skin is principally due to exposure to direct sunlight. Skin exposure is significantly modified by clothing, which generally provides a high degree of protection. Thus, parts of the body not normally clothed, such as the face and hands, tend to receive much higher cumulative exposures, and are consequently subject to more damage. However, an important exception is that malignant melanoma appears to be associated with intermittent intense exposure of normally unexposed skin.

Biological Responses

Acute exposure to UV may produce deterministic effects, such as increased pigmentation, skin reddening (erythema), swelling (edema), and corneal sensitivity (photokeratitis). In addition, chronic exposure can induce degenerative changes, such as wrinkling and elastosis of the skin, and cataract formation in the eyes; retinal degeneration is also associated with solar exposure. Chronic exposure may also elicit stochastic effects, including both melanoma and nonmelanoma skin cancers. The induction of immunosuppression, which may occur following acute exposure, could be relevant to skin carcinogenesis and infectious disease. Such effects, however, have not been established in human populations.

Dermal effects

The most common adverse response of the skin to UV is erythema (sunburn), and the skin is most sensitive in the 250 nm to 300 nm range. The erythemal response, a vascular reaction involving vasodilation and increased blood volume, ranges from a slight reddening to severe blistering, depending on the dose and spectral content of the incident radiation, the pigmentation and exposure history of the skin, and the thickness of the stratum corneum. The erythemal response starts from 2 to 4 hours after exposure, reaches a peak at 14 to 20 hours, and lasts for up to 2 days. The threshold dose for erythema (15–50 mJ/cm^2) applies to lightly pigmented skin that has not recently been exposed to UV radiation (not tanned). Defensive reactions taken by the skin on exposure, melanogenesis and skin thickening subsequent to hyperplasia, increase the threshold required to produce the same degree of reddening.

Some chemicals found in medications, plants, or occupational environments are photosensitizing agents. Photosensitivity includes two types of reactions: phototoxicity and photoallergy, with phototoxicity being more common. It affects all individuals when the UV dose or the dose of the photosensitizer is high enough. Photoallergy is an acquired altered reactivity in the exposed skin resulting from an immunologic response. Photosensitizing agents include many medications, some sunscreen agents, plants (e.g., figs, parsley, limes, parsnips, and pinkrot celery), and industrial photosensitizers including coal tar, pitch, anthracene, naphthalene, phenanthrene, thiophene, and many phenolic agents.

Three types of skin cancers are of concern with UV exposure: squamous cell carcinomas (SCC) and basal cell carcinomas (BCC) [referred to jointly as nonmelanoma skin cancer (NMSC)] and cutaneous malignant melanoma (CMM). The American Cancer Society (ACS) estimated that about 800,000 new cases of NMSC are diagnosed annually.[1] Four variables have been implicated in NMSC: *(1)* lifetime sun exposure; *(2)* the intensity and duration of the UV-B component in sunlight; *(3)* genetic predisposition; and *(4)* other factors unrelated to sunlight, such as exposure to ionizing radiation and polycyclic aromatic hydrocarbons. The carcinogenic action spectrum for humans is known to include the UV-B region, but may extend throughout the UV-A region. The incidence of cutaneous malignant melanoma has increased rapidly in the U.S. and worldwide over the past 40 years, with about 40,000 new cases of CMM and more than 7000 deaths anticipated each year.[1]

Ultraviolet exposure depresses both the systemic and local immunologic response. Changes have been observed in Langerhans cells, and the density of these cells is reduced after exposure. Langerhans cells, located above the basal membrane of the epidermis, are not protected by the melanocytes, and thus effects may be independent of skin pigmentation.

Ultraviolet exposure also produces some beneficial or therapeutic effects, including vitamin D_3 synthesis and therapy for skin conditions including vitiligo, psoriasis, mycosis fungoides, acne, eczema, and pityriasis rosea. In some treatments, photosensitizing agents are used to enhance the effect of UV radiation.

Ocular effects

The eye (Fig. 10–2) is adapted to focus visible radiation but will also focus other optical radiations including UV, and the consequent increase in irradiance within the eye increases its sensitivity to the harmful effects of UV exposure. The cornea absorbs UV strongly, particularly at shorter wavelengths, with over 90% of incident radiation below 300 nm being absorbed. Transmission of UV-A by the human lens is greatest in young people, falling from about 75% under the age of 10 years to around 20% in adults. The human lens absorbs strongly

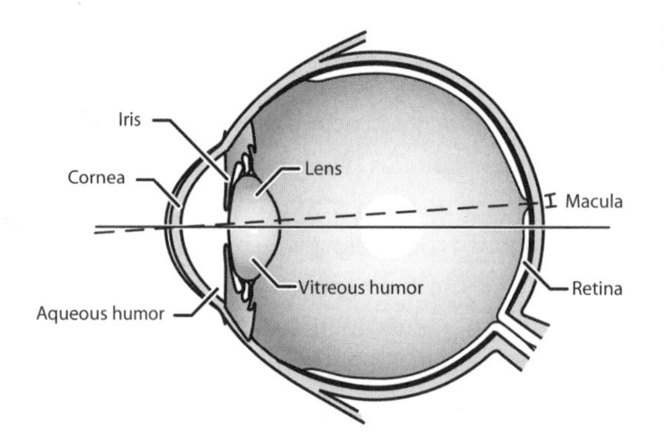

FIGURE 10–2. Components of the human eye.

throughout the UV-A and blue light regions. As the wavelength of the radiation increases, progressively more penetrates to the posterior eye, and in particular to the retina, with an increase in irradiance of over 10^5-fold. The combination of carotenoid and other pigments and a highly oxygenated environment, particularly in the central macula, can result in damage as a consequence of the photosensitized generation of reactive oxygen species (ROS).

The cornea and conjunctiva are the primary absorbers of UV-B and UV-C. Corneal transmission ranges from 60% to over 80% in the UV-A band, with much of the energy absorbed by the lens. Photokeratitis and photoconjunctivitis result from acute, high-intensity exposure to UV-B and UV-C. Injury results from exposure of the unprotected eye to a welding arc or other artificial sources rich in UV-B and UV-C. Natural solar radiation exposure produces these effects only when environments have highly reflective surfaces, such as snow (snow blindness) or sand. Symptoms of UV damage include lacrymation and photophobia, accompanied by a sensation of grit in the eye and severe pain. These symptoms become evident from 2- to 12-hours postexposure, and persist for up to 48 hours, usually without residual damage. Tissue damage depends on the total dose, and not the dose rate.

The only eye-lens (lenticular) effect linked with UV exposure, primarily solar radiation, is the cataract. In the U.S., estimates of the number of cataract operations are about 1 million annually, and cataracts are the third leading cause of blindness. Predisposing factors include age, gender, family history, nutritional status, and certain medical conditions and medications. The mechanism for UV-induced cataracts may be photochemical in the 295 to 320 nm range, and thermal at longer wavelengths.

Epidemiological studies of human populations have sought associations between sunlight exposure and the occurrence of cataracts, specifically senile cataracts, using diverse exposure surrogates, such as UV-B levels, hours of sunlight exposure, and geographic location. Relative risks ranged from 1.3 to 5.8, demonstrating a consistent association between UV exposure and cataracts.[2] The estimated threshold for cataracts is daily exposures of 7 to 90 mJ/cm^2 for UV-B and 0.4 to 98 J/cm^2 for UV-A.[3]

Exposure to UV-A and UV-B, primarily from solar radiation, has been implicated as an etiologic agent in solar retinitis, cystoid macular edema (CME), and senile macular degeneration (SMD). In adults, transmission of these wavelengths through the ocular media is minimal, except in an absence of the lens. Although originally thought to be a thermal injury, solar retinitis (also known as eclipse blindness) is a photochemical lesion resulting from absorption of UV-A and blue wavelengths.

Protective measures

Protective measures for UV radiation must address both skin and eye. Personal protection includes clothing, sunscreens and sun blocks, and the use of protective eyewear.

Most common materials transmit little UV. Common window glass (2.4 mm thick) transmits almost no UV below 300 nm; around 330 nm the transmission increases to about 50%. Little radiation at 308 nm is reflected from the surface of glass at incident angles of less than 60°. For greater angles the degree of reflection is greatly increased.

Lamp enclosures may be interlocked, such as self-extinguishing mercury vapor lamps. These lamps stop operating within 15 min of breakage of the outer of the two envelopes. In the U.S., the FDA requires that self-extinguishing mercury vapor lamps be marked with the letter "T". If the lamp is not self-extinguishing, the FDA requires that such lamps be marked with the letter "R".

In recent years, the use of sunblocks and sunscreens to reduce cutaneous UV exposure from solar radiation has greatly increased. Sunblocks reduce exposures by reflecting and scattering the incident radiation. Zinc oxide and titanium dioxide reflect up to 99% of the radiation both in the UV and visible regions, possibly into the IR region. While effective, sunblocks are viewed as presenting an unattractive appearance.

Sunscreens absorb UV over a limited wavelength range in the UV-B and UV-A regions, and are considered to be drugs by the FDA. The agents include para-aminobenzoic acid (PABA) and its esters, benzophenones, salicylates, cinnamates, and anthranilates. When used in a gel or cream, the preparations have good coverage. They bind to the stratum corneum, and resist removal by perspiration during heavy activity or by water when swimming. All provide protection in the UV-B range; while the benzophenones and anthranilates also provide some protection in the UV-A region. PABA preparations can discolor clothing and can cause contact-type, eczematous dermatitis. The body's natural photoprotector, melanin, absorbs strongly in the UV-A.

While sunscreens are designed to protect against UV-induced erythema and sunburn, their efficacy in reducing the risk of cancer and immunologic effects has not been established. The sun protection factor (SPF) is the measure of effectiveness of these agents; SPF equals the ratio of the UV-B dose required to produce erythema with protection to that required without protection. To achieve a product's SPF rating, it is important to apply the proper amount of sunscreen to the skin. Also, sunscreens provide less protection in the outdoor environment than suggested by label values because of the changing ratio of UV-B to UV-A with changes in the angle of the sun throughout the day.

Quick-tanning preparations containing β-carotene or carthoxanthine produce a "tan" by coloring the skin but offer no protection against UV. Since their effectiveness in preventing melanoma has not been established, other protective measures such as hats and protective clothing, and avoidance of exposure during peak hours should be used. Factors affecting UV protection of fabrics include weave, color, stretch, weight, quality, and water content.

VISIBLE RADIATION

Sources of Visible Light

The sun is the major source of visible light, along with various lamps, projection systems, welding arcs, and lasers (see Table 10–2). The luminance of the noon-day sun is 1.6×10^5 candelas per centimeter squared (cd/cm^2), and the time necessary for blue-light injury is about 90 seconds. Luminance from welding arcs can be hundreds to ten thousands cd/cm^2.

Xenon short-arc lamps emit relatively high levels (10^4 to 10^5 cd/cm^2) of blue light, while low-pressure fluorescent lamps emit relatively low levels. For potential blue-light exposures to photoflood lamps used in TV studios and theaters, acceptable exposure duration varies from 1 min to 3 hours at distances between 2.25 and 10 m.

Biological responses

Dermal. Above 400 nm, high-intensity exposure to visible wavelengths can lead to thermocoagulation of skin similar to that produced by electrical or thermal burns. Several variables influence the threshold for and the amount of damage: absorption and scattering by the skin, the incident intensity, exposure duration, area of skin exposed, and degree of vascularization of the irradiated tissue. Some photosensitizing agents may have action spectra that reach into the visible region.

Ocular. Since the human eye is relatively transparent to light that enters through the pupil, it is transmitted through the ocular media to the retina with minimal absorption. In the retina, these photons initiate a photochemical chain reaction in light-sensitive absorbers, resulting in the sensation of vision. The light

TABLE 10–2. Common Exposures to Optical Radiation Sources

SOURCES	SPECTRAL REGIONS OF CONCERN	POTENTIAL EXPOSURES
Sunlight	UV, visible, near-IR	Farming, construction, landscaping, life guarding, other outdoor work
Arc lamps	UV-visible, near-IR	Photoreproduction, optical laboratories, entertainment
Germicidal lamps	Actinic UV	Hospitals, laboratories, medical clinics, maintenance
Hg-HID lamps (broken envelope)	UV-A, blue light actinic UV	Maintenance, industry, warehouses, gymnasiums
Carbon arcs	UV, blue light	Laboratories, search lights
Industrial IR sources	IR	Steel mills, foundries, glassmaking, drying equipment
Metal halide UV-A lamps	Near-UV, visible	Printing plants, maintenance, integrated circuit manufacturing
Sunlamps	UV, blue light	Tanning parlors, beauty salons, fitness parlors
Welding arcs	UV, blue light	Construction, repair and maintenance, bypassers

IR, infrared; UV, ultraviolet; HID, high-intensity discharge.

intensity at the retina is a factor of 10^4 to 10^6 greater than that incident on the pupil (the optical gain).

Retinal effects occur through four interaction mechanisms: *(1)* thermal; *(2)* photochemical; *(3)* elastic or thermoacoustic transient pressure waves; and d) nonlinear responsiveness. However, the latter two mechanisms are significant only with laser light.

The absorption of light by tissue produces heat. At sufficient intensities, a rapid rise in temperature can denature proteins and inactivate enzymes. The thermal mechanism is the primary damage mechanism for high intensity exposure durations (1 ms to 10 sec). Long-term (>10 to 100 sec) exposure to light levels above normal environment levels may produce photochemical damage in the retina. The action spectrum mimics the spectral absorption of melanin through the lower end of the visible (500 to 400 nm) region down into the UV-A region. Photochemical damage can be enhanced by the thermal mechanism that predominates in the 500 to 1400 nm range, although there is no sharp cutoff point between the two.

Exposure to intense light sources, such as the sun, carbon arc, or welder's arc, without proper protection may produce temporary or permanent retinal blind spots. Reports of injuries from observing solar eclipses date back as far as Hippocrates (460 to 370 B.C.). Factors affecting the degree of retinal hazard include the size, type, and spectral intensity of the source, the pupil size, retinal image quality, and the spectral transmittance of the ocular media, the spectral absorption of the retina and choroid, and the exposure duration.

Glare may produce visual discomfort, often due to squinting in an effort to screen out light. If glare is substantial or frequently induced, it may result in fatigue, irritability, possibly headache, and a decrease in work efficiency. Glare can be differentiated into veiling glare, discomfort glare, or blinding glare (flash blindness). Although all three are present in the case of high-intensity light, the effects of the first two are primarily evident only when the source is present. Blinding glare is especially significant where it produces afterimages that persist. The glare source can cause discomfort or affect visual performance, or both. The visual discomfort or annoyance from glare is well understood. People sometimes become more physically tense and restless under glare conditions. Although the cause is physical, the discomfort brought about by glare is often subjective. The evaluation of discomfort relies upon subjective responses as criteria. Flash blindness is a temporary effect in which visual sensitivity and function are decreased severely over a short time period. This normal visual response, whose complex mechanism is not well understood, is related to the eye's adaptive state and the size, spectral distribution, and luminance of the light source.

INFRARED RADIATION

Biological Responses

Sources

Most of the sources discussed under visible radiation also emit IR radiation. Also, a number of IR lasers and optical wireless communications systems use IR light-emitting diodes (LEDs).

Dermal

The damage to skin from IR exposure results from a temperature increase in the absorbing tissue. The increase depends on the wavelength, the parameters involved in heat conduction and dissipation, the intensity of the exposure, and the exposure duration. The most prominent effects of near-IR include acute skin burn, increased vasodilation of the capillary beds, and an increased pigmentation that can persist for long periods of time. With continuous exposure to high-intensity IR, the erythematous appearance due to vasodilation may become permanent.

Many factors affect IRs ability to produce a skin burn. The rate at which the temperature of the skin is permitted to increase is of prime importance. High levels of far-IR, often referred to as radiant heat, are encountered in glassblowing, foundries, and furnaces. This IR exposure can be a significant contributor to thermal stress in the work environment.

Ocular

Infrared produces thermal effects in the eye. The cornea is highly transparent to IR-A, has water absorption bands at wavelengths of 1.43 and 1.96 μm, and becomes opaque to IR above 2.5 μm. Acute corneal damage can range from epithelial haze to corneal erosion with a focused beam incident on a miotic (contracted) pupil. Chronic corneal exposure to subthreshold doses may lead to "dry-eye," characterized by conjunctivitis and decreased lacrymation.

Moderate IR doses can result in constriction of the pupil (miosis), hyperemia, and the formation of aqueous flares. More severe exposures may lead to muscle paralysis, congestion with hemorrhage, thrombosis and stromal inflammation. Within a few days, necrosis of the iris may cause bleached atrophic areas to form.

Damage to the lens of the eye from IR has been investigated for many years. The occupational groups at risk include glassblowers, foundry and forge workers, cooks, and laundry workers, as well as those who work in sunlight. The mechanism for IR associated cataractogenesis has long been debated. Some results appear to support the hypothesis that the iris must be involved in IR- or heat-induced cataractogenesis, at least with regard to acute exposure conditions.

The retina is susceptible to near-IR since the ocular media are relatively transparent to these wavelengths. For extended exposures, the corneal irradiance required to produce a minimal retinal lesion at 1064 nm is almost three orders of magnitude greater than that at 442 nm. Absorption of IR by the retinal pigment epithelium produces heat. If the heat is not dissipated rapidly and the temperature of the tissue rises about 20°C, irreversible thermal damage will result from the denaturation of protein and other macromolecules.

LASER RADIATION

Laser radiation is UV, optical or IR radiation that propagates in the form of a beam and has some special properties. While radiation emitted from conventional sources is usually broad-band and spreads out in all directions as it propagates away from the source, most lasers emit light in a very narrow bandwidth, which is described as monochromatic (i.e., a single wavelength or color). Laser radiation also propagates in a highly directional manner with little divergence, and is characterized by a high energy density. Coherence means that the wavelengths of laser radiation are in phase both in space and time.

Lasers may operate continuously (called continuous wave or CW) or be pulsed (normal pulse, Q-switched, or mode-locked). Continuous wave lasers emit a "temporally constant power of laser light." Pulsed lasers may emit single pulses or repetitive pulses. The innate human aversion response time to bright light, including visible laser light, is assumed to be within 0.25 sec. However, the aversion response does not occur with exposure to invisible optical radiation such as UV and IR. With this in mind, if an optical laser emits radiation for a time greater than or equal to 0.25 sec, it is defined as a CW laser. It follows that pulses are noncontinuous emissions in which the duration of each pulse is shorter than 0.25 sec. Pulse widths, however, may be much shorter than the aversion response time. Q-switching produces pulses on the order of a few nanosecond to microseconds, while mode-locked pulses are even shorter, in the picosecond domain. Special pulsing techniques can produce pulses on the order of femtoseconds.

In some applications, such as information management with bar-code scanners, the laser beam may be scanned. In scanning, the output is spatially distributed (often in some form of a linear pattern) in a manner that makes it physically impossible for the entire output to enter the eye. This reduces the retinal irradiance compared to an unscanned beam.

Exposures to laser radiation may be direct (primary beam) or indirect (scattered or diffusely reflected). Most direct exposures will be to a small beam or point source of light. Reflections may be specular or diffuse, or a combination of the two. Specular reflections, which may be regarded as a type of direct viewing, occurs when the beam is incident on a mirrorlike surface. In the United States, the ANSI standard requires that eyewear must be marked with an attenuation factor called the optical density (OD) and wavelength, so users can select the proper protection.[4]

Lasers are classified according to their output power and intended use. Typical keychain and pointer type lasers are Class 1 lasers. Class 1 lasers are those that cannot emit radiation at levels that can be hazardous. However, no laser beam should be viewed directly.

Laser beams at wavelengths that are not visible to the eye can be viewed using various phosphor image converter materials. These are often in the form of a "viewing card." The cards absorb the invisible radiation, then emit at wavelengths that are visible through protective eyewear. Since there may be significant reflections from viewing cards that are laminated with high-gloss plastics, it is best to purchase viewing cards with diffusing finishes, or to place matte-finish tape over the laminate.

RADIO FREQUENCY AND MICROWAVE RADIATION

The radio frequency (RF) spectral region extends from 300 GHz to 3 kHz. Usually, microwave radiation is considered a subset of RF radiation, although an alternative convention treats radiowaves and microwaves as two spectral regions. In the latter context, microwaves occupy the spectral region between 300 GHz and 300 MHz, while radiowaves include 300 MHz to 3 kHz.

Various order-of-magnitude band designations (Table 10–3) have been assigned to the RF and sub-RF portion of the spectrum. Frequencies in these bands are allocated for various uses, including navigation, aeronautical radio, broadcasting, and citizens' radio. In addition to band designations, specific frequencies are designated for industrial, scientific, and medical uses.

Sources

Sources of RF waves can be natural (sun, galaxies, lighting, human body) or anthropogenic. Sources include antennas, leakage sources, or a combination. Leakage may be the consequence of poor design, lack of maintenance, or improper maintenance. Information on selected sources is contained in Table 10–4.

The microwave beam emitted from radar antennas is highly directional and, in some cases, a very narrow beam is produced. Some antennas move horizontally (scan) or vertically (elevation), and most units are pulsed at relatively high peak powers. The combination of scanning, elevation, and pulsing (duty cycle < 1) usually results in brief exposures for individuals irradiated by the beam. Evaluations of commercial radar (airport surveillance and approach traffic control), aircraft, marine, and police traffic-control radars have not demonstrated overexposures during normal operation. However, exposure to airport radar and aircraft units may be of concern during maintenance activities.

Broadcasting types and frequencies are in Table 10–5. Broadcast towers may support a single antenna or multiple, stacked antennas (FM and TV), or be a dedicated antenna (AM radio). If an antenna occupying a high position on the tower

Table 10–3. Nomenclature of Radio Frequency Band Designations

FREQUENCY RANGE	DESIGNATION	ABBREVIATION
< 30 Hz[a]	Sub-extremely low frequency	Sub-ELF
30–300 Hz[a]	Extremely low frequency	ELF
300–3000 Hz[a]	Voice frequency	VF
3–30 kHz	Very low frequency	VLF
30–300 kHz	Low frequency	LF
300–3000 kHz	Medium frequency	MF
3–30 MHz	High frequency	HF
30–300 MHz	Very high frequency	VHF
300–3000 MHz	Ultra high frequency	UHF
3–30 GHz	Super high frequency	SHF
30–300 GHz	Extremely high frequency	EHF

[a]The IEEE definition of band designations does not include VF, and defines ELF as 3–3000 Hz, and < 3 Hz as ultralow frequency (ULF).

TABLE 10–4. Information on Some Important Radio Frequency Sources

SOURCE	FREQUENCIES (MHZ)	USES	SYSTEM COMPONENTS
Dietectric heater	10–70 many at 27.12	Heat, seal, weld, emboss, mold, or cure dietectric materials	Power supply, RF generator, tuning circuitry, press, electrodes (die)
Induction heater	0.250–0.488	Heat conductive materials via electromagnetic induction	Power supply, RF generator, transmission line, induction coil
Plasma processors	0.1–27 many at 13.56	Chemical milling; nitriding of steel; synthesis of polymers; modifying polymeric surfaces; deposition (sputtering) and hardening of coatings and films; and etching, cleaning, or stripping photoresist	RF generator, transmission line, reactor vessel, RF tuning and control module, vacuum pump, gas storage, and gas delivery system
Radar	EHF, SHF, UHF	Detection, tracking, ranging	Transmitter, waveguide, antenna, receiver, display
Broadcasting	See Table 10–5	Radio, TV transmission lines, tower, antennas	Transmitter
Communications	HF, VHF, UHF	Fixed position and mobile systems used for voice/data transmission	Transmitter, receiver, transmission lines, antennas
Video display terminals	VLF, LF	Visual imaging component of information processing systems	Cathode-ray-tube VDTs have been the focus of most evaluations
Diathermy	Microwave (915 or 2450) or shortwave (13.56 or 27.12)	Heat therapy	Generator, control console, transmission line, applicators
Electrosurgical units	0.5–100	Cauterizing of coagulating tissues	Generator, transmission line, surgical probe, current return cable

RF, radio frequency; EHF, extremely high frequency; SHF, super high frequency; UHF, ultra high frequency; HF, high frequency; VHF, very high frequency; VLF, very low frequency; LF, low frequency; VDT, video display terminal.

TABLE 10–5. Broadcast Frequency Allocation

TYPE	CARRIER FREQUENCY (MHZ)
AM radio	0.535–1.605
FM radio	88–108
Low-band VHF-TV	54–72, 76–88
High-band VHF-TV	174–216
UHF-TV	470–806

VHF, very high frequency; UHF, ultra high frequency.

must be serviced, it is possible that maintenance workers may be exposed to fields from energized antennas located lower on the tower. The hands and feet of climbing personnel may also receive high exposures, especially if the transmission line is located near the ladder.

Mobile and portable communication systems may produce relatively high RF levels very near the antennas. Hence, when the antenna is located very near the head, exposure may result in relatively high local values. Radio frequency currents on metallic parts of a radio case may also produce relatively high levels of exposure to the face.

Diathermy units may operate continuously or be pulsed, and some may be amplitude modulated or have a ripple at ELF frequencies. The leakage field of the applicator depends on the type of applicator.

Evaluations of solid-state and spark-gap electrosurgical units (ESUs) demonstrated that field strengths increased with increasing output power and levels were higher for solid-state units. Levels near the probe and unshielded leads may exceed exposure criteria.

Other common sources of RF radiation include emissions from microwave ovens (2.45 GHz) and cellular telephones, which operate between 800 and 900 mHz.

Characterization of Quantities and Units

Electric-field strength (E) and magnetic-field strength (H) are vector quantities, but only the magnitude is reported in safety evaluations. E fields are generated by electric charges and are measured in terms of the electric potential (V) over some distance. The unit is the volt per meter (V/m). Since power is related to the square of the voltage, E^2 (V^2/m^2) is often used in exposure guidelines or in describing the output of measurement instruments.

Magnetic fields are generated by moving electric charges, such as a current (I) moving through a long, thin wire. The flux density (B) of the magnetic field generated by a current I at some distance (r) from the wire is

$$B = I/2\pi r \qquad (10\text{–}2)$$

Radio frequency magnetic fields are generally represented by H, the magnetic field strength. H has units of amperes per meter (A/m). Since power deposition in tissues is related to current squared H^2 (A^2/m^2) may also be used. (To convert between B and H, use $\mu = B/H$, where μ is the magnetic permeability. For fields in air, $\mu = 1.257 \times 10^{-6}$ henry/meter.) Power density (W) represents the time-averaged energy flow across a surface, and typically is used when measuring microwave radiation. The unit of power density is watts per meter squared (W/m^2), although the use of milliwatts per centimeter squared (mW/cm^2) in hazard evaluation is common. (Conversion: 1 W/m^2 = 0.1 mW/cm^2.)

Radio frequency fields can induce currents within exposed tissues. These induced currents (I_I) flow through the body to ground, with a common path through the foot, which is called the *short-circuit* or *foot current*. The unit of electric current is the ampere (A), although the milliampere (mA) is the magnitude usually addressed in safety evaluations. In an environment where there are RF fields, it is possible for contact with conductive objects to result in currents that flow into the body at the point of contact, which is usually the hand. If this occurs, exposure guidelines may require evaluation of contact currents (I_o) in mA.

Physical Characteristics

Understanding certain properties of an RF field is necessary for hazard evaluation. These include near and far fields, plane waves, impedance, polarization, modulation, gain, and duty cycle.

Radio frequency energy is radiated by an antenna on which a time varying current is imposed. RF energy passes through the near field then into the far field. The space immediately surrounding the antenna contains the reactive near field. Here, the E- and H-field components exist in a complex temporal and spatial pattern, and the energy is "stored." A short distance from the antenna the fields begin to radiate. This is the radiating near field, characterized by both energy storage and propagation (radiation). Beam intensities near the antenna may increase or decrease with distance or may remain unchanged. Beyond a transition zone is the far field, where there is propagation, and the power density follows the inverse square law, that is the magnitude of the power density (W) is inversely proportional to the square of the distance from a point source.

The magnetic and electric field strengths are related by the impedance, Z, of free space. It is the quotient of E/H. In the near-field this relationship is complex and must be determined. However, in the far field the free-space wave impedance is a constant value, 377 ($120\,\pi$) ohms (Ω), at a given point in space.

Combining the expressions for power density and impedance for a plane wave yields:

$$W\ (\mathrm{mW/cm^2}) = E^2/3770 \qquad (10\text{–}3)$$

and

$$W\ (\text{mW/cm}^2) = 37.7H^2 \tag{10–4}$$

which are useful formulas for conversions involving field strength and power density.

Polarization is that property of an electromagnetic field describing the direction and amplitude of the time-varying electric-field vector. A field may be polarized linearly, circularly, or elliptically, or it may be unpolarized.

Modulation is the process by which some characteristic of a carrier wave (a carrier of information) is varied by imposing an overlaying signal wave. The modulating signal, which is lower in frequency than the carrier, superimposes information on the carrier wave. When the signal modifies the amplitude of the carrier wave, the wave is amplitude modulated (AM). When the frequency or phase of the carrier is modified by the signal, then the wave is frequency modulated (FM) or phase modulated, respectively. AM and FM are used in broadcasting, while FM and phase modulated are used in communications. Other modifications known as digital modulations and code-division multiple-access are also used in modern communication.

Some industrial and medical RF sources may be amplitude modulated, with the modulating signal in the ELF spectral region. This occurs because the electric circuitry allows the imposition of the fundamental or a higher harmonic of the power frequency (50 or 60 Hz) on the RF carrier.

Gain is a measure of the directional properties of an antenna. For a point-source antenna, emission is uniform over all directions and the gain equals 1. When a reflector is used it changes the radiation pattern increasing the energy in one direction at the expense of another. The collimation or focusing increases the gain in that direction.

Some sources may exhibit a cyclic or intermittent operation, where RF is emitted for only a fraction of the total time of operation, the "on-time," in an operational cycle. The ratio of on-time to the total time of operation is called the duty factor or duty cycle (DC). Duty cycle is also the product of the pulse repetition frequency (PRF) in pulses per second (Hz) and the pulse width or duration (PW) in seconds (PRF $\times$ PW).

Duty cycle measures time on and time off and must be known to determine average power. Most exposure guidelines are expressed in terms of average power. Sources that typically have a duty cycle less than 1 include radar, dielectric sealers, induction heaters, RF welding units, some communication devices, and medical diathermy units.

Biological Responses

Human data on biological effects from RF are limited and present no clear exposure-response trends, so scientists have relied on effects in animal models;

these effects have been extrapolated to humans and used in setting exposure limits. Animal studies have found effects in the nervous, neuroendocrine, reproductive, immune, and sensory systems. In general, the absorption results in thermal energy deposition in the tissues. The rate at which energy is absorbed is called the specific absorption rate (SAR) which is measured in W/kg.

Interaction with tissues

Tissues can interact with the RF field and absorb energy. Radio frequency energies are more highly absorbed in tissues of high water content (e.g., muscle) than in tissues with low water content (e.g., fat). Radio frequency interaction with tissues may be complex, with standing waves formed at the interface of tissues with different dielectric properties, such as skin–fat or fat–muscle interfaces.

In general, short-wavelength RF has only a relatively shallow penetration depth into tissues, such that at frequencies of more than a few gigahertz, absorption is in the skin. Longer wavelengths may penetrate more deeply, and the body is relatively transparent to long-wavelength magnetic fields. Thus, penetration depth affects risk to organs or systems. Radio frequency energies clearly produce thermal effects, although some nonthermal effects have been reported.

Radio frequency exhibits three modes of tissue interaction at the molecular level: polar molecule alignment, molecular rotation and vibration, and the transfer of kinetic energy to free electrons and ions. Alignment of polar molecules with the field results in frictional heating.

Behaviorial and nervous system effects

Exposure guidelines are based on a few well-established effects observed in test animals. One of these is reversible behavioral changes in short-term studies, a sensitive measure of RF exposure. In general, behavioral changes are thermal effects attributed to significant increases in body temperature due to absorbed RF energy. Radio frequency workers with certain nonspecific symptoms associated with the nervous system may have clinical signs extending to the cardiovascular system, called radiowave illness or microwave sickness following acute overexposure to microwaves. In addition to behavioral effects, combined interactions of RF fields with neuroactive drugs and chemicals have been reported in test animals.

Reproduction and development

Teratogenic effects have been demonstrated at 27.12 MHz with rats, when the whole-body average SAR was relatively high, around 10 to 11 W/kg. Developmental abnormalities were observed in rodents at 2450 MHz.

Ocular effects

Effects have been reported to the cornea, iris vasculature, lens, and retina. Cataracts are of concern because the avascular nature of the lens increases its susceptibility to heat-induced change. However, no cataracts were observed with far-field exposure of unrestrained animals, even when exposures were almost lethal. Studies of cataracts in people with purported RF exposure do not support a causal link, although an occupational study suggested an aging effect on the lens.

Cancer

Animal data have been inconclusive in this regard. Epidemiological studies have provided some suggestive evidence that RF energies are carcinogenic to human beings. One study reported a link between exposure of Polish military personnel to pulsed RF and an increased incidence of cancers of the alimentary canal, brain, and hematopoietic and lymphatic systems.[5] Another study categorized possible RF exposure of Air Force personnel on the basis of job title. An increase (39%) in brain cancer was observed, which was marginally statistically significant.[6] However, the human studies to date have a number of limitations, typically the absence of information on doses, dose-response, or duration of exposure. Others include the classification of possible exposures on the basis of job title, a small number of cases or small sample size, little control for confounding factors, and no consistency in findings in the studies reporting statistically significant positive associations. However, because of some suggestive findings, further study is needed.

Other concerns

Exposure to radio-frequency fields may cause perturbation of the field by metallic implants (e.g., metal staples, cochlear implants) or metallic objects that are worn (e.g., jewelry, watches, metal-framed spectacles). Radio frequency fields may also interfere with electronic devices such as sampling devices, medical electronics (e.g., cardiac pacemakers). In some chemical sample preparation methods, microwaves have been reported to superheat solutions, which may lead to melting of reaction vessels or to explosions.

REFERENCES

1. American Cancer Society. Cancer Facts and Figures-1996. Atlanta: American Cancer Society, 1996.
2. Pitts, D.G., Cameron, L.L., Jule, J.G., and Lerman, S. Optical Radiation and Cataracts. In: Optical Radiation and Visual Health. Boca Raton, FL: CRC Press, Inc., 1986, pp. 5–41.
3. Waxler, M. Long-Term Visual Health Problems: Optical Radiation Risks. In: Optical Radiation and Visual Health. Boca Raton, FL: CRC Press, Inc., 1985, pp. 183–204.

4. American National Standards Institute. American National Standard for the Safe Use of Lasers (ANSI Z136.1–1993). Orlando, FL: Laser Institute of America, 1993.
5. Szmigielski S. Cancer morbidity in subjects occupationally exposed to high frequency (radiofrequency and microwave) electromagnetic radiation. Sci. Total Env. 180:9–17, 1996.
6. Grayson, J.K. Radiation exposure, socioeconomic status, and brain tumor risk in the U.S. Air Force: A nested case-control study. Am. J. Epidemiol. 143:480–486, 1996.

11

Ionizing Radiation and Environmental Radioactivity

Naturally occurring ionizing radiation has always pervaded the biosphere, although this was only recognized a little more than a century ago. Ionizing radiation is electromagnetic or particulate radiation that is so named because it produces ion pairs in any material it traverses. An ion pair is a pair of charged particles, usually consisting of a negatively charged electron that has been separated from an atom, and the residual positively charged atom. Ionization occurs when the radiation transfers sufficient energy to the electron to enable it to separate and move away from the positive atom. If too little energy is given to the electron for it to move completely away from the residual atom, the ions can quickly recombine. If still less energy is transferred, the interaction will not produce ion pairs, but simply result in an atom that has more energy than normal, or an "excited atom."

Since the least strongly bound electron in an atom requires about 11 eV (see Table 11–1 for definitions of units) of energy to move away from the atom, radiation with less energy cannot cause ionization. Environmental ionizing radiation consists of high energy photons that travel at the speed of light ($c = 3 \times 10^{10}$ cm/sec), or charged atomic, or subatomic particles.

Natural radioactivity was discovered by Henri Bequerel in 1896. He was studying the phosphorescence of uranium by exposing the uranium containing rock to light and then recording the stimulated light on film. He found, however, that the

TABLE 11–1. Definitions

Sources

Activity: The quantity of a radioactive source is defined by its "activity" or the rate of spontaneous nuclear transformation (Table 11–2).

The unit of activity is the becquerel (Bq):

$$1 \text{ Bq} = 1 \text{ s}^{-1}$$

Thus, 1 Bq represents one transformation, or disintegration, per second.

The conventional unit of activity is the curie (Ci):

$$1 \text{ Ci} = 3.7 \times 10^{10} \text{ s}^{-1} \text{ (exactly)}$$

Note: the Ci was originally defined as 1 gram of radium. In 1950 the current definition was set. Most environmentally relevant amounts are small and require the use of a prefix such as mCi, μCi, nCi, pCi (10^{-3}Ci, 10^{-6}Ci, 10^{-9}Ci, 10^{-12}Ci). The picocurie (pCi) represents 2.22 disintegrations per minute.

To convert between Ci and Bq note that:

$$1 \text{ nCi} = 37 \text{ Bq and } 1 \text{ Bq} = 27 \text{ pCi}$$

Radiation

Exposure is a measure of the quantity of X or gamma radiation. It is defined by the electric charge the radiation produces as it traverses an air mass. Exposure does not have a special unit in the SI system but combines the basic units of charge in coulombs (C) and mass in kilograms (kg).

The units of exposure are C kg^{-1}.

The conventional unit of exposure is the roentgen (R):

$$1 \text{ R} = 2.58 \times 10^{-4} \text{ C kg}^{-1} \text{ (exactly)}$$

Thus, 2.58×10^{-4} C is the charge of the ions of one sign produced in one kg of air by one roentgen of X or gamma radiation.

Energy: Corpuscular radiation is generally defined by stating the particle identity and its kinetic energy. The SI unit of energy is the joule, but conventional units in multiples of the electron volt (eV) are used almost exclusively. Common multiples are keV (10^3 eV) and MeV (10^6 eV). One eV is the kinetic energy acquired by an electron accelerated through a potential difference of 1 volt.

$$1 \text{ eV} = 1.602 \times 10^{-19} \text{ J}$$
$$= 1.602 \times 10^{-12} \text{ ergs}$$

Note: Particle rest mass is sometimes expressed in units of energy through the transformation $E = mc^2$. Based on this transformation 1 atomic mass unit is equal to 931 MeV.

Dose

Absorbed Dose: Dose is the energy transferred to the absorber by the ionizing radiation.

The SI unit of absorbed dose (D) has been given the special name, the gray (Gy)

$$1 \text{ Gy} = 1 \text{ J kg}^{-1}$$

(*continued*)

TABLE 11–1. *(continued)*

The conventional unit of absorbed dose is the rad, which is equal to 100 ergs per gram of absorber.

$$1 \text{ rad} = 10^{-2} \text{ Gy}$$

Equivalent Dose: There is a special unit for use in radiation protection called the Equivalent Dose (H_T). It is the product of the average absorbed dose in a specified organ or tissue ($D_{T,R}$) and a radiation weighting factor (W_R) that accounts for biological effectiveness of the ionizing radiation producing the dose. Thus, equivalent dose is:

$$H_T = W_R D_{T,R}$$

where: $D_{T,R}$ = the absorbed dose in a specified tissue

W_R = the radiation weighting factor.

The value of W_R for x and gamma rays is 1, for alpha particles it is 20. For other radiations (e.g. neutrons, protons, fission fragments, etc.) see NCRP No. 116, or ICRP No. 60. The unit of equivalent dose (H_T) is the sievert (S_v).

$$1 \text{ Sv} = 1 \text{ J kg}^{-1}$$

The conventional unit is the rem

$$1 \text{ rem} = 10^{-2} \text{ J kg}^{-1}$$

Effective dose (or effective dose equivalent): There is a special unit for use in radiation protection called the effective dose (E). It is the product of the equivalent dose (H_T) to specific organ or tissue and a weighting factor (w_T) that expresses the contribution of the specific organ to the risk of a fatal cancer. This is a unit used for limiting the total risk of fatal cancer in an individual.

$$E = \sum_T w_T H_T$$

Where: w_T = a tissue weighting factor

H_T = the equivalent dose received by tissue T

The unit of effective dose (E) is the sievert (S_v).

$$1 \text{ Sv} = 1 \text{ J kg}^{-1}$$

The conventional unit is the rem

$$1 \text{ rem} = 10^{-2} \text{ J kg}^{-1}$$

film was exposed even when rock and film were stored in a dark drawer so that there could have been no phosphorescence, and realized that rays that could penetrate matter were emitted from the material itself.

Madam Marie Curie tested many elements to see if others might have similar properties. She discovered these properties in thorium. Her continued studies revealed some ores with higher radioactivities than could be accounted for by their U or Th content. She recognized that the source could not have been a known element because she had examined all of them. Her husband Pierre joined her in a search for new, highly radioactive elements. She named the first one they discovered, in July of 1898, polonium in honor of her native Poland, and named the second radium when it was discovered in December of the same year. The following year, Ernest Rutherford examined the nature of the particles emitted from uranium and found that they were alpha and beta particles. By that time, X-rays produced by deceleration of electrons (Bremmstrahlung) had also been discovered by Wilhelm Roentgen.

BASIC CONCEPTS

There are three separate entities to consider when studying ionizing radiation. These are the source, the radiation, and the absorber (Fig. 11–1). Sources include: *(1)* man made generators such as those used to produce medical X-rays, or linear accelerators; *(2)* extraterrestrial objects such as the sun, which send streams of radiation to earth; and *(3)* radioactive materials, which contain unstable atomic nuclei that eject a portion of their energy in order to become more stable. To discuss the size of a source, or amount of radioactivity, a unit was needed to describe the amount or quantity of activity. The original unit (Table 11–1), named for M. Curie, was the number of decays per second that occurred in one gram of radium. The System International (SI) unit, defined later, was named in honor of H. Becquerel.

The radiation is the particle or packet of energy that is transmitted from the source to an absorber. This may be a particle, or a photon of electromagnetic radiation. If is travelling through a vacuum it will continue on a straight course outward from the source without losing any energy.

The absorber is the material, or object, in which the radiation will deposit energy by ionization and excitation of the atoms. Thus, it absorbs the energy that is carried by the radiation. It is here that we require the concept of dose, which is a quantity of energy absorbed, or transferred to, a unit mass of the absorbing material by the radiation. Dose is determined by measuring the amount of ionization that occurs in the absorber.

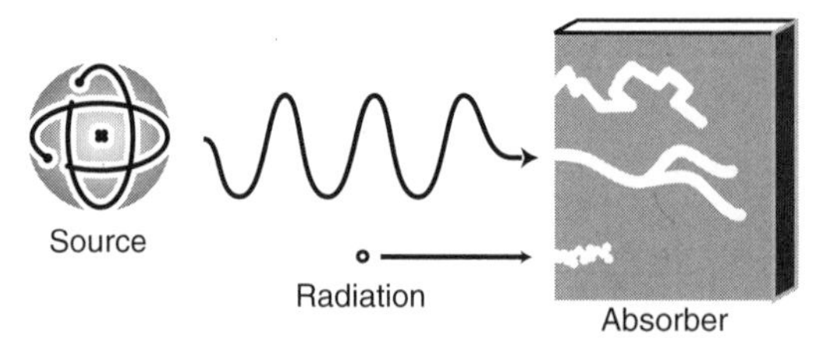

FIGURE 11–1. The pattern of ionization in an absorber depends on the source, nature of the radiation (α, β, γ) and its energy level.

Convenient measurement units such as the curie, roentgen and rad (Table 11–1) were developed over the years by scientists working with ionizing radiation. As knowledge and measurement processes improved, the historical units were occasionally re-evaluated and standardized. A new, coherent, set of units consistent with the SI was adopted in 1975 as a result of international agreement.[1,2] A few important units in Table 11–1 apply to: *(1)* the magnitude of a source; *(2)* the quantity and energy of the radiation; and *(3)* the dose, or energy deposited by the radiation in an absorber. In examining the potential effect of sources of radiation to the public, the concept of collective dose is sometimes used. The collective dose is the sum of the individual doses in an exposed population. The table lists both historical and SI units.

Radioactivity

Except for high voltage X-ray units (e.g., therapy, diagnosis, industrial) and high energy physics research and applications, environmental radiation originates from nuclear processes. Nuclear reactions that take place in the cosmos shower the earth with high energy charged particles. These extraterrestrial particles, known as cosmic rays (primarily protons), produce secondary particles that penetrate to ground level (mostly muons and electrons). On earth, all nuclei with atomic numbers (Z) greater than 82 are naturally radioactive. These nuclei are unstable because interactions of the particles (protons and neutrons) within the nucleus can result in a packet of excess energy that will be ejected from the nucleus. The transformation or decay, of a nucleus is a spontaneous random event (Table 11–2). It is not possible to identify which of a group of identical atoms will decay in any given time period. The process will always take place in the same way for any particular isotope; that is, the same particles and photons will be emitted, and the time it takes for half of the atoms to decay will always be exactly the same.

The physical properties of the emitted radiation determine both the biological significance of the radiation and various requirements for sampling and detection. The most common corpuscular radiations are alpha or beta particles. Nuclear decay also produces electromagnetic radiation in the form of high energy photons called gamma rays.

Alpha particles

Alpha particles are helium nuclei. They are emitted mainly from nuclei with high atomic mass leaving behind an atom with atomic number reduced by 2, and mass reduced by 4 mass units. Alpha particles emitted from a given nuclear species are monochromatic; that is, they all have the same kinetic energy. Their energies range from about 2 to 11 MeV. Alpha particles are massive enough so that they are not easily deflected as they traverse matter, and typically their paths

TABLE 11–2. Radioactive Decay

The transformation, or decay, of a nucleus is a random process so that if there are a large number (N) of identical radioactive atoms, the rate at which they decay (dN/dt) in a given time period will be a constant fraction of N.

$$\frac{dN}{dt} = -\lambda N \qquad (11\text{–}1)$$

where: dN = the number of unstable nuclei which transform in a time interval dt

λ = the proportionality constant or the fraction which decay per unit time.

λ is known as the decay constant and is characteristic of a given nuclide or atomic species. dN/dt is the "activity" of a source. Decay is a stochastic or random process; thus, Equation 1 only applies to sufficiently large samples of a nuclide.

Integration of Equation 11–1 from time $t = 0$ to t yields the number of nuclei which survive to time t:

$$N = N_o e^{-\lambda t} \qquad (11\text{–}2)$$

where: N_o = the number of nuclei at $t = 0$

N = the number present at time t.

The time (T) at which half the nuclei will have transformed or decayed ($t = T$ when $N/N_o = 1/2$) is then:

$$T = \frac{0.693}{\lambda} \qquad (11\text{–}3)$$

where:

T = the half-life of the species and is a characteristic time which is always the same for a particular nuclide.

are straight lines. The double charge and relatively high mass causes dense ionization along the track. A 5.0 MeV alpha particle, for example, will cause several thousand ion pairs per micrometer (μm) of water, or tissue, transferring about 100 keV of energy per μm to the molecules of the absorber.

The rate at which energy is transferred per unit path length of an absorber is called the linear energy transfer (LET). Alphas are classified as high LET particles. They can only traverse a few cm of air or a few μm of tissue before losing all of their initial kinetic energy. This very limited range prevents alpha particles from penetrating the skin. Unless an alpha particle source (i.e., a radioactive alpha emitting particle) is inhaled or ingested, significant irradiation of internal tissue cannot occur. Any absorber in the path of an alpha particle will significantly reduce its energy. Absorption within the source itself can be substantial.

Beta particles

Beta particles are positive or negative electrons. When an atom decays by beta emission, the atomic number changes by $\pm$ 1, but the atomic mass does not change if an electron (e^-) is emitted, since an orbital electron will replace the lost mass. If a positron (e^+) is emitted, the atomic mass is reduced by twice the mass of an electron. When a nucleus decays by beta emission, a neutrino or antineutrino is also emitted and the energy loss is shared between the particles. Thus, betas from a given species are emitted with a range of energies up to a maximum that is specific to the nuclear transition. The average share of the energy carried off by the beta particle (from a collection of the same atoms) is about one-third of the total energy of the nuclear transition. Typical energies range from 10 keV to 4.0 MeV. Beta particles are easily deflected by interactions with orbital electrons because they have the same mass, so they travel erratic paths, causing ionization and excitation of atoms as they pass until all of their initial kinetic energy has been transferred to the absorber. The trail of ion pairs left behind will be much less dense than that of an alpha particle. Beta particles will typically lose energy to the absorber at a few keV per micrometer and are thus low LET radiation. Positrons will ultimately interact with an electron causing both to annihilate with the emission of two 0.511 MeV gamma rays. Beta particles, depending on energy, may travel from a few cm to 10 or 15 m in air, or a few μm to about 2.0 cm in tissue.

Gamma rays

Gamma rays are photons and exhibit both wave and particle properties. The energy (E) is proportional to the frequency (f) of the radiation; $E = hf$. The proportionality constant h is Planck's constant ($h = 6.626 \times 10^{-34}$ Js^{-1}). Photons from a particular nuclear transition are monochromatic, but some nuclear decays result in emission of several different photons. Typical energies range from a few keV to a few MeV. The manner in which high energy photons, or gamma rays, interact with matter to ionize atoms in the absorber varies with energy and the specific properties of the absorbing material. The energy of a beam of gamma radiation will be attenuated exponentially because interactions between the gamma rays and the atoms of the absorber are stochastic. Gamma rays do not exhibit a finite range but the mean free path, i.e., the average distance a photon will travel before having a collision, gives a measure of the penetration. The mean free path is also known as the relaxation length. The mean free path in air for a 1.0 MeV gamma ray is about 120 m; in water or tissue, it is approximately 14 cm.

Other emissions

A variety of particles other than alpha particles, beta particles and gamma rays are emitted less commonly in nuclear transformations. These include protons, neutrons, conversion electrons, Auger electrons, and X-rays.

Decay Rate

As seen in Table 11–2, the decay of a radioactive isotope is exponential. The half–life (T) of any nuclide is specific and can be used to identify the isotope.

Half-lives range from microseconds to billions of years. Half of the initial material will be gone when the time period equal to 1 half-life has elapsed, and 1/4 will be gone after 2 half-lives; after 7 half-lives less than 1% of the original material will remain. Thus, the shorter the half-life the less mass is needed to produce a certain amount of activity. For example, 1 g of ^{226}Ra (T = 1602 yrs), will have an activity of 1 Ci, but the same amount activity is present in less that 1 mg of ^{32}P (T = 14.3 days) and 167 ng of ^{42}K (T = 12.4 hrs). It is useful to remember that more than 99% of a radioactive isotope will decay in 7 half-lives. This can be helpful when considering waste disposal or contamination cleanup, but of course the utility depends on the time span involved.

HUMAN EXPOSURE

All people are subject to routine exposure to naturally occurring nuclides and cosmic radiation. In addition, human activity may redistribute, or concentrate, a natural nuclide causing increased exposure to a limited population. Such sources are known as enhanced naturally occurring radioactive materials (NORM). The average annual dose to people in the U.S. from natural background is approximately 3 mSv (300 mrem); specific exposure sources are detailed below. While there is no evidence that any radiation dose is safe for people, this value can serve as a frame of reference when considering the potential effects of various exposures to which people may be subjected.

In the middle of the twentieth century the discovery and development of nuclear fission created a new set of radioactive nuclides. Some were distributed worldwide by the detonations of nuclear weapons and led to some small exposures to the general public, particularly during weapons testing prior to the nuclear test ban treaty of 1963. Other exposures to the general public are generally limited to those that may occur from routine operation of the nuclear fuel cycle, and from the incorporation of useful radionuclides into consumer products and applications in nuclear medicine.

A few additional radioactive materials needed for medical uses or for experimental purposes are now produced in specialized accelerators. Production usually involves only small quantities and there is little potential for these nuclides to enter the ecosystem.

Accidental releases of man made radioactive nuclides also occur. The result may be negligible exposures to a very few people, or there may be very substantial releases causing widespread population exposure. Although it is not possible to predict accidents or the resultant exposure, this chapter includes information derived from events such as the disastrous 1986 fire at the Chernobyl reactor in the Ukraine (former USSR). A new problem that is becoming more pervasive involves so-called "Orphan Sources." These are abandoned or discarded medical or industrial radiation sources.

Occupational exposures may also be experienced by people who work with radiation. However, the doses represent only a small fraction of the total collective effective dose for the entire U.S. population.

This chapter focuses on exposure of the public (Table 11–3). Much of the information is derived from NCRP reports and many of the values for doses noted in this text are based on measurements and calculations described in detail in those Reports.[6–10]

NATURAL BACKGROUND RADIATION

Primordial Radionuclides

Non-series nuclides

Several dozen naturally occurring nuclides are radioactive. Most are found in soils and rocks. They have half-lives (T) at least the same order of magnitude as

TABLE 11–3. Relative Contributions to the Dose to the U.S. Public from Various Sources of Ionizing Radiation

RADIATION SOURCE	NUMBER OF PEOPLE EXPOSED (MILLIONS)	AVERAGE ANNUAL EFFECTIVE DOSE (mSv)	RANKING
Cigarettes	48	13	1
Indoor radon (primarily from the soil beneath homes)	260	2	2
Medical radiation X-rays and radiopharmaceuticals	260	0.5	3
Internally deposited naturally occurring radionuclides	260	0.4	4
Cosmic radiation	260	0.3	5
Terrestrial radiation	260	0.3	6
Building materials	125	0.07	7
Domestic water supply (radon)	100	0.05	8
Weapons testing fallout	260	0.02	9
Agricultural fertilizers	260	0.02	10
Secondhand smoke from cigarettes	150	0.01	11
Airline travel	160	0.01	12

(*Source*: Moeller, D.M., 1998.)[24]

the estimated age of the earth (4.5×10^9 years), which is why they are still present. Shorter lived nuclides that may have been formed with the earth have all decayed to stable offspring. Those with still detectable radioactivity constitute what is known as the primordial inventory. Of these, approximately 15 are not significant as sources of human exposure because of a combination of factors that reduce their potential for exposing humans, such as their abundance or half-lives. Two, ^{40}K and ^{97}Rb, are directly significant. ^{40}K ($T = 1.28 \times 10^9$ years) makes up 0.0118% of natural potassium. U.S. Department of Transportation regulations define a radioactive material as one which has a specific activity in excess of 0.002 μCi/g; this is only 2.5 × that of natural K. Since K is a relatively abundant tissue component, and a fairly significant percentage of it is radioactive, it contributes about half the annual radiation dose people receive from natural radioactive nuclides contained in the body (0.18 mSv/year; 18 mrem/year). ^{97}Rb is also a natural body component, but the dose it delivers is less that 2% of that delivered by ^{40}K.

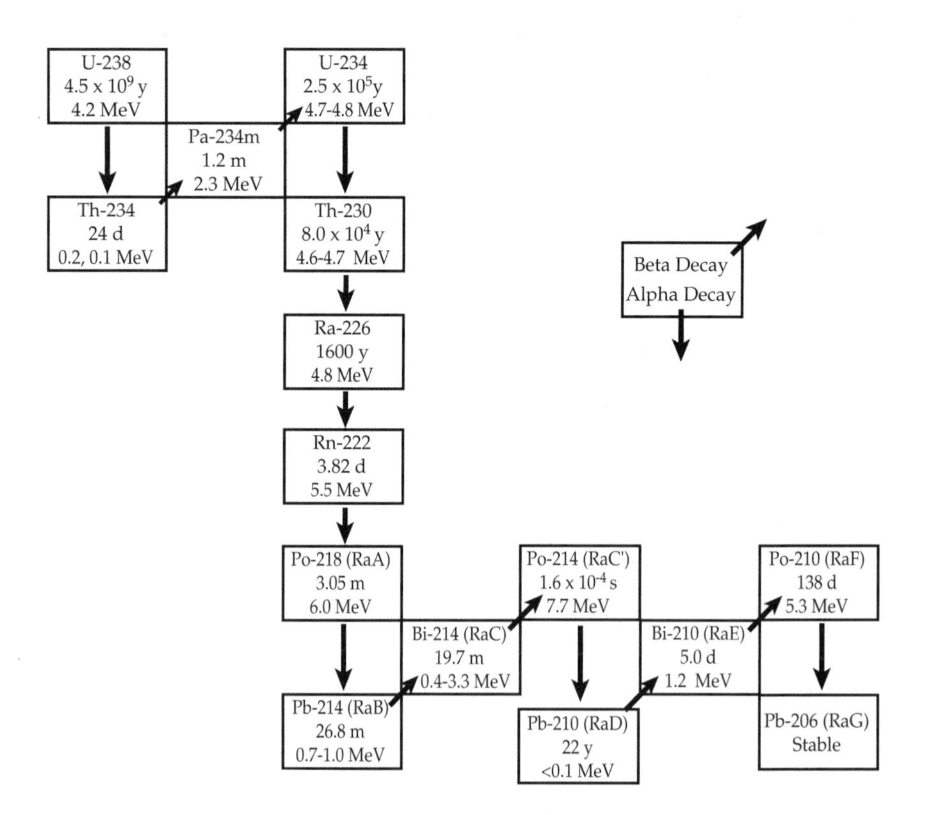

FIGURE 11–2. Decay scheme of the uranium-238 series.

Radioactive series

Among the most important primordial nuclides from the point of view of people are the three that are the initial parents of a series of radioactive progeny. These are ^{238}U, ^{232}Th, and ^{235}U. The radioactive series are shown in Figures 11–2, 11–3, and 11–4. Each square represents the specific nucleus shown by symbol and atomic weight. Also shown are the half-life (T) in common units.

The most abundant of these are ^{238}U and ^{232}Th. The crustal abundance (by mass) of ^{232}Th averages about three times that of ^{238}U but the activity concentrations are about equal because of the much longer half-life of ^{232}Th. Generally the mass concentration in rocks is about 4 ppm_w for ^{232}Th, and 1 ppm_w ^{238}U. The activity is about the same for both however, about 10 Bq/kg (0.3 pCi/g), by virtue of the shorter half-life of ^{238}U. The half-life of ^{235}U is much shorter and its abundance is only about 0.72% that of ^{238}U.

Many of the decay products that are created along these series are of dosimetric significance to people. Most of them are present in soils and rocks in equilibrium with the parent. Their presence produces a field of external radiation to which we are all subjected. The average annual equivalent dose to people from this terrestrial source is about 0.28 mSv (28 mrem). While most of the isotopes

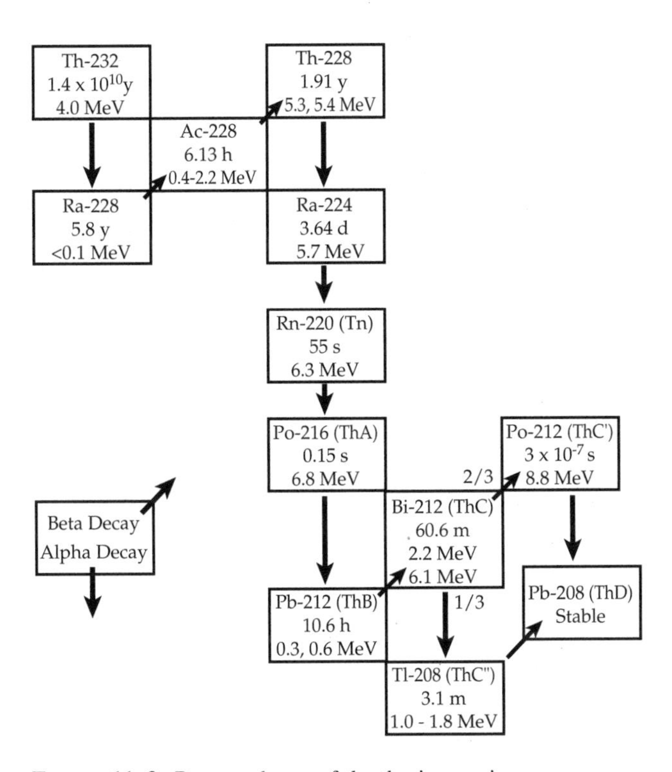

FIGURE 11–3. Decay scheme of the thorium series.

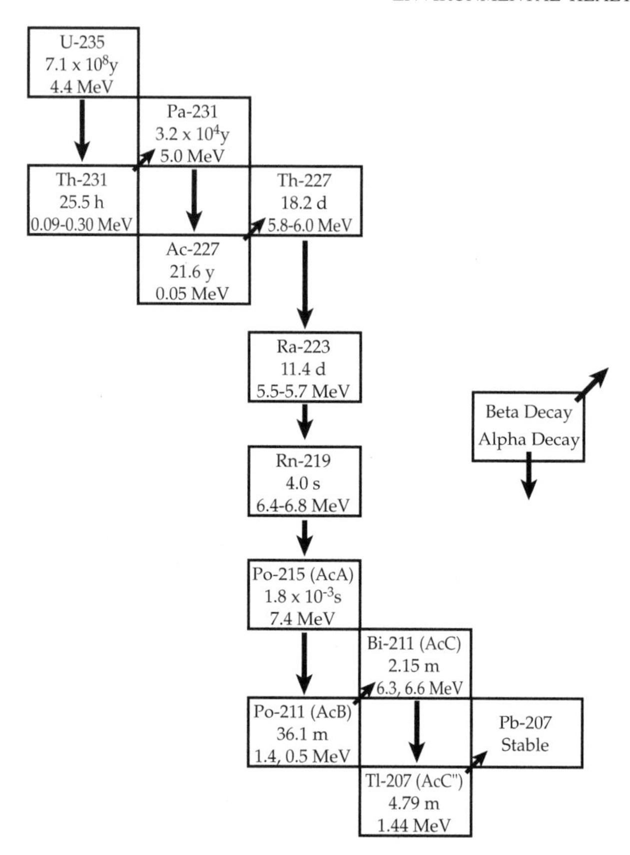

FIGURE 11–4. Decay scheme of the uranium-235 series.

in the decay chain remain at the location at which they are formed, some move through the biosphere in ways that are based on their chemical properties. The chemical behavior, of course, changes with each transformation into a new element. The solubility in water particularly influences the movement of elements, especially if they are formed in porous rock or in the presence of groundwater. Some, such as radium dissolved in water, may eventually be ingested by people. Some enter the food chain in other ways. These ingested nuclides are incorporated into body tissue and deliver a dose that averages about 0.16 mSv/years (16 mrem/years).

In some cases, human activity separates offspring from the parent nuclides, resulting in a set of materials collectively referred to as enhanced NORM. The processing of ores for example may divide groups of radioactive elements. Phosphate mining will split groups of elements depending on the separation chemistry, while extraction of uranium from enriched ore leaves the radioactive progeny in the mine tailings. Tailings piles have, in the past, been used for fill when homes are built. This practice results in greater than normal concentrations of the offspring series of nuclides in the subsoil of the home. Table 11–4 lists these sources. The most notable exposure to people from an enhanced natural source results from the natural accumulation of ^{210}Pb and ^{210}Po, progeny of radon gas decay, in tobacco leaves. Inhalation of cigarette smoke containing ^{210}Pb and ^{210}Po produces a greater collective radiation dose to the public than any other source of ionizing radiation.

Radon

From a human exposure viewpoint, the most important radioactive element produced in these decay series is radon (Rn). Radon is a radioactive noble gas produced about halfway along each of the three series as a decay product of radium (^{219}Rn, ^{220}Rn, ^{222}Rn). Because radon is a gas it is less likely than its solid precursors to remain where it was formed. Some of it diffuses to the ground surface and becomes distributed throughout the atmosphere. The short-lived progeny of radon, or "daughter" atoms, attach to very small airborne particles and eventually settle to earth. Since this takes time, the T values determine which of the three series produced radon isotopes is most dispersed in the air, and also which of the subsequent progeny remain airborne.

The most significant isotope with respect to exposure of people to background radiation is ^{222}Rn from the ^{238}U decay series. Its half-life of 3.82 days allows time for substantial diffusion to the atmosphere. ^{220}Rn (thoron), with a half-life of 55 sec, contributes less significantly to the airborne inventory of radon. ^{219}Rn (actinon), both because of its short half-life (3.96 sec), and because the content of ^{235}U in crustal matter is less than 1% that of ^{238}U, is the least abundant isotope and of little dosimetric significance.

The atmospheric concentration of ^{222}Rn far exceeds that of ^{220}Rn. Also the radiation dose that results from exposure to ^{220}Rn is only about 1/3 as great as that from an equal activity concentration of ^{222}Rn. This is because of the decay scheme and the half-lives of subsequent progeny. For special circumstances (e.g., geological formations with highly elevated thorium concentrations or manufacturing processes utilizing thorium), thoron exposure may be significant.

Radon, along with its short-lived progeny, is inhaled by people and the small airborne particles with the attached progeny are deposited on the airway epithelium. The radiation emitted as the "daughters" continue to decay, is known to cause cancer in uranium and other underground miners. Radon is also present at elevated concentrations in many homes and workplaces. Although exposure in most homes is low, measurements have demonstrated radon levels in some homes high enough to deliver a radiation dose to the bronchial epithelium equal to that known to produce cancer in underground miners. Radon and its short lived progeny contribute approximately 2 mSv/year (200 mrem/year) to the average person in the U.S. This amounts to 55% of the

Table 11–4. Exposures to Enhanced Sources of Naturally Occurring Radioactive Material and Radiation—Sources, Quantities, Characteristics, and Exposures

SOURCE	DESCRIPTION	AVERAGE RADIONUCLIDE CONCENTRATION (pCi/g)	INDIVIDUAL EXPOSURES (mrem/YR)	COLLECTIVE EXPOSURES (EDE) (PERSON REM/YR)
Uranium mining overburden	The overburden, low grade ore, and spoils associated with uranium mining contains slightly elevated levels of naturally occurring radioactivity	Approximately 38 million MT per year is produced containing an average of 25 pCi/g of Ra-226	*	*
Phosphate waste Phosphogypsum Slag Scale	The mining of phosphate rock for phosphate for fertilizers, detergent, and numerous phosphate products generates huge volumes of tailings containing elevated levels of naturally occurring radioactivity	Approximately 50 million MT per year containing an average Ra-226 content of about 35 pCi/g with some scale containing over 1000 pCi/g	*	*
Phosphate fertilizers	Fertilizer contains elevated levels of naturally occurring radionuclides	Approximately 5 million MT are produced per year containing an average of 8.3 pCi/g of Ra-226		
Coal ash Fly ash Bottom ash and slag	Very large volumes of coal ash are produced each year containing elevated levels of naturally occurring radionuclides	Approximately 61 million MT are produced per year containing an average of about 3.7 pCi/g of Ra-226	*	*

Oil and gas scale and sludge	Large volumes of scale and sludge are produced in the oil and gas industry	Approximately 260,000 MT per year are produced with an average Ra-226 concentration of about 90 pCi/g	*	*
Water treatment Sludges Radium selective resins	Sludges produced in water treatment systems contain elevated levels of naturally occurring radionuclides	Approximately 300,000 MT are produced per year containing an average Ra-226 concentration of 16 pCi/g. However, radium selective resins can have Ra-226 concentrations as high as 35,000 pCi/g	*	*
Metal mining and processing Rare earths	The overburden, low grade ore, and spoils associated with metal mining contains slightly elevated levels of naturally occurring radioactivity	Approximately 1×10^9 MT are produced per year containing an average Ra-226 concentration of about 5 pCi/g, with some material containing 900 pCi/g	*	*
Geothermal energy wastes		Approximately 54,000 MT per year of geothermal waste is produced containing an average Ra-226 concentration of 132 pCi/g	*	*

(*continued*)

TABLE 11–4. Exposures to Enhanced Sources of Naturally Occurring Radioactive Material and Radiation—Sources, Quantities, Characteristics, and Exposures (*continued*)

SOURCE	DESCRIPTION	AVERAGE RADIONUCLIDE CONCENTRATION (pCi/g)	INDIVIDUAL EXPOSURES (mrem/YR)	COLLECTIVE EXPOSURES (EDE) (PERSON REM/YR)
Tobacco products	Naturally occurring Pb-210 and Po-210 accumulate on tobacco leaves and are transported to and deposited in the lungs, where they deliver relatively high localized radiation doses.	NA	Approximately 16,000 mrem/yr to lung tissue of smokers	NC
Air travel	Elevated exposure to pilots, flight attendants, and passengers due to the higher levels of cosmic radiation at high altitudes	NA	Approximately 0.6 mrem/hr of flight at 35,000 ft. During solar flares, 10 mrem/hr of flight at 41,000 ft. Air crews receive 20–910 mrem/yr	
Building materials	Living in structures made with naturally occurring uranium, thorium, and potassium in wall board, cement and other building products	NA	7 mrem/yr EDE	8.4×10^5
Road construction materials	Exposure of travelers to roadways made of material with elevated levels of natural radioactivity		4 mrem/yr EDE	2×10^4

Mining and agricultural products	Fertilizer contains elevated levels of naturally occurring radionuclides, and people who handle fertilizer can receive elevated exposures. Also the fertilizer distributed in the environment can increase external exposures and internal exposures from radionuclides in food		0.5–5 mrem/yr EDE	$< 2 \times 10^5$
Combustible fuels: coal, oil, natural gas, and LPG	Coal and coal ash contain elevated levels of natural radionuclides, which are distributed into the environment in the airborne and liquid effluents and in solid wastes. Oil represents a much smaller source of exposure. Natural gas use in the home represents a source of indoor radon, but which is small compared to radon normally present in homes	Approximately 9 pCi/g of U-238 in coal fly ash	< 1–1 mrem/yr EDE	Approximately 1×10^5

*Dose and risk assessments associated with these large volumes of bulk material containing slightly elevated levels of naturally occurring radionuclides, primarily Ra-226, are being performed by EPA.

EDE, effective dose equivalent (Table 11–1); MT, megaton; NA, not available.

(*Source*: Mauro, J.J. and Cohen, N., 2000.)

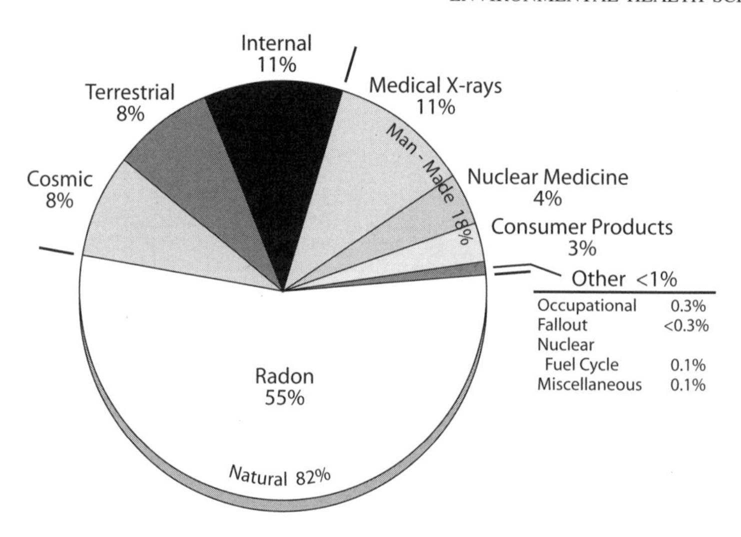

FIGURE 11–5. Percent contributions of various radiation sources to the total average effective dose equivalent in the U.S. population. [*Source*: Adapted from NCRP Report No. 93, Ionizing Radiation Exposure of the Population of the United States (1987).]

total annual dose equivalent (Fig. 11–5), and two-thirds of the average annual dose from natural radiation.

Detailed information on concentrations of the radon isotopes, sources, emanation rates, atmospheric mixing and transport, the radiation dose resulting from exposure and the measurement of radon and radon daughters in air can be found in a series of reports produced by the NCRP[7,12,13] and Cohen, 2001.[14] Access to several informative radon web sites is available via www.epa.gov.

COSMIC RAY-PRODUCED RADIOACTIVITY

The cosmic rays that continuously bombard the earth may interact with atoms in the atmosphere to produce radioactive nuclides. A cosmic ray may cause parts of a nucleus to break away (spallation) leaving behind a radioactive nucleus, or a cosmic particle may be captured by an atmospheric nucleus resulting in a radioactive nuclide. These new nuclides are collectively known as cosmogenic radionuclides. Spallation will produce nuclides equal to or lighter than the target atom. An important example is ^{7}Be (T = 53.3 days) produced by spallation of ^{16}O, ^{12}C, or ^{14}N. Neutron capture produces a radionuclide that is one mass unit heavier than the target for example, ^{14}C (T = 5730 years) produced from interactions with N and O. Tritium (^{3}H) and ^{22}Na are also major cosmogenic nuclides.

The four cosmogenic radionuclides noted above, three of which are major body constituents, contribute a measurable dose of about 0.01 mSv/year (1 mrem/year) to people.

Cosmogenic radionuclides will also be produced in people and materials travelling above the earth's atmosphere, and one estimate lists approximately 22 such radionuclides that would be induced in an astronaut after a two-day flight.

Direct irradiation by cosmic rays is ongoing and delivers an annual dose of about 0.27 mSv (27 mrem). Dose increases with elevation, since there is less protective atmosphere above. A round trip subsonic flight from New York to Los Angeles will add approximately 2 μSv (0.2 mrem); from New York to Paris will add about 3 μSv (0.3 mrem).

MAN-MADE RADIATION SOURCES

Nuclear Fission

The products of nuclear fission are mid atomic number nuclei; some are induced by neutron reactions with normal components of the atmosphere. The half lives range from fractions of a second to over 100 years. Which nuclides are significant to people depends strongly on their yield, the quantity produced, half-lives and chemical behavior. The half-life determines which will survive long enough to complete a path to people, and the pathway is determined by the chemical properties of the isotopes. Also important are the metabolic properties. The three most significant fission-product nuclides are ^{131}I, ^{137}Cs and ^{90}Sr.

A chain of circumstances causes ^{131}I to be one of the most important radionuclides immediately following an release of fission products. Although its half life is only 8.1 days and it soon decays to a stable isotope of xenon, the fission yield is high and it is volatile. Thus, it is easily released and widely distributed. The ^{131}I will ultimately deposit on the earth's surface and should it land on a field in which dairy cattle graze, it will be ingested by the cattle and concentrated in milk. If the milk is distributed while fresh, not much time has elapsed to allow radioactive decay, so the ^{131}I content may be substantial. Since iodine is concentrated by the thyroid, it can deliver a significant dose to the thyroid, particularly in young children, who are important consumers of fresh milk. This scenario occurred after the Chernobyl accident in 1986, when a disastrous fire took place at a nuclear power reactor. Unlike power reactors used in the U.S., the Chernobyl reactor did not have a containment structure. Much of the area surrounding and downwind of the plant was contaminated with radioactive material. Exposures of the public to ^{131}I and to ^{137}Cs (see below) were extensive. As a result, an increase in thyroid abnormalities is already notable in the population that lived in the heavily contaminated region, especially among children who were 0–5 years of age at the time of the accident. It is possible to mitigate this potential exposure after a release of fission product by using only stored dried milk. The fresh milk immediately produced after an event need not be discarded, but can be dried and stored until the ^{131}I decays. When the dried milk is used after a sufficient delay there will be no exposure from this route. Had this been done at Chernobyl, there would not be the large number of thyroid irregularities now being uncovered in children in the fallout region who consumed fresh milk.

Cesium, because of its volatility, can also be widely distributed in a fission release accident and can then be an important source of external radiation. Studies of the contaminated area after the Chernobyl release showed that the most important external source of radiation to the population was ^{137}Cs (T = 30 y) and ^{134}Cs (T = 2.046 years).

The ^{137}Cs and ^{90}Sr (T = 27.7 years) can enter the food chain and, in addition to ^{131}I, are the most critical internal emitters for long-term effects. This is because the half lives are of the same order of magnitude as a human lifespan, and because each is a chemical congener of an important body component. ^{90}Sr behaves like Ca and will be deposited and stored in bone, and ^{137}Cs behaves like K, an important component of muscle. With control of contaminated areas, exposures to these elements is very limited for most populations.

The consequences of the incident in 1979 at the U.S. Three Mile Island reactor in Pennsylvania, in which a portion of a the reactor core was destroyed, stand in marked contrast to the Chernobyl incident. In the former case, a minimal amount of radioactivity was released because the fission products remained within the containment structure. The highest dose to the maximally exposed individual among people living nearby was less than the average annual dose from background radiation.

Weapons Complex and Fallout

The immense scale of the nuclear weapons complex that has been revealed to the public since the end of the cold war has been well described:[11]

> The Nuclear Weapons Complex is an industrial complex consisting of a collection of enormous factories devoted primarily to research, development, and production of nuclear weapons. It has resulted in a legacy of radioactive contamination and radiation exposure to radiation workers and the general public that began in the 1940s and continues today. In many respects, the nuclear weapons production process is similar to the nuclear fuel cycle; i.e., it involves the mining and milling of uranium, uranium enrichment, fuel fabrication, operation of production reactors, and the management of spent fuel, high level waste, and low level waste. Some of the important differences between the commercial nuclear fuel cycle and weapons production include the following:
>
> 1. The weapons production program continued throughout the cold war, and national security was an important consideration in the management of the program.

2. The program required a large investment in research and development, which greatly exacerbated the potential for worker exposure and environmental contamination.
3. By its very nature, weapons production is associated with the production of large quantities of very long-lived transuranic wastes, which must be isolated from the accessible environment virtually indefinitely.
4. The program required weapons testing, . . . which resulted in elevated levels of radiation exposure near the test sites and globally as a result of global fallout, traces of which are still detectable in the environment.
5. Our knowledge of the fate and effects of radioactivity was limited until the program matured, which, in retrospect, resulted in elevated exposures and environmental contamination that could have been minimized or avoided.

The extent of the complex, and the occupational and public exposures attributable to it and its legacy, has been estimated. For the public, data for 1986 revealed organ doses ranging from a few μSv/year to a maximum of 0.25 mSv/year (25 mrem/year), with collective doses ranging from less than 0.01 to 6.7 person Sv/year (1 to 670 person-rem/year). There is public concern that there may have been episodic releases of activity that delivered doses higher than routine exposures noted above. Also there is concern that there may be future exposures resulting from inadvertent release of existing inventories of radioactive materials. These concerns are being addressed by a large environmental management program within the U.S. Department of Energy.

Atmospheric testing of nuclear weapons resulted in the widespread dissemination of fission products, and deposition of nuclear products on the earth's surface beginning in 1945. The doses attributable to fallout have been decreasing since 1962. At present, doses are extremely small, amounting to less than 0.01 mSv/year (1 mrem/year); only a small fraction of the average annual background exposure.

The Nuclear Fuel Cycle

Nuclear fission offers the possibility of a cheap, clean and renewable source of power. The development of nuclear power production, however, has been troubled with a whole complex of problems ranging from accidental releases to questions about the long term storage of spent fuel. It is not possible to know whether or when nuclear power will fulfill a major part of the needs of society. A number of nations have chosen to utilize nuclear power reactors to varying degrees (Fig. 11–6). In the United States, there are about 110 commercial nuclear reactors generating about 20% of its electrical power. In France, nuclear plants produce more than 75% of the electrical power.

The major potential for exposure to fission products is from accidental releases from nuclear reactors, and fallout from weapons, but the remainder of the nu-

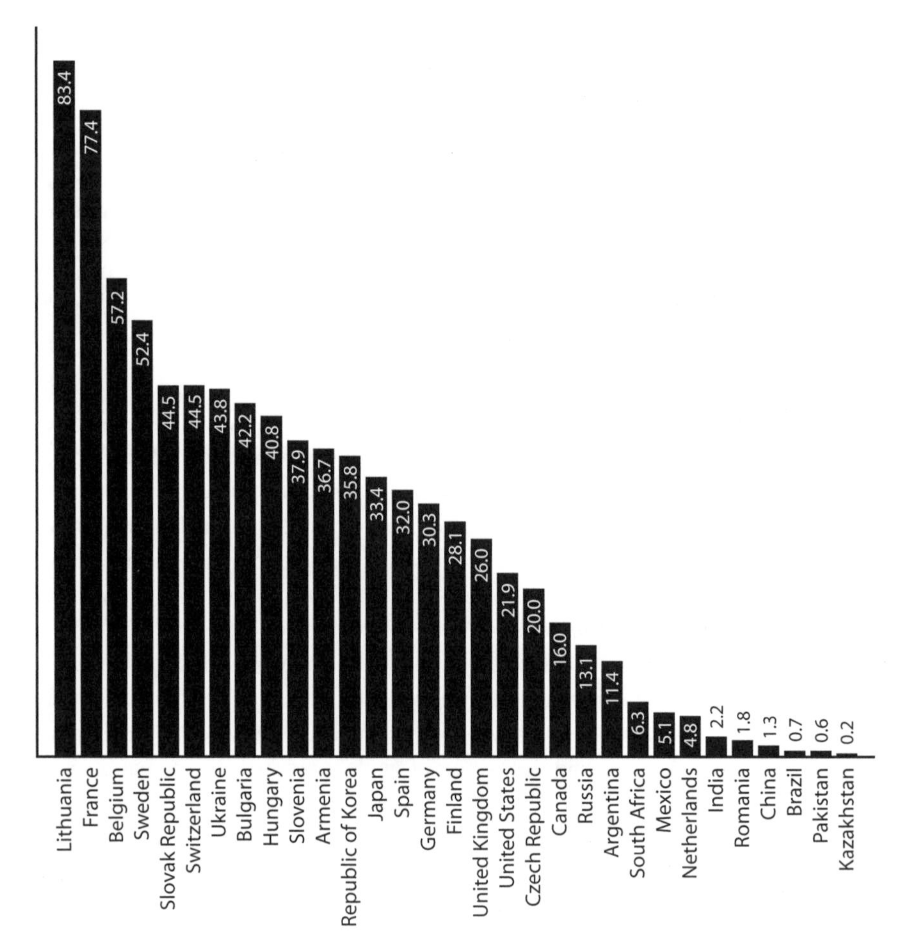

FIGURE 11–6. Share of electricity generated by nuclear power in January 1997. (*Source*: Adapted from IAEA Bulletin 39 #3 1997.)

clear fuel cycle is also of some interest. Initial hopes were that the spent fuel from power reactors would be processed to recover unspent ^{235}U and fissionable materials (i.e., ^{239}Pu produced when the ^{238}U in the fuel captures a neutron) for an ongoing power source. This process is not in use in the U.S. at this time, so the fuel cycle is not really a cycle, but a linear process.

The nuclear fuel cycle begins with the mining of uranium, and proceeds through milling of the ore, refineries, fuel fabrication, reactors, and waste handling. The decommissioning and decontamination of reactors when they are taken out of service has recently come to be considered a part of this process. Extensive consideration has been given to the potential exposure of people all along the pathway that begins with removing uranium containing ore from the ground, through the production of power, and ending with the ultimate decommissioning of a nuclear power facility. Possible exposure pathways from the various steps are shown in Figure 11–7. These routes, direct exposure, inhalation, and ingestion, are those that in general can lead to human exposure to contaminants. Those shown are: *(1)* direct irradiation such as could occur during transportation of spent nuclear fuel rods; *(2)* inhalation exposure; *(3)* ingestion via food; and *(4)* ingestion via drinking water.

With the exception of a release of nuclear fission products leading to inhalation or ingestion, there is very little potential for exposure of people from the remainder of the nuclear fuel cycle. Estimated exposures from each part of the process are available.[4,5] Although there is some potential exposure of people from each portion of the cycle, the exposures are extraordinarily low, amounting to an average annual dose of less than 10 μSv/year (1 mrem/year) (Table 11–5) in the U.S.

Consumer Products

A large variety of consumer products are available that may emit ionizing radiation. These consist of electronic products which may produce X-radiation as a

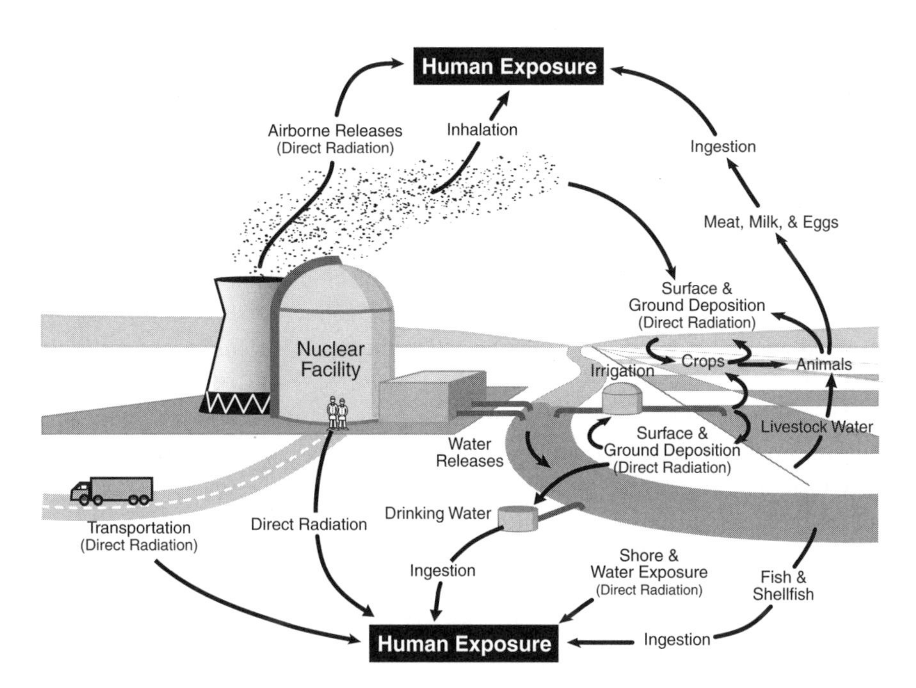

Figure 11–7. Pathways of releases from nuclear facilities to human exposures. [*Source*: Adapted from NCRP Report No. 92, Public Radiation Exposure from Nuclear Power Generation in the United States (1987).]

TABLE 11–5. Annual Estimated Effective Dose Equivalent for a Member of the Population of the United States

SOURCE	DOSE (mrem/YEAR)	DOSE (mSv/YEAR)	PERCENT OF TOTAL
Natural			
Inhaled	200	2.0	55
Cosmic	27	0.27	8
Cosmogenic	1	0.01	0.15
Terrestrial	28	0.28	8
Internal	39	0.39	11
Total natural (rounded)	**300**	**3**	**82**
Artificial			
Medical X-ray	39	0.39	11
Nuclear medicine	14	0.14	4
Consumer products	10	0.1	3
Other			
Occupational	0.9	< 0.01	< 0.3
Nuclear fuel cycle	< 1	< 0.01	< 0.03
Fallout	< 1	< 0.01	< 0.03
Miscellaneous	< 1	< 0.01	< 0.03
Total artificial	**63**	**0.63**	**18**
Total artificial and natural (rounded)	**360**	**3.6**	**100**

(*Source*: Adapted from National Council on Radiation Protection and Measurements Report. No. 93 Ionizing radiation exposure of the population of the United States, NCRP 1987.[9])

byproduct, such as television receivers, and some products used for their radiation, such as airport luggage inspection systems. These specific sources are local and controlled by strict standards so that there is very little exposure to an individual.

Other products incorporate radioactive materials. These include luminous timepieces, smoke detectors, power sources, and others. In addition natural radioactive materials are present in many materials, such as building materials, and tobacco products, and also contribute to the annual dose to people.

The NCRP[6] has divided these products into 3 groups as follows:

Group I involves a large number of people and the individual dose equivalent is relatively large. The most notable are those containing radon progeny, i.e., tobacco products and domestic water supplies. Others include building materials, mining and agricultural products, combustible fuels, glass and ceramics (including dental prostheses) and ophthalmic glass.

Group II involves many people but the dose equivalent is relatively small or is limited to a small portion of the body. None of them compares to those in group I in terms of the population dose contribution. They include items such as television receivers, radioluminous products and airport inspection systems; also gas and smoke detectors, highway and road construction materials, aircraft transport of radioactive materials, spark gap irradiators and electron tubes, and thorium products such as fluorescent lamp starters and gas mantles.

Group III involves relatively few people and the collective dose equivalent is small. It includes thorium products such as welding rods, and check sources. Neither of these contributes much to the collective effective dose to the population.

If tobacco products are omitted the overall annual average effective dose from consumer products is about 0.05 to 0.13 mSv (5 to 13 mrem).

Orphan Sources

Orphan sources are radioactive sources that are no longer in use that have escaped institutional controls. These include medical radiotherapy and industrial sources, frequently ^{60}Co, ^{226}Ra and ^{137}Cs, that are no longer useful to the original owner. Some may have been stored because of the unavailability or expense of recycling. Others are illegally disposed of in dumps or sold for scrap. Abandoned teletherapy units have caused serious accidents as in Juarez, Mexico in 1983 and Goiania, Brazil in 1987. Additional serious exposures have occurred from sources accidentally recycled into steel, then used in construction or consumer products.

The accident in Goiania involved the release of over one thousand curies of ^{137}Cs into an urban environment from a piece of surplus medical equipment. A teletherapy unit that contained 51 TBq (1375 Ci) of ^{137}Cs in the form of $CsCl_2$ powder was left in an abandoned medical clinic. The abandoned source was vandalized, with the resultant spread of the cesium powder throughout the neighborhood ultimately causing 4 deaths due to acute radiation injury.[7]

The International Atomic Energy Agency (IAEA) and national agencies in the U.S. and elsewhere are working to track down abandoned, or scrapped sources. Records may be lost for many of the so-called "disused" sources, which then become abandoned or lost.

It has been reported that there were 2300 instances of radioactive materials found in scrap yards in the United States in 1997.[8] In the former Soviet Union, weapons sources have been lost or dumped. The European Community estimates that of an accountable 110,000 sources in its member countries, 27% are disused. It has been estimated that the equivalent figure in the United States could be up to 500,000, although the figure is not actually known. However even 10% of this would mean 50,000 sources. If these sources are mishandled the consequences can be serious, and efforts are increasing to limit the risk.

HEALTH EFFECTS OF IONIZING RADIATION

The health impact of ionizing radiation is based on cellular interactions of an ion pair produced by the radiation with cellular components. This has been well described by the 1995 report of the Organization for Economic Cooperation and Development (OECD) Nuclear Energy Agency (NEA).[9]

> As ionising radiation passes through the body, it interacts with the tissues transfering energy to cellular and other constituents by ionisation of their atoms. This phenomenon has been extensively studied in the critical genetic material, DNA, which controls the functions of the cells. If the damage to DNA is slight and the rate of damage production is not rapid, i.e., at low dose rate, the cell may be able to repair most of the damage. If the damage is irreparable and severe enough to interfere with cellular function, the cell may die either immediately or after several divisions.
>
> At low doses, cell death can be accommodated by the normal mechanisms that regulate cellular regeneration. However, at high doses and dose rates, repair and regeneration may be inadequate, so that a large number of cells may be destroyed leading to impaired organ function. This rapid, uncompensatable cell death at high doses leads to early deleterious radiation effects which become evident within days or weeks of exposure, and are known as "deterministic effects". These deterministic effects can be life-threatening in the short term if the dose is high enough.

The effects of ionizing radiation on people differ with the dose range to which they are exposed; as is the case with chemical toxicants, the "dose makes the poison." In the event of massive or high level exposures, such as might be experienced following a nuclear catastrophe, acute effects will occur that involve the malfunction of organ systems. The blood and the gastrointestinal system are especially sensitive. Systemic effects can ultimately result in death if the dose is extremely high. For doses of several Sv, (several hundred rem) death will occur in 50% of the exposed population in 2–6 weeks. For doses over 10 Sv (1000 rem) vomiting will usually occur within 30 minutes and death within a few hours up to 2 days.

In the normal course of events, it is the biological response to low levels of radiation that are of interest. Again, as described in the NEA report cited above:

> Lower doses and dose rates do not produce these acute early effects, because the available cellular repair mechanisms are able to compensate for the damage. However, this repair may be incomplete or defective, in which case the cell may be altered so that it may develop into a cancerous cell, perhaps many years into the future, or its transformation may lead to heritable defects in the long term. These late effects, cancer induction and hereditary defects, are known as "stochastic effects" and are those effects whose frequency, not severity, is dose dependent. Moreover, they are not radiation-specific and, therefore, cannot be directly attributed to a given radiation exposure.

For this reason, low dose health effects in humans cannot be measured and, therefore, risk projections of the future health impact of low-dose ionizing radiation exposure have to be extrapolated from measured high-dose effects. The assumption was made that no dose of ionising radiation is without potential harm and that the frequency of stochastic effects at low doses would be proportional to that occurring at high doses. This prudent assumption was adopted to assist in the planning of radiation protection provisions when considering the introduction of practices involving ionising radiations. The ICRP has estimated the risk of fatal cancer to the general population from whole-body exposure to be 5 per cent per sievert.

These potential low dose effects were intensively evaluated and summarized by the Committee on the Effects of Ionizing Radiation of the National Academy of Sciences in 1990.[10] The committee concluded that the long-term effects include: *(1)* the development of cancer in the exposed organism; *(2)* heritable effects which had not yet clearly been demonstrated in people; and *(3)* mental retardation in offspring whose mothers were exposed at 8–15 weeks of gestation.

There is a group of scientists who propose that low doses of ionizing radiation result in stimulatory, adaptive and beneficial effects,[11] but this view is not accepted when determining radiation protection criteria. At the time of this writing, a U.S. National Academy of Sciences committee has been convened to review information on the biological effects of ionizing radiation (BEIR) that has become available since the 1990 BEIR V report, and work is in progress on an updated report, Health Risks from Exposure to Low Levels of Ionizing Radiation BEIR VII.

SUMMARY

Natural sources of ionizing radiation have always been present in the environment. An inventory of naturally occurring radioactive isotopes combines with cosmic radiation to deliver an average annual radiation dose to people of about 3 mSv. Since the middle of the twentieth century, human activities, particularly the use of nuclear fission and fission products, have added to the world's inventory. While the increase in the average exposure of the overall population is small, there are opportunities for significantly increased exposures to a limited number of individuals, and such exposures have taken place. The potential effects of small increases in doses to large populations are almost impossible to demonstrate. Studies of large populations exposed to somewhat elevated amounts of background radiation have not been able to demonstrate any adverse health effects. This is reassuring, yet because effects at low doses are stochastic, it is prudent to avoid excess exposures within reasonable limits. The effects of radiation on individuals exposed to large doses have been used in various ways to estimate the effects of low doses on people. Current radiation protection philosophy assumes that any exposure to ionizing radiation, no matter how small, can have a deleterious effect, and regulations for limiting exposure are based on this philosophy. There are great benefits to individuals and society from the use of ionizing radiation and radioactive materials. When they are utilized, exposures below certain prescribed limits are considered acceptable as long as there is a commensurate benefit, and exposures are kept as low as reasonably achievable. Over 100 years have passed since the first uses of ionizing radiation for medical treatment, and the discovery of radioactivity. However, as is the case with many new chemical compounds, society has not yet come to a comfortable determination of how to balance potential benefits with potential detriments.

REFERENCES

1. International Commission on Radiological Protection. Fundamental Quantities and Units for Ionizing Radiation ICRU Report 51. ICRP, 7910 Woodmont Avenue, Washington, DC 20014, 1993.
2. International Commission on Radiological Protection. Fundamental Quantities and Units for Ionizing Radiation ICRU Report 60. ICRP, 7910 Woodmont Avenue, Washington, DC 20014, 1998.
3. National Council on Radiation Protection and Measurements. A Handbook of Radioactivity Measurement Procedures, 2nd Ed. NCRP Report No. 58. NCRP, Bethesda, MD, 1985.
4. Knoll, G.F. Radiation Detection and Measurement, 2nd ed. New York: John Wiley and Sons, Inc., (1989).
5. Firestone, R.B., Shirley, V.S., Baglin, C.M., Chu, S.Y.F., and Zipkin, J. (Eds.) Table of Isotopes. New York: John Wiley and Sons, Inc., 1996.
6. National Council on Radiation Protection and Measurements. Exposure of the U.S. Population from Occupational Radiation. NCRP Report No. 101. NCRP, Bethesda, MD, 1989.
7. National Council on Radiation Protection and Measurements. Evaluation of Occupational and Environmental exposures to Radon and Radon Daughters in of the U.S. Population from Occupational Radiation. NCRP Report No. 78. NCRP, Bethesda, MD, 1984.
8. National Council on Radiation Protection and Measurements. Public Radiation Exposure from Nuclear Power Generation in the United States. NCRP Report No. 92. NCRP, Bethesda, MD, 1987.
9. National Council on Radiation Protection and Measurements. Ionizing Radiation Exposure to the Population of the United States. NCRP Report No. 93. NCRP, Bethesda, MD, 1987.
10. National Council on Radiation Protection and Measurements. Radiation Exposure of the U.S. Population from Consumer Products and Miscellaneous Sources. NCRP Report No. 95. NCRP, Bethesda, MD, 1987.
11. Mauro, J.J. and Cohen, N. Manmade ionizing radiation and radioactivity; sources, levels and effects. In: M. Lippmann (ed.), Environmental Toxicants: Human Exposures and Their Health Effects, 2nd Ed. New York: Wiley-Interscience, 2000, pp. 523–561.

12. National Council on Radiation Protection and Measurements. Exposures from the Uranium Series with Emphasis on Radon and Its Daughters. NCRP Report No. 77. NCRP, Bethesda, MD, 1984.
13. National Council on Radiation Protection and Measurements. Measurement of Radon and Radon Daughters in Air. NCRP Report No. 97. National Council on Radiation Protection and Measurements, Bethesda, MD, 1988.
14. Cohen, B.S. Radon and Its Short-Lived Decay Product Aerosols. In: K. Willeke and P.A. Baron (eds.), Aerosol Measurement: Principles, Techniques, and Applications. New York: J. Wiley and Sons, 2001, pp. 799–815.
15. National Council on Radiation Protection and Measurements: Exposure of the Population in the United States and Canada from Natural Background Radiation. NCRP Report No. 94. National Council on Radiation Protection and Measurements, Bethesda, MD, 1987.
16. Health Physics, Volume 60, 1991.
17. Reuters/PlanetArk: Interview 05/21/99.
18. Lubenau and Yusko. Editorial HPS Newsletters V 28, #7, July 2000, p. 6.
19. NEA 1995 Chernobyl Ten Years on Radiological and Health Impact. An Assessment by the NEA Committee on Radiation Protection and Public Health. November 1995.OECD NUCLEAR ENERGY AGENCY http://www.nea.fr/html/rp/chernobyl/chernobyl.html).
20. International Commission on Radiological Protection: Radiation Protection: 1990 Recommendations of the International Commission on Radiological Protection. ICRP Publication 60. Annals of the ICRP, 21(1–3). Elmsford, NY: Pergamon Press, 1991.
21. Beir V. Committee on the Biological Effects of Ionizing Radiations. Health Effects of Exposure to Low Levels of Ionizing Radiation. Washington, DC: National Academy Press, 1990.
22. Luckey, T.D. Radiation Hormesis, CRC Press, 1991.
23. IAEA (International Atomic Energy Association) Bulletin. 40 year Anniversary Edition 39:3, 1997.
24. Moeller, D.M. Radiation in perspective. The Health Physics Society's Newsletter. V 26. #6, June 1998, p. 18.

12

Contamination Criteria and Exposure Limits: Guidelines and Standards

Excessive levels of chemical contaminants can clearly produce adverse health effects and degradation of environmental quality. Since the extent and frequency of the effects vary with the magnitude and duration of the exposure, it follows that the effects can be eliminated, or at least reduced in frequency and severity, by reducing the exposures.

Eliminating exposures entirely can sometimes by accomplished by banning the use or consumption of a material, as was done by the federal FDA ban on the artificial sweetener, cyclamate. Since cyclamate is not found in nature, human exposures gradually fell toward zero as inventories were depleted. The ban was readily accepted by the public, in part because of the availability of a "safe" alternative artificial sweetener, i.e., saccharin. When a ban on saccharin was proposed by FDA in 1977, there was a much greater reluctance on the part of the public to accept this action, and implementation was forestalled by an Act of Congress.

The alternative to a ban on the use of a toxic material is a permissible or acceptable content or level of exposure. As an example, there are permissible levels or "tolerances" for the carcinogen aflatoxin in peanuts and peanut products, for coliform organisms in dairy products, for rodent hair and feces in bakery products and for mercury in fish. A low level of contamination is acceptable for such food products, because a societal judgment has been made that a total ban on their consumption is unacceptable. In practical terms, a contamination level is acceptable as long as it produces no observable adverse effects. Acceptable levels are changed periodically to reflect a wider range of observations of effects and to reflect shifting societal values on what actually are acceptable effects.

Standards or Guidelines for the degree of quality for air, food, or water that are expected to ensure protection of the public health and/or prevent environmental degradation are known as exposure limits or contamination criteria (e.g., air-quality criteria, water-quality criteria, etc.).

In broad terms, Guidelines are nonbinding recommendations prepared by knowledgeable professionals to assist other professionals and public health authorities in evaluating the nature and extend of health risks associated with exposures to chemical agents. They are an essential part of the process that has become known in recent years as risk assessment (see Chapter 13). By contrast, concentration limits or emission limits having the force of law behind their enforcement are commonly known as Standards. Such standards are generally established and enforced by regulatory agencies in national governments. However, there are also "Consensus Standards" established by the ISO and/or affiiliated national standards organizations that only have the force of law behind them when they are also adopted by regulatory authorities. There are also Standards that are recommendations of professional societies. For example, the American Society of Heating, Refrigeration, and Air Conditioning Engineers (ASHRAE) has published guidelines for indoor air quality that they have called Standards. Some of these are legally binding in those parts of the United States that have included them in local codes.

In terms of exposure limits on the international level, the lead agency is the WHO, which has, through its worldwide headquarters office in Geneva, established Guidelines. The purpose of WHO Guidelines is to provide a basis for protecting public health from adverse effects of pollution and for eliminating, or reducing to a minimum, those contaminants that are known or likely to be hazardous to human health and well being.

While Guidelines should provide background information for standard setting, their use is not restricted to this. In moving from Guidelines to Standards, prevailing exposure levels and environmental, social, economic and cultural conditions can be taken into account. For example, WHO explicitly acknowledges that, in certain circumstances, there may be valid reasons to pursue policies that will result in pollutant concentrations above or below the guideline values.

It is generally accepted that a Standard is a description of a level of pollution that is adopted by a regulatory authority as enforceable. At its simplest, an environmental quality Standard should be defined in terms of one or more concentrations and associated averaging times. In addition, information on the form of exposure and monitoring, which are relevant in assessing compliance with the Standard, as well as methods of data analysis and Quality Assurance and Quality Control requirements, should be parts of a Standard.

In some countries a Standard is further qualified by defining an acceptable level of attainment or compliance. Levels of attainment may be defined in terms of the fundamental units of definition of the Standard. Percentiles have been used: for example, if the unit defined by the Standard is the day, then a requirement for 99% compliance allows 3 days exceedance of the Standard in the year. The cost of meeting any Standard is likely to critically depend on the degree of compliance required.

It is important to remember that the development of standards is only a part of an adequate environmental quality management strategy (see Chapter 14). Legislation, identification of authorities responsible for enforcement of emission Standards and penalties for exceedances are all also necessary.

The process by which contamination criteria and exposure limits are established and subsequently modified is inherently difficult, slow, and contentious. There are generally conflicting forces at play, with major economic interests, public health and environmental quality concerns, and professional reputations at stake. The available effects data are always inadequate, sometimes pathetically so. The standards-setting process, once begun, can seldom be delayed sufficiently to await the availability of more or better data. Laboratory studies of informative biological effects generally are expensive and time consuming. Similarly, large-scale surveys of environmental quality or public-health parameters are frequently very expensive, even when the measurement technology is adequate. Often, however, successful field evaluations require the prior development of better measurement techniques, and such developments often take many years. Criteria and limits are, therefore, heavily dependent upon "informed judgment"; they are, in the end, educated guesses by well-informed professionals who have considered and weighed the available data and the views of the interested advocacy groups.

While tolerance limits for contaminants in food have been established in the U.S. by the federal government for more than 60 years, it is only within the past 30 years that it has become heavily involved in standards setting in other aspects of the environment. Occupational exposure limits were initially proposed by professional society committees and/or by consensus-type standards-setting organizations. These recommendations usually were incorporated into code limits by local governments. Air and water contaminant limits were also established by state and municipal governments. As a result, there were different standards in different jurisdictions and relatively little real incentive to enforce those that existed. Nearly all standards setting in the U.S. is now being done by the federal government, and the procedures have become much more formalized and elaborate.

BASES FOR ESTABLISHING CONTAMINATION CRITERIA AND EXPOSURE LIMITS

There are many possible bases for the establishment of contamination criteria and the setting of exposure limits. These include: *(1)* epidemiological studies of populations exposed in their occupations, or through contamination of food, drinking water or community air. Such studies can provide statistically significant associations between contaminant levels and reported effects; *(2)* toxicologic studies, i.e., studies of groups of animals intentionally exposed in controlled laboratory experiments where it is possible to define the doses, their frequency of application, and their route of administration. Such studies can provide more complete information on metabolic pathways, storage depots, and the types and degrees of biological damage that the agents produce, including information on whole body effects; *(3)* extrapolation of available epidemiological and toxicological data on other related materials to the material in question, based on their similarities in chemical structure and metabolism, and perhaps their effects in simplified biological test systems, such as bacteria and cell or organ tissue cultures.

Existing contaminant limits were not all designed to protect human health. Lower limits may sometimes be needed to prevent health effects in domestic and wild animals than the limits needed for the protection of public health. Some materials, such as ethylene gas, which are essentially nontoxic to mammalian species, can produce severe damage to rooted plants and trees. Controls on the levels of aerosol mass have been based on the soiling properties of particles and the attendant costs of cleaning and earlier replacement of clothing, building materials, etc. On a broader spatial scale, the effects of submicrometer particles on atmospheric visibility and the effects of aerosols and carbon dioxide on atmospheric temperature may provide a basis for controlling their airborne concentrations.

Epidemiological Studies

The primary advantage of epidemiological data for establishing safe limits for human exposure is that they are not complicated by the uncertainties of interspecies variations inherent in the interpretation of animal data. On the other hand, the number of materials whose standards can be set on the basis of measured adverse health effects in human populations is, fortunately, quite limited. Intentional exposures of humans to known or potentially toxic materials are severely constrained by ethical and legal considerations and, therefore, controlled studies in animals are generally needed in place of, or to supplement, available human data.

The application of available epidemiological data in the standards-setting process is also limited by either poor quality or other inherent failings. This is less a reflection on the epidemiologists than on the materials that are generally available to them. As discussed in Chapter 6, the populations at risk may be hard to define in terms of their number; their exact ages; ethnic and educational backgrounds; prior smoking habits; occupational and residential histories; the number, extent, and severity of prior diseases and medical treatments; their past and current consumption of alcohol or drugs; their past and current dietary practices; etc. These factors can affect the reported incidence of many of the reportable diseases of nonspecific etiology, and may affect the recognition of a disease frequency being influenced by the environmental factor in question. One of the most important and difficult tasks in designing an epidemiologic study is the selection of a suitable control population. Ideally, it should share all of the pertinent characteristics of the study population, with the single exception of the exposure of interest.

Another major problem is the characterization of the health endpoint. While death is a generally reliable and easily definable statistic, its cause(s) may be more difficult to ascertain. At a minimum, it is necessary to locate the place of death and have access to the death certificate. However, the reporting physician may not have entered the secondary causes, and these may be the most informative for the study in question. A sandblaster with advanced silicosis may die of a heart attack; but it is important to know that the lung disease was present, since it put a great strain on the heart. The influence of contributory factors, such as cigarette smoking, on mortality are more difficult to obtain than are data on the death certificate, and few investigations have the resources to do so.

Morbidity statistics have additional complications. There is a lack of consistency in the criteria for defining cases of disease and/or dysfunction. Data collected for other purposes are generally not usable. While physicians must report deaths of patients in their care, they are under no obligation to report cases of most diseases. Furthermore, they tend to differ on the severity of symptoms needed to classify an individual as diseased. In addition to the individual variability in the reporting of disease in a given geographic area, there are also regional and national differences in reporting criteria.

The utility of both mortality and morbidity studies is often limited by the absence or poor quality of the data on the exposure of the population of interest and/or the control population to the agent under study. In some cases, no environmental measurement data are available at all. In others, measurement data are available for the recent past, but not for exposures in earlier times. In any case, the environmental parameters measured may not be the most appropriate ones. In many community pollution problems, the evidence for health effects may be an increase in the incidence of a chronic nonspecific disease, and the specific causative agent, if any, may not be known. Finally, even if the measurements are made on the appropriate chemical species and are accurate, they still may not be indicative of the population exposure. For example, the relation between the concentration of an air contaminant as measured on the roof of a public school building, and the actual concentration in the breathing zones of various individuals in the community, is uncertain and variable. There are spatial variations in the outdoor environment, and there may be large differences between indoor and outdoor concentrations because of differences in air exchange rates, particle sizes, chemical reactions between infiltrating pollutants and airborne chemicals and surfaces indoors.

Epidemiologic studies on community air and water contaminants are generally not definitive with respect to cause and effect, and only rarely establish reliable dose–response relationships. This should not be surprising, considering the extraordinary difficulty of characterizing population exposures, and the fact that most diseases associated with exposure to chemical contaminants can also be caused or exacerbated by smoking and other factors. Epidemiologic studies of working populations can more frequently establish cause and effect and dose–response, because industrial exposures to chemical agents may be much higher than community exposures. They are, therefore, more likely to produce clear-cut symptoms and/or lesions, including many not commonly seen in the general population. Also, the populations exposed are more easily defined, and their exposure levels and intervals can be more easily determined. Furthermore, supplementary indications of exposure and biological effects can frequently be obtained by physiological testing and collection and analysis of samples of blood, urine, hair, exhaled air, etc. Information may also be available on other factors that affect their vital statistics, for example, smoking histories, preexisting diseases, residential locations, ethnic backgrounds, etc.

The major problems with epidemiologic data on occupational groups are generally the relatively small population sizes at risk for any given exposure, and the reluctance of most managements to publish data which might increase their legal and financial liabilities. The problem of limited population size can sometimes be overcome by establishing industry-wide studies, although these generally can only be performed by the NIOSH or by organizations acting for NIOSH under the authority of the Occupational Safety and Health Act of 1970.

The limited amount of reliable human health effects data available on occupationally exposed populations are of considerable value in establishing exposure limits for workers. Fortunately, there aren't very many materials that have adversely affected enough workers and, therefore, most occupational exposure limits have been based on studies in experimental animals.

In any case, the human health effects data from occupational exposures are of limited value in establishing safe limits for general community exposures. Community exposure limits are almost always much lower than occupational exposure levels for a variety of reasons. Among the more important of these are:

1. Intermittent vs. Continuous Exposure: Employee groups are exposed during working hours, and generally have at least 16 hours per day of essen-

tially negligible exposure between their workday exposures. During this time, some of the accumulated dose can be eliminated and other fractions can be neutralized or immobilized. Community exposures to some contaminants are, on the other hand, essentially continuous.

2. Selected vs. Total Population: Working populations are inherently more resistant to environmental stresses since they do not include most of the more vulnerable segments of the overall population, such as young children, the aged and infirm, and those people with chronic diseases or disabilities too severe to permit them to work.
3. Voluntary vs. Involuntary Exposure: While working populations are entitled by right and by law to safe and healthy working environments, there will always be some risk of accidents and excessive chemical exposures due to unknown or unanticipated events and toxicities of materials. In accepting employment, each employee implicitly accepts some risks. The people in the surrounding community, on the other hand, seldom obtain direct benefits from contaminants emitted into their air and water and therefore, are much less willing to accept any significant risk. At most, the risk should be proportionate to the indirect benefits of the activities generating the contaminant releases, for example, a healthy local economy and minimal rises in the cost of living.

To the above, one may add an additional practical reason for different standards for the same chemicals between occupational and community exposures. This is the probability of a detectable incidence of measurable effects. As indicated earlier, industrial populations exposed to a particular chemical under defined conditions are generally relatively small and seldom exceed a few thousand. Thus, considering population variations, conditions that elevate the number of cases of, for example, emphysema, lung cancer, liver cirrhosis, or heart disease by 1 in 1000 will seldom, if ever, be detected. On the other hand, an increase in the incidence of a significant disease by 1 in 1000 in the total U.S. population would result in more than 200,000 excess cases, and would be considered a major public-health catastrophe.

Toxicological Studies

A major advantage of toxicological data for establishing safe exposure limits is that the experimental design and protocols are set by the investigator, and the number of uncontrolled variables can be minimized. Another is that the lifespans of most test species are relatively short, and life term studies can be conducted within reasonable time limits.

Some other specific advantages include:

1. Statistical uncertainties can be reduced by using large numbers of animals in each test group.

2. Inherent interindividual variability can be held down by *(a)* using inbred strains of test animals, *(b)* using animals of one gender, and *(c)* using animals of essentially the same age.
3. The effects of extraneous environmental factors can be limited by: *(a)* providing a diet compatible with the study objective and one constant over time; *(b)* maintaining a uniform temperature and humidity in the housing and dosing facilities; *(c)* using well trained and highly motivated animal handlers who will keep the facility clean and free of infectious agents and other contaminants.
4. The effects of the exposure protocols themselves can be compensated for by giving sham exposures to control animals.
5. The exposures can be made quite uniform in each test group with respect to the manner and amount of administered dose to each individual animal and with respect to the number of doses and the intervals, if any, between them.
6. The observations, test, and lab evaluations on each animal can be made in a systematic manner to avoid biased results.
7. The kinds of observations and tests to be performed on each animal, and the periods of exposure, testing, and follow-up can be selected to optimize the prospects of achieving the study objectives.

To the extent that an animal test system is idealized, it becomes somewhat unrealistic as a model for human exposure. Many of the effects that environmental agents produce in humans are seen primarily in people who have preexisting diseases and/or physiological dysfunctions. There are animal models available that mimic some human diseases, but the extent of the correspondence is often debatable. In any case, purebred strains can have very different responses or sensitivities to some chemicals than other strains in the same species, and there can be substantial further variations among the common animal test species.

There are well-established reasons for much of the interspecies variability. Many materials are not very toxic themselves, but undergo biotransformation into more toxic chemicals. The enzymes that catalyze these transformations and, hence, the products of metabolism, may vary substantially among species.

Thus, even with animal test data that are consistent and reliable, the degree of confidence with which they can be extrapolated to indicate the potential effects in humans is always fairly limited. It is generally desirable to have data on several different species, and to have some other information to indicate which species most closely resemble humans in terms of metabolism of the chemicals in question.

Table 12–1 lists the animal species most commonly used for toxicological evaluations, some of their more important characteristics, and the kinds of tests most frequently performed. These species are readily available, at reasonable cost, from

TABLE 12–1. Animal Species Commonly Used for Biological Testing

SPECIES	APPROXIMATE ADULT WEIGHT (kg)	APPROXIMATE LIFE-SPAN (YEARS)	MAJOR USAGE IN TOXICOLOGICAL EVALUATIONS					
			TOXICOLOGICAL EFFECTS				PHYSIOLOGICAL EFFECTS	CARCINOGENESIS
			FEEDING	SKIN	EYE	INHALATION		
Mouse	0.03	2	X	X		X		X
Hamster (Syrian)	0.1	2	X			X		X
Rat	0.3	4	X	X		X		X
Guinea pig	0.6	7				X	X	
Rabbit	3	6		X	X			
Monkey	5	15	X	X		X	X	
Dog (beagle)	10	15				X	X	

well-established breeding colonies. Because these animals are so widely used, their anatomy, physiology, pathology, and pharmacology are well-characterized. This knowledge is important in experimental studies, where the effects produced by the toxic materials under investigation may be minor or subtle, and would be difficult to distinguish against an unknown or variable pattern in the control animals.

For most studies, the more commonly used laboratory animals listed in Table 12–1 provide adequate models for human toxicity or physiological effects studies. When they do not, studies can be performed on other animal species which have the desired similarities in anatomic, physiologic, metabolic, histologic, biochemical, and disease progression patterns. Frequently, such patterns can be found in large domestic animals, for example, swine, sheep, cattle, donkeys, horses, etc. Swine are similar to humans in skin characteristics and airway branching patterns. Equines are good models for studies of pulmonary function and pathology. Comprehensive reviews of anatomic, physiologic, and metabolic similarities and dissimilarities between humans and experimental animals, the uses of some common animals in research studies, and of the more uncommon, uniquely useful animal models are available, and are provided in the Appendix.

In evaluating the toxicity of a newly synthesized chemical, a standardized pattern of testing is generally employed. Table 12–2 lists the kinds of evaluations that may be needed. Carcinogenic testing usually involves an exposure interval of at least 18 months, and observations throughout the natural life of the animals. The standard kinds of observations and examinations of animals are listed in Table 12–3.

The tests, observations, and procedures used are not all performed on all chemicals, and the degree of postexposure follow-up is quite variable, depending on the objectives and persistence of the investigator. Thus, the absence of observed effects does not necessarily mean that there was no toxicity, and animal tests can never provide absolute certainty that a chemical is safe for its intended uses. They are, however, essential screening steps for any chemical for which either industrial workers or the general public can be expected to receive significant exposures.

Extrapolation of Health Effects Data

Chemical contaminants in the environment can be found in almost all possible molecular and ionic forms, and many form isomers with different geometric configurations. They can vary from monomers, to dimers, to polymers, and can also have varying degrees of hydration. These differences in structure and charge levels can have major effects on the expression of toxicity. It is obviously impossible to perform toxicity tests on all of the forms of a chemical in the environment. Thus, frequent use is made of the available toxicity data, in conjunction with available information on the effects of physical form and structure as

Table 12–2. Outline of Animal Toxicologic Tests

I. Acute Tests (single dose)
  A. LD_{50} determination (24-hour test and survivors followed for 7 days)[a]
    1. Two species (one that is not a rodent)
    2. Two routes of administration (one by intended route of use if other than by topical contact)
  B. Topical effects on rabbit skin (if intended route of use is topical; evaluated at 24 hours and at 7 days)

II. Prolonged Tests (daily doses)
  A. Duration—three months
  B. Two species (usually rats and dogs)
  C. Three dose levels
  D. Route of administration according to intended route of use
  E. Evaluation of state of health
    1. All animals weighed weekly
    2. Complete physical examination weekly
    3. Blood chemistry, urinalysis, hematology, and function tests performed on all ill animals
  F. All animals subjected to complete autopsy including histology of all organ systems

III. Chronic Tests (daily doses)
  A. Duration—one to two years
  B. Species—Selected from results of prior prolonged tests, pharmacodynamic studies on several species of animals, possible single dose human trial studies. Otherwise use two species, one of which is not a rodent.
  C. Two dose levels
  D. Route of administration according to intended route of use
  E. Evaluation of state of health
    1. All animals weighed weekly
    2. Complete physical examination weekly
    3. Blood chemistry, urinalysis, hematologic examination and function tests on all animals at six-month intervals and on all ill or abnormal animals
  F. All animals subjected to complete autopsy including histologic examination of all organ systems

IV. Special Tests
  A. For potentiation with other chemicals
  B. For effects on fertility
  C. For teratogenicity
  D. For carcinogenicity

[a]The LD_{50} (median lethal dose) is the dose at which 50% of the exposed population will die within a specified time.

modifiers of biological effects, to develop estimates of acceptable levels of those forms not tested.

Many concentration limits for air, water, and food may appear to be specific, but actually are generic. This is especially true for the metals. The toxicity may vary considerably among the various compounds, but the only distinction made,

TABLE 12–3. Signs and Symptoms Obtainable by Observation and Physical Examination of Animals Undergoing Toxicologic Tests

OBSERVATION	PHYSICAL EXAMINATION
Bizarre physical positions	Altered muscle tone
Bizarre tail positions	Catatonia
Exploratory behavior	Muscle tremors
Aggressiveness toward some species	Aggressiveness toward experimenter
Inactivity	Coma
Convulsions, spontaneous	Convulsions to touch
Dyspnea	Alterations in cardiac rate and rhythm
Sedation	Paralysis
Nystagmus	Change in pupillary size
Cyanosis	Sensitivity to pain
Abnormal excreta	Skin lesions
Salivation	Corneal opacities
Nasal discharge	Pacing reflexes
Piloerection	Righting reflexes
Phonation	Grasping reflexes
	Pinnal reflexes
	Death

if any, will be between "soluble" and "insoluble" forms, or between organic and inorganic compounds. In such cases, experimental data on one or several compounds have, in effect, been extrapolated to cover related materials.

In one particular field, i.e., the development of standards for internally deposited radionuclides, essentially all of the exposure limits are based upon extrapolations. This was the case because it was necessary to estimate potential health effects at doses which were orders of magnitude below the lower limit of actual human experience, and are delivered over long periods of time.

The one exception involved radium, where there were data from low-level, long-term exposures of radium dial painters during World War I and the following two decades. For radium, the critical organ, i.e., the organ receiving the highest radiation dose, is bone; the biological effects were bone cancer and bone degeneration. Using knowledge of the measured body burdens in the survivors and in tissues of the deceased, and a knowledge of radium metabolism, it was possible to relate the internally deposited radiation dose to the biological effects. It was concluded that no effects would be observed among workers for a critical body burden of 0.1 μg of ^{226}Ra. Except for standards for bone seekers, which are all based upon radium, current standards are based upon extrapolation from experience with many different sources of ionizing radiation, obtained largely since World War II.

The first standards were based solely upon X-ray exposure. The extension of standards to new sources and types of radiation was made possible by the use of units that allowed comparison of radiation doses from different sources.

The unit of emitted radiation is the Roentgen, while the conventional unit for absorbed radiation dose is the rad (R), which is equivalent to 100 ergs per gram of tissue. To compare the biological effects of different types of radiation having differing energies, a unit of equivalent dose was adopted. The rem, later redesignated in terms of Sieverts (Sv), is equal to the product of two factors. These are: *(1)* the absorbed dose; and *(2)* a radiation weighting factor, determined by the type of radiation and the pattern of its energy deposition in tissue. Recommendations on allowable doses of external radiation and internal emitting radionuclides for workers and the general public have been made by the International Commission on Radiological Protection (ICRP).[1]

The deposition of energy in tissue from the decay of internally deposited radionuclides depends on many factors. One is the type of radiation. Some heavy elements, such as radium, uranium, and plutonium, decay by the emission of alpha (α) particles, which are helium nuclei. These heavy decay particles leave a dense track of ionization in tissue, but have a very limited linear range. Most lighter radionuclides decay by emitting beta (β) particles (electrons) and gamma (γ) rays (high-energy electromagnetic radiation). The β particles produce a less-dense ionization track and penetrate further than the α-particles, and γ-rays penetrate further still. Thus, the βs and γs affect more cells, but deposit less energy in each. Also the damage caused by α-irradiation is more concentrated and may be more irreversible than that produced by β and γ irradiation. These differences are recognized by the use of the radiation weighting factor.

The present system of radiation protection is based on the following general principles: the application must be justified, that is, it must have a positive net benefit; the application must be optimized, that is, all exposures must be kept as low as reasonably achievable (ALARA), with economic and social factors taken into account; and doses to individuals must not exceed established limits. Considering specific organ radiosensitivities, the ICRP occupational exposure standards recognize that some organs may receive a greater dose than permissible for whole-body exposure. Thus, while occupational limits are 50 mSv (per year) for whole body, they can be 500 mSv for the skin, hands, and feet. The exception is for the embryo or fetus, whose dose may not exceed 0.5 mSv.

Much greater safety factors are built into exposure limits for the general population, on the basis that this is a nondiscretionary risk, that a small increase in mutation of genetic material in a large population can be of great significance, and upon the assumption of no threshold for genetic effects.

A major factor affecting the pattern of energy deposition is metabolism. Radionuclides follow the same metabolic pathways as do nonradioactive nuclides of the same element. Thus, a knowledge of the element's metabolism can be used, in conjunction with a knowledge of the rate of intake into the body, to predict the concentration of the nuclide of interest in each particular organ of the body. With knowledge of the organ burden, and mode and rate of radioactive decay, one can calculate the energy deposition in that organ.

If certain simplifying assumptions are made, the basic dose considerations outlined in the preceeding discussion can be used to generate specific permissible concentrations for all of the radionuclides. For occupational exposure limits the basic premises are:

1. That exposure begins at age 18 or greater, and continues at a constant rate for 50 years.
2. That one consumes 2×10^7 cm^3 of air and 2200 mL of water per day, half of that occurring during an eight-hour workday.

The National Committee on Radiation Protection (NCRP) has tabulated values of q, f_a, and f_w for most of the nuclides of interest. They have also calculated and tabulated MPC_a and MPC_w values for both 8-hr/day and 24-hr/day exposures.

At the current time in the U.S., there are serious inconsistencies in the manner of implementation of radiation limits, involving orders-of-magnitude differences in the lifetime risks associated with the currently permissible limits for exposures to technologically enhanced, naturally occurring radiation sources (such as indoor radon), for short-term and long-term exposures of population groups to artificial sources, for exposures resulting from liquid and airborne releases to the environment from nuclear power plants, and for potential exposures from operation of the proposed deep geologic repository for disposal of high-level radioactive wastes (see Fig. 12–1).

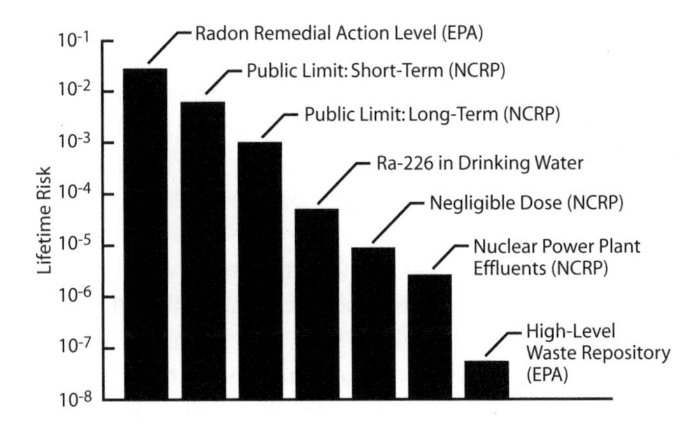

FIGURE 12–1. U.S. criteria for exposures to various sources of ionizing radiation, 1995. (*Source*: Moeller, 1997.)

CONTAMINATION AND EMISSION LIMITS FOR CHEMICALS IN THE ENVIRONMENT

The ultimate goal of chemical contamination criteria and exposure limits is to protect people and other environmental receptors from exposures to chemicals that can produce adverse effects. Adverse health effects include not only excess mortality and morbidity, but also significant degrees of dysfunction. Human welfare effects that can be considered adverse include soiling and reduced quality, value, or lifetime of clothing, building materials, artworks, recreational resources, visibility reduction, etc., as well as economic losses from reduced quality or yields of crops, forest products, or livestock. Adverse ecological impacts can include loss of habitat, biodiversity, species extinctions, etc.

Exposures of concern can take place via one dominant pathway, such as inhalation, ingestion, or surface contamination, or by a combination of pathways, and one limitation of our current environmental quality criteria is that they are generally based on protecting excessive exposures via a single pathway.

Excessive exposures can be controlled by enforcing concentration limits in environmental media (air, water, foods), by enforcing emission limits (into ambient air and surface waters and onto land) or a combination of both. Concentration limits are generally most appropriate for monitoring exposures to chemicals arising from multiple and widespread sources (often including natural background sources), while emission limits are generally most appropriate for identifiable point sources that can produce important local impacts downwind or downstream.

When concentration limits are exceeded, control agencies generally will need to conduct an emissions inventory in order to determine which specific sources or source categories are causing the elevated exposures, and then to impose emission restrictions on those sources or source categories that are responsible for the excesses.

Concentration limits established by the U.S. EPA to control atmosphere contamination that are directly related to human health are known as "primary standards." Those that are based upon recognized adverse effects on animals, vegetation, or building materials, economic losses, or evidence of aesthetic degradation of surface air or water are considered to be effects upon "public welfare", and are known as "secondary standards."

In some cases, the evidence used to establish secondary standards is better defined and more susceptible to realistic cost accounting than that used to establish standards based on human-health effects. It is not as difficult or time consuming to estimate the impact of air contaminants on the soiling of clothing, home furnishings, and building materials; on the reduction in their useful lives; and on their maintenance and replacement costs. Similarly, direct economic impacts due to damage to crops and livestock can readily be calculated. On the other hand, there are some effects whose costs are more intangible. These include, for example, the limitation of tree and ornamental plant species that can be grown in contaminated airsheds, and the limitation or alteration of aquatic species that live in contaminated surface waters. An example of intangible costs which, however poorly defined, are deemed unacceptable by many are effects on the survival of natural species. The successful pressures on EPA to ban general U.S. usage of DDT were based largely on its effects on the viability of the eggs of wild birds. The potential of DDT and its metabolites to produce human-health effects were, and still are, quite speculative.

BASES FOR ESTABLISHING EMISSION LIMITS AND SOURCE CONTROLS

Contaminant concentration limits provide a standard of comparison for measured ambient levels. When ambient levels exceed the limit, the focus of concern shifts to the reduction in source strengths or elimination of major sources of the contaminant of interest. When one source is dominant, for example, fluoride contamination downwind of a fertilizer manufacturing plant, that source may be held accountable for whatever problems result from the contamination. Typically, the ambient contaminant level is due to many sources, and excessive levels can only be effectively reduced by: *(1)* an across-the-board reduction in emissions by all sources; or *(2)* by eliminating or greatly reducing the source strengths of a limited number of major sources.

The attainment of reduced exposure levels through effective control of emissions requires the establishment of rational and enforceable emission limits. The first step is generally an inventory of sources and their strengths. It is also important to know the location of the discharge point and the temporal pattern of emissions, since the latter affects contaminant dispersion. Other important factors are the technological and economic feasibility of the application of controls. Finally, it is important that there be some positive incentives for the installation and maintenance of controls and/or penalties for not installing them or maintaining their effectiveness. For example, the effectiveness of the manufacturer-supplied motor-vehicle emission controls has often been considerably less than their potential because of improper maintenance and some deliberate disconnections and alterations of the system components. In some states, there are no requirements for mandatory inspection or maintenance of auto-emission controls.

Other types of emission controls have been, predictably, more effective. These include those for lead, achieved through the phased elimination of the lead content of gasoline, and SO_2, achieved through reductions in the sulfur content of fossil fuels used in boilers and motor vehicles. In practice, it is much easier to obtain compliance of standards from the relatively small number of suppliers than from the relatively large number of consumers.

ESTABLISHMENT OF CONTAMINATION CRITERIA AND EXPOSURE LIMITS

Exposure levels have considerable temporal variability. Some toxic effects are determined primarily by cumulative exposure, while others are influenced more by peak levels of exposure. As a result, several different kinds of exposure limits are needed, some based on overall intake or accumulation, and some based on rate of intake. Another basic factor affecting the choice of a numerical standard is the degree of protection that is desired. As discussed previously, lower limits are generally set for general population exposures than for occupational exposures. Within the occupational environment, it may be desirable to have relatively high emergency limits as well as routine or regular exposure limits. Such emergency limits are usually based on brief single exposures at levels that may be expected to produce clearly demonstrable, but largely reversible, adverse effects. The rationale for accepting such effects is that it permits actions that can prevent more serious consequences. These actions include rescue of injured or unconscious workers, fire fighting, and gaining access to equipment or controls in order to halt releases of toxic or explosive materials.

Occupational Health

In the first half of the twentieth century the greatest need for exposure limits for chemical contaminants was in occupational health protection, where clear-cut cases of chemical intoxication and chronic diseases were very common. In response to this need, the first organized and continuing mechanisms for establishing hygienic limits were begun by groups of concerned professionals.

In 1940, the American Standards Association (ASA) formed its Z37 Committee to formulate allowable air concentrations of carbon monoxide, lead dust, and various solvent vapors. This organization is a voluntary, consensus type group, consisting of representatives from industry, labor, insurance companies, and governmental agencies. Since October, 1969, the organization has been known as the ANSI. Its standards currently are known as "maximum acceptable concentrations" (MACs) and are interpreted as upper bounds on the excursions of air concentrations at industrial operations. Since ANSI is a consensus-type organization, standards are adopted by unanimous approval. While this led to careful consideration, it also ensured that the process could only advance slowly. During the period from 1941 until 1969, when MACs were being established, the output was limited to 24 chemicals.

An alternate source for occupational exposure limits has been the ACGIH. For more than 50 years, its Threshold Limits Committee for Chemical Substances has annually updated and expanded its list of recommended TLVs; these values refer to airborne concentrations of substances. The original (1947) list contained approximately 140 listings, while the 2001 list has more than 800.[2] The lists also contain guidance on the interpretation of occupational exposures to carcinogens, substances of variable composition, mixtures, nuisance particles, and asphyxiants.

Full membership in the ACGIH is limited to professionals in industrial hygiene and coordinate disciplines who are employees of governmental agencies or universities. The members of the TLV Committee have been people close to the problems who are not directly concerned with the economic consequences to industry. They have made their recommendations as "best estimates." By and large, their work has been well received and has stood the test of time.

Until 1963, all TLVs were defined as time-weighted average (TWA) concentrations over the course of the workday, representing conditions under which it was believed that nearly all workers may be repeatedly exposed daily without any adverse effect. Since 1964, some listings have been given a "C," or ceiling, notation which, in effect, makes them equivalent to a MAC, i.e., an absolute upper limiting value below which all concentrations should fluctuate. Ceiling values apply to chemicals having a prompt response. For most compounds, where the response develops relatively slowly, the TWA concentrations are more appropriate to hazard evaluations.

In 1976, the TLV Committee of ACGIH introduced the concept of a short-term exposure limit (STEL) to supplement its TWA TLVs. These STEL values were defined as maximal concentrations to which workers can be exposed for a period up to 15 minutes continuously without suffering from: *(1)* irritation; *(2)* chronic or irreversible tissue damage; or *(3)* narcosis of sufficient degree to increase accident proneness, impair self-rescue, or materially reduce work efficiency. The provisos are that no more than four excursions per day are permitted, with at least 60 minutes between excursion periods, and that the daily TLV-TWA is not exceeded The STEL should be considered a maximum allowable concentration, or absolute ceiling, not to be exceeded at any time during the 15-minute excursions. ACGIH also specifies that a STEL value should not be used as an engineering design criterion or considered as an emergency exposure level.

The MACs and the TLVs were conceived of as guidelines for use by professionals who understood their nature and limitations. The application of TLVs to novel work schedules has been discussed in several sources. Various authors[3–6] have developed guidelines for modified TLVs for work schedules which depart significantly from the 8 hours per day, 5 days per week schedule assumed as normal by the TLV Committee.

Special consideration is given to some TLVs by the added notation "skin." The substances involved are those for which there is a substantial potential contribution to the overall exposure by the cutaneous route, including mucous membranes and eye, either via air, or more particularly, by direct contact with the substance. Many solvents can alter skin absorption. This attention-calling designation is intended to suggest appropriate measures for the prevention of cutaneous absorption so that the threshold limit is not invalidated.

While enforcement of airborne concentration limits is generally the best approach to control of occupational overexposures, there are many situations where it is difficult to characterize airborne exposure, and where routes other than inhalation are important to the overall exposure. This is frequently the case for maintenance workers, whose irregular schedules and work locations may be difficult to characterize or keep track of. Among the other means which may be useful in determining the extent of exposure are Biological Exposure Indices (BEIs). These values represent limiting amounts of substances (or their effects) to which the worker may be exposed without hazard to health or well-being as determined by analysis of his tissues and fluids or exhaled breath. The biologic measurements on which the BEIs are based can furnish two kinds of information useful in the control of worker exposure: a measure of the individual worker's overall exposure or a measure of the worker's individual and characteristic response. Measurements of response furnish a superior estimate of the physiologic status of the worker, and may be made of: *(1)* changes in amount of some critical biochemical constituent; *(2)* changes in activity of a critical enzyme; or *(3)* changes in some physiologic function. Measurement of exposure may be made by: *(1)* determining the amount of a substance to which the worker was exposed, by analysis of blood, urine, hair, nails, and other body tissues and fluids; *(2)* determination of the amount of the metabolite(s) of the substance in tissues and fluids; *(3)* determination of the amount of the substance in exhaled breath. The biologic limits may be used as an adjunct to the TLVs for air, or in place of them. The BEIs, and their associated procedures for determining compliance, should thus be regarded as an effective means of providing health surveillance of the worker.

FEDERAL OCCUPATIONAL HEALTH STANDARDS

The TLVs and MACs are stated as numbers with one or, at most, one and one-half significant figures. The epidemiological and/or toxicological data base is generally inadequate, especially in view of inherent intersubject variability, to establish more precise limits. Thus, they were not intended to provide fine lines separating safety and hazard or to provide a basis for regulatory control. For many years, the TLV preface included a disclaimer to the effect that the list was not intended nor suitable for inclusion in legislative codes. However, by the late 1960s most states had established codes for permissible occupational exposure levels based on TLVs, primarily because numerical standards were needed for code enforcement, and no other reasonably comprehensive and authoritative recommendations were available.

While almost all states based their codes on TLV lists, states still varied considerably in permissible limits, because their codes were based on the limits recommended in the years preceding the adoption of the code, and the frequency of periodic updating varied considerably among the states. As the list was continually updated and expanded, many states were left with outdated exposure limits.

Some of the confusion of varying state exposure limits was eliminated by the Occupational Safety and Health Act of 1970. Under this Act, the Secretary of Labor was directed to promulgate uniform federal standards. Since Congress recognized that permanent standards–setting would be time-consuming, provision was made for the adoption of interim standards.

Twenty-two MACs are being used as interim standards on the basis that where consensus-type standards exist, it is the policy of the federal government to favor them over all other external recommendations. Where TLVs existed, but not MACs, as was the case for approximately 280 other materials having interim standards, the 1968 TLVs were adopted. The rationale was that the U.S. Department of Labor had already incorporated the 1968 values in regulations pertaining to occupational health and safety for federal government contractors under provisions of the earlier Walsh-Healey Act.

The interim standards were to be replaced, in due time, by permanent standards The procedure for establishing permanent federal occupational health standards begins with NIOSH, an agency within the U.S. Department of Health and Human Services (DHHS). NIOSH, or a NIOSH contractor, prepares a draft criteria document. After internal and external reviews by qualified personnel and representatives of professional societies, there are public hearings. The responses are weighed by NIOSH and a modified criteria document is prepared and, with the endorsement of the Secretary of DHHS is transmitted to the Secretary of the U.S. Department of Labor (DOL). After further consideration within OSHA, and further public hearings, the Secretary of Labor may promulgate a permanent standard.

In practice, the process has advanced quite slowly. Even as late as June 1997, there were only 204 substances governed by OSHA Standards, and a majority of these resulted from an accelerated collaborative effort with NIOSH. The OSHA permissible exposure limits (PELs) can be found in Tables Z-1, Z-2, and Z-3 of the OSHA General Industry Air Contaminants Standard (29 CFR 1910.1000). It should be noted that, in July 1992, the 11th Circuit Court of Appeals in its decision in *AFL-CIO v. OSHA*, 965 F.2d 962 (11th Cir., 1992) vacated more protective PELs set by OSHA in 1989 following an accelerated process that relied heavily on ACGIH TLVs of the late 1980s. These covered 212 substances. As a result, OSHA had to go back to PELs established in 1971. The appeals court also vacated new PELs for 164 substances that were not previously regulated. Although OSHA is currently enforcing exposure limits in Tables Z-1, Z-2, and Z-3 of 29 CFR 1910.1000, which were in effect before 1989, violations of the "general duty clause" as contained in Section 5(a)(1) of the Occupational Safety and Health Act may be considered when worker exposures exceed the 1989 PELs for the 164 substances that were not previously regulated. Thus, in the first three decades following the passage of the Occupational Safety and Health Act, it had not been possible to develop a viable mechanism for the timely promulgation of PELs that reflected current knowledge on the health risks posed by occupational exposures to chemical agents.

In the meantime, it is instructive to compare historic and current TLVs with current NIOSH RELs, OSHA PELs, and German MAKs (Table 12–4).

OCCUPATIONAL HEALTH STANDARDS IN OTHER NATIONS

The ACGIH's TLVs have been used as a pattern for standards-setting by many countries throughout the world. Other countries, especially those in the European Union, have adopted the MAKs (Maximale Arbeitsplatz-Konzentration) values developed in Germany by the Commission for the Investigation of Health Hazards of Chemical Compounds in the Work Area. The TLVs and MAKs differ in some respects, but were in general agreement in most respects. However, exposure standards developed in the Soviet Union and in the countries that followed their lead were quite different, and frequently much lower, than the corresponding TLVs or MAKs. The Russian standards, which are all ceiling values, are based primarily on neurophysiological responses in experimental animals and on behavioral responses in humans. The standards are set at the no response level. On the other hand, the Russian standards have not, in practice, been treated as limits to be enforced, but rather as goals and as design criteria for new facilities. In general, occupational health professionals in the United States have rejected the Russian approach. Discussions of occupational health standards used in various countries are available.[7–9]

AIR CONTAMINATION GUIDELINES AND STANDARDS

Historical Backgrounds

The air pollution episode that occurred in Donora, Pennsylvania, in 1948 was found, in retrospect, to have resulted in an estimated 20 excess deaths and in other health effects among 43% of a total population of 13,800. The team of engineers and physicians dispatched by the U.S. Public Health Service to investigate this disaster was drawn from the staff of its Division of Occupational Health.

TABLE 12–4. Recommended Air Concentration Exposure Limits (ppm) and Standards for Some Airborne Vapors

	RECOMMENDATIONS				STANDARDS	
	ACCIH			NIOSH	OSHA	FRG
	1946	1968	2001	1999	1999	2000
SUBSTANCE	MAC	TLV	TLV	REL	PEL	MAK
Acetone	500	1000	500	250	1000	500
Acrolein	0.5	0.1	0.1^{c}	0.1	0.1	LA^{A_2}
Ammonia	100	50	25	25	50	20
Benzene	100	25^{s}	0.5^{A_1}	0.1^{A_1}	10, 50^{c}	LA^{A_1}
Chloroform	100	50^{c}	10^{A_3}	2^{c}	50^{c}	10^{A_2}
Ethyl alcohol	1000	1000	1000	1000	1000	500
Ethylene oxide	100	50	1^{A_2}	$< 0.1, 5^{c}$	1	$LA^{A_2,s}$
Formaldehyde	10	5^{c}	$0.3^{c,A_2}$	$0.1^{c,A_2}$	0.75	0.3^{A_2}
Hexane	500	500	50,*500	50	500	50*,200
Nitroglycerin	0.5	$0.2^{c,s}$	0.05^{s}	0.1^{s}	$0.2^{c,s}$	0.05^{s}
Ozone	1	0.1	$0.1^{\neq}$	0.1^{c}	0.1	LA^{A_2}
Sulfur dioxide	10	5	2^{A_4}	2	5	0.5
Trichloroethylene	200	100	50^{A_5}	LA^{A_2}	100,200^{c}	LA^{A_1}

ppm = Concentration in parts per million parts of air (by volume)

LA = No specific limit—lowest attainable level

* = Limit for n-hexane only (ACGIH limits for other hexanes remain 500 ppm)

≠ = For light work only; 0.08 ppm for moderate work; 0.05 ppm for heavy work

s = Skin absorption caution

c = Ceiling value, rather than time-weighted average concentration

A_1 = Known human carcinogen

A_2 = Suspected human carcinogen

A_3 = Animal carcinogen-unknown relevance to humans

A_4 = Not classifiable as a human carcinogen

A_5 = Not suspected as a human carcinogen

MAC, MAK = Maximum allowable concentrations—time-weighted average values for 8- to 10-hr work day

TLV = Threshold limit value—time weighted average values for 8- to 10-hr work day—unless indicated by c for ceiling value

REL = Recommended exposure limit

PEL = Permissible exposure limit—time-weighted average values for 8- to 10-hr work day—unless indicated by c for ceiling value

FRG = Federal Republic of Germany

OSHA = Occupational Safety and Health Administration

NIOSH = National Institute for Occupational Safety and Health

ACGIH = American Conference of Governmental Industrial Hygienists

At that time there was no air pollution group in the Public Health Service, indicative of the fact that air pollution was not considered a significant health problem at the national level.

In the early 1950s, the Public Health Service formed the nucleus of an air pollution research program. The federal government's involvement grew substantially over the years and, since 1970, has been carried forward by the U.S. EPA.

In 1948, air contamination was still a local concern, and was considered more of a nuisance problem than a health hazard. In eastern and midwestern cities it was primarily a soot problem, involving soiling and light extinction. In Los Angeles, people were beginning to wonder why their eyes smarted at midday on 10 to 20 days a year in the summer and fall months in air enriched in strong oxidants, as opposed to the reducing agents in traditional air pollution. In both cases, contaminants in the air were causing the effects, but it was not at all clear what the specific offending chemicals were, or what the threshold levels were for their effects.

The only community air contamination standard that was in widespread use in 1948 was an emission standard for black smoke from point sources. This was the Ringelmann Chart, named after the French engineer who developed it in 1895. It consisted of a row of squares having 20%, 40%, 60%, and 80% in coverage with black ink (Fig. 12–2).

The Ringelmann chart was simple, inexpensive, easy to use, and unambiguous in interpretation. A smoke inspector would hold it up as he looked at a smokestack. All one had to do was decide which square was closest in blackness to the plume from the stack. Ringelmann charts were still used as enforcement tools into the late 1970s.

One other index of air pollution that had widespread use in 1948 was dustfall. Dustfall is the weight of the particles that fall into an open pot in 1 month, normalized for the cross-sectional area of the entrance to the pot. The results were reported in terms of tons/sq. mile/month, and were useful in gauging trends, provided that there were no transient sources, like construction activities, and no significant changes in airflow patterns around the sampling site. Dustfall is an index of very large contaminant particles, but is useless as an index of health risk. Particles small enough to be inhaled do not fall into the pot.

Since air contamination was considered to be a local problem, standards for contaminant levels that did exist were established for local jurisdictions such as

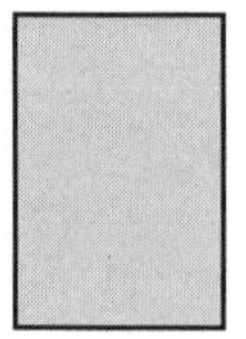

2) 40% Black

FIGURE 12–2. Modified Ringelmann's scale for grading smoke density.

cities, counties, and states. Different jurisdictions regulated different air contaminants and often had different standards for the same contaminants. The most frequently regulated contaminants were smoke, carbon monoxide, and sulfur dioxide.

With the passage of the Air Quality Act of 1967, air pollution control in the U.S. became a federal responsibility to be shared with states that developed control programs meeting federal standards. Since air contaminant problems were not confined to single political jurisdictions, provision was made to establish Air Quality Control Regions based in part on airshed configurations. Other provisions of the Act directed the Secretary of the Department of Health, Education and Welfare (DHEW) to issue Air Quality Criteria and Control Technology documents covering specific contaminants. Following official notice of the release of these documents by announcement in the Federal Register, the governors of states with designated air-quality control regions within their boundaries had 90 days to notify the Secretary of DHEW that they intended to adopt air-quality standards for the contaminants. They then had 180 days to hold public hearings and adopt standards, and another 180 days to adopt plans for enforcement. The standards adopted by the states are subject to review and approval. In the event no local standard was approved, DHEW had the right to impose one.

Other provisions of the Air Quality Act of 1967 included: *(1)* the establishment of the President's Air Quality Advisory Board, the Advisory Committee on Criteria, and the Advisory Committees for the various contaminants, comprised of experts from industry, academia, and other agencies outside the federal government, to assist in developing Criteria and Control documents; *(2)* the conducting of comprehensive cost studies to assess the economic impact of air standards on industry; *(3)* the expansion of research and development programs for air pollution control; *(4)* the study of emissions from aircraft and national emission standards; and *(5)* the registration of fuel additives.

Criteria and control documents were issued in 1969 and 1970 for particulate matter, sulfur oxides, carbon monoxide, photochemical oxidants, hydrocarbons, and nitrogen oxides, the chemicals designated as criteria air pollutants. These documents were relied upon in 1971 by the newly established EPA in setting the initial suite of National Ambient Air Quality Standards (NAAQS). Since then, lead was designated as a criteria air pollutant, and hydrocarbons were removed from this pollutant category. Table 12–5 summarizes the main specifications for the NAAQS pollutants that have been in place since July of 1997.

The EPA has had primary. responsibility for the enforcement of federal air pollution legislation since 1970. The 1970 Clean Air Act amendments were also concerned with: *(1)* controlling existing mobile or stationary sources of contaminants to bring air quality to levels defined by the NAAQS; *(2)* setting national emission standards for new or existing hazardous air contaminants for which ambient air quality standards were not applicable, for example, asbestos, beryllium,

TABLE 12–5. National Ambient Air Quality Standard in Effect Since 1997

	PRIMARY (HEALTH RELATED)		SECONDARY (WELFARE RELATED)	
POLLUTANT	TYPE OF AVERAGE	STANDARD LEVEL CONCENTRATION[a]	TYPE OF AVERAGE	STANDARD LEVEL CONCENTRATION
CO	8-hour[b]	9 ppm (10 mg/m^3)	No secondary standard	
	1-hour[b]	35 ppm (40 mg/m^3)	No secondary standard	
Pb	Maximum quarterly average	1.5 μg/m^3	Same as primary standard	
NO_2	Annual arithmetic mean	0.053 ppm (100 μg/m^3)	Same as primary standard	
O_3	1-hour[c]	0.12 ppm (235 μg/m^3)	Same as primary standard	
	8-hour[d]	0.08 ppm (157 μg/m^3)	Same as primary standard	
PM_{10}	Annual arithmetic mean	50 μg/m^3	Same as primary standard	
	24-hour[e]	150 μg/m^3	Same as primary standard	
$PM_{2.5}$	Annual arithmetic mean[f]	15 μg/m^3	Same as primary standard	
	24-hour[g]	65 μg/m^3	Same as primary standard	
SO_2	Annual arithmetic mean	0.03 ppm (80 μg/m^3)	3-hour[b]	0.50 ppm (1300 μg/m^3)
	24-hour[b]	0.14 ppm (365 μg/m^3)		

[a]Parenthetical value is an approximately equivalent concentration.

[b]Not to be exceeded more than once per year.

[c]Not to be exceeded more than once per year on average.

[d]3-year average of annual 4th highest concentration.

[e]The preexisting form is exceedance-based. The revised form is the 99th percentile.

[f]Spatially averaged over designated monitors.

[g]The form is the 98th percentile.

(*Source*: Section 40 Code of the Federal Register, Part 50.)

and mercury; *(3)* setting nationwide performance standards for new or modified stationary air contaminant sources. A primary purpose of the 1970 amendments was to prevent the general occurrence of new air contamination problems by requiring the installation of the best controls during initial construction, when the installation of such controls is least expensive. The new standards were not, however, to be applied to existing sources.

In the amendments, "standard of performance" was defined as "a standard for emissions of air pollutants which reflects the degree of emission limitation achievable through the application of the best system of emission reduction which (taking into account the cost of achieving such reduction) . . . has been adequately demonstrated." A "new source" was defined as "any stationary source, the construction or modification of which is commenced after the publication of proposed regulations for that source type." "Modification" is defined as "any physical change in the method of operation of a stationary source which increases the amount of any air contaminant emitted by the source or which results in the emission of any air contaminant not previously emitted." Examples of the source categories for which EPA has promulgated standards of performance are fossil fuel fired steam generators, municipal incinerators, Portland cement plants, nitric acid plants, and sulfuric acid plants.

Source controls for CO, NO_X, and hydrocarbons were initially focused on the internal combustion engine. Pre-1968 automobiles, which had no emission controls, gave off 8.7 grams per mile (gm/mi) of hydrocarbons, 87 gm/mi of CO, and 3.6 gm/mi of NO_X. With the introduction of evaporative controls, positive crankcase ventilation, and exhaust-gas recirculation, the corresponding emissions of 1973–1974 automobiles were down to about 3.0, 78.0, and 3.1 gm/mi, respectively. With the addition of oxidation catalysts on the exhaust line, most 1975-model cars had emissions reduced to 1.5, 15.0, and 3.1 gm/mi, respectively. The tighter standards for the 1978-model year specified in 1970 were not met by the auto industry, and were replaced by less-restrictive standards in the 1977 Clean Air Act amendments.

By the mid 1990s, the emission standards for automobiles were down to 0.15 gm/mi for hydrocarbons, 2.11 gm/mi for CO, and 0.24 gm/mi for NO_X, but the benefits of these tighter limits were not fully realized because of the increasing preference of the public for sport utility vehicles (SUVs). Sport utility vehicles had only to meet the less stringent requirements for light trucks. In 1999, the EPA mandated that the sulfur content of motor vehicle fuels be drastically reduced.

The 1977 amendments also clarified several issues of concern not specifically addressed in the earlier legislation. One was the prevention of significant deterioration in areas that were cleaner than the NAAQS. Areas having the purest air were designated as Class I; this designation was mandatory for national wilderness sites. Areas where the air was not as pure as the Class I regions, but is cleaner than national standards, were classified as Class II. Allowable contaminant levels were highest in Class III areas. A state may reclassify any area other than a mandatory Class I area by following a procedure set out in the Act amendments.

The Act also provided for limited allowable increments. An "allowable increment" is the permissible increase in contaminant levels in any Class I, II, or III area. The smallest increments are allowed in Class I, the next largest in Class II, and the largest increments are allowed in Class III areas.

However, a variance above the established Class I increment can be granted by a State Governor (8% above the allowable increment for low-terrain areas and 15% for high-terrain areas). The President of the United States is made arbitrator regarding approval of a variance in cases where there is a disagreement between the state and the federal land manager.

Another area of concern addressed by the 1977 amendments was the leeway granted to EPA when air-quality goals were not attained. The 1977 amendments endorsed EPA's "offset" policy for new or modified major sources of air contaminants in areas that do not meet air-quality standards. The offset policy allows new development if the net effect is an improvement in overall air quality due to decreases from other sources. However, the Act also provided for waivers of offset requirements where the state has an adequate program for incremental reductions in emissions that would assure attainment of the standards by the deadlines (1982 for contaminants other than those that were auto-related; 1987 for those that were auto-related).

The 1977 CAA amendments required the EPA to apply different levels of stringency to airborne emissions in areas that met the existing air quality standards (attainment areas) versus those that did not (nonattainment areas). Furthermore, to ensure that pollution would not increase in attainment areas, the 1977 amendments incorporated a "prevention of significant deterioration" requirement. New stationary sources in such areas were required to use the best available control technology (BACT). At the same time, the amendments required the EPA to take into account the costs of compliance. Existing sources in nonattainment areas were required to use "reasonably available control technology" (RACT), which represented a lesser level of control that could be achieved at lower cost.

For certain air contaminants called "toxic air pollutants", or "air toxics" (primarily substances that tests have shown to be carcinogenic) the establishment of standards has been difficult. A primary question is whether there are threshold concentrations below which they have no biological effects and, if not, how much risk to the public can be considered acceptable.

One of the important changes in the 1990 CAA amendments was the separation of emission standards into several classes. These included risk-based standards designed to protect public health, technology-based standards requiring application of various levels of control technology, and technology-forcing standards designed to ensure that industry develop and apply the very best control technology. In many respects, these changes amplified the requirements mandated under the 1970 amendments. At the same time, Congress mandated the regulation of 189 toxic air pollutants.

The 1990 CAA amendments also mandated further reductions in motor vehicle emissions, as well as a 50% reduction in power plant emissions of SO_2 and NO_x, and called for the establishment of a new permit system consolidating all applicable emission control requirements, and mandated a production phaseout by the year 2000 of the five most destructive ozone-depleting chemicals.

The traditional approach to mobile sources has been to require that pollution controls be incorporated into the product by the manufacturer. In contrast, the primary approach for limiting airborne emissions from stationary sources (for example, major manufacturing facilities) has been to apply a combination of controls, such as RACT or BACT, and to enforce the requirements through the granting of operating permits. To assure successful control, Congress mandated that each state develop an implementation plan describing how the federally specified standards would be met.

Among the new approaches incorporated into the 1990 CAA amendments was a provision that permits the buying and selling of air pollution emission allowances. The goal is to encourage those industries that can remove pollutants at minimal cost to sell their polluting allowances to industries whose costs are higher. Setting a limit on the total amount of pollution that can be released enables companies to trade their emission allowances at market prices.

The market for SO_2 allowances has already worked very well. As discussed in Chapter 14, reduced emissions have been achieved at a much lower overall cost than using any other approach, and the market has functioned very well. Economic considerations also led Congress to mandate cost–benefit analyses under the 1990 CAA Amendments. A retrospective cost–benefit analysis for the Clean Air Act for 1970–1990 has been completed, and prospective analyses of the costs and benefits of the 1990 CAA Amendments are in progress. The findings of the retrospective analysis are summarized in Chapter 15.

WATER CONTAMINATION STANDARDS

Contamination criteria for water have been more narrowly focused than those for air, which is reasonable, considering the basic differences in contaminant dispersion in the two media. The atmosphere is one large and continuous mantle, whose motion distributes contaminants released into it in all directions. Contaminants dispersed in the ambient air can be inhaled by all air-breathing creatures, including humans. Surface water, on the other hand, flows only downhill, and generally within confined channels. Thus, the water supplies used for drinking water or other specific purposes can be selected on the basis of their freedom from excessive contamination, or can be purified to specified quality criteria prior to delivery for the desired use.

Historically, there have been three types of standards established by public agencies for the maintenance of environmental water quality: drinking-water standards, surface-water standards, and effluent-quality regulations. There are also specific industry standards that define the quality factors required of water supplies for cooling and process operations.

In the U.S., standards for toxic chemicals in drinking water in the various states have been based on the recommendations of the Federal Government. The 1975 U.S. standards, which also included limits for a variety of chlorinated hydrocarbon pesticides, were set under the Safe Drinking Water Act (SDWA) of 1974. The Act was also designed to protect underground sources of drinking water by prohibiting waste-water disposal in areas which rely upon aquifers as a principal drinking-water source.

Under the SDWA, the EPA establishes national drinking-water quality standards, including the specification of maximum contaminant levels (MCLs) for specific substances in water. The MCLs are set at a level to prevent known or anticipated adverse health effects. Some limits are risk based, and others are technology based. EPA may either establish a maximum contaminant level for a specific substance or prescribe a technique for its control. In the former case, the limiting technology may be the ability to detect the contaminant in the water. When the technology for monitoring the level of a contaminant at the required sensitivity is readily available, establishment of an MCL is generally the preferred approach. Since the feasibility of achieving a specified MCL or of implementing a given treatment will change with advancing technology, the act requires the EPA to revise and update the regulations on a continuing basis.

The 1977 SDWA amendments recognized the finite nature of the nation's water supplies and the need to assess present and future supplies and demands. It included requirements for an analysis of the projected demand for drinking-water, the extent to which other uses would compete with drinking water needs, the availability and use of methods to conserve water or reduce demand, the adequacy of present measures to assure adequate and dependable supplies, and the problems (financial, legal, or other) requiring resolution in order to assure the availability of adequate quantities of safe drinking water for the future. The emphasis on conserving water and reducing demand was part of a growing recognition of the need to manage the nation's limited natural resources in a sustainable manner.

Also reflected in the 1977 SDWA amendments were concerns about the potential health effects of by-products that occur in drinking water as a result of the use of disinfectants, such as chlorine. The EPA was directed to study the reactions of chlorine with humic acid (a common natural ingredient in surface waters), and to evaluate the potential health effects, including any possible carcinogenic nature, of the new chemical products that result.

The SDWA was amended in 1986 and 1996 to specify additional contaminants to be regulated and acceptable treatment techniques for each such contaminant. The amendments further required disinfection of all drinking-water supplies, prohibited the use of lead products in drinking-water conveyances, and emphasized the need for protection of groundwater sources. A major stimulus for the 1996 amendments was the recognition that many water suppliers were not analyzing for some of the emerging contaminants, such as *Cryptosporidium*. The new amendments required that such analyses be performed, and that consumers be provided with data on the concentrations of contaminants in their supplies. They also required that over a period extending to 2005, EPA would examine and update, as necessary, guidance and rules on approximately 85 drinking water contaminants.

Water-quality criteria define levels of contaminants for the maintenance of specified water uses. Maximum levels are set by the federal government for some elements in water that is to be used for irrigation. Standards for surface-water quality have, however, traditionally been established by state governments, and generally on the principle of assigned best usage.

The individual states assess the quality of their waters by determining if their waters attain state water quality standards. Water quality standards consist of beneficial uses, numeric and narrative criteria for supporting each use, and an antidegradation statement: Designated beneficial uses are the desirable uses that water quality should support. Examples are drinking water supply, primary contact recreation (such as swimming), and aquatic life support. Each designated use has a unique set of water quality requirements or criteria that must be met for the use to be realized. States may designate an individual waterbody for multiple beneficial uses. Numeric water quality criteria establish the minimum physical, chemical, and biological parameters required to support a beneficial use. Physical and chemical numeric criteria may set maximum concentrations of pollutants, acceptable ranges of physical parameters, and minimum concentrations of desirable parameters, such as dissolved oxygen. Numeric biological criteria describe the expected attainable community attributes and establish values based on measures such as species richness, presence or absence of indicator taxa, and distribution of classes of organisms.

Narrative water quality criteria define, rather than quantify, conditions and attainable goals that must be maintained to support a designated use. Narrative biological criteria establish a positive statement about aquatic community characteristics expected to occur within a waterbody; for example, "Ambient water quality shall be sufficient to support life stages of all indigenous aquatic species." Narrative criteria may also describe conditions that are desired in a waterbody, such as, "Waters must be free of substances that are toxic to humans, aquatic life, and wildlife."

Antidegradation statements protect existing designated uses and prevent high-quality waterbodies from deteriorating below the water quality necessary to maintain existing or anticipated designated beneficial uses.

The Clean Water Act provides primary authority to states to set their own standards but requires that all State beneficial uses and their criteria comply with the "fishable and swimmable" goals of the Act. At a minimum, state beneficial uses must support aquatic life and recreational use. In effect, States cannot designate "waste assimilation" as a beneficial use, as some states did prior to 1972.

Where possible, states identify the pollutants or processes that degrade water quality and indicators that document impacts of water quality degradation. Pollutants include sediment, nutrients, and chemical contaminants (such as dioxin and metals). Processes that degrade waters include habitat modification (such as destruction of streamside vegetation) and hydrologic modification (such as flow reduction). Indicators of water quality degradation include physical, chemical, and biological parameters. Examples of biological parameters include species diversity and abundance. Examples of physical and chemical parameters include pH, turbidity, and temperature.

The Clean Water Act of 1972 and its amendments are the driving force behind many of the water quality improvements we have witnessed in recent years. Key provisions of the Clean Water Act provide the following pollution control programs.

Water Quality Standards and Criteria

States adopt EPA-approved standards for their waters that define water quality goals for individual waterbodies. Standards consist of designated beneficial uses to be made of the water, criteria to protect those uses, and antidegradation provisions to protect existing water quality.

Effluent Guidelines

The EPA develops nationally consistent guidelines limiting pollutants in discharges from industrial facilities and municipal sewage treatment plants. These guidelines are then used in permits issued to dischargers under the National Pollutant Discharge Elimination System (NPDES) program. Additional controls may be required if receiving waters are still affected by water quality problems after permit limits are met.

Total Maximum Daily Loads

The development of Total Maximum Daily Loads, or TMDLs, establishes the link between water quality standards and point/NPS source pollution control actions such as permits or Best Management Practices (BMPs). A TMDL calculates allowable loadings from the contributing point and nonpoint sources to a given waterbody and provides the quantitative basis for pollution reduction necessary to meet water quality standards. States develop and implement TMDLs for high-priority impaired or threatened waterbodies.

Permits and Enforcement

All industrial and municipal facilities that discharge waste water must have an NPDES permit and are responsible for monitoring and reporting levels of pollutants in their discharges. EPA issues these permits or can delegate that permitting authority to qualifying states. The states and EPA inspect facilities to determine if their discharges comply with permit limits. If dischargers are not in compliance, enforcement action is taken. In 1990, EPA promulgated permit application requirements for municipal sewers that carry storm water separately from other wastes and serve populations of 100,000 or more and for storm water discharges associated with some industrial activities. The EPA is developing regulations to establish a comprehensive program to regulate storm sewers, including requirements for State storm water management programs.

Nonpoint Source Control

The EPA provides program guidance, technical support, and funding to help the states control nonpoint source pollution. The states are responsible for analyzing the extent and severity of their nonpoint source pollution problems and developing and implementing needed water quality management actions.

Control of Combined Sewer Overflows

Under the National Combined Sewer Overflow. Control Strategy of 1989, States develop and implement measures to reduce pollution discharges from combined storm and sanitary sewers. The EPA works with the states to implement the national strategy. The CWA also established pollution control and prevention programs for specific waterbody categories, such as the Clean Lakes Program. Other statutes that also guide the development of water quality protection programs include:

The Safe Drinking Water Act, under which states establish standards for drinking water quality, monitor wells and local water supply systems, implement drinking water protection programs, and implement Underground Injection Control (UIC) programs.

The Resource Conservation and Recovery Act, which establishes State and EPA programs for ground water and surface water protection and cleanup and emphasizes prevention of releases through management standards in addition to other waste management activities.

The Comprehensive Environmental Response, Compensation, and Liability Act (Superfund Program), which provides EPA with the authority to clean up contaminated waters during remediation at contaminated sites.

The Pollution Prevention Act of 1990, which requires EPA to promote pollutant source reduction rather than focus on controlling pollutants after they enter the environment.

The maintenance of water quality depends on the control of noxious discharges. Prior to 1971, the control of contaminant effluents was entirely up to the states. However, in that year, a federal court ruled that with the enactment of the National Environmental Policy Act, the permits required for discharges into navigable waterways under the 1899 Refuse Act had to be accompanied by an environmental impact statement. As a result, the Army Corp of Engineers had to immediately assume responsibility for evaluating and regulating the impact of toxic effluents on streams. The confusion that resulted was partially ended with the passage of the Federal Water Pollution Control Act of 1972. A major feature of this Act was its emphasis on effluent limitations. The overall goals of the Act were to eliminate discharge of contaminants into navigable waters by 1985, to achieve high water quality by July 1, 1983 (later changed by the 1977 Clean Water Act to 1984), and to eliminate the discharge of specific toxic contaminants. The regulations provided for: *(1)* a NPDES, which required that point sources which discharge contaminants into waterways obtain discharge permits; *(2)* Effluent Guidelines and Standards; *(3)* Pretreatment Standards; *(4)* Oil and Hazardous Substances Rules; *(5)* Ocean Dumping Rules; and *(6)* Toxic-Pollutant Standards. The EPA requests that NPDES applicants have a preapplication conference with EPA at least 24 months before the discharge starts. This period provides EPA with additional time to prepare an environmental impact statement, if required.

The Act mandated that effluent guidelines and standards be established for industrial plants. These standards are end-of-pipe limitations expressed as either pound of contaminant per 1000 pounds of product, or as milligram of contaminant per liter of effluent.

Regulations apply to "liquid effluents" discharged from "point sources" into "navigable waters." The broad definition applied to these terms makes the Effluent Guidelines and Standards virtually all-inclusive. Liquid effluents include every type of water, from process wastes to uncontaminated stormwater. A point source is a discharge through any type of conveyance (pipe, channel, etc.). A navigable water is any water other than groundwater. Effluent Guidelines and Standards are issued in three increasing levels of restrictiveness: *(1)* the Best Practical Control Technology Currently Available (BPCTCA), which existing plants had to meet by July 1, 1977; *(2)* the Best

Available Demonstrated Control Technology (BADCT), which new plants had to meet upon startup; and *(3)* the Best Available Control Technology Economically Achievable (BACTEA), which all plants were to meet originally by July 1, 1983. Thus, these guidelines are technology-based effluent limits that are developed following appraisal of the treatment technologies available to a particular industrial category, and the economic consideration associated with the installation of such technology for the particular industry. Current effluent guidelines are applied for BOD, COD, total suspended solids (TSS), pH, and some other waste water constituents.

The intent of the Act was to use the progressive restriction on the discharge of contaminants to approach the goal of zero discharge by 1985.

Zero discharge means no discharge of contaminants; therefore, an effluent stream containing substances not harmful to the receiving body of water is compatible with the goal.

The Effluent Guidelines and Standards and the Pretreatment Standards are closely related. Pretreatment Standards apply to discharges into municipal sewers rather than directly into waterways. This sewer discharge could cause the contaminants to interfere with the operation of the waste treatment facility. These standards eliminate the economic advantages of plants changing their discharge from a navigable water to a municipal system. This economic disincentive is achieved by having the numerical limits virtually identical to the BPCTCA and BADCT levels of the Effluent Guidelines and Standards.

The July 1, 1977, deadline for the application of the Best Practical Control Technology Currently Available was not met by about 15% of the major industrial discharges, nor by about 70% of the municipal sewage treatment jurisdictions. The 1984 and 1985 target dates specified in the Act also proved to be too optimistic. However, the Act made it possible to achieve substantial progress in water pollution control.

Some chemicals are so highly toxic and impose such severe risks to humans or aquatic life that they warrant a special regulatory mechanism to control their presence in waterways. Under the Clean Water Act, the EPA may set up special effluent standards for these toxic contaminants. In 1977, final regulations were prepared by EPA to control direct discharges of DDT, aldrin/dieldrin, endrin, toxaphene, benzidine, and PCBs.

Furthermore, pursuant to a 1976 settlement with the National Resources Defense Council, Inc., and Citizens for a Better Environment, the EPA was committed to a program to investigate 65 designated contaminants that represent substantial concern related to their potential health or environmental effects; these include both organic and inorganic agents, many of which are recognized or potential carcinogens, mutagens, or teratogens. The goal established was development of water-quality criteria for each of these by June, 1978, and control of their discharge based upon these criteria.

The 1987 amendments to the Clean Water Act significantly changed the thrust of enforcement, by increasing the attention paid to the monitoring and control of toxic constituents in waste water, and to discharges of polluted runoff from city streets, farmland, mining sites, and other "nonpoint" sources. The 1987 amendments also changed the NPDES program by requiring much stricter discharge limits and expanding the number of chemical constituents that must be monitored in pollutants that reach waterways. Thus, the Clean Water Act emphasizes a permitting system for the release of pollutants into lakes and streams. Polluters can apply for discharge permits that specify the required control technology, as contrasted to specifying limits on the concentrations of specific pollutants in the receiving bodies of water. Technology-based, as opposed to harm-based, standards are emphasized.

FOOD CONTAMINATION

The FDA is responsible for establishing tolerances, i.e., permissible levels of contamination in food. Table 2–5 lists some tolerance levels for pesticides in food. Tolerance levels have also been established for some carcinogenic contaminants, for example, 20 ppb_w for aflatoxin in peanuts and corn.

In the Food Quality Protection Act of 1996, a major concern was the adequacy of food contaminant limits for the protection of children, on the basis that they may have greater percentage uptake and dose to target tissues than adults consuming the same food products. The EPA was directed to add an additional safety factor of 10 for pesticide chemicals if it could not demonstrate that such an additional margin of safety was not needed. In order to address this issue, the Agency initiated an internal review process on its hazard assessment and risk assessment procedures used to establishing acceptable residue levels. It also set up mechanisms for their review by other federal agencies (U.S. Department of Agriculture, the Food and Drug Administration, etc.) and by its own external Scientific Advisory Panel. They also established a policy that when assessing dietary (food) risks from pesticides, they will use a 10-fold factor unless, based on a weight-of-the-evidence evaluation of available and reliable data, it concludes that this factor should be modified or not used. In the reviews conducted in the first few years after passage of the act, it chose to use no additional, or less than a 10-fold extra, safety factor for most of the chemicals that were re-evaluated. Needless to say, the topic remains controversial.

REFERENCES

1. ICRP Task Group. Human Respiratory Tract Model for Radiological Protection. ICRP Publication 66, Tarrytown, NY: Elsevier, 1994.

2. ACGIH. 2001 TLVs and BEIs, Cincinnati, American Conference of Governmental Industrial Hygienists, 2001.
3. Brief, R.S. and Scala, R.A. Occupational exposure limits for novel work schedules. *Am. Ind. Hyg. Assoc. J.* 36:467–469, 1975.
4. Mason, J.W. and Dershin, H. Limits to occupational exposure in chemical environments under novel work schedules. *J. Occup. Med.* 18:603–606, 1976.
5. Calabrese, E.J. Further comments on novel schedule TLVs. *Am. Ind. Hyg. Assoc. J.* 38:443–446, 1977.
6. Hickey, J.L.S. and Reist, P.C. Application of occupational exposure limits to unusual work schedules. *Am. Ind. Hyg. Assoc. J.* 38:613–621, 1977.
7. Hatch, T.F. Permissible levels of exposure to hazardous agents in industry. *J. Occup. Med.* 14:134–137, 1972.
8. AIHA. An international review of procedures for establishing occupational exposure limits. Am. Ind. Hyg. Assoc., Fairfax, VA, 1996.
9. Vincent, J.H. International Occupational Exposure Standards: A Review and Commentary. *Am. Ind. Hyg. Assoc. J.* 59:729, 1998.

13

Risk Assessment

The human race has always faced certain dangers. Risk is an inescapable fact of life. At the same time, enlightened societies have traditionally sought to minimize avoidable risks. The greatly increased life expectancy now enjoyed by populations in the industrialized world attests to the success with which modern civilization has been able to reduce some environmental risks to human health and safety.

By the early 1980s, it had become clear to leaders in public health and environmental protection that there were myriad risks to public health and welfare from the various chemical and physical agents being released as a result of anthropogenic activities, and that their aggregate resources for mitigating risks were limited. In order to develop a strategic approach to risk characterization and management, William Ruckelshaus, then Administrator of the U.S. EPA, requested a study of options for this task from the National Research Council (NRC). The report prepared by the NRC Committee[1] proposed a new paradigm for risk assessment and risk management that was largely adopted by EPA and other agencies. Its major recommendations are summarized in Figure 13–1. It called for a distinct separation between the process described in Table 13–1 that it called risk assessment, which is largely based on the acquisition and interpretation of scientific principles and data, from the process it called risk management. Risk management is based on decisions that recognize the nature and limitations of the

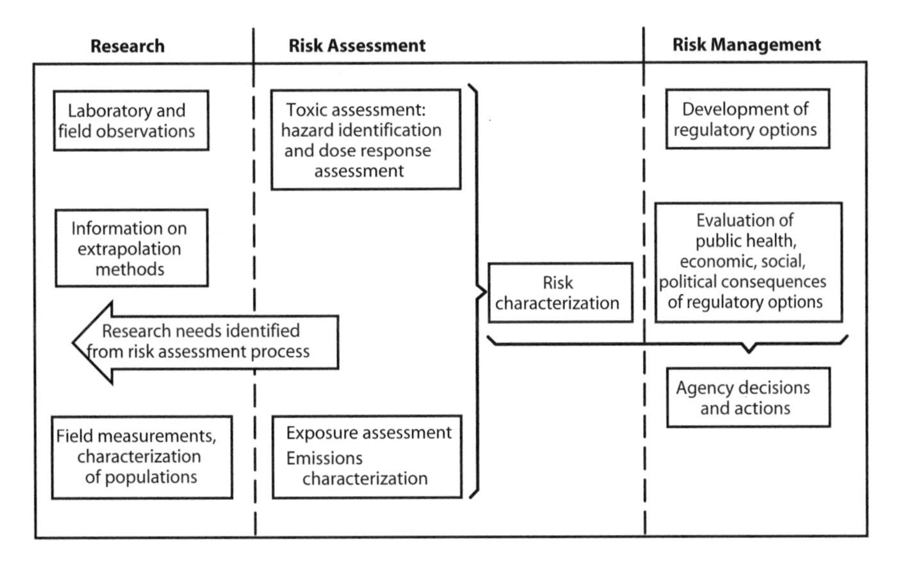

FIGURE 13–1. Risk assessment relies on evaluation techniques. [*Source*: Science and Judgment in Risk Assessment (NRC, 1994a). Reprinted with permission.]

TABLE 13–1. The "Red Book" Paradigm: The Four Steps of Risk Assessment

STEP	DEFINITION
1. Hazard identification	A review of the relevant biologic and chemical information bearing on whether an agent may pose a carcinogenic hazard and whether toxic effects in one setting will occur in other settings.
2. Dose–response assessment	The process of quantifying a dosage and evaluating its relation to the incidence of adverse health effects response.
3. Exposure assessment	The determination or estimation (qualitative or quantitative) of the magnitude, duration, and route of exposure.
4. Risk characterization	An integration and summary of hazard identification, dose-response assessment, and exposure assessment presented with assumptions and uncertainties. This final step provides an estimate of the risk to public health and a framework to define the significance of the risk.

(*Source*: National Research Council, Committee on the Institutional Means for Assessment of Risks to Public Health. Risk Assessment in the Federal Government: Managing the Process. Washington, DC: National Academy Press, 1983.)

scientific risk assessment, but is also influenced by the constraints imposed by legislative mandates, the capabilities and costs of implementation of available control options, and the anticipated acceptibility of these options in a sociopolitical and legal context. The implication was that scientists with appropriate expertise are best equipped to perform risk assessments, but should have no special or dominant role in selecting the means or schedule for the implementation of risk mitigation options. The latter are reserved for public officials, who can be held accountable by the public and the court system.

As indicated in Table 13–1, environmental risk assessment is based on: *(1)* hazard identification; *(2)* dose–response assessment; *(3)* exposure assessment to determine population distributions of exposures to an environmental stress; and *(4)* risk characterization, which establishes an estimate of the risk for overall populations and for subsegments of the overall population that may be especially sensitive when exposed, each with associated uncertainties.

This chapter reviews environmental risks to human health from two standpoints: the risk to the individual and the risk to the community. Considered in this context are scientific bases for assessing such risks, the relative magnitudes of different environmental risks as evaluated by knowledgeable experts, the contrasting perspectives in which risks may be perceived by different members of the public, and difficulties in risk communication that complicate societal efforts to protect health and the environment. Options for reducing risks at the individual and community levels are discussed in Chapter 14.

The technical means of assessing human exposures to chemical toxicants were discussed in detail in Chapter 8, and to physical agents in Chapters 9, 10, and 11. The means for establishing exposure-response relationships for human health effects were discussed in broad terms in Chapter 6 for chemical agents and in Chapters 9, 10, and 11 for physical agents. Thus, this chapter is largely confined to a discussion of how risk assessments are performed, and how technical risk assessment may differ from risk perception among segments of the overall public.

THE NATURE OF RISK

Risk is commonly defined as "hazard, peril, or exposure to loss or injury." The term *environmental risk to health* is taken herein to mean the probability of an adverse effect on human health resulting from exposure to a particular environmental agent or combination of agents. Such a risk may be expressed in various ways, depending on the context in which it is considered; for example, average annual risk per individual, average lifetime risk per individual, average number of individuals affected annually in a given population, average loss of life expectancy in affected individuals, etc.

For certain types of health effects, such as pollutant-induced cancers, the risk may also be expressed either as an absolute risk (i.e., absolute increase in the number or probability of cancer incidence) or as a relative risk (i.e., a relative increase in the background frequency of cancer). Depending on the baseline frequency, or background rate, a small increase in relative risk may be equivalent to a large increase in the number of individuals affected. Conversely, merely a few additional cases of an otherwise rare disorder may result in a large increase in the relative risk.

The importance attached to a given risk depends on the severity as well as the frequency of the effect in question. Determinants of severity include such factors as the extent to which the effect is or is not symptomatic, painful, disfiguring, incapacitating, reversible, progressive, lethal, etc., these being the properties that determine its impact on the affected individual and on his or her loved ones, descendants, co-workers, neighbors, and community. In the broadest context, therefore, the measures of severity have many ramifications, including esthetic, psychosocial, ethical, and economic impacts, as well as impacts on health per se.

Apart from objective measures of the frequency and severity of environmental risks to health, other qualitative characteristics, such as those listed in Table 13–2, can be important in determining how risks are perceived. Nonscientists often not only fail to understand the technical basis for evaluating a given risk, but actually distrust and reject it. It has been suggested, therefore, that the definition of an environmental risk should include these nontechnical aspects that may be of concern to the public, i.e., its "outrage" factors. The importance of such nontechnical factors is illustrated by the marked degree to which public perceptions of a given risk may differ from those of informed experts (Table 13–3).

TABLE 13–2. Psychosocial and Cultural Characteristics Affecting the Perception of Risk

CHARACTERISTICS OF A RISK THAT TEND TO INCREASE ITS ACCEPTABILITY	CHARACTERISTICS OF A RISK THAT TEND TO DECREASE ITS ACCEPTABILITY
Voluntary	Involuntary
Familiar	Unfamiliar
Immediate impact	Remote impact
Detectable by individual	Nondetectable by individual
Controllable by individual	Uncontrollable by individual
Fair	Unfair
Noncatastophic	Catastrophic
Well understood	Poorly understood
Natural	Artificial
Trusted source	Untrusted source
Visible benefits	No visible benefits

TABLE 13–3. Perceived as Compared with Real Risks Associated with 30 Widespread Activities and Technologies

ACTIVITY OR TECHNOLOGY	TECHNICAL ESTIMATES (DEATHS/YEAR)[a]	GEOMETRIC MEAN FATALITY ESTIMATES, AVERAGE YEAR		GEOMETRIC MEAN MULTIPLIER, DISASTROUS YEAR	
		LOWV[b]	**Students[c]**	**LOWV[b]**	**Students[c]**
Smoking	150,000	6900	2400	1.9	2.0
Alcoholic beverages	100,000	12,000	2600	1.9	1.4
Motor vehicles	50,000	28,000	10,500	1.6	1.8
Handguns	17,000	3000	1900	2.6	2.0
Electric power	14,000	660	500	1.9	2.4
Motorcycles	3000	1600	1600	1.8	1.6
Swimming	3000	930	370	1.6	1.7
Surgery	2800	2500	900	1.5	1.6
X-rays	2300	90	40	2.7	1.6
Railroads	1950	190	210	3.2	1.6
General (private) aviation	1300	550	650	2.8	2.0
Large construction	1000	400	370	2.1	1.4
Bicycles	1000	910	420	1.8	1.4
Hunting	800	380	410	1.8	1.7
Home appliances	200	200	240	1.6	1.3
Fire fighting	195	220	390	2.3	2.2
Police work	160	460	390	2.1	1.9
Contraceptives	150	180	120	2.1	1.4
Commercial aviation	130	280	650	3.0	1.8
Nuclear power	100[d]	20	27	107.1	87.6
Mountain climbing	30	50	70	1.9	1.4
Power mowers	24	40	33	1.6	1.3
School and college football	23	39	40	1.9	1.4
Skiing	18	55	72	1.9	1.6
Vaccinations	10	65	52	2.1	1.6
Food coloring	[e]	38	33	3.5	1.4
Food preservatives	[e]	61	63	3.9	1.7
Pesticides	[e]	140	84	9.3	2.4
Prescription antibiotics	[e]	160	290	2.3	1.6
Spray cans	[e]	56	38	3.7	2.4

[a]Based on assessments by technical experts.

[b]League of Women Voters.

[c]College students.

[d]Geometric mean of estimates, which ranged from 16 to 600 per year.

[e]Estimates were unavailable.

IDENTIFICATION AND QUANTIFICATION OF RISKS

Assessment of an environmental risk to human health involves a sequence of interrelated steps, beginning with identification of the causative agent or exposure situation, and culminating in an evaluation of the number of persons who are ultimately affected and the severity of their effects.

Hazard Identification

The first of the above steps, hazard identification, consists of identifying potentially harmful agents to which persons may be exposed, regardless of the level of exposure. For this purpose, reliance has traditionally been placed primarily on clinical and epidemiological evidence. For most environmental agents of interest, however, toxicity to humans cannot be evaluated adequately from the limited data that are available.[2,3] Instead, the evaluation must depend on toxicological approaches, including systematic analysis of pertinent molecular structure-activity relationships, results of in vitro short-term tests, and biological activity in short-term or long-term whole-animal bioassays. Principles and procedures for utilizing such methods in predicting toxicity to humans have been developed, and will be discussed further in subsequent sections of this chapter, but the diversity of toxic reactions caused by different agents is so large, and the variations in reactivity among different species so great, that the reliability of this approach is limited.[3] For most of the chemicals in commercial production, moreover, the available toxicological data do not suffice to enable adequate evaluation (Fig. 13–2).

Dose–Response Analysis

In the second step, dose–response analysis, the mathematical relationship between the dose of the agent of interest and any health effects that it may cause, is evaluated in order to estimate the nature and magnitude of risks attributable to the agent at the levels of exposure encountered in practice. Since ambient exposure levels are typically many times lower than the levels at which any toxic effects may have been documented previously, formulation of the desired risk estimate often requires extrapolation over a broad range of doses and/or animal species, necessitating the use of a dose–response model that may be of uncertain validity.

Although thresholds are known to exist for many, if not most, types of toxic reactions, no threshold is known or presumed to exist for the mutagenic and carcinogenic effects of certain toxicants. For such agents, therefore, an appropriate dose–response model must be employed for estimating the magnitude of any risks they may pose to exposed populations, selection of which is fraught with uncer-

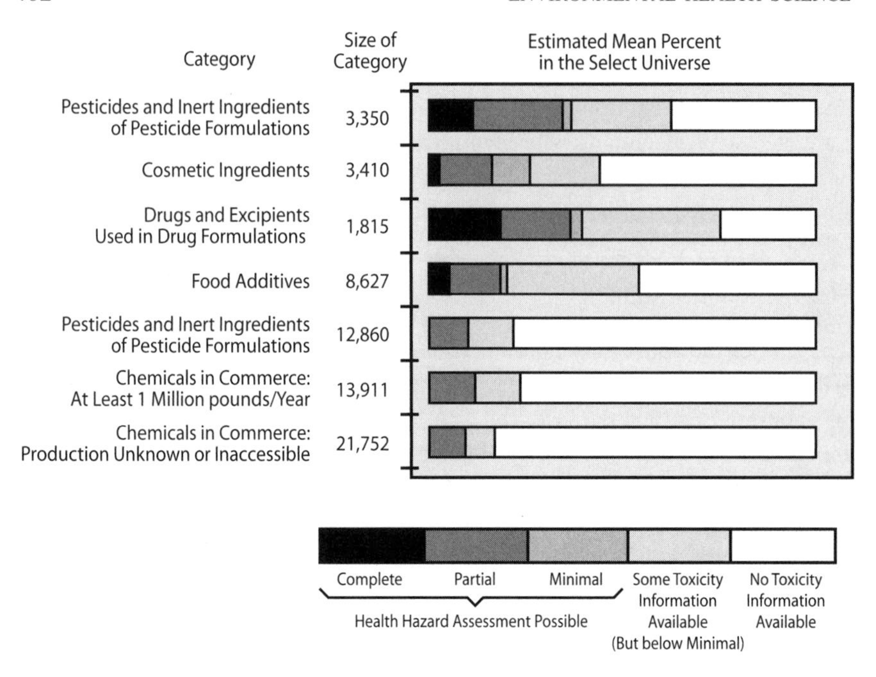

FIGURE 13–2. For most chemicals in commercial productions, toxicological date is not sufficiently available for adequate evaluation.

tainty. Again, the problem is complicated by a paucity of relevant dose–response data. Even in the relatively few instances where human data are available to provide anchor points from which to extrapolate, the data do not suffice to define the dose–response relationship in the low-dose domain. In the use of dose–response data from laboratory animals, moreover, there is uncertainty both about the choice of the model for extrapolation to low doses and of the model for extrapolation to humans.[4] Extrapolation options are depicted in Figure 13–3.

Another major source of uncertainty stems from the fact that, in the human environment, agents are usually, if not always, encountered in combination with many other agents, rather than in the pure form in which they have been evaluated in most clinical or toxicological studies. Because synergistic or other complex interactions among agents may occur under such conditions, the combined effects of mixtures of agents can seldom be confidently predicted from what is known about the toxicological effects of any given agent acting alone.[5,6]

Exposure Assessment

The third step, exposure assessment, consists of evaluating the extent to which persons are, or are likely to be, exposed to a particular environmental agent or combination of agents. For the most part, assessments of exposure have relied

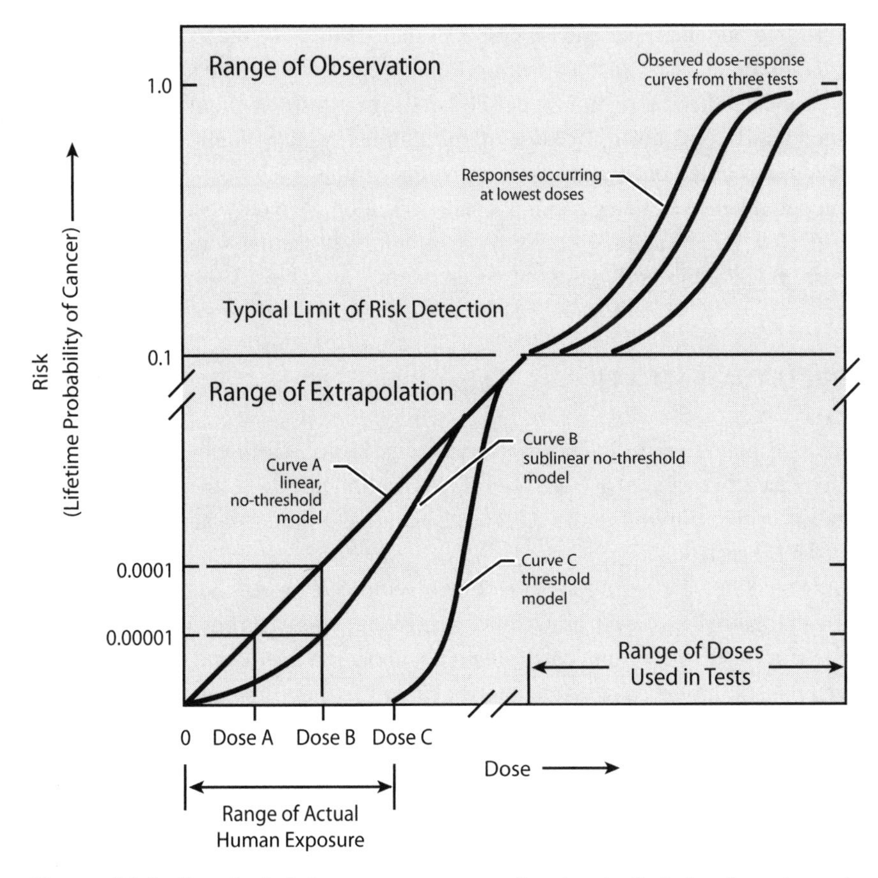

FIGURE 13–3. Hypothetical dose–response curves for chemically-induced carcinogenicity, showing measured dose–response curves from three studies (*top right quadrant*) and some possible ways those curves might behave in the low dose–low risk region (*lower left quadrant*, in The Range of Extrapolation). Note: Not to scale, *lower left quadrant* greatly expanded to illustrate extrapolation options.

thus far largely on data from unvalidated exposure models or from the monitoring of some relevant exposure media (air, water, soil, food, etc.). Monitoring of human beings themselves has been limited, in part because of the lack of suitably sensitive, reliable, and practicable methods and measures of exposure. Recent advances in analytical techniques, however, and in the development of biomolecular markers, such as DNA adducts, give promise of future improvements in this area.

Risk Characterization

In the fourth step, risk characterization, the information generated in the first three steps is integrated to derive an estimate of the numbers of persons who may be affected and the types and severities of their effects. To the extent that the information obtained in each of the preceding steps is constrained by uncertainty, the final characterization of risk derived in the fourth step will, of course, be correspondingly constrained. Because of the complexity, data requirements, and cost of each step in the process, as well as the uncertainties inherent therein, detailed and comprehensive attempts at risk characterization have only been made for relatively few environmental problems. Examples illustrating some of the uncertainties involved in such assessments are shown in Table 13–4.

RISK COMMUNICATION

People respond to risks as they perceive them. Hence, since experts trained and experienced in evaluating risks often fail to communicate their assessments adequately to the public, efforts to protect health and the environment are sometimes misdirected.[7]

As noted above, perceptions of risk involve nontechnical condiderations ("cultural rationality") as well as technical considerations ("technical rationality"). Hence, in order to communicate effectively about the nature and magnitude of a given risk, both types of considerations (Table 13–5) must be taken into account. Because the nontechnical considerations are rooted in cultural, anthropological, and ethical traditions, they vary among different groups in society. For communicating a given risk to all audiences, therefore, no single message is likely to be adequate.

Furthermore, for optimal effectiveness in risk communication, the process should involve a two-way, iterative exchange of information between the technical risk assessor and any stakeholders who may be directly or indirectly affected. Ideally, moreover, such an exchange should begin as early as possible in the process of risk assessment, so that those who may bear the risks can participate fully in the derivation of the assessment itself. Trust between all who are involved is also critical to the success of risk communication, and it is best fostered through the mutual exchange of information in an open, participatory, consensual process.

In contrast to other risks in daily life (such as various types of accidents, the frequencies of which are well documented in recorded statistics), many environmental risks to health are not known precisely and can be estimated only on the basis of unproven assumptions and extrapolations. As noted above, such assessments are complicated at virtually every step by large uncertainties in: *(1)* the numerical values of measurements or other quantities affecting the risks; *(2)* the modeling of exposure and/or toxic responses; *(3)* temporal, spatial, and inter-individual differences in exposure and/or susceptibility; and *(4)* the comparison of societal and personal measures of risk. To the extent that these sources

TABLE 13–4. Major Sources of Uncertainty in Risk Assessment

HAZARD IDENTIFICATION	DOSE–RESPONSE ASSESSMENT	EXPOSURE ASSESSMENT	RISK CHARACTERIZATION
Different study types: Prospective, case-control, bioassay, *in vivo* screen, *in vitro* screen Test species, strain, sex, system Exposure route, duration	Model selection for low-dose risk extrapolation Low-dose functional behavior of dose–response relationship (threshold, sublinear, supralinear, flexible) Role of time (dose frequency, rate, duration, age at exposure, fraction of lifetime exposed) Pharmacokinetic model of effective dose as a function of applied dose Impact of competing risks	Contamination scenario characterization (production, distribution, domestic and industrial storage and use, disposal, environmental transport, transformation and decay, geographic bounds, temporal bounds) Environmental fate model selection (structural error) Parameter estimation error Field measurement error	Component uncertainties Hazard identification Dose–response assessment Exposure assessment
Definition of incidence of an outcome in a given study (positive–negative association of incidence with exposure)	Definition of "positive responses" in a given study Independent vs. joint events Continuous vs. dichotomous input response data	Exposure scenario characterization Exposure route identification (dermal, respiratory, dietary) Exposure dynamics model (absorption, intake processes)	
Different study results Different study qualities Conduct Definition of control populations Physical–chemical similarity of chemical studied to that of concern	Parameter estimation Different dose–response sets Results Qualities Types	Integrated exposure profile Target population identification Potentially exposed populations Population stability over time	
Unidentified hazards	Extrapolation of tested doses to human doses		
Extrapolation of available evidence to target human population			

TABLE 13–5. Comparison of Factors Relevant to the Cultural Rationality, as Opposed to the Technical Rationality, of Risk

TECHNICAL RATIONALITY	CULTURAL RATIONALITY
Trust in scientific methods, explanations, democratic process	Trust in political culture and evidence
Appeal to authority and expertise	Appeal to folk wisdom, peer groups, and traditions
Boundaries of analysis are narrow and	Boundaries of analysis are broad and include the use of analogy and historical precedent
Risks are depersonalized	Risks are personalized
Emphasis on statistical variation and probability	Emphasis on the impacts of risk on the family and community
Appeal to consistency and universality	Focus on particularity; less concerned about consistency of approach
Where there is controversy in science, resolution follows expertise, status	Popular responses to science; the differences do not follow the prestige principle
Those impacts that cannot be measured are less relevant	Unanticipated or unarticulated risks are relevant

of uncertainty limit the reliability of a risk assessment, each must be made explicit if the comprehensibility, credibility, and utility of the assessment are not to be jeopardized.

Because, as noted, the perception of risk is a complex process, risk is difficult to communicate in a way that places it in proper perspective. Comparisons of quantitative risk estimates, such as have often been presented for the purpose (e.g., Tables 13–6 and 13–7), or attempts to weight risks solely on the basis of their impacts on life expectancy, on the quality of life as in Figure 13–4, or on their economic costs, are likely to be inadequate by themselves.[8] Instead, the strategy for risk communication must take into account the known dynamics of risk perception, which involve the following principles: *(1)* unfamiliar risks tend to be less acceptable than familiar risks; *(2)* involuntary risks are less acceptable than voluntary risks; *(3)* risks controlled by others are less acceptable than risks that are under one's own control; *(4)* inapparent and undetectable risks are less acceptable than risks that are apparent and detectable; *(5)* risks that are perceived to be unfair are less acceptable than risks that are perceived to be fair; *(6)* risks that do not permit individual protective action are less acceptable than risks that do; *(7)* dramatic and dreadful risks are less acceptable than undramatic and commonplace risks; *(8)* unpredictable risks are less acceptable than predictable risks; *(9)* cross-

TABLE 13–6. Situations or Activities Involving a One-in-a-Million Risk of Death

EXPOSURE OR ACTIVITY	CAUSE OF DEATH
Smoking 1.4 cigarettes	Cancer, heart disease
Drinking 1/2 L of wine	Cirrhosis of the liver
Spending 1 hour in a coal mine	Black lung disease
Spending 3 hours in a coal mine	Accident
Living 2 days in New York or Boston	Air pollution
Traveling 6 min by canoe	Accident
Traveling 10 miles by bicycle	Accident
Traveling 300 miles by car	Accident
Flying 1000 miles by jet	Accident
Flying 6000 miles by jet	Cancer caused by cosmic radiation
Living 2 months in Denver	Cancer caused by cosmic radiation
Living 2 months in an average masonry building	Cancer caused by natural radioactivity
One chest X-ray	Cancer caused by radiation
Living 2 months with a cigarette smoker	Cancer, heart disease
Eating 40 tablespoons of peanut butter	Liver cancer caused by aflatoxin B_1
Drinking Miami, Florida drinking water for 1 yr	Cancer caused by chloroform
Drinking 30 12-oz. cans of diet soda	Cancer caused by saccharin
Living 5 years at the boundary of a nuclear plant	Cancer caused by radiation
Eating 100 charcoal-broiled steaks	Cancer caused by benzopyrene

(*Source*: Wilson, R. Analyzing the risks of daily life. *Technol. Rev*. 81:41–46, 1979.)

hazard comparisons tend to be unacceptable; and *(10)* risk estimation is inherently of less interest to people than risk reduction, and neither is likely to be of interest in the absence of real concern about the risk, or risks, in question.

HAZARD IDENTIFICATION AND DOSE–RESPONSE ASSESSMENT

Historically, many hazards were identified and quantitated in observational studies in human populations, especially in groups of workers having similar high levels of exposure. With sufficient characterization and quantitation of their exposures and sufficient data on the frequency of health related responses as a function of exposure level, it was possible to identify and, based on professional judgement of what effects or degrees of responses were deemed to be adverse health responses, one could establish a no observable adverse effect level (NOAEL), or a lowest observable adverse effect level (LOAEL). There is, presumably, a threshold level for adverse response somewhere between the two. Threshold levels of exposures that were selected generally included some safety

Table 13–7. Ranking the Risks from Possible Carcinogens on the Basis of Their Estimated Potencies

HAZARD INDEX: HERP (%)[a]	DAILY HUMAN EXPOSURE	CARCINOGEN DOSE PER 70-kg PERSON
	ENVIRONMENTAL POLLUTION	
0.001	Tap water, 1 L	Chloroform, 83 μg (US Avg)
0.004	Well water, 1 L contaminated (worst well in Silicon Valley)	Trichloroethylene, 280 μg
0.0004	Well water, 1 L contaminated, Woburn	Trichloroethylene, 267 μg
		Chloroform, 12 μg
		Tetrachloroethylene, 21 μg
0.0002		
0.0003		
0.008	Swimming pool, 1 hr (for child)	Chloroform, 250 μg (Avg. pool)
0.6	Conventional home air (14 hr/day)	Formaldehyde, 2.2 mg
		Benzene, 155 μg
0.004		
2.1	Mobile home air (14 hr/day)	Formaldehyde, 2.2 mg
	PESTICIDE AND OTHER RESIDUES	
0.0002	PCBs: daily dietary intake	PCBs, 0.2 μg (U.S. Avg.)
0.0003	DDE/DT: daily dietary intake	DDE, 2.2 μg (U.S. Avg.)
0.0004	EDB: daily dietary intake (from grains and grain products)	Ethylene dibromide, 0.42 μg (U.S. Avg.)
	NATURAL PESTICIDES AND DIETARY TOXINS	
0.003	Bacon, cooked (100 g)	Dimethylnitrosamine, 0.3 μg
0.006		Diethylnitrosamine, 0.1 μg
0.003	Sake (250 ml)	Urethane, 43 μg
0.03	Comfrey herb tea, 1 cup	Symphytine, 38 μg (750 μg of pyrrolizidine alkaloids)
0.03	Peanut butter (32 g; one sandwich)	Aflatoxin, 64 ng (U.S. Avg., 2ppb)
0.06	Dried squid, broiled in gas oven (54 g)	Dimethylnitrosamine, 7.9 μg
0.07	Brown mustard (5 g)	Allyl isothiocyanate, 4.6 mg
0.1	Basil (1 g of dried leaf)	Estragole, 3.8 mg
2.8	Beer (12 oz, 354 ml)	Ethyl alcohol, 18 ml
4.7	Wine (250 ml)	Ethyl alcohol, 30 ml

(*continued*)

TABLE 13–7. *(continued)*

HAZARD INDEX: HERP (%)[A]	DAILY HUMAN EXPOSURE	CARCINOGEN DOSE PER 70-kg PERSON
	FOOD ADDITIVES	
0.06	Diet cola	Saccharin, 95 mg
	DRUGS	
[0.3]	Phenacetin pill (Average dose)	Phenacetin, 300 mg
16	Phenobarbital, one sleeping pill	Phenobarbital, 60 mg
17	Clofibrate (Average daily dose)	Clofibrate, 2000 mg
	OCCUPATIONAL EXPOSURE	
5.8	Formaldehyde: Average daily intake	Formaldehyde, 6.1 mg
140	EDB: Average daily intake (high exposure)	Ethylene dibromide, 150 mg

[a]Possible hazard: the amount of rodent carcinogen indicated under carcinogen dose is divided by 70 kg to give milligram per kilogram equivalent of human exposure, and this human dose is given as the percentage of TD_{50} in the rodent (in milligrams per kilogram) to calculate the human-exposure/rodent potency index (HERP).

(*Source*: Ames B.N., Magaw, R., and Bold, L.S. Ranking possible carcinogenic hazards. *Science* 236:271–280, 1987.)

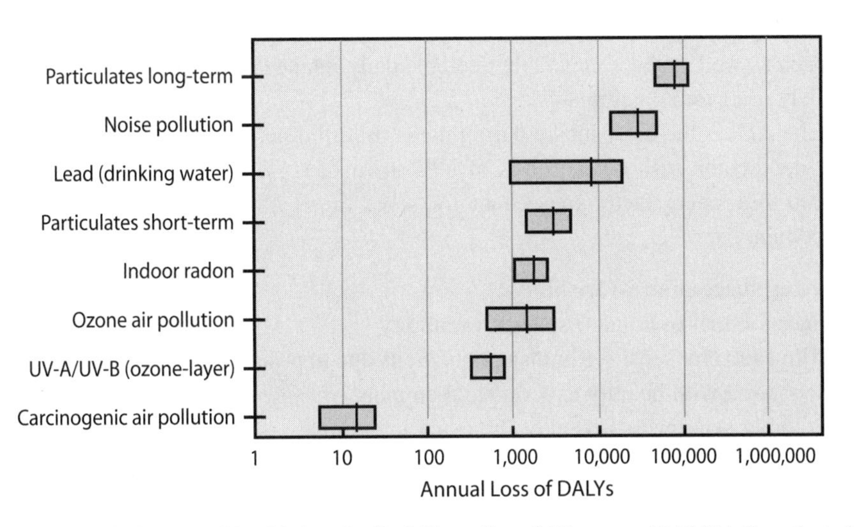

FIGURE 13–4. Annual health loss in disability-adjusted life years (DALYs) for selected environmental exposures in the Netherlands.

factor (margin of safety) in recognition of uncertainties in the data and the likelihood that other populations would be likely to include individuals with greater susceptibility to adverse responses than the population(s) initially studied.

Toxicological Approach

As numerous new chemicals entered commerce during and after World War II, it was recognized that their potential for producing adverse health effects in production workers or in the users and consumers of products containing these chemicals needed to be evaluated prospectively, using laboratory animals as surrogates for humans. The basic nature of toxicity testing in laboratory animals was reviewed in Chapter 6. This chapter covers the approaches that have developed in recent decades for extrapolating the results of toxicity testing in laboratory animals to human health risk assessment.

The formal use of safety factors began in the U.S. in the mid-1950s for food additives in the FDA. It was based on the concept that a safe level of food additives or contaminants could be derived from a chronic NOAEL (in mg/kg of diet) from animal studies divided by a 100-fold safety factor. This approach was also adopted by the Joint Food and Agriculture Organization and World Health Organization (FAO/WHO) Expert Committee on Food Additives (JECFA) and the Joint Meeting of Experts on Pesticides Residues (JMEPR) of the WHO/FAO in 1961. The safe level that was adopted was called the acceptable daily intake (ADI), expressed in mg/kg body weight per day. The procedure involved collecting all relevant data, ascertaining the completeness of the available dataset, determining the NOAEL using the most sensitive indicator of toxicity, and applying an appropriate safety factor to derive the ADI for humans. The ADI approach as well as the comparable tolerable daily intake (TDI) approach, are now widely used for contaminants.

The ADI is the daily intake during the entire lifetime that appears to be without appreciable risk on the basis of all known facts. It has generally included a 100-fold safety factor to account for some or all of the following areas of uncertainty:

- Intrasubject human variability
- Inter (animal to human)-species variability
- Allowance for sensitive human populations due to prior or current illness when compared with healthy experimental animals
- Possible synergistic action of the many intentional and unintentional food additives or contaminants
- Differences in body size of the laboratory animals vs. humans
- Differences in diet varying with age, sex, activity level, and environmental conditions

- Differences in water exchange between the body and its environment among species
- The fact that the number of animals tested is small compared with the size of the human population that may be exposed
- The difficulty in estimating the human ingestion intake, and its variability

The purpose of the safety factor is to allow for uncertainties in knowledge based on toxic responses of a small number of rather homogeneous laboratory animals in establishing safe doses for a heterogeneous human population, and it should be reconsidered periodically. When setting an ADI, various test data and judgmental factors should be considered and are needed to be taken into account, for example, nature of the effects, adequacy of data base, age-related effects, metabolic and pharmacokinetic data, and available human data.

The FDA has recommended an additional factor of 10 when estimating an ADI from short-term toxicity data, and the Food Quality Protection Act of 1996 mandates that an additional safety factor of 10 be considered for exposures of children.

The Reference Dose Concept

In 1988, the U.S. EPA formally adopted, subject to a number of modifications, the ADI approach in its regulatory measures for reducing environmental pollution. Instead of the terms ADI and safety factor (SF), the terms reference dose (RfD) and uncertainty factor (UF) respectively, have been used for noncancer endpoints. The RfD is derived from the NOAEL by the consistent application of generally one order-of-magnitude UFs that reflect the various types of data sets used to estimate RfDs. UFs generally consist of:

- A 10-fold factor to account for human variation in sensitivity
- A 10-fold factor to account for uncertainties in interspecies extrapolation
- A 10-fold factor to adjust for the use of the NOAEL obtained from a subchronic animal study rather than a chronic study
- A 10-fold factor to adjust for the use of the LOAEL in the absence of the NOAEL
- A 10-fold factor that considers the adequacy of the total database

In addition, a modifying factor (MF) ranging from less than 1 to up to 10 is applied when the database includes, for example, a very small number of animals per dose level.

Calabrese and Gilbert[9] suggested modifications of UFs because of the lack of independence of these factors. The interspecies UF is generally recognized as providing an extrapolation from the average animal to an average individual assuming that humans may be 10-fold more sensitive. The intraspecies UF assumes that most human responses fall within approximately a 10-fold range. Calabrese and Gilbert proposed that the use of a 10-fold intraspecies UF should begin with the average human and extend to cover the higher-risk segments of the population. Consequently, a UF of 5 would be expected to protect most humans. However, an UF 10 should be used when the limit is based on an occupational epidemiological study, because this type of study does not consider the most sensitive humans.

The factor used when a semichronic study is used includes an age-dependent factor that is comparable in some respects to the age-dependent factor in the intraspecies uncertainty factor. The age component in the intraspecies uncertainty factor concerns the age differential response over the entire lifetime span, whereas the age differential of the less-than-lifetime uncertainty factor concerns only the age-related differences that the end of the study to the end of the normal life span. High susceptibility is not exclusive for young animals. In certain circumstances, susceptibility may be greater in adulthood than in the young and may further increase in elderly animals. Assuming that age differences account for 50% of the intraspecies variation, they stated that this factor could be reasonably apportioned as 60% for prior to weaning and 40% for after weaning. If a 24-month rodent exposure accounts for 40% of age effects, then it would be reasonable to reduce the age component of the intraspecies variation by the proportion described to age. If the intraspecies factor is 5 as recommended, then this reduces the factor to 4. Table 13–8 provides the uncertainty factors recommended by Calabrese and Gilbert in light of the above considerations.

The Benchmark Dose Concept

The NOAEL is defined as the highest dose level at which no statistically significant effects occur (for all endpoints that are considered toxicologically relevant).

TABLE 13–8. Recommended Modifications in Current Uncertainty Factors on the Concept of Independence and Interdependence of Uncertainty Factors

EXTRAPOLATION STEP	UNCERTAINTY FACTOR
Animal to human	10
Interindividual	
Less-than-lifetime animal study	5
Animal study with normal experimental lifetime	4
Occupational epidemiological study	10
Environmental epidemiological study (normal lifespan)	5
Use of LOAEL instead of NOAEL	10
Less-than-lifetime	10

LOAEL, lowest observable adverse effect level; NOAEL, no observable adverse effect level.

[*Source*: Calabrese, E.J. and Gilbert, C.E. Lack of total independence of uncertainty factors (UFs): Implications for the size of the total uncertainty factor. *Regulat. Toxicol. Pharmacol.* 17:44–51, 1993.]

It is important to keep in mind that the NOAEL is not the same as the $NAEL_{true}$ and that, although the NOAEL could be considered an estimate of the true threshold dose, the quality (precision) of the estimate cannot be assessed.

Objections against the use of the NOAEL have been raised. In general, there is a need for consideration of the dose-response relationship as a whole. One of the alternatives proposed has been the benchmark approach.

The benchmark approach to a regression function fitted to response data can be used to estimate the dose at which adverse effects can be detected.[10] Using regression models for describing the dose-effect relation has two advantages. First, an HMF to account for the steepness of a dose–effect curve is redundant, and second there is no need to extrapolate a LOAEL to a NOAEL. The latter may be considered as a major advantage because there is no scientific justification for the use of an assessment factor for LOAEL–NOAEL extrapolation.

In the benchmark concept, one needs to postulate a critical effect size (CES). The CES for a critical endpoint is defined as the value of effect-size below which there is no reason for concern, and the associated critical effect dose (CED) is defined as the dose at which the average animal shows the (postulated) critical effect–size defined for a particular endpoint.

A drawback of using dose–effect curves for the evaluation of toxicity is that current toxicological and biological knowledge does not provide a sufficient basis to unequivocally establish the break point between nonadverse and adverse effect size for most health-effect endpoints. Because a single universal CES does not seem a realistic option, a value must be chosen for each separate endpoint. A widespread implementation and acceptance of the value of CES for each of the (most relevant) endpoints would require a broad concensus.

The CED is a true, unknown value, which can only be estimated, to some definable degree of precision, when suitable data for the endpoint of concern are available. The true no-adverse-effect-level ($NAEL_{true}$) may then be defined as the lowest CED of all endpoints, i.e., $NAEL_{true} \equiv$ minimum of all CEDs.

The definition of the NAEL refers not only to an unknown, but also to a rather theoretical value, because it is unknown to what endpoint it is associated. In practice, one can never be sure whether information on all relevant endpoints for the compound studied is present. Furthermore, the lowest CED in two situations (e.g., animal vs. human) may not refer to the same endpoints. For example, rats may be most sensitive to endpoint A, but humans to endpoint B. A drawback to the use of dose–response modeling from a practical point of view is that most toxicity data are not suitable for curve-fitting procedures. A typical study design as agreed on in, for example, OECD toxicity testing guidelines, considers three dose groups and a control. Ideally, more dose groups should be used with each dose group comprising less animals.

When data are available for a particular endpoint that allow for fitting a regression function, the CED may be estimated. Depending on the quality of the data, this estimate has a certain degree of imprecision. The complete uncertainty distribution can be estimated by bootstrapping; once a regression model has been fitted, Monte Carlo sampling is used to generate a large number of new data sets from this regression model, each time with the same number of data points per dose group as observed animals in the real experiment. For each generated data set the CED is reestimated. Taking all these CEDs together results in the required distribution.

Human Limit Values

Because there will be a certain distribution over all endpoints and substances for each effect, it is possible to extrapolate any CED from one situation to another. Thus, instead of choosing a single (most sensitive) endpoint from the animal data, each CED distribution that is associated to a relevant endpoint can be extrapolated to the distribution of the associated CED in the sensitive human ($CED_{sens.human}$) by probabilistic combination with the distributions of each effect. This results in a series of distributions for $CED_{sens.human}$, each related to another endpoint. Then this complete set of distributions can be considered as a basis for deriving a human limit value (HLV), for example, by choosing the lowest of each distribution's critical percentile. It has been assumed that there is a complete independence of the various distributions of effects, but this worst-case assumption may not have been valid.[9] When correlations can be demonstrated and quantified, the method allows for these by introducing correlation coefficients.

The approach, as discussed above, differs from the benchmark approach in various ways. Crump[11] introduced the benchmark dose level (BMDL), defined as the lower 95% confidence limit of the CED, as a starting point for extrapolation to the (sensitive) human. By dividing the BMDL by assessment factors for interspecies and intraspecies variation (default values of ten), an HLV can be derived. Instead of this, Vermeire et al.[10] proposed to use the entire distribution of the CED instead of the lower 95% confidence limit of the CED. Secondly, they proposed to combine this CED distribution with distributions of extrapolation factors in a probabilistic way. The result of the probabilistic combination of distributions is in the form of an assessment distribution, so that the degree of conservatism is quantifiable in any particular assessment. Their approach allows for deriving a HLV as a function of an a priori chosen degree of conservatism. In addition, it allows for estimating the lower and upper bounds for possible health effects in the sensitive population at a given exposure level.

USE OF EPIDEMIOLOGIC DATA IN RISK ASSESSMENT

Epidemiologic data may play a prominent role in hazard identification and dose–response assessment, and may also be used in exposure assessment and risk characterization. Hazard identification is inherently integrative, drawing on all relevant lines of evidence, as do the criteria for causality that are widely applied for interpeting epidemiologic findings. In fact, there are no guidelines for interpretation of epidemiologic data in risk assessments that go beyond the conventionally applied criteria for causality. Because epidemiologic data come from humans, they are usually given strong weighting if they are positive in indicating an adverse effect. On the other hand, in commenting on toxic air pollutants, the NRC report, Science and Judgement in Risk Assessment,[3] gave preference to toxicologic data collection over epidemiologic data collection, citing the cost of epidemiologic research and the ambiguity of findings of some observational studies. However, there are numerous examples of evidence from epidemiologic research that provide definitive identification of hazards, including such well-known causal associations as radon and lung cancer, asbestos and mesothelioma of the lung, vinyl chloride and angiosarcoma of the liver, and active and passive cigarette smoking and lung cancer.

Once a hazard is identified, the second component—the dose–response assessment—is initiated to establish the quantitative relationship between dose or exposure and response. While the dose–response relationship is of prime interest in risk assessment, epidemiologic studies more typically address the exposure–response relationship. Exposure refers to contact with material, while dose is the material actually entering the body. An exposure measure may be considered as a surrogate for dose or may be used to estimate dose. For the purpose of risk assessment, characterization of the exposure–response relationship in the range of relevant human exposures is needed. For some agents, such as environmental tobacco smoke, data on risks are available in the exposure range of interest; for many others, data for estimating dose–response relationships often come from studies of workers and may only be available for levels of dose or exposure above usual environmental levels. For such exposures, exposure–response relationships estimated at the higher exposures are extended downward along an assumed model for the relationship between exposure and dose. When biologic understanding of the mechanism of action is sufficiently certain, a biologic model of the relationship between exposure or dose and response may be assumed for analysis of either toxicologic or epidemiologic data. for example, in developing risk models for radon and lung cancer, the Biological Effects of Ionizing Radiation (BEIR) VI Committee assumed a linear no-threshold relationship based on biologic considerations.[12] Alternatively, the epidemiologic data may be used in analyses to determine the best-fitting relationship between exposure or dose and response.

For the purpose of risk assessment, epidemiologic data may be used to quantify the dose–response relationship or to guide the selection from among alternative models for the relationship between dose and response. The ability to estimate precisely the quantitative relationship between dose and response may be limited by the extent of the data available and by exposure or dose misclassification. Exposure and dose are often estimated from incomplete information or with the use of surrogates, and comprehensive data in all biologically relevant time windows may not be available. Consequently, misclassification of exposure may bias the description of the exposure–response relationship and confidence intervals may be wide, perhaps with substantially different policy implications from the risks at the lower and upper bounds.

In analyzing epidemiologic data on the dose–response relationship, researchers typically have *a priori* interest in determining if a dose–response relationship can be shown to be statistically significant and in characterizing the shape of the relationship. Initially, the shape of the dose–response relationship may be explored descriptively, but inevitably statistical models are used to quantify the change in response with increasing exposure. There has been a general reliance on linear models without a threshold, particularly for carcinogens. For some agents, for example, alpha radiation, a relatively strong basis exists for assuming a linear model, whereas for other agents, the selection of a linear no-threshold relationship reflects a policy default that is viewed as "conservative" in protecting public health because of the model assumption that any level of exposure conveys some risk.

Epidemiologic data may also be fit with alternative models of the dose–response relationship if there is uncertainty about the most appropriate shape of this relationship (see Fig. 13–3). Model fit may be used to guide the identification of the "best" model. However, epidemiologic data are rarely sufficiently abundant to provide powerful discrimination among alternative models, and sample size requirements for comparing fits of alternative models having different public health implications may be very high. For policy-making purposes, the shape of the dose–reponse relationship at the lower exposure levels experienced by the population is critical, but epidemiologic data are often very limited or lacking at these levels.

For the purpose of risk assessment, information is needed on full distribution of exposures in the population. Measures of central tendency may be appropriate for estimating overall risk to the population, but use of central measures alone may hide the existence of more highly and unacceptably exposed individuals. Thus, the upper end of the exposure distribution may also be of interest, as set out in the EPA's Guidelines for Exposure Assessment.[13] Driven largely by the needs of risk assessment, exposure assessment has matured and become a field largely separate from epidemiology. Modern exposure assessment is based on a conceptual framework that relates pollutant sources to effects through multimedia paths of exposure, which ultimately determine the dose. The concept of total personal exposure is central; that is, for health risk assessment, exposures received by individuals from all sources and media need to be considered. To date, epidemiologic data have not played prominent roles in exposure assessments for risk assessments. However, epidemiologic data may contribute and also serve to validate exposure models.

USES OF HEALTH RISK ASSESSMENTS

The use of risk assessment has become central in many activities of state and federal regulatory agencies and of the private sector since the publication of the Red Book.[1] Risk assessment is used by regulatory agencies to: *(1)* set priorities for the regulatory agenda; *(2)* develop regulatory exposure limits, emission standards, or cleanup standards; and *(3)* set priorities for research. In the non-regulatory setting, the information generated by risk assessment is used by a wide variety of groups including industry, labor unions, and consumers.

Federal agencies that use risk assessment prominently are the EPA, the OSHA, and the Consumer Product Safety Commission (CPSC). Statutes requiring the assessment of health risks include the Clean Air Act, the Federal Insecticide, Fungicide, and Rodenticide Act, the Toxic Substances Control Act, the Occupational Safety and Health Act, the Federal Food, Drug, and Cosmetic Act, the Safe Drinking Water Act, and the Comprehensive Environmental Response, Compensation and Liability Act (Superfund).

Within the agencies, the use of risk assessment may be dictated by statute and may vary even by sections within a statute. For example, Section 108 of the Clean Air Act requires the EPA to establish and periodically review NAAQS for pollutants labeled "criteria" pollutants (ozone, carbon monoxide, nitrogen dioxide, particulate matter, lead, and sulfur dioxide) through the preparation of a comprehensive criteria document. The standard is required to protect the public health with an adequate margin of safety, without regard to cost. By contrast, Section 112 of the Clean Air Act as applied to point-source pollutants, is technology-driven in its first phase, requiring Maximum Available Control Technology (MACT) for 189 substances without regard to health risk. Approximately 8–9 years after the application of control technology, EPA must then determine whether more stringent standards are required to protect public health "with an ample margin of safety." This risk-driven phase requires that EPA establish such standards for carcinogens that present an excess cancer risk greater than one-in-a-million, even with MACT controls installed. In a third example of the use of risk assessment within the Clean Air Act, the EPA Administrator is required to identify not fewer than 30 of the 189 toxic substances that present the greatest threat to public health in the largest number of urban areas. The Administrator is then required to schedule actions that substantially reduce the public health risks from hazardous air pollutants, and by these actions to achieve a reduction in the incidence of cancer attributable to exposure to hazardous air pollutants emitted by stationary sources by at least 75%. Other statutes are similarly specific in the use of risk assessment.

Since the publication of the NRC's Science and Judgement in Risk Assessment,[3] recognition has grown of the need to use risk assessment in framing research questions—and thereby improve the relevance of research findings for risk assessment—for example, What is the risk to children? Are there sensitive subpopulations? What are the major pathways of exposure? The risk assessment paradigm developed by the NRC in 1983 was instrumental in the 1995 reorganization of the Office of Research and Development at EPA into national laboratories on effects, exposure, and risk management, and into national centers on risk assessment and exploratory research and quality assurance. This organizational structure is intended to provide a logical, appropriate framework for conceptualizing and conducting research to best address uncertainties in risk assessment.

In addition to federal and state agencies, private industry uses risk assessment techniques. For example, some companies use risk assessment principles to set occupational exposure limits for substances that may not be covered by regulations. The ACGIH[14] recommends TLVs, which, while non-binding, also serve as guidelines for safe occupational exposures. These TLVs usually assume a dose–response relationship with a threshold separating safe and unsafe exposures. Short-term tolerable exposure limits (usually based on acute effects) have also been developed for emergency responses. Frequently, these exposure guidelines/limits are based on results of occupational epidemiology studies. Risk assessment techniques are also applied increasingly to the environmental arena, where the effects of effluent exposure on non-human receptors (e.g., fish, wildlife, and flora) are of concern.

INFLUENCE OF JUDICIAL REVIEWS ON REGULATORY RISK ASSESSMENTS

The adoption of new regulatory mandates by a federal agency in the U.S. often leads to challenges in the courts by affected or interested parties. Some of the most notable examples, listed below, affected not only the particular regulatory action at issue, but also the ways and rates of future decisions on related issues.

1980—Benzene Decision

In a case involving the OSHA exposure standard for benzene, the Supreme Court held that OSHA must provide an estimate of the actual risk associated with a toxic substance. Although only OSHA was involved in this case, the decision provided a de facto mandate for quantitative risk assessment at all regulatory agencies. The Court recognized that OSHA may use assumptions (i.e., science policy) in risk assessment, but only to the extent that those assumptions have some basis in reputable scientific evidence.

1987—Vinyl Chloride Decision

In this litigation involving EPA's air emissions standard for vinyl chloride, the U.S. Supreme Court interpreted the Clean Air Act (CAA) to require EPA to first determine a "safe" level of exposure for air pollutants before considering economic or technological feasibility of achieving reduced emissions. The rule was remanded to EPA and, in the subsequent, rulemaking, EPA decided to emphasize quantitative risk assessment in the establishment of CAA standards.

1992—OSHA Air Contaminants Decision

In this case, the U.S. Supreme Court struck down PELs for 428 toxic substances on the basis that assumptions used by OSHA in the risk assessments supporting the PELs were not substantiated by the available scientific evidence. This case reiterates the lesson of the Benzene decision that, although science policy is clearly permissible in risk assessment, science policy decisions must have some basis in fact. Through this rulemaking, OSHA was attempting to update standards that had been set more than twenty years earlier. By requiring a better substantiated scientific basis for assumptions—a requirement which may not be practical or possible—this case may effectively block OSHA's ability to update many of the earlier standards, particularly *en masse*.

2001—Particulate Matter and Ozone Standards Decision

In this case, the Supreme Court dismissed a claim that the Congress' delegation of Authority to EPA to set ambient air quality standards was unconstitutional, and that EPA had made appropriate use of the available scientific information to establish a new standard for $PM_{2.5}$. However, it referred back to the EPA the question of whether a PM_{10} limit was a suitable air quality index for the control of exposures to the coarse fraction of thoracic particulate matter ($PM_{10-2.5}$).

INTERNATIONAL ASPECTS OF RISK ASSESSMENT

Formal risk assessment procedures are being used increasingly by international regulatory bodies. Some of these procedures use different methods for the dose–response step. For example, Maynard et al.[15] suggest a risk assessment procedure based on the use of NOAELs and "uncertainty factors" for carcinogens, along with subsequent risk management steps. Similarly, Hunter et al.[16] have described the European Union's process for setting occupational exposure limits, and mention the NOAEL/uncertainty factor approach for noncarcinogens, but do not recommend a prescriptive method for carcinogens. Other countries, such as the Netherlands and Canada, rely on a mathematical modeling approach in the dose–response step. While the exact procedures used in the dose–response step vary between countries and for different health outcomes, a common theme is the preference for basing risk assessments on high-quality epidemiologic data, if available. Despite this preference, relatively few risk assessments use epidemiologic data in the hazard-identification and dose–response steps.

REFERENCES

1. National Research Council. Risk Assessment in the Federal Government: Managing the Process, Washington, DC: National Academy Press, 1983.
2. National Research Council. Toxicity Testing: Strategies to Determine Needs and Priorities. Washington, DC: National Academy Press, 1984.
3. National Research Council. Science and Judgement in Risk Assessment. Washington, DC: National Academy Press, 1994.
4. Rodricks, J.V. Calculated Risks. Cambridge: Cambridge University Press, 1992.
5. National Research Council. Complex Mixtures: Method for In Vivo Toxicity Testing. Washington, DC: National Academy Press, 1988.
6. Mauderly, J.L. Toxicological approaches to complex mixtures. *Environ. Health Perspect. Suppl.* 101(4):155–164, 1993.
7. National Research Council. Understanding Risk. Informing Decisions in a Democratic Society. Washington, DC: National Academy Press, 1996.
8. National Research Council. Improving Risk Communication. Washington, DC: National Academy Press, 1989.
9. Calabrese, E.J. and Gilbert, C.E. Lack of total independence of uncertainty factors (UFs): Implications for the size of the total uncertainty factor. *Regulat. Toxicol. Pharmacol.* 17:44–51, 1993.
10. Vermeire, T., Stevenson, H., Pieters, M.N., Rennen, M., Slob, W., and Hakkert, B.C. Assessment factors for human health risk assessment: A discussion paper. *Crit. Rev. Toxicol.* 29(5):439–490, 1999.
11. Crump, K.S. A new method for determining allowable daily intakes. *Fundam. Appl. Toxicol.* 4:854–871, 1984.
12. National Research Council. Health effects of exposure to radon (BEIR VI). Committee on Health Risks of Exposure to Radon, et al. Washington, DC: National Academy Press, 1998.
13. U.S. Environmental Protection Agency. Guidelines for exposure assessment. Washington, DC: Office of Health and Environmental Assessment (Publication No. EPA/6002-92/001 FR57:2288–22938), 1997.
14. ACGIH. Threshold Limit Values for Chemical Substances and Physical Agents, and Biological Exposure Indices, Cincinnati American Conference of Governmental Industiral Hygienists, 1999.
15. Maynard, R.L., Cameron, K.M., Fielder, R., et al. Setting air quality standards for quantitative carcinogens: An alternative to mathematical qualitative risk assessment. *Hum. Toxicol.* 14:175–186, 1995.
16. Hunter, W.J., Aresini, G., Haigh, R., et al. Occupational exposure limits for chemicals in the European Union. *Occup. Environ. Med.* 54:217–222, 1997.

14

Risk Management

Risk management is a process by which responsible authorities take actions to reduce or eliminate risk factors. It is carried out at many different levels. Individuals make risk management decisions every day through their dietary choices, use of medications, personal habits and types and levels of exercise, use of personal and mass forms of transportation, crafts and hobbies, household maintenance, and, to some extent, in the ways that they perform their tasks at work or school. Their choices in each of these activities are likely to involve exposures to chemicals or physical agents that could affect their health. Individuals have only limited control over some aspects of factors that affect their exposures, dependent as they are on the contents of the foods, beverages, and consumer products that they buy and use, and on the concentrations of some of the pollutants in the air they breathe. However, through their attention to product labels and other forms of public health and consumer product information, they can make choices that can minimize their exposures.

Employers have more clearly defined obligations and legal requirements to minimize employee exposures to workplace stressors, both physical and chemical. Workplace health and safety standards, if followed, should ensure a low order of risk of harm to employees. Legally mandated effluent emission limits, if followed, should be protective of the public downwind or downstream of such effluents or of waste storage sites or repositories. Manufacturers are also responsible for the safety of the products they sell. Product liability lawsuits and the costs of worker's compensation claims awarded are further stimulants to industry to maintain safe workplaces and products. Unfortunately, not all industrial companies have been good, law-abiding public citizens, as documented by the continuing high toll of occupational disease and the huge public and corporate expenses being devoted to the clean up of abandoned waste repositories and contaminated work sites.

Governmental agencies are responsible for the effective enforcement of public statutes enacted to protect workers and the public from exposures to chemical and physical agents, for developing a knowledge base for identifying and evaluating risk management options, and for providing information to the public about the residual risks that remain from exposures that result from uncontrolled sources of toxicants. In the U.S., the EPA has, as its primary mission, the management of environmental risks. This task has multiple dimensions. For determination of the nature and extent of the risks, EPA's vision for risk management is depicted in Figure 14–1. It involves starting with risk assessment, and extends into technical means of control, regulatory options, and risk communication to concerned segments of the public. Other considerations arise in terms of resource allocation. A flow sheet for these aspects has been recommended to EPA by its Science Advisory Board (See Fig. 14–2). It indicates that follow-up and reassessment is periodically needed.

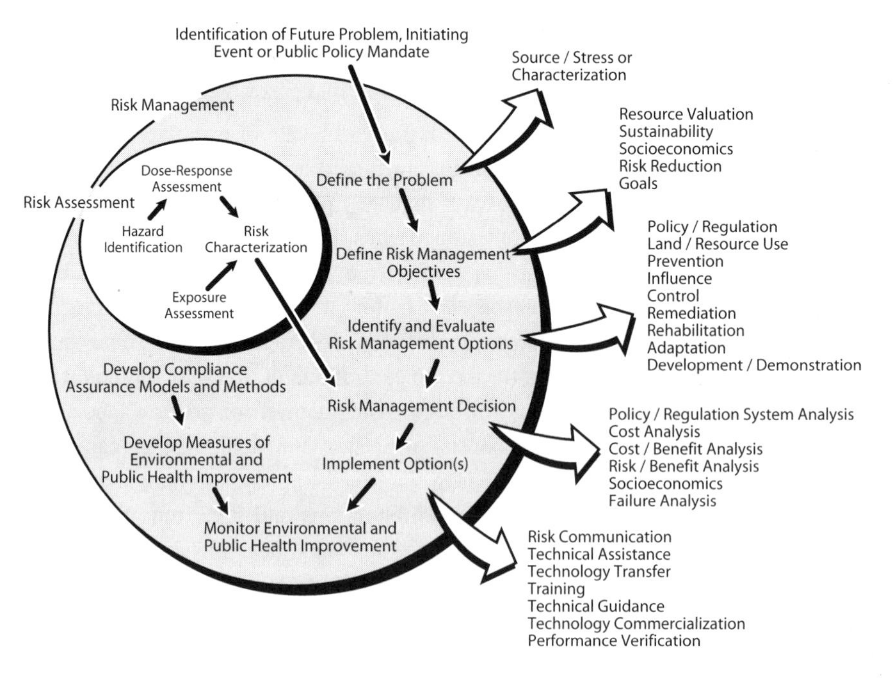

FIGURE 14–1. Risk management/risk assessment paradigm.

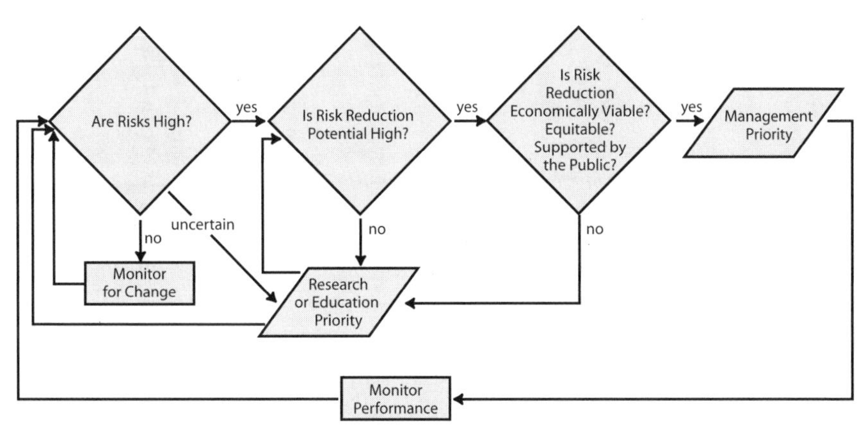

FIGURE 14–2. Iterative nature of risk management processes at EPA.

Educational institutions and the media can affect the management of risks by informing the public about the nature and extent of the risks and what can be done to reduce them by actions at both the individual citizen's level and by actions taken by the executive and legislative arms of government. Examples of options for risk reduction that can be accomplished by individuals, groups, industry, and others are illustrated in Table 14–1.

This chapter emphasizes technical means of controls that are or can be applied to minimize emissions from sources and exposures to people at work and in the general environment, but also introduces legislative and regulatory actions that can have a major impact on human exposures. It ends with a brief discussion of the role of individuals in controlling their own and their fellow citizens exposures and risks.

REGULATORY CONTROLS

A total ban on usage of a material may be appropriate when: *(1)* such usage is not essential, but rather one of marginal economic consequence or personal preference, such as fluorocarbon propellants in spray cans of household products; or *(2)* less hazardous materials are available that are equal to or better than the hazardous material for the purpose. A ban on lead-based white pigments in indoor paint was feasible because of the availability of titanium-based pigments to replace them.

When a material has unique properties and cannot readily be replaced without introducing or increasing other hazards, its usage must be rigorously controlled. An example is the use of asbestos for fireproofing steel beams. Asbestos had been sprayed onto the beams at the construction site, with resulting excessive

TABLE 14–1. Examples of Risk Reduction Activities[a]

	INDIVIDUALS	GROUPS[b]	INDUSTRY	OTHER INSTITUTIONS[c]
Preventing pollutant generation	Energy and water conservation	Car pooling	Raw material substitution	Purchase of biodegradable products
	Purchase non-hazardous household products	Integrated past management	Process redesign	Purchase of recycled products
	Organic gardening	Land acquisition for environmental protection	Product redesign	Zoning to protect critical resources
Recycling and reuse	Reuse of paint cleaners	Community solid waste recycling	Solvent reclamation	Paper recycling
	Trade in used car batteries	Oil recycling	Use of scrap iron in steel making	Commercial glass recycling
	Donate unused paint to school art department	Community hazardous waste recycling	Kraft process for chemical and energy recovery in pulp making	Use composted yard waste for fertilizer
Treatment and control	Asbestos removal	Water supply treatment	Solid and hazardous waste incineration	Co-composting sludge and solid waste
	Auto inspection and maintenance	Community composting	Air pollution control devices	Wastewater treatment
	Heating system maintenance	Landfill wood chipping	Accident prevention programs	Chemical inventory, audit and control systems
Reduce residual exposure	Home ventilation for radon, gas stoves	Proper sanitary landfill	Secure chemical landfill	Smoke free work areas
	Home water filtration devices	Land use planning	Pollutant dispersion technologies	Proper building ventilation
	Don't fish in polluted waters	Household hazardous waste collection	Controlled pesticide application	Purchase bottled water

[a]Many of these strategies, e.g., energy conservation, can be employed by all.

[b]Communities, community groups.

[c]Federal and state government, academia, health care institutions, commercial business, etc.

exposures of construction workers and passersby to airborne fibers. It was later applied in a matrix that assured coverage without significant airborne dispersion. As asbestos usage declined due to legislative restrictions on its availability, other, less hazardous, insulating materials were used.

There are several levels of regulatory controls. In some areas, states and local governments retain significant regulatory authority. However, to an increasing extent, the basic authority for governmental regulation comes from a series of federal acts that created new programs or expanded existing ones, and directed that certain objectives be achieved and maintained. The key federal legislation affecting the control of chemical contamination in the environment is briefly summarized in Table 14–2. As shown in Figure 14–3, the pace of federal legislation was greatest in the 1970s, and has tapered off since then.

Under the enabling legislation passed by Congress, each of the federal agencies charged with environmental-control responsibilities promulgates regulations that are published in the Federal Register. These regulations have the force of law and, unless overruled by court actions, are enforced by the appropriate agencies.

As discussed in Chapter 12, regulations may be of several different types as appropriate to the specific task. They can specify standards or permissible levels of contamination in community and workroom air, in drinking water supplies and streams, or in foods and packaging materials. They can also specify effluent standards and work practices. The regulatory standards involving numerical concentration limits may also require specific types of analytical measurement techniques, as discussed in Chapter 8.

Federal regulations that establish numerical standards provide a uniform frame of reference and goals to be achieved and maintained, putting all parties involved on an equal basis and giving them due notice of what is required. These regulations free industry and local authorities from the need to make technical judgements as to the levels that are toxic or may produce environmental damage. Such judgements, as previously discussed, are very difficult ones, and when made for a particular situation on a local basis, are likely to differ substantially from place-to-place and time-to-time.

Governmental regulations may also specify requirements for work practices and the maintenance of records on effluent discharges and the exposures and medical histories of employees. Such regulations may, therefore, affect the manner in which industry achieves control of exposures through both administrative and technical controls.

TECHNOLOGICAL CONTROLS

Implicit in the discussions of the previous chapters was that ways and means existed to eliminate or control contaminant sources when the exposures that they

Table 14–2. Major Federal Legislation Pertaining to Control of Chemicals

AIR CONTAMINANTS

1955 Air Pollution Control Research and Technical Assistance Act

Provided temporary authority and funding for five years for a federal program of research in air contamination, and technical assistance to local governments. (Extended in 1959 for an additional four years.) Regulatory agency: HEW

1963 Clean Air Act

Granted permanent authority for federal air pollution control activities. Provided for *(1)* federal grants to state and local air pollution control agencies to establish and improve their control programs, *(2)* federal action to abate interstate air contamination through a system of hearings, conferences, and court actions, *(3)* an expanded federal research and development program with particular emphasis on motor-vehicle exhaust and sulfur oxide emissions from coal and fuel-oil combustion.

1965 Amendments to Clean Air Act

Provided for *(1)* the promulgation of national standards relating to motor-vehicle exhaust, *(2)* cooperation with Canada and Mexico to abate international air contamination.

1967 Air Quality Act (amending the 1963 Clean Air Act)

Declared a national policy of air-quality enhancement and provided a procedure for designation of air-quality control regions and setting of standards by cooperation between federal and state governments; provided for registration of fuel additives.

1969 Further Amendments to Clean Air Act

Extended authorization for research on low-emission motor vehicles and cleaner fuels.

1970 Further Amendments to Clean Air Act

Provided for *(1)* the establishment of national ambient air quality standards and their achievement through the implementation plans of air-quality control regions and states, *(2)* a 90% reduction from 1970 levels of hydrocarbon and carbon monoxide emissions from automobiles by the 1975-model year, and 90% reduction from 1971 levels in nitrogen oxide emissions by the 1976-model year (with one-year extensions if necessary); *(3)* studies of aircraft emissions. Regulatory agency: EPA

1977 Amendments to Clean Air Act

Required EPA to apply different levels of stringency to emission controls on new sources for criteria pollutants in areas meeting existing National Ambient Air Quality Standards (NAAQS), i.e., best available central technology (BACT), than in areas exceeding the NAAQS. For these nonattainment areas, existing sources were required to use reasonably available control technology (RACT).

EPA was mandated to increase the promulgation of National Emissions Standards for Hazardous Air Pollutants (NESHAPs), and to re-examine the adequacy of the NAAQS every five years.

(*continued*)

TABLE 14–2. *(continued)*

AIR CONTAMINANTS

EPA was mandated to establish a Clean Air Scientific Advisory Committee (CASAC) to conduct public reviews of the criteria to be used as a basis for NAAQS revisions, and to advise the EPA Administrator on research needs for ambient air pollutants.

1990 Amendments to Clean Air Act

Required a phase in of 50% reductions in emissions of sulfur dioxide and nitrogen oxides from stationary sources.

Required technology based emission controls for 189 specific hazardous air pollutants, and assessments of residual risks after the application of such controls.

Required tighter emission controls for motor vehicles.

Required a production phase-out of stratospheric ozone-depleting chemicals.

WATER CONTAMINANTS

1899 "Refuse Act of 1899" (part of River and Harbor Act of 1899)

Prohibited discharges into navigable rivers.

1912 Public Health Service Act

Authorized investigation of water contamination in relation to human diseases.

1924 Oil Poilution Act

Prohibited discharge of oil by any means, except in emergency or by accident, into navigable waters of the U.S.

1948 Water Pollution Control Act

Provided five-year authorization to fund research studies, low-interest loans for construction of sewage- and water-treatment works, and a Federal Water Pollution Control Advisory Board. Authorized the Department of Justice to bring suits against individuals or firms, but only after notice, hearing, and consent of the state involved. (Extended in 1952 for an additional three years.)

1956 Amendments to Water Pollution Control Act

Provided for *(1)* permanent authority, *(2)* grants for construction of sewage-treatment plants, *(3)* abatement of interstate water contamination by federal enforcement through a conference public-hearing court-action procedure.

1961 Federal Water Pollution Control Act

Permitted the Secretary of Health, Education and Welfare (HEW), through the Department of Justice, to bring court suits to stop contamination of interstate waters without seeking permission of the state. Extended pollution abatement procedures to navigable intrastate and coastal waters, with permission of state. Authorized seven regional laboratories for research and development in improved methods of sewage treatment and control. Authorized funds for grants to local communities for sewage-treatment plants.

(continued)

TABLE 14–2. Major Federal Legislation Pertaining to Control of Chemicals (*continued*)

WATER CONTAMINANTS

1961 Oil Pollution Act

Enacted to implement provisions of the International Convention for the Prevention of the Pollution of the Sea by Oil, 1954.

1965 Water Quality Act

Declared a national policy of water-quality enhancement. Established the Federal Water Pollution Control Administration (FWPCA). Provided for the states to adopt water-quality standards for interstate waters and plans for implementation and enforcement, to be submitted to the Secretary of HEW (later to Secretary of Interior after FWPCA was transferred to the Department of the Interior) for approval as federal standards; authorized the Secretary to initiate federal actions to establish standards if the state criteria were inadequate. Authorized grants for research and development to control storm water and combined sewer overflows and authorized funds for sewage treatment plant grants.

1966 Clean Water Restoration Act

Provided for grants for research and development of advanced waste-treatment methods for municipal and industrial wastes. Authorized grants for construction of treatment plants. Amended the Oil Pollution Act of 1924 by transferring responsibility to Secretary of the Interior and provided for suits against "grossly negligent, or willful spilling, leaking, pumping, pouring, emitting or emptying of oil."

1970 Water Quality Improvement Act

Strengthened federal authority to deal with sewage discharges from vessels, hazardous contaminants, and contamination from federal and federally related activities. Provided for liability for oil spills from onshore- and offshore-drilling facilities and from vessels.

1972 Marine Protection, Research, and Sanctuaries Act (Ocean Dumping Act)

Regulation of the ocean dumping of materials which may be hazardous to human health and welfare. Regulatory agency: EPA

1972 Ports and Waterways Safety Act

Regulations relating to prevention or mitigation of damage to the marine environment due to transport of oil and other hazardous materials. Regulatory agency: Department of Transportation

1972 Water Pollution Control Act (Clean Water Act)

Extended national water pollution program to intrastate waters. Established *(1)* a system of national eflfluent limitations with goals of best practicable water pollution control technology by mid-1977 and best available technology by mid-1983, *(2)* national performance standards for new industrial and publicly owned waste treatment plants, *(3)* a national system of permits for discharge of contaminants. Authorized funds for treatment facilities. Regulatory agency: EPA

(*continued*)

TABLE 14–2. *(continued)*

WATER CONTAMINANTS

1974 Safe Drinking Water Act (amendment to Public Health Service Act)

Authorized EPA to establish federal drinking-water standards for protection from all harmful contaminants, applicable to all public water supplies in the United States. Established a joint federal-state system for compliance with standards and protection of underground sources of drinking water.

1977 Amendments to Water Pollution Control Act of 1972

Delayed installation of best available control technology until 1984. Continued federal grants for sewage-treatment plants. Added 65 chemicals and classes of chemicals to list of toxic agents.

1978 National Ocean Pollution Planning Act

Establishes comprehensive five-year plan for federal ocean pollution research and development and monitoring programmes, and co-ordinates research on Great Lakes and estuaries of national importance.

1988 Ocean Dumping Ban Act

Prohibits issuance of new permits for dumping of sewage sludge or industrial waste into ocean waters; phases out existing permits by 31 December 1991.

1986 Safe Drinking Water Act and Amendments

Provision of maximum limits for contaminants in public drinking water and techniques for their removal.

1996 Safe Drinking Water Act and Amendments

Requirements for specific analyses for emerging contaminants, such as *Cryptosporidium*; provides a revolving fund to help state and local authorities improve drinking-water systems.

SOLID WASTES

1965 Solid Waste Disposal Act

Began a national research, development, and demonstration program for solid wastes. Provided financial assistance to interstate, state, and local agencies for planning and establishing solid-waste disposal programs. Regulatory agency: EPA

1970 Resource Recovery Act

Provided for *(1)* research into new and improved methods to recover, recycle, and reuse wastes, and *(2)* financial assistance to states in the construction of solid-waste disposal facilities.

(continued)

Table 14–2. Major Federal Legislation Pertaining to Control of Chemicals (*continued*)

SOLID WASTES

1976 Resource Conservation and Recovery Act

Promulgates regulations for treatment, storage, and ultimate disposal of hazardous solid wastes. Regulatory agency: EPA

1980 Comprehensive Environmental Response, Compensation and Liability Act ("Superfund")/Superfund Amendments and Reauthorization

Imposes notification and public disclosure requirements on persons who handle, store or dispose of hazardous substances: establishes national hazardous substance response plan, including methods of determining priorities among releases, and provides for liability for response costs incurred by government; imposes financial liability on companies for direct damage to individuals and natural resources.

PESTICIDE CONTAMINATION & FOOD ADDITIVES

1938 Federal Food, Drug, and Cosmetic Act

Provided for the establishment of tolerances for pesticide residues in food.

1947 Federal Insecticide, Fungicide, and Rodenticide Act

Provided for *(1)* registration of "economic poisons" by the U. S. Department of Agriculture for products marketed in interstate commerce and *(2)* seizures of adulterated, misbranded, unregistered, or insufficiently labeled pesticides.

1954 Miller Amendment to the Federal Food, Drug, and Cosmetic Act

Provided for condemnation of raw agricultural commodities containing pesticide residues in excess of tolerances as fixed by the Secretary of HEW.

1972 Federal Insecticide, Fungicide, and Rodenticide Act

Gave EPA authority to regulate uses of pesticides so as to prevent environmental damage.

1996 Food Quality Protection Act

Repeal of Delaney clause; eases regulation of processed foods and tightens regulation of raw foods.

OCCUPATIONAL ENVIRONMENT

1936 Walsh-Healey Act

Enabled Federal Government to set standards for safety and health in work places engaged in activities relating to Federal contracts.

1969 Coal Mine Health and Safety Act

Directed the Secretary of Labor to set standards for exposure to coal mine dust and to compensate miners for coal workers pneumoconiosis resulting from past exposures.

(*continued*)

OCCUPATIONAL ENVIRONMENT

1970 Occupational Safety and Health Act

Established National Institute for Occupational Safety and Health to conduct research and training, develop exposure standards, and make inspections relevant to the protection of the health and safety of workers. Regulatory agency: OSHA

1973 Mine Safety and Health Act

Created the Mine Safety and Health Administration within the Labor Department to establish standards for occupational exposures of workers in metal and non-metal mines and associated ore processing mills.

RADIOACTIVE WASTES

1954 Atomic Energy Act (plus amendments)

Regulates release of radioactive was{es into the environment. Regulatory agency: Nuclear Regulatory Commission (NRC)

1978 Uranium Mill Tailings Radiation Control Act

Requirements for remediation of former uranium mill processing and disposal sites.

1982 Nuclear Waste Policy Act

Requirements for disposal of high-level radioactive wastes.

1985 Low-Level Radioactive Waste Policy Amendments Act

Requirements for disposal of low-level radioactive wastes.

GENERAL

1966 Freedom of Information Act

Provides public access to government-held information.

1969 National Environmental Policy Act

Declared a national policy for the environment to encourage harmony between man and his environment, to promote efforts that will prevent or eliminate damage to the environment, and to enrich the understanding of ecological systems and natural resources important to the nation. Established a three-member Council on Environmental Quality, in the Executive Office of the President, charged with making studies and recommendations to the President and with preparing an annual Environmental Quality Report. Directed that all agencies of the Federal Government include in every recommendation or report on proposals for legislation and other major Federal actions significantly affecting the quality of the human environment, a detailed statement on: *(1)* the environmental impact of the proposed action, *(2)* any adverse environmental effects which cannot be avoided should the proposal be implemented, *(3)* alternatives to the proposed action,

(*continued*)

TABLE 14–2. Major Federal Legislation Pertaining to Control of Chemicals (*continued*)

GENERAL

(4) the relationship between local short-term uses of the environment and the maintenance and enhancement of long-term productivity, and *(5)* any irreversible and irretrievable commitments of resources which would be involved in the proposed action should it be implemented.

1970 Environmental Quality Improvement Act

Establishes national policy of enhancement of environmental quality though state and local governments, encouraged and supported by the Federal Government.

1972 Coastal Zone Management Act

Makes federal funds available to encourage states to develop comprehensive management programmes to increase effective management, beneficial use, protection and development of coastal zones.

1975 Hazardous Materials Transportation Act

Regulates handling and transportation in commerce of hazardous materials (amended in 1976).

1975 Energy Policy and Conservation Act

Requires states to prepare energy conservation plans in order to receive financial assistance for eligible programmes; sets energy conservation standards for appliances; authorizes Secretary of Energy to make grants for energy inspections and audits of, and instruction of energy conservation improvements in, schools and hospitals.

1976 Toxic Substances Control Act

Provided for regulation of new chemicals or new uses for existing chemicals to prevent adverse effects upon human health or the environment. Provides for chemical testing, as well as authority to delay use of or ban specific chemicals or uses of chemicals. Regulatory agency: EPA

1986 Emergency Planning and Community Right-to-Know Act (Title III of 1986 Superfund amendments)

Requires owners and operators of facilities containing extremely hazardous substances to notify state emergency response commission and requires joint preparation of emergency plan.

1990 Pollution Prevention Act

Establishes waste management hierarchy, with preferenece for source reduction.

1992 Energy Policy Act

Requirements for improvements in the energy efficiency of a wide range of items, including transportation vehicles and industrial and home appliances, and promotion of the use of renewable resources.

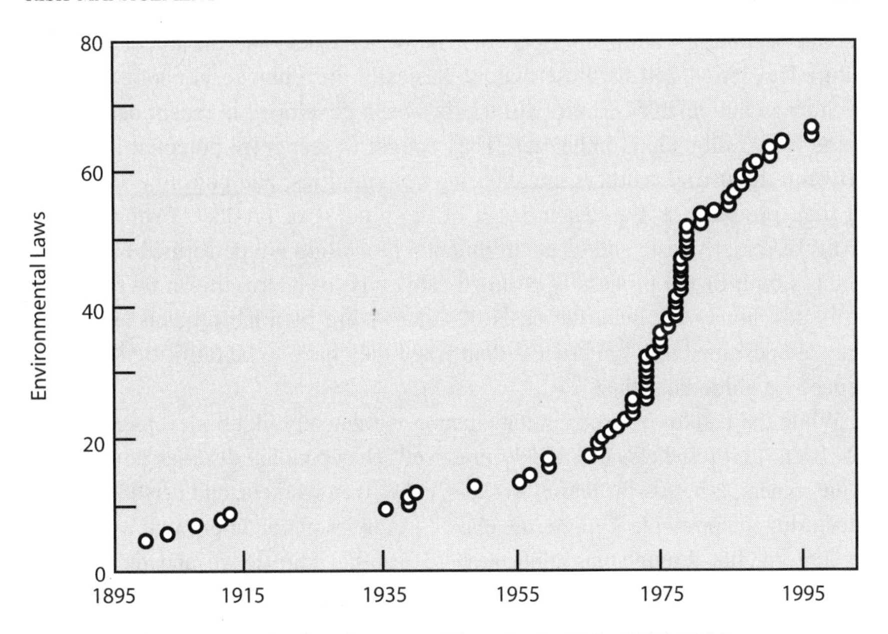

FIGURE 14–3. The growth of environmental laws in the U.S., 1899–1996.

caused were deemed to be excessive. One may expect that the administrative and technical skills and ingenuity displayed in creating the technologies that generate contaminants could also be employed in controlling them. By and large, this expectation is realistic. When the motivation is provided, whether by enlightened self interest or legislative mandate, it has been possible to achieve substantial control over ambient levels of chemical contaminants.

Unfortunately, there has been, in practice, too little application of existing control technology. The installation and maintenance of controls on automobile exhaust, process equipment in industry, and liquid and gaseous waste streams from industrial operations may be very costly. In the absence of clear-cut standards and regulations for effluent discharges, or the lack of evidence for damage to human health or environmental quality associated with such discharges, there has often been too little incentive for voluntary application of contaminant controls. One of the major benefits of the recently developing consciousness of the impact of environmental contamination on human health and welfare, exemplified by the substantial body of environmental legislation (Table 14–2), has been a major impetus toward the application of existing technology, as well as the development of new and improved technologies, for the prevention and/or control of contaminant effluents.

Responses to damaging conditions in the environment will always continue to generate needs for controls. In future years, alleviation of preexisting conditions should become a diminishing part of control activities, and the major focus of future legislation will be those that are basically preventative in nature.

Such an anticipatory control attitude has been developed in recent decades by some more enlightened industries. They sought to recognize potential problems affecting industrial workers, neighboring communities, and consumers or users of their products, at the design stage of the process or product. Evaluations in terms of toxicity tests and/or environmental modelling are performed before the plant is built or the process is installed. This type of approach can be economically advantageous, since the costs of controls are invariably much less when they are designed into the process than when they have to be retrofitted onto the process at some later date.

While the pattern of problem anticipation is relatively highly developed, it has not been, unfortunately, too widely practiced. Occupational diseases among uranium miners, asbestos-insulation workers, coke-oven workers, and personnel manufacturing the pesticide Kepone, are classic examples of conditions that were readily preventable through the application of existing knowledge and technology. Similarly, the damage to aquatic life and the restrictions of commercial seafood harvests resulting from releases of mercury, PCBs, Kepone, and Mirex to surface waters, could also easily have been prevented. Much of the recent environmental legislation has, in fact, been spurred by public reaction to the failure of industry to recognize their own interests in the application of preventive controls.

Control Approaches

When a decision has been made that an imminent or serious potential hazard exists due to the presence of a chemical contaminant in the environment, and there is a need to control its further release or usage, choices must be made concerning the means by which control is to be achieved.

One approach involves outright bans, specification of permissible usages, permissible times for operation and discharge of effluents, and permissible concentrations and amounts of effluents. These are all examples of control by the regulatory process.

Another approach, which is largely restricted to the occupational environment, is to control access to potentially hazardous conditions and environments. Management may be able to restrict access of personnel to contaminated areas, or to obtain the cooperation of its employees in using personal protective devices, so as to limit the duration and/or the intensity of exposures.

A third approach is known as engineering control. In this approach, controls are built into the process itself in order to reduce the formation and release of chemicals into the environment. This may be achieved through appropriate design and selection of materials, processes, and equipment; the intent is to depend as little as possible on the individual actions of plant personnel or consumers.

Engineering controls can be subdivided into process controls and source (or effluent) controls. The former emphasize the reduction or diminution of contaminant formation, while the latter act to reduce or prevent the release to the environment of any contaminants that are formed.

A fourth approach involves control via dilution in the ambient air and water.

Administrative Controls for Workers

Administrative controls of contaminant emissions and exposures depend upon the ability of management to motivate and control the personnel whose actions affect contaminant release, dispersion, and accessibility of themselves and others to contaminated areas.

The most effective means of administrative controls are those achieved through programs of education and motivation. Personnel whose actions affect their own exposures, or the extent of contaminant releases to the community environment, should be aware of the potential consequences of the resulting exposures and of the effects that their own work practices have on the extent of the releases. They should be thoroughly familiar with the intended functions, proper operating parameters, and maintenance procedures for the process equipment in their unit and for any control devices associated with its operation, so that substandard equipment performance may be recognized and controlled. These people should also be trained to cope with malfunctions and emergencies, including safe procedures for shutting down process operations, and to be thoroughly familiar with evacuation routes and procedures.

Personnel training programs are also needed for the proper use of personal protective devices, such as gloves, aprons, coveralls, eye-protectors, hearing protectors, and respiratory protective devices. These programs should include the criteria for the selection of the particular devices provided, when and how they should be worn or used, the degree of protection that they provide, their useful life and replacement schedules, and the conditions under which they should be maintained and stored between periods of use.

Management's role goes beyond education and encouragement of employee participation. Other aspects include human engineering of equipment, incentives for positive efforts, and disincentives or penalties for poor performance. In terms of human engineering (known as ergonomics), the provision of process controls and protective equipment within easy reach, which can be readily operated with natural motions, will usually increase effective performance. On the other hand, the lure of special incentives or the threats of penalties are not usually very effective in achieving a uniformly high level of employee performance.

Management also has a responsibility to limit the access of personnel to contaminated areas when unlimited access would result in overexposures. This type of control can take several forms. One involves the designation of personnel into those who shall have access to certain areas and those who shall not. The former category may include employees who have been fitted with personal protective devices. It may also include personnel without protective equipment, but whose work-time within the contaminated area will be sufficiently brief that their cumulative exposures will still be well within the permissible daily limits.

Among those for whom management is obligated to restrict access to contaminated areas are people who may be hypersensitive, have preexisting conditions, or accumulated prior exposures that would place them at special risk. The information needed for the identification of such personnel can be obtained at preemployment and periodic medical examinations and, for some conditions and materials, by special screening tests.

Engineering Controls

The most effective controls of contaminant release are those that are built into the process itself, and do not normally require the attention or assistance of operating personnel. There are four basic approaches to engineering control: material substitution, process modification, and isolation (which are all techniques of process control), and source control.

Material substitution

Substitution of materials can ensure against exposure and contamination due to a particular chemical by eliminating it from the process entirely and replacing it with another chemical that is less toxic or offensive. This technique is usually practical where the material in question is used as a solvent, pigment, thermal or electrical insulator, or for other applications where there are a number of alternate materials having similar properties that may be used. Some notable examples of materials substitution that have substantially reduced occupational disease incidence and/or environmental contamination are presented in Table 14–3.

Process modification

The control of contaminant discharges by modification of process procedures and equipment involves using process elements that provide a greater degree of enclosure, and/or the combination of a series of process operations in a single step. Both of these techniques are generally used in switching from batch-processing operations to continuous processing. The loading, unloading, and transfer of materials from one batch-processing vessel to another provides ample opportunity for uncontrolled releases, and these are minimized in continuous operations. Some notable examples of process substitutions that have substantially reduced contaminant release are also presented in Table 14–3.

TABLE 14–3. Applications of Control by Substitution

I. Substitution of Less-Toxic Materials

ORIGINAL MATERIAL	LESS-TOXIC SUBSTITUTE(S)	APPLICATIONS
Yellow phosphorus	Red phosphorus	Safety-match heads
Carbon tetrachloride	Perchloroethylene	Cleaning solvent
	Methylene chloride	Degreasing solvent
Benzene	Toluene, cyclohexane	Chemical raw material, solvent
Lead	Titanium, zinc	Interior paint pigments
Mercury nitrate	Various materials	Caroting fur for hats
Beryllium	Calcium phosphate	Phosphors for fluorescent lamps
Asbestos fibers	Glass fibers	Insulating materials
Sand	Silicon carbide	Abrasive cutting and shaping
Radium	Tritium	Luminous phosphors in dials

II. Substitution of Equipment or Processes That Disperse Less Contaminant

ORIGINAL EQUIPMENT OR PROCESS	LESS-CONTAMINATING EQUIPMENT OR PROCESS	APPLICATIONS
Spraying	Dipping	Painting of parts and products
Sandblasting	Hydroblast; chemical etching	Cleaning of parts
Soldering or welding	Riveting, crimping, or adhesive bonding	Joining of parts
Batch charging	Continuous feeding	Addition of materials
Diesel engines	Battery-powered electric engines	Fork-lift and delivery vehicles
Flanged piping	Welded pipe	Transfer lines
Mercury gauges	Mechanical gauges	Instrumentation

Isolation

When the generation of contaminants cannot be completely eliminated, the next best thing is to prevent contact of the contaminants with people and the environment. This can be done by isolating the contaminant source or, occasionally, by isolating the people to be protected from the source. It is generally easier and less expensive to isolate the source; usually this is done by enclosing it within a box or shell that will eliminate or reduce the escape of the material. On the other hand, when the sources are numerous and the people to be protected are few, it may be less expensive to isolate the people and create a clean artificial environment for them. This is frequently done, for example, in foundries, where the crane operator works within a cab provided with clean breathing air; the operator moves, within the cab, through dusty air above the foundry operations.

Source controls

When processes generate contaminants that must be controlled, the most economical and effective controls are those that exert their action closest to the source. It becomes more difficult and expensive to collect a chemical from a waste stream as process volume increases and the concentration decreases, such as following dilution by ambient air or water, and as the number of other constituents increases. Cocontaminants may produce interferences in the separation procedures and may also increase the cost of, or limit the freedom for, ultimate disposal of the extracted material. The use of process controls may act to concentrate contaminants in a small volume of air or water, thus decreasing the cost of any source cleaning devices, as well as increasing their efficiency.

Effluent controls include the removal of contaminants from waste streams, and recycling of the extracted materials back into the process, or disposal in an environmentally acceptable manner. When recycle or sale of the extracted material is feasible, it will usually be necessary to segregate waste streams according to their content and to treat some separately in order to avoid mixing and dilution of materials. On the other hand, where the material is simply to be disposed of, it may be possible to combine various waste streams in ways favoring the neutralization of one waste with another. For example, an acidic liquid waste can be mixed with an alkaline waste to produce a neutral salt. It may also be possible to bubble boiler-flue (smokestack) gases containing carbon dioxide to neutralize alkaline liquid wastes.

Control by dilution

In the past, it was often stated that "dilution is the solution to pollution." As time went on, this old adage became harder to justify. There will, however, always be some suitable application of control by dilution, such as for contaminants with short residence times in the environment and for those whose degradation products are innocuous. For contaminants that persist, or that are degraded in the environment into persistent chemicals, control by dilution is inappropriate. Also, what was acceptable when there were few sources may become unacceptable when the number of sources increases.

In the air environment, toxic chemicals from power plants and industrial operations may be vented through high stacks. Such stacks can penetrate normal inversion layers and, as discussed in Chapter 4, the maximum ground-level concentrations decrease approximately as the square of the effective stack height. Some power plants and industrial operations depend on dilution via tall stacks most of the time, but switch fuels or process operations to control effluent levels on those days when stack dispersion will not be adequate.

In the water environment, dilution rates depend on stream flow, and industrial operations frequently utilize detention basins on site to hold some of the wastes for periodic discharge during times of high stream flow.

In the occupational environment, dilution ventilation is sometimes used to reduce air concentrations from levels slightly above to slightly below acceptable limits, especially when there are multiple small sources, and where the material is considered more of a nuisance or housekeeping problem than a toxic hazard. Where the sources are few and well defined, or where toxicity is involved, source control by local exhaust ventilation is usually preferred over dilution ventilation.

Local exhaust ventilation and dilution ventilation in the occupational environment

Local exhaust ventilation is one of the key techniques for controlling air contaminant levels within the occupational environment. The principle is to create sufficient suction in the zone of active contaminant release to draw essentially all of the contaminant into a hood enclosure, along with a minimum volume of workroom air. The contaminant stream is then generally guided through a duct system to an air-cleaning device, fan, and discharge stack. Various exhaust-hood designs for specialized industrial and laboratory operations have evolved over the last 60 years.[1] Examples of some local exhaust hood designs are illustrated in Figures 14–4 and 14–5.

A special consideration in ventilation control of air contaminant concentrations in industry is the cost of supply make-up air. For each volume of contaminated air exhausted, it is necessary to supply an equivalent volume of clean air, and this latter air will usually have to be cooled or heated to maintain the desired temperature in the workroom. With the increasing costs of energy, the relatively large volume requirements of dilution ventilation make it increasingly less attractive as a contaminant control technique. This is, however, still a major technique used in underground mines.

Wet operations

A widely used technique for source control of industrial dusts is to wet the dust generated in operations such as crushing, grinding, cutting, and drilling. Dust generation may be greatly reduced by spraying a water mist or a stream of water onto the working face of the machine or tool.

Personal Protective Devices

Personal protective devices play an important role in occupational health protection. Chemical contaminants in the workplace can be systemically absorbed through the skin, eyes, lungs, and gastrointestinal tract, or can affect these portals directly.

Gloves, aprons, face shields, goggles, and various kinds of protective clothing can provide effective barriers against skin and eye contact, provided the proper materials are selected for their construction.

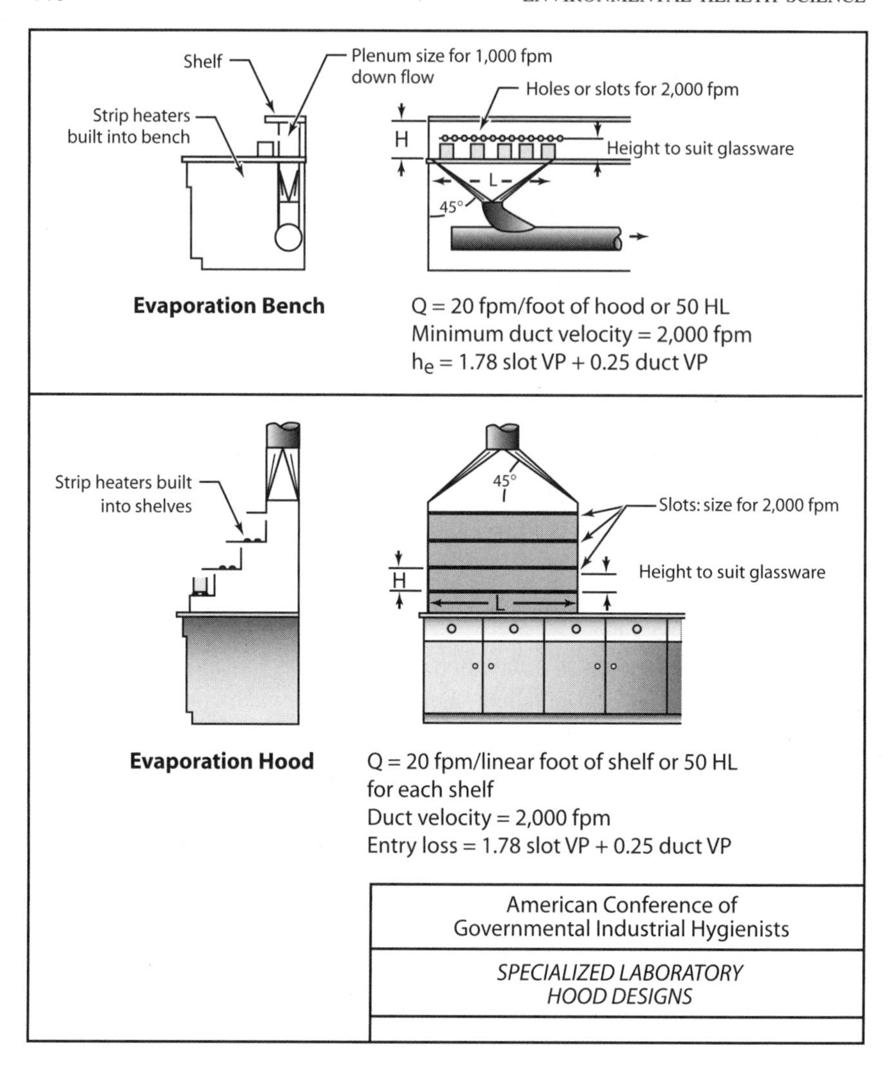

FIGURE 14–4. Specialized laboratory exhaust-hood designs.

The direct ingestion of chemicals in industry usually occurs from poor personal hygiene practices, such as touching food or cigarettes with contaminated hands. When contaminated cigarettes are burned, the chemicals on them, or their thermal degradation products, can be inhaled.

Respiratory protective devices provide a last resort defense against the inhalation of airborne contaminants. There are two basic types of devices: air-supplying and air-purifying respirators. In the former type, an excess of clean air is introduced into or around the nose or mouth. The air can be supplied by a portable tank under pressure, as in scuba diving, or by an air hose from a fixed tank or

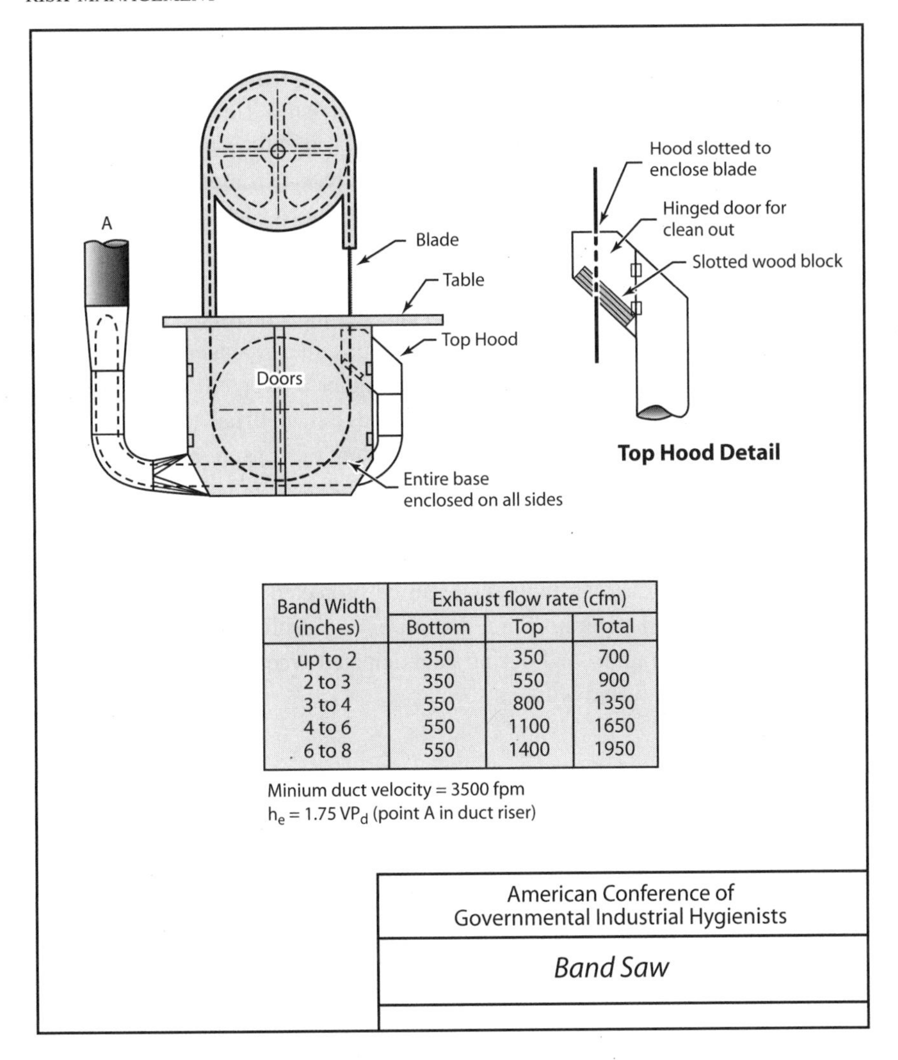

Band Width (inches)	Exhaust flow rate (cfm)		
	Bottom	Top	Total
up to 2	350	350	700
2 to 3	350	550	900
3 to 4	550	800	1350
4 to 6	550	1100	1650
6 to 8	550	1400	1950

Figure 14–5. Hood design for a band saw.

pump located out of the contaminated air. Portable tanks can only contain enough air or oxygen for brief periods, while air hoses limit mobility and freedom of action.

In air-purifying respirators, the contaminated air passes through a canister containing a filter and/or bed of adsorbing granules that extract the contaminants and pass the air. One type uses a battery-powered fan to push the air through the canister and thereby deliver it at positive pressure to the interior of a face mask or hood. It, therefore, resembles the air-supply type of device, in that leakage is outward.

By contrast, in most air-purifying respirators, the driving force to move the air through the canister is provided by the wearer's lungs; the pressure inside the mask is lower than that outside, and leakage is inward. Thus, even with complete contaminant removal from the air passing through the canister, the inhaled air will be partially contaminated if there is any leakage through or around the seal between the mask and the face. There is always resistance to flow through the canister, and this resistance generally increases with increasing collection efficiency and increasing flow.

For maximum protection, the correct air canister must be used. This is one that is rated for the particular contaminant in the exposure atmosphere and within its concentration and time limits. If it is used at higher concentrations, or if its adsorptive capacity is exceeded by prolonged usage, it will fail to be protective. Also, no canister can compensate for a deficiency of oxygen. Selection of respirators and canisters should be limited to those that have been tested and approved for the particular duty by NIOSH.

With a well-fitted mask, the appropriate air-purifying canister, and the motivation to use it properly, an individual can be protected from the inhalation of contaminated air, and respirators are, therefore, very useful for protection during infrequent brief operations and during unanticipated emergencies when used by well trained and motivated workers.

Control of Effluents Affecting Community Air Quality

The effective control of ambient air quality ultimately depends upon the control of source emissions. For the criteria air contaminants, i.e., PM, lead (Pb), SO_2, CO, NO_2, and O_3, the first step in their control was to construct an inventory of sources, source strengths, and patterns of dispersion so that control priorities could be set up. The original inventories established that PM and SO_2 were primarily attributable to stationary fossil fuel combustion sources, that CO and O_3 were primarily derived from mobile sources, and that NO_2 was attributable in similar measure to both of these source categories.

Most noncriteria air contaminants that are regulated are primarily of industrial origin, and have been controlled by the specification and enforcement of effluent standards.

While source controls are preferable in most cases, there still remain times when satisfactory levels of air quality can be maintained most economically by adequate dilution of the contaminants in the atmosphere. Since the mixing characteristics of the atmosphere are quite variable, dilution is frequently coupled with specifications on intermittent discharge.

Source controls

Source controls are discussed first in terms of air-cleaning techniques. This will be followed by a discussion of the application of available technology to the specific control of air contamination from mobile and stationary combustion sources.

Air-Cleaning Techniques. The process of removing contaminants from an air stream is known as air cleaning. It can involve extraction of the material from the air, or its conversion to less objectionable forms. An example of the latter method is the burning of toxic organic compounds producing CO_2 and H_2O.

Gases and vapors can be extracted from an airstream by condensation, adsorption, and absorption in gas washers and scrubbers. Particles can also be efficiently captured in some scrubbers. They can also be captured in dry collection systems on the basis of their diffusional and inertial displacements during passage through filters or specialized collectors, and by electrostatic precipitation. The basic mechanisms of dry-particle collection are illustrated in Figure 14–6, and those used to collect gases and vapors, and in some cases particles by scrubbing, are illustrated in Figure 14–7.

The selection of any particular cleaning method depends on the contaminants, the degree of removal required, the volumetric rate of flow to be processed, and the availability of suitable and economical means of disposal of the materials extracted from the air or of the secondary products formed during the control process.

Combustion. The simplest and generally the most economical way to dispose of organic wastes or other combustible contaminants in air is to burn them. If combustion is complete, all wastes are converted into CO_2 and H_2O. The burning of so-called "sour" waste gases, i.e., containing H_2S and organic sulfur compounds, in refineries results in SO_2 in the effluent, but this SO_2 is generally much less of a problem than the original compounds. In most cases, the amounts of SO_2 and NO_x in the effluent of a waste-gas combustion system will be negligible in comparison to the other anthropogenic sources of these contaminants.

Two methods are widely used for the combustion of effluents. These are the flame method and the catalytic method. In the former, an external gas supply is generally needed to maintain a flame temperature sufficiently high to ensure complete combustion. An example is a refinery flare tower used to dispose of hydrocarbon vapors. The other method is based on catalytic oxidation, and is generally used for low-concentration streams. Such devices are used on post-1975 cars to reduce the carbon monoxide and hydrocarbon content of exhaust gases.

Adsorption and Condensation. Contaminant gases and vapors can be removed by passing the airstream through a bed of granules whose surfaces will adsorb and retain the contaminants that reach them by diffusion. For example, activated carbon is often used to adsorb organic vapors. Since the surfaces eventually become saturated, the adsorption bed must either be periodically replaced

Brownian Separator
The Brownian Separator removes particles in the size range from 0.01 to 0.05 μm. This device consists of filaments, usually glass, arranged so that the space between them is less than the mean free path of the particle to be collected. Thus, the particle must collide with one of the filaments, where it is captured.

Filtration
The panel-type filter is limited to relatively light dust loadings because cleaning is time-consuming and costly. The baghouse, on the other hand, can be used with heavy loadings. These units are made up of a large number of cylindrical bag filters, which may be cleaned automatically to provide continuous operation. The baghouse should not be used for oily, hygroscopic or explosive dusts. Gas temperature is limited by the composition of the filter medium.

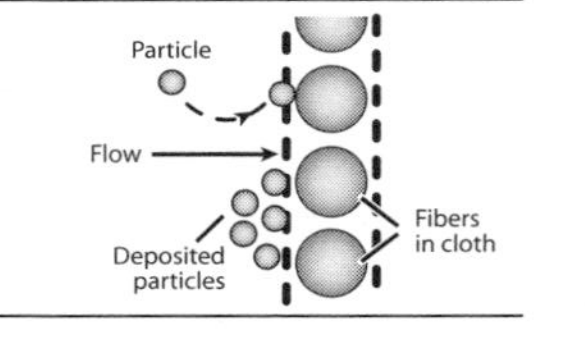

Electrostatic Precipitator
In this common collecting device, a high voltage is imposed on a relatively slow-moving gas stream. Charged particles are attracted to the grounded electrode, where they are periodically removed by rapping, vibration or washing. Conventional precipitators are quite bulky because of low air velocities. They have the advantage of providing dry collection, generally down to the 0.2 to 0.5 μm range. Theoretically, there is no minimum limit to the size of particles that can be collected.

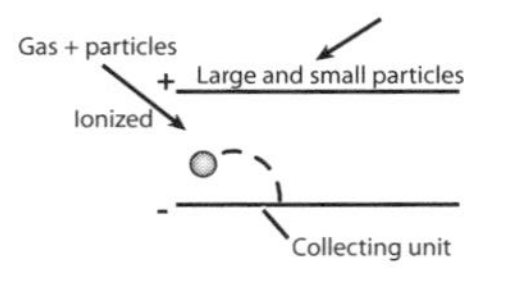

Centrifugal Collectors
Avalilable in a number of different designs, cyclone separators rely on centrifugal force to drive particles to the wall of the chamber where they drop out of the gas steam into a collector. They are useful for relatively coarse separations. A large-diameter cyclone will remove particles 15 μm and larger. Small-diameter units usually connected in parallel are effective down to the 10-μm range.

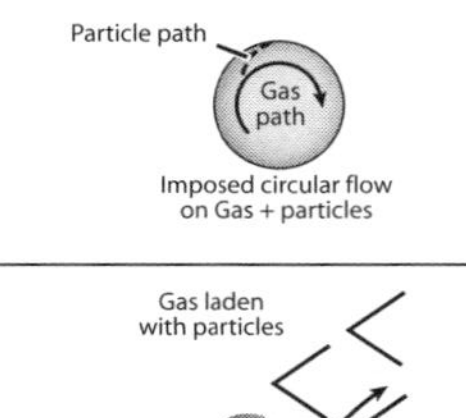

Inertial Separators
A variety of dry mechanical collectors are based on inertial impaction of particles on baffles arranged in the gas stream. Because there is a practical limit on how closely together the baffles can be placed, these devices are best for separations above 20 μm. However, some designs can achieve 5 to 8 μm separations.

Gravity Settling
The oldest and simplest means of particle separation is the gravity setting chamber, in which particles fall onto collecting plates. These are useful for removing course dusts above 40 μm, and may be placed ahead of other separation equipment.

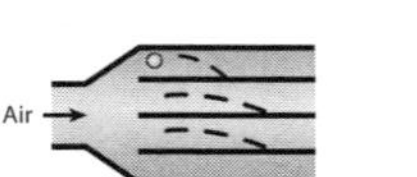

FIGURE 14–6. Basic methods for dry-particle collection.

Spray Towers
In spray towers the gas stream passes at low velocity through water sprays created by pressure nozzles. These units are simple, but only moderately effective. They will remove particles down to the 10 to 20 μm range and absorb very soluble gases.

Wet Cyclones
In this version of the cyclone separator, swirling gas flows through water sprays. Droplets containing dusts and absorbed gas are separated by centrifugal force and collected at the bottom of the chamber. Wet cyclones are more effective than spray towers. They will absorb fairly soluble gases and remove dusts down to the 3 to 5 μm range.

Venturi Collectors
The venturi design relies on high gas velocities on the order of 100 to 500 ft./sec. through a constriction where water is added. The impact breaks the water into droplets, with the fineness of spray determined by gas velocity. Venturis collect particles to the 0.1 μm level and recover soluble gases.

Perforated Impingement Trays
Here, gas flows through small orifices at 40 to 80 ft./sec. and hits a liquid layer to form spray. The liquid captures particles and gases, and is collected on impingement baffles. Performance is relatively good with particle collection possible down to 1 μm and absorption of fairly soluble gases.

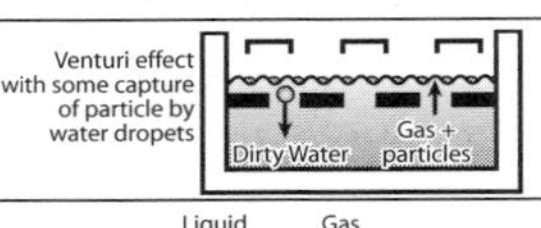

Packed Towers
Packed towers were primarily created for gas absorption. With some new designs, they can also be used for dust removal. Gas-liquid flow may be concurrent, cocurrent or crossflow. Two kinds of mass and particulate transfer are possible, depending on the packing. Extended surface packings provide absorption by spreading the liquid surface, and collect particles by cyclonic action. Recovery is limited to 10-μm sizes and larger. With filament packing, absorption by surface renewal is twice as effective and particles to 3 μm are separated by inertial impact. A cross-flow tower gives the highest solids handling capability with the lowest pressure drop.

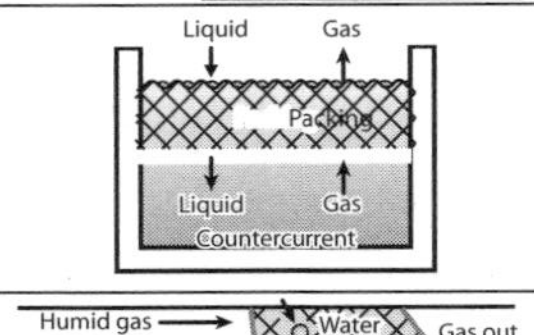

Nucleation Scrubber
This process grows submicron particles, down to 0.01 μm, by condensation. it collects grown particles on filament-type packing by inertial impact at low energy. At the same time, absorption occurs as in a conventional cross-flow packed tower.

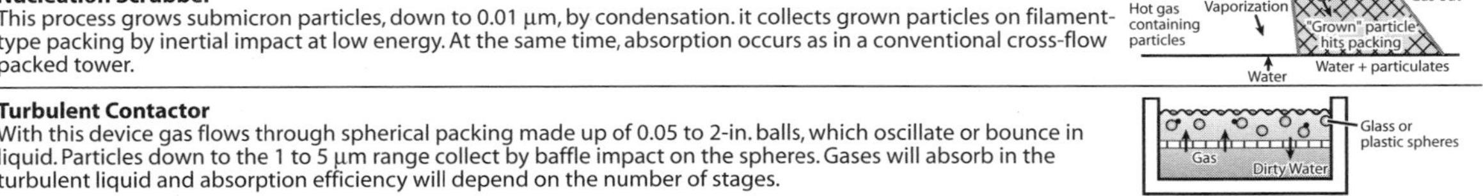

Turbulent Contactor
With this device gas flows through spherical packing made up of 0.05 to 2-in. balls, which oscillate or bounce in liquid. Particles down to the 1 to 5 μm range collect by baffle impact on the spheres. Gases will absorb in the turbulent liquid and absorption efficiency will depend on the number of stages.

Wet Filters
This is an open filter whose efficiency is improved by spraying with water. Its absorption ability is limited to those gases that are very soluble.

Chromatographic Recovery
The chromatographic unit contains inexpensive extended surface solids with a mono-to-termolecular coating of an active reagent. Thus the solute gas need only diffuse to the surface of the solid where it reacts either by ionic or molecular reaction. Where the reaction is ionic, the absorption is generally irreversible. Where the reaction is molecular, the absorption can be reversible, and the solute gas can be stripped off in essentially pure form.

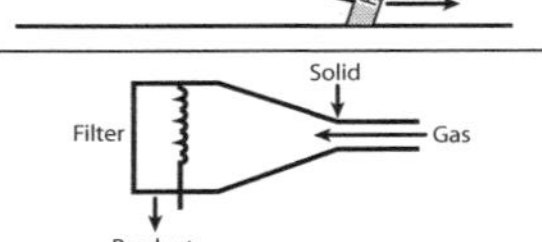

FIGURE 14–7. Basic equipment that may be used for both particle and gas collection.

or reconditioned, and provisions must be made for the disposal of the bed or the materials collected on and stripped from the bed during its reconditioning.

Adsorbants may be impregnated with various materials (Table 14–4) to convert the contaminant to less-harmful forms (e.g., CO into CO_2) or to promote a reaction that results in a form that may be more readily collected.

Some gas-phase contaminants may be removed by use of cold surfaces within or lining the flow path. Similar considerations concerning reconditioning apply here as well. Organic vapors are often controlled using this technique.

Scrubbing. Liquid streams and droplets can be used to extract gases and vapors from airstreams in devices known as scrubbers. The gases and vapors are removed by absorption into the liquid phase. The removal efficiency depends on both the solubility and the degree of saturation within the liquid, and also on the contact time between the contaminant in the gas phase and the surfaces of the liquid phase. Table 14–5 summarizes contaminants commonly removed by scrubbing and the scrubbing media used.

Scrubbers can also be used to collect particulate matter. Particles that contact a liquid surface are collected, with removal due to impaction, diffusion, and in some cases, electrostatic precipitation. Not surprisingly, collection efficiency is strongly dependent on particle and droplet sizes.

TABLE 14–4. Some Adsorbent Impregnations for Gaseous Contaminants

ADSORBENT	IMPREGNANT	CONTAMINANT	ACTION
Activated alumina	Potassium permanganate	Easily oxidizable gases, e.g., formaldebyde	Oxidation
	Sodium carbonate or bicarbonate	Acidic gases	Neutralization
Activated carbon	Bromine	Alkenes, e.g., ethylene	Conversion to dibromide
	Iodine	Mercury	Conversion to HgI_2
	Lead acetate	Hydrogen sulfide	Conversion to PbS
	Oxides of Cu, Cr, V, etc.; noble metals (Pd, Pt)	Oxidizable gases, including H_2S and mercaptans	Catalysis of air oxidation
	Phosphoric acid	Ammonia; amines	Neutralization
	Sodium carbonate or bicarbonate	Acidic vapors	Neutralization
	Sodium silicate	Hydrogen fluoride	Conversion to fluorosilicates
	Sodium sulfite	Formaldehyde	Conversion to addition product
	Sulfur	Mercury	Conversion to HgS

TABLE 14–5. Some Widely Used Scrubbing Media for Gaseous Contaminants

CONTAMINANT	SCRUBBING MEDIA
Chlorine (Cl_2)	H_2O, NaOH, NH_3
Hydrogen chloride (HCl)	H_2O, NaOH, NH_3, $Ca(OH)_2$, $Mg(OH)_2$
Hydrogen sulfide	(H_2S)NaOH, Na_2CO_3, KOH, K_2CO_3
Nitrogen oxides	(NO_x)$Ca(OH)_2$, $Mg(OH)_2$, $Na_2SO_3 - NaHSO_3$, urea
Sulfur dioxide (SO_2)	NaOH, Na_2CO_3, Na_2SO_3, KOH, K_2CO_3, K_2SO_3, CaO, $Ca(OH)_2$, $CaCO_3$, NH_3

Scrubbers, such as the Venturi type, which break up the liquid into very small droplets, may have relatively high collection efficiencies for small particles. However, these devices consume much more energy in the process than do gas washers such as the spray tower or packed tower.

The contaminants contained within the scrubbing liquids will generally require special handling in terms of treatment and disposal. Considerations in the handling of such contaminated liquids are discussed later in this chapter, under water-treatment techniques.

Bag Filters. Fibrous-filter media formed into cylindrical sleeves or bags are the most widely used type of dry-particle collector for air cleaning. By appropriate selection of fiber type, diameter, and packing density, fiber-mat thickness, and total surface, a high degree of collection efficiency may be achieved under a wide variety of operating and ambient conditions, and for aerosols having a broad range of characteristics.

Filtration in bag filters is similar in some respects and different in others to that occurring in air-sampling filters. The face velocity across a bag filter is generally only a few centimeters per second and, therefore, collection seldom depends on impaction deposition. Furthermore, the filtration occurs in the accumulated dust layer as well as in the filter mat itself. By contrast, in air sampling, the dust loadings are generally much lower, and a major portion of the sampled volume may be drawn through the filter before a significant dust layer accumulates. The clean filter must, therefore, be an efficient particle collector.

As dust accumulates on a bag filter, the flow must pass through the dust layer; the resistance to flow, therefore, increases, and will eventually impose a great burden on the air mover used. An analogous situation occurs in canister-type home vacuum cleaners that use a permanent-type felt bag, which must periodically be emptied. When the bag is emptied, some dust clings to the felt, and, therefore, the pressure drop and collection efficiency never return to the original new-bag levels. The same considerations apply to industrial bag filters, which are emptied and reused many times before they develop tears or other defects that lead to their replacement.

Two typical configurations for bag-type industrial air cleaners are illustrated in Figure 14–8. In these devices, numerous identical bags hang vertically within an enclosure called a bag house. The bags are closed at one end. Particle-laden air enters the housing at the top or bottom, and flows through the felt surfaces of the bags and out of the center of each bag into the clean-air plenum. The particles accumulate on the outsides (pressure-jet type) or the insides (traveling-ring type) of the bags, until the pressure drop across the bag reaches the preselected action level. In the pressure-jet device, the dust cake is periodically removed by a pressure pulse created by air-jet discharges. The pulse makes the bags expand,

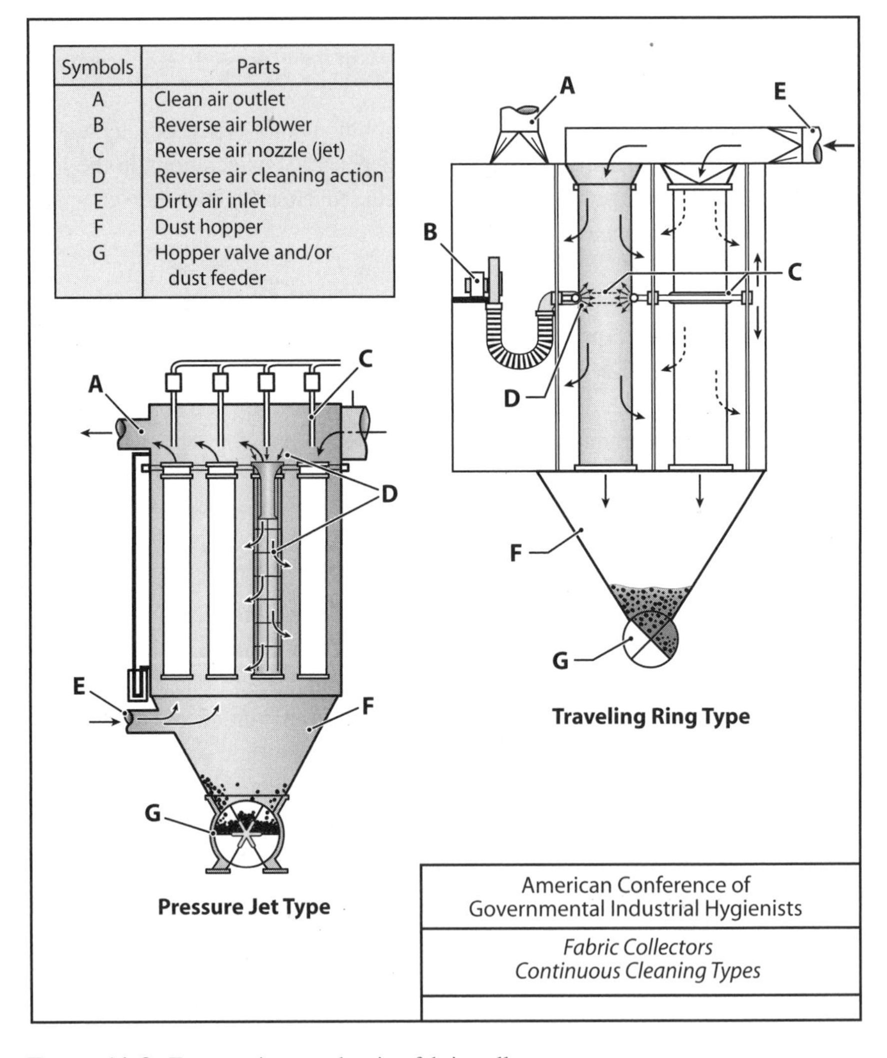

FIGURE 14–8. Two continuous-cleaning fabric collectors.

and the dust layer falls off and down into the collection hopper. Between cleaning cycles, the dust reaccumulates on the bags. In some bag filters, the cleaning is done by mechanical shaking. In the traveling-ring type, a doughnut-shaped ring with small air jets on its inner surface travels slowly up and down each bag to dislodge the dust.

Bag-filter control devices are available with an enormous variety of design features, numbers, sizes and shapes of bags, efficiency ratings, and operating conditions, and can be used for many, but not all, air-cleaning applications. They cannot be used effectively at very high temperatures without special high-temperature fiber mats, nor for dusts that tend to gum, or accumulate moisture excessively.

Electrostatic Precipitators. Electrostatic precipitators used for air-cleaning applications are generally single-stage types, in which both the charging and collection of the particles take place in the same electrode configuration.

A negative high voltage is applied to the corona wires, creating a bipolar glow region around each wire, and a unipolar stream of negative air ions that migrate toward the collecting plates on each side. Particles in the airstream passing through are charged and accelerated toward the collecting plates.

The collecting plates must be periodically cleaned in order to maintain a high overall collection efficiency, since the resistivity of the dust cake affects the voltage gradient and corona current and, thereby, the performance of the precipitator; the resistance to air flow does not change appreciably with dust accumulation. The plates can be cleaned by any of several techniques, as appropriate to the precipitator and the dust. They can be mechanically shaken, or periodically washed. Alternatively, the plates can be continually wetted by a falling film of water, and thereby maintain a more constant operating characteristic.

High-voltage power supplies and electrodes for precipitators are very costly to install, and precipitators are generally not economically competitive with bag filters, except for very large installations. However, for high-temperature, high collection efficiency air-cleaning applications, precipitators may be the only types of air cleaners available. They are widely used to clean coal-fired power-plant effluents.

Inertial Separations. When particles larger than approximately 1 to 2 μm in diameter are suspended in a moving stream of air, their motion will deviate less than that of the carrier air when the stream is turned or deflected. If particle displacement within the stream is sufficient to bring them into contact with a surface, they can be collected. The probability of collection increases rapidly with increasing particle size, air velocity, and sharpness of the directional change in the flow. Two types of inertial air cleaners, the baffle type and the cyclone, are illustrated in Figure 14–6.

In the cyclone, dusty air enters tangentially, and the particles are projected onto the outer walls as the stream follows a descending spiral. As dust accumulates in an air-cleaning cyclone, it migrates in flocs along the wall toward the collecting hopper at the bottom. Part of the way down the conical section, the descending air spiral containing the fine particle fraction turns inward and upward, and leaves the axial exit pipe on a tighter spiral.

Their simplicity of construction and operation, and their relatively low power requirements, make inertial collectors relatively inexpensive to purchase and operate. However, they are of limited value for controlling the release of particles having health significance, because of their inability to capture particles smaller than approximately 5 μm. These devices are, however, frequently used to collect nuisance-type dusts having large particle sizes. They are also used as precleaners upstream of more efficient and expensive particle collectors, such as bag filters, electrostatic precipitators, or Venturi scrubbers. When the mass median particle size is large, an inertial precollector can remove a substantial fraction of the total mass at low cost, reducing the loading on the more expensive second-stage air cleaner.

Mobile-source controls

The control of mobile-source (motor vehicle) emissions was mandated by Congress in stages. The sequence of steps was intended to permit adequate lead time for the development and testing of control technology. The entire industry adopted essentially the same technology for the control of evaporative losses of fuel and gaseous leakage around the pistons, but chose several different approaches to the control of tailpipe emissions of CO and hydrocarbons. Most adopted the catalytic converter to more completely oxidize exhaust gases; others initially elected to achieve more complete combustion within the engine, some with electronic ignition systems, and others with different combustion chamber designs such as the stratified-charge engine. As emission requirements became more stringent, essentially all auto manufacturers installed catalytic converters on their cars.

Stationary combustion source controls

The effluents from industrial and utility boilers fired by coal and heavy oil contain substantial quantities of ash, sulfur dioxide, and nitric oxide. Up until the 1960s, the only exhaust-gas cleaning that was commonly done was removal of most of the ash, using either electrostatic precipitators or bag filters. Neither type of air cleaner removed any significant amount of the gas-phase contaminants.

The initial focus of stationary-source control under the Clean Air Act of 1970 was the reduction of SO_2 emissions by: *(1)* reducing the average sulfur content of the fuel burned; and *(2)* extracting SO_2 from the effluent gas before it leaves the stack. Most utilities having an adequate supply of low-sulfur fuel chose the former approach. The increased fuel costs could be passed directly to the power consumers. The alternative was to incur the additional expenses required for land acquisition and plant construction and operation for a stack gas-cleaning system. Some utilities sought permission for a third alternative, i.e., dilution via high stacks, but EPA refused to approve control by dilution, and this position has been upheld in the courts. Since there is not enough low-sulfur fuel to accomodate the demand, some utilities installed flue-gas desulfurization (FGD) processes to clean their effluents.

In the United States, six types of FGD systems have been used for controlling full-scale utility boilers. Most of the operating capacity involved lime- or limestone-slurry, or sodium carbonate scrubbing techniques. These are known as "throwaway" processes, since the SO_2 is removed in a form that is discarded. On the other hand, the magnesium oxide and Wellman-Lord processes produced salable sulfur products, such as elemental sulfur, sulfuric acid, or liquid sulfur dioxide.

In concept, lime- or limestone-slurry scrubbing processes are very simple. In practice, however, the chemistry and the system design for a full-scale operation can become quite complex.

The overall absorption reaction taking place in the scrubber and the hold-tanks for a limestone-slurry system produces hydrated calcium sulfite:

$$CaCO_3 + SO_2 + 1/2\ H_2O \rightarrow CaSO_3 \cdot 1/2\ H_2O + CO_2 \tag{14–1}$$

With a lime-slurry system, the overall reaction is similar, but yields no CO_2:

$$CaO + SO_2 + 1/2\ H_2O \rightarrow CaSO_3 \cdot 1/2\ H_2O \tag{14–2}$$

(The actual reactant in Eq. (14–2) is $Ca(OH)_2$, since CaO is slaked in the slurrying process.)

In practice, some of the absorbed SO_2 is oxidized by oxygen absorbed from the flue gas; the resultant product appears in the slurry as either gypsum ($CaSO_4 \cdot 2H_2O$) or as a calcium sulfite/sulfate mixed crystal. The slurry is recycled around the scrubber to obtain the high liquid-to-gas ratios required.

Lime- and limestone-slurry scrubbing systems can be engineered for almost any desired level of SO_2 removal. Commercial utility systems are generally designed for 80% to 95% removal; however, some systems have, at times, achieved removal efficiencies as high as 99%.

Some low-sulfur coals contain large amounts of alkaline metal oxides (e.g., CaO, MgO) in the ash that results from combustion. These coals appear particularly suitable to SO_2 control by scrubbing the waste gases with a slurry of the alkaline fly ash. There are two ways to add the ash to the system: *(1)* collecting the fly ash in an electrostatic precipitator upstream of the scrubber and then slurrying the dry fly ash with water so that it can be pumped into the scrubber circuit; and *(2)* scrubbing the fly ash directly from the flue gas by the circulating slurry of fly ash and water.

"Throwaway" FGD systems depend, of course, on having a suitable place to throw the waste away. The enormous amounts of impure gypsum slurry produced by lime- and limestone-process plants must be piped to large settling and evaporation ponds. These FGD processes are, therefore, economically feasible only where land for such ponds is available close by and at low cost. The sodium carbonate process produces a solution of Na_2SO_4, which has no commercial value, and cannot be readily disposed of except in some desert areas.

The magnesium oxide process differs from the above techniques in that it is a "regenerable" or "salable product" process; the SO_2 removed from the flue gas is concentrated and used to make marketable H_2SO_4 or elemental sulfur. This process employs a slurry of MgO or $Mg(OH)_2$ to absorb SO_2 from the flue gas in a scrubber, and yields magnesium sulfite and sulfate. When dried and calcined, the mixed sulfite/sulfate produces a concentrated stream (10–15%) of SO_2 and regenerates MgO for recycle to the scrubber. Carbon added to the calcining step reduces any $MgSO_4$ to MgO and SO_2.

In commercial applications, the scrubbing and drying steps would normally take place at the power plant. The regeneration, and the sulfur or H_2SO_4 production steps, might be performed at a conventional sulfuric acid plant. Alternatively, a central processing plant could produce sulfur from mixed magnesium sulfite/sulfate brought in from other desulfurization locations.

The Wellman-Lord (W-L) process is also a regenerable system. When coupled with other processing steps, it can make salable liquid SO_2, H_2SO_4, or elemental sulfur.

The W-L process employs a solution of Na_2SO_3 to absorb SO_2 from waste gases in a scrubber or absorber, converting the sulfite to bisulfite:

$$Na_2SO_3 + SO_2 + H_2O \rightarrow 2\ NaHSO_3 \tag{14–3}$$

Thermal decomposition of the bisulfite in an evaporative crystallizer can regenerate sodium sulfite for reuse as the absorbent:

$$2\ NaHSO_3 \rightarrow Na_2SO_3 + SO_2 + H_2O \tag{14–4}$$

The evaporative crystallizer produces a mixture of steam and SO_2 and a slurry that contains sodium sulfite/sulfate plus some undecomposed $NaHSO_3$ in solution. As water condenses from the steam/SO_2 mixture, it leaves a wet SO_2-enriched gas stream to undergo further processing for recovery of salable sulfur.

Dilution and intermittent discharge

Dilution is a control technique only in the sense that it depends on turbulent diffusion in the atmosphere to reduce the concentration of the effluents to acceptable levels. It may also depend on the ability of the normal processes in the atmosphere to degrade, transform, or remove the contaminants, so that they do not accumulate excessively within the atmosphere. Consideration of the acceptability of control by dilution may even extend to the effects of the accumulation of airborne contaminants on the land, in surface waters, and in the biosphere. The technical considerations in determining the extent of dilution of contaminants discharged into the atmosphere were covered in some detail in Chapter 4.

Intermittent discharge is, as previously discussed, a useful adjunct to dilution in the atmosphere. Since effective dilution varies with the atmospheric lapse rate and wind velocity, control by dilution is better justified when there are means of stopping or reducing effluent discharges during periods when dilution factors are unfavorable. The most notable example of voluntary effluent reductions during periods of poor atmospheric dispersion is the use of reserve supplies of natural gas or low-sulfur fuel for industrial and utility boilers as a means of limiting the build-up of ambient SO_2 levels.

CONTROL OF SURFACE WATER QUALITY

Background

By the beginning of the twentieth century, the concentration of people in metropolitan areas and the increasing use of sewer systems that discharged directly into surface waters resulted in the frequent appearance of floating fecal matter and attendant problems of odor and visual blight. Thus, until about mid-century, water pollution control was primarily concerned with sewage and other wastes having similar properties. The installation of primary treatment facilities was generally sufficient to alleviate the immediate problem. This stage of treatment involves removal of larger suspended and floating solids, and oil and grease, generally by mechanical means.

Primary treatment, however, only removed part of the oxygen demand of the waste, and the continuing increase in the total amount of sewage led to frequent depletion of the dissolved-oxygen levels in surface waters around major metropolitan areas. Oxygen depletion, in turn, led to fish kills and odors associated with putrefaction. The general solution to this problem was the installation, beginning on a large scale in midcentury, of secondary-treatment facilities to supplement the primary treatment. Secondary treatment generally is synonomous with biological treatment. In this process, the liquid waste is contacted with bacteria, which consume most of the organic material in the waste during their metabolism. The actual reduction in oxygen demand achieved depends upon the ability of the bacteria to use the organics in the waste, and the contact time of the contaminants with the bacteria.

Depending upon their biodegradability, nonsewage chemical contaminants in waste streams may be partially removed by the bacteria in secondary-treatment facilities. Some chemical contaminants, however, present serious problems to sewage treatment plant operations in that they are toxic to the bacteria. If too many bacteria are killed, the operation of the treatment plant can be seriously disrupted, and it may take many days for the reestablishment of an effective bacterial colony in the facility.

Primary-treatment steps are frequently needed to modify the waste to the extent that it will be amenable to biological treatment. Conditions calling for such preliminary treatments are listed in Table 14–6.

In recent decades, concern shifted from the oxygen demand to the toxicity and carcinogenicity of contaminants in surface waters. This concern has led to an acceleration in the development of a variety of advanced physical and chemical treatment techniques (also known as tertiary treatment) for the removal of many chemicals from waste streams. Much of this modern technology has been based on adaptations of the process technology of chemical engineering that has been used to recover materials from industrial-process waste streams. However, applications of these techniques to large-volume municipal-waste streams of extremely heterogenous composition is a greater challenge.

The kinds of waste water-treatment processes used, and their sequence, are illustrated in Figure 14–9. The various treatment schemes accomplish different levels of removal, and as the degree of treatment increases, the cost also rises. Note that there is some overlap in techniques used in the different stages of water treatment. The contaminants for which the various processes are effective are presented in Table 14–7.

Control of Chemical Contamination from Point Sources

Stream manipulation

Segregation of Waste Streams. When there are numerous waste streams, with many having similar characteristics, it may be desirable to have two or more

Table 14–6. The Concentration of Contaminants That Make Primary Treatment Necessary

CONTAMINANT	LIMITING CONCENTRATION
Acidity	Free mineral acidity
Alkalinity	0.5 lb alkalinity as $CaCO_3$/lb BOD removed
Suspended solids	> 125 mg/L
Oil, grease	> 50 mg/L
Dissolved salts	> 16 gm/L
Organic-load variation	> 4:1
Trace metals	> 1 mg/L
Sulfides	> 100 mg/L
Phenols	> 70–160 mg/L
Ammonia	> 1.6 gm/L

BOD, biochemical oxygen demand.

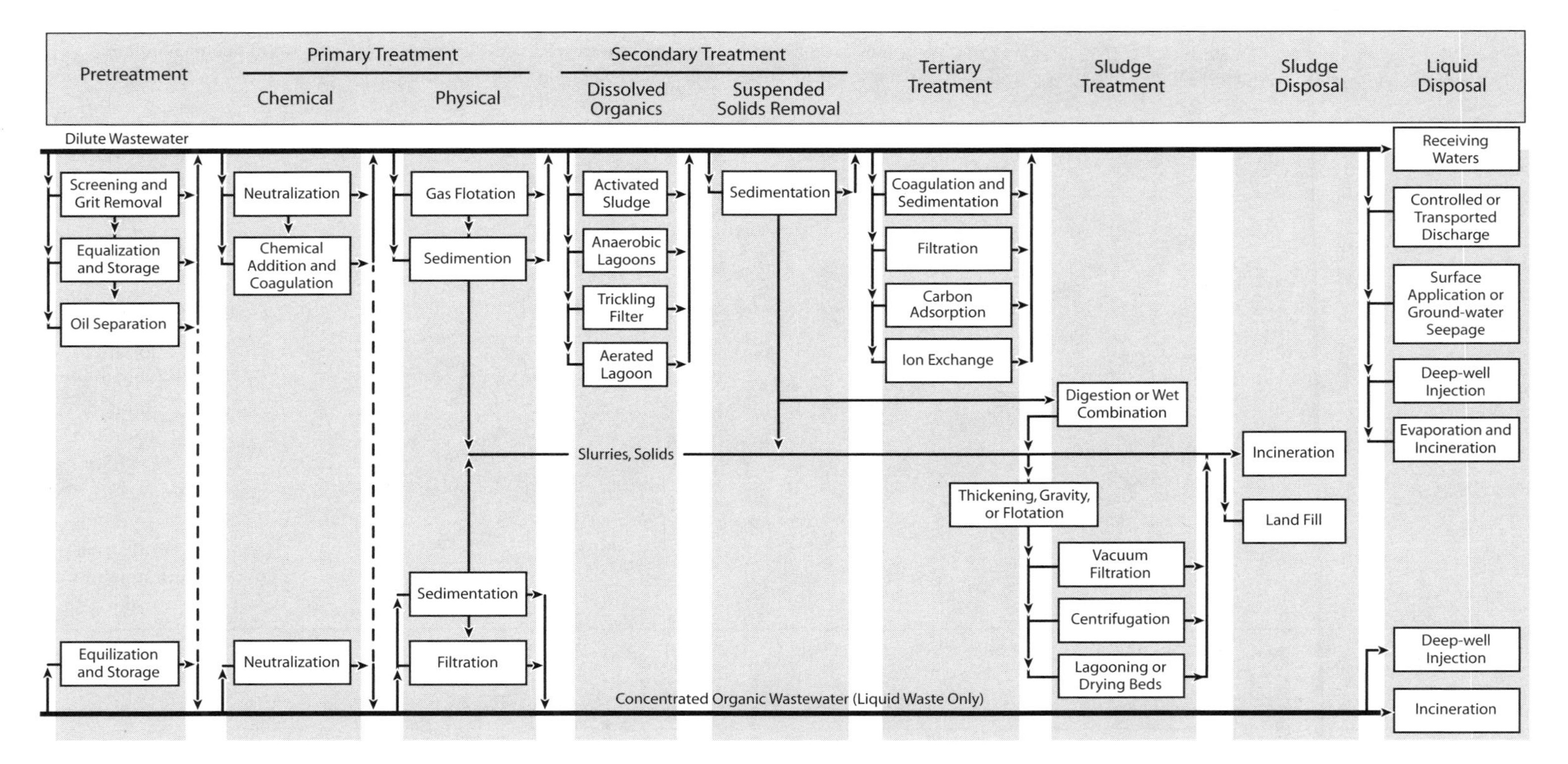

FIGURE 14–9. Waste water-treatment sequence. Very often, one process may be substituted for another, or a variety of different processes may be needed for treatment of specific contaminants. (Pretreatment is usually considered to be part of the primary treatment of waste water.)

TABLE 14–7. Typical Applications of Wastewater Treatment Processes

PROCESS	CONTAMINANT											
	ACIDS	ALKALIES	TOTAL DISSOLVED SOLIDS	SUSPENDED SOLIDS	NITRATE	PHOSPHATE	TRACE METALS	ORGANIC MATERIAL (BOD)	OILS	PERSISTENT PESTICIDES	COLOR	TASTE AND ODOR
Filtration				X			X					
Sedimentation				X					X			
Clarification				X		X	X	X	X			
Flotation				X					X			
Neutralization	X	X										
Biological treatment					X	X		X			X	X
Lagooning				X	X	X		X	X		X	X
Chemical oxidation or reduction											X	X
Emulsion breaking									X			
Adsorption				X				X		X	X	X
Ion exchange			X		X	X	X					
Reverse osmosis			X	X	X	X		X				
Electrodialysis			X		X	X						

BOD, biochemical oxygen demand.

[*Source*: Compiled from: Paulson, E.G. Water pollution control programs and systems. In H.F. Lung (ed.), Industrial Pollution Control Handbook. New York: McGraw-Hill, 1971; and Metcalf and Eddy, Inc. Wastewater Engineering: Collection, Treatment, Disposal. New York: McGraw-Hill, 1972, pp. 611–627.]

separate waste systems, for example, one for oily wastes, one for inorganic chemicals, one for storm drainage. In some cases, it may not be necessary to clean the storm drainage at all, and keeping it out of the chemical-waste system will help to avoid flow surges that can overwhelm the capacity of the waste-treatment facilities.

Mixing of Waste Streams. Under some circumstances, it is better to mix waste streams than to segregate them for separate treatment. If, for example, one stream is acidic and another is basic, one waste can neutralize the other, producing a salt solution that may require no further treatment. Even when the salt is insoluble and requires collection and disposal, the net effect may still be beneficial, and the purchase of chemicals for intentional neutralization can be minimized. The economic benefits of complementary wastes frequently lead neighboring industries to exchange waste streams or to share in the costs of operating a combined waste-treatment facility.

The mixing of streams can also be beneficial in terms of equalization of the strength of the waste, especially when one or more of the major sources are intermittent. The mixing of streams within the sewer system or preliminary-treatment steps may prevent concentration peaks that could adversely affect subsequent biological treatment or advanced chemical processes.

Reduction of waste volumes

Reduction of waste volumes involves both decreases in the amount of contaminant and the amount of dilution water; both can generally be achieved by a good preventive maintenance program that detects and corrects leakage. Improvements in process design, equipment, and operating procedures may also make it possible to maintain or improve process output with reduced amounts of waste materials.

Water treatment techniques

Screening. Screening is a mechanical process that separates suspended particles on the basis of size. There are several types of devices that may have static, vibrating, or rotating screens. Openings in the screening surfaces range from several centimeters down to approximately 20 μm.

Screens are used for treating raw water, storm water, and waste waters from certain industries that produce large volumes of solids, such as food-process plants, textile mills, and pulp and paper mills. The amount of solids removal depends upon screen size and characteristics of the water or waste water being treated. For example, fine-mesh microstrainers, with screen apertures of approximately 20 μm, remove solids, such as various forms of plankton and general microscopic debris; coarse bar screens that have metal bars spaced approximately 25 to 50 mm apart are used to remove the large suspended solids. The screens are periodically cleaned, generally by automatic equipment.

Comminutors, or large circular garbage grinders, may be used to grind into smaller pieces those solids that penetrate the coarse screens.

Centrifugal Separation. Hydrocyclones are used to remove relatively dense suspended solids from a liquid stream; a common application is for separating grit from storm water or waste water. Figure 14–10 shows their operation. Fluid-pressure energy is used to create rotational fluid motion in a cyclone. This motion causes relative movement of materials suspended in the fluid, and permits separation of these materials from the fluid. The bulk of the fluid is removed through a top outlet, and the separated solids are discharged through a second outlet located in an axial position at the bottom.

Smaller particles can be separated using centrifuges, but such separations are much more expensive, both in terms of capital outlay and operating costs.

Neutralization. When there is an excess of acid or base in the wastes, it may be necessary to treat the waste stream with sufficient basic or acidic chemicals to produce neutralization. For small volumes of acidic wastes, sodium hydroxide is used, and the resulting salts will usually not present any significant disposal problem. Lime and ground limestone are much less expensive per unit of basicity, but produce insoluble neutralization products that will usually require separate disposal.

Alkaline wastes can be neutralized with sulfuric or hydrochloric acids. Relatively inexpensive neutralizations can be achieved by bubbling flue gas containing CO_2 through the waste stream.

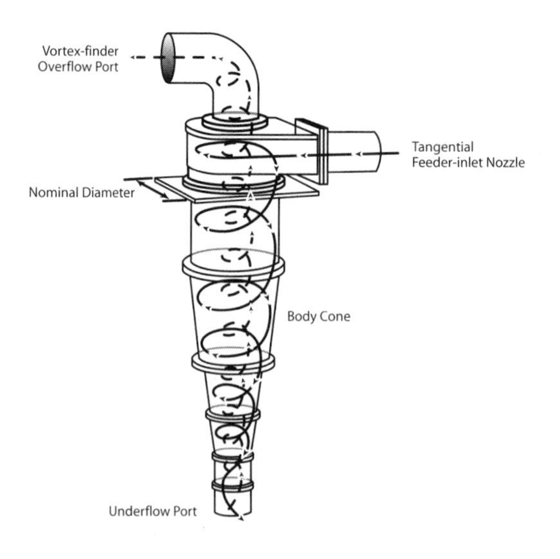

FIGURE 14–10. Hydrocyclone.

Precipitation. Precipitation reactions are often carried out in water and waste treatment. Lime is frequently used to precipitate calcium carbonate and magnesium hydroxide in water treatment. In waste-treatment operations, the precipitation of metallic hydroxides from plating, metallurgical, and steel mill wastes and also from acid mine drainage is commonplace. Wastes that contain phosphates may also be treated to precipitate calcium or aluminum phosphate. Lime or limestone is used for the precipitation of calcium sulfite or sulfate from stack-gas scrubber water.

Essentially, every reaction is carried out with the stoichiometric amount of precipitant and at the optimum pH. If the solubility of a compound exceeds the required effluent concentration, an excess of the precipitant may be added to reduce the solubility.

Precipitation reactions are usually carried out in the presence of previously formed sludge. This minimizes supersaturation, and also results in more rapidly settling precipitates because precipitation occurs on existing slurry particles.

Flocculation and Coagulation. Flocculation is the process of bringing together fine particles, for example, colloids, so that they agglomerate, forming larger particles (flocs) that will settle more rapidly. Mechanical stirring or air injection may be used to cause the suspended particles to collide. Alternatively, a chemical coagulant may be used; these cause suspended solids to agglomerate by reducing colloidal charge levels. When a metallic cation such as aluminum, for example, as aluminum sulfate (alum), or iron, for example, as ferric chloride, is used, particulate metallic hydroxides are initially formed, which adsorb the colloids.

Synthetic polymers are often used as coagulants or as coagulant aids. Polymers may be cationic, and adsorb a negatively charged particle; anionic, which permit bonding between a colloid and polymer; or nonionic, which adsorb flocculates by hydrogen bonding between the solid surfaces and the polar groups of the polymer.

Separation by Density Differences. Separation by density differences involves the removal of suspended solids or oils when the specific gravity difference from water causes settling or rising of the solids or oils during passage through a tank under suitably quiescent conditions.

Static conditions that affect such separations are: *(1)* water temperature, which affects both viscosity and density of the water; *(2)* specific gravity of the oil or suspended solids; *(3)* size and shape of suspended oil droplets and of particles; and *(4)* solids concentration, which results in free or hindered settling.

Sedimentation is the removal of suspended solids via gravity settlement, and is usually performed in tanks (known as settling tanks) having a continuous flow and a detention time of several hours. The settling velocities of particles will change with time and depth, as particles agglomerate and form larger floc sizes.

Settling tanks are divided into four zones: *(1)* inlet zone, to provide a smooth transition from the influent flow to a uniform steady flow desired in the settling zone; *(2)* outlet zone, to provide smooth transition from settling zone to the effluent flow; *(3)* sludge zone, to receive and remove settled material and prevent it from interfering with the sedimentation of particles in the settling zone; and *(4)* settling zone, to provide tank volume for settling, free of interference from the other three zones. Settling tanks which follow preliminary treatment such as screening are known as primary clarifiers. Typical primary-clarifier units are shown in Figure 14–11.

The surface area of a settling tank is one of the most important factors that influence sedimentation. The tank should be designed so as to produce a clarified effluent at minimum water temperature, and to allow for separating floc particles that may not be of maximum size or density. This latter problem may be due to either partial deflocculation in the inlet zone, or to partially ineffective coagulation. Tanks are generally approximately 30 m in diameter and approximately 4–5 m deep.

If the release of entrained air might cause floating floc, or if floating solids may be present, a scum baffle plus a scum skimmer mechanism are usually installed. Sludge removal from the tank bottom may be performed manually, or by a continuous belt-drive system.

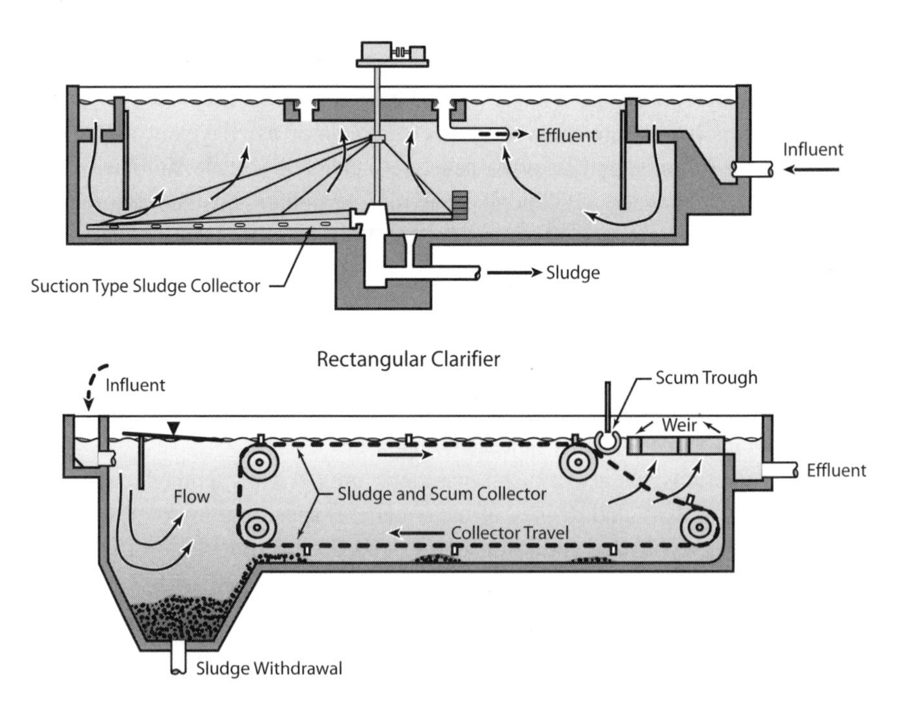

FIGURE 14–11. Typical clarifier units.

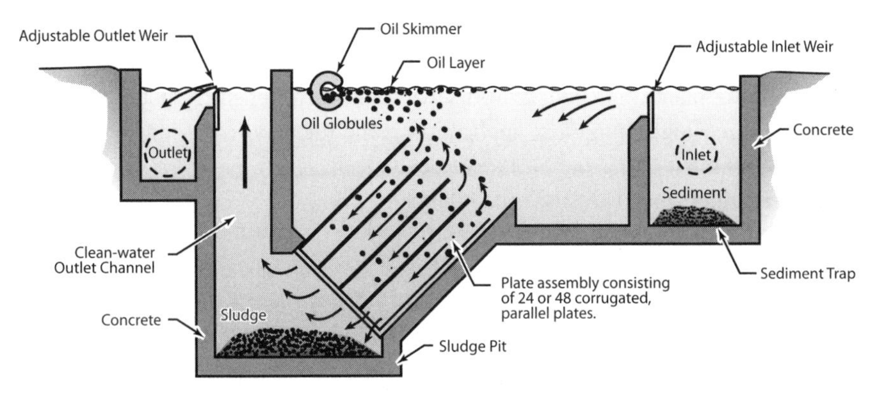

FIGURE 14–12. Corrugated-plate interceptor separator.

An oil/water separator is used to separate free oil from refinery waste water. This type of unit will not separate soluble substances, or break emulsions.

A corrugated-plate interceptor for oil is shown in Figure 14–12. Waste water enters a separator bay and flows downward through corrugated plates arranged at an angle of 45° to the horizontal. Oil collects on the underside of the plates and rises to the surface where it is skimmed. Solids settle into a sludge compartment, with the now-clarified waste discharging into an outlet channel.

In dissolved air flotation, illustrated in Figure 14–13, air is intimately contacted with an aqueous stream at high pressure, dissolving the air. The pressure on the liquid is reduced through a back-pressure valve, thereby releasing micrometer-sized bubbles that sweep suspended solids and oil from the contaminanted stream to the surface of the air-flotation unit. Applications of this tech-

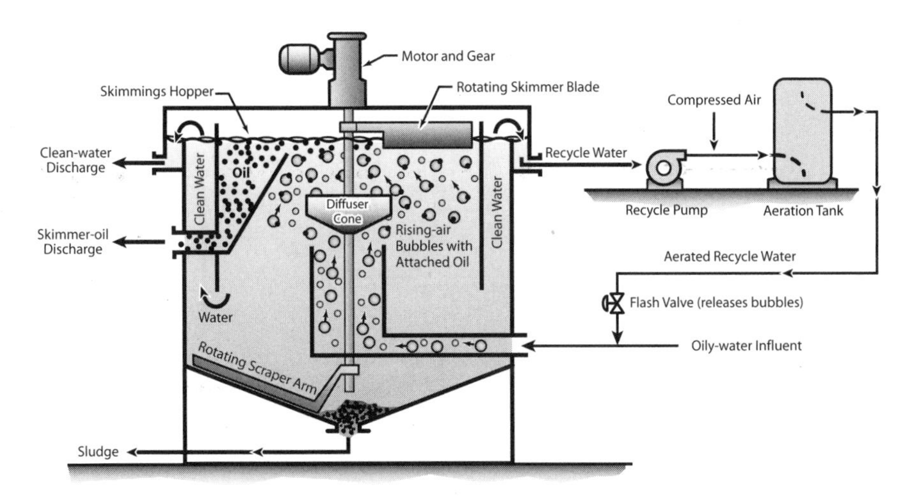

FIGURE 14–13. Dissolved-air flotation unit.

nique include treating effluents from oil refineries, metal-finishing processes, pulp and paper mills, cold-rolling mills, poultry processing, grease recovery in meat-packing plants, and cooking-oil separation from french-fry potato processing. An increasingly important application is the thickening of sludge.

The attachment of gas bubbles to suspended solids or oily materials occurs by several mechanisms. The suspended-solids/gas mixture is carried to the vessel surface after: *(1)* precipitation of air on the particle; *(2)* collision of a rising bubble with a suspended particle; *(3)* trapping of gas bubbles, as they rise, under a floc particle; and *(4)* adsorption of the gas by a floc formed or precipitated around the air bubble.

Flocculants, such as synthetic polymers, may be used to improve the effectiveness of dissolved-air flotation. Also, coagulants, such as alum, may be used to break emulsified oils and to agglomerate materials for improved flotation recovery.

Flotation can also be achieved by induced air, as illustrated in Figure 14–14. Air drawn into the flotation cell by action of the rotor is mixed with the water and transformed into minute bubbles. Oil particles and suspended solids attach themselves to the gas bubbles and are borne to the surface of the water. Skimmer paddles push the contaminated froth from the top of the cell into collection launders. The tank is designed with sloping sides at the lower part to recirculate the water for continuous purification. The conical shape of the dispenser hood, with its perforated surface, acts to quiet the liquid surface.

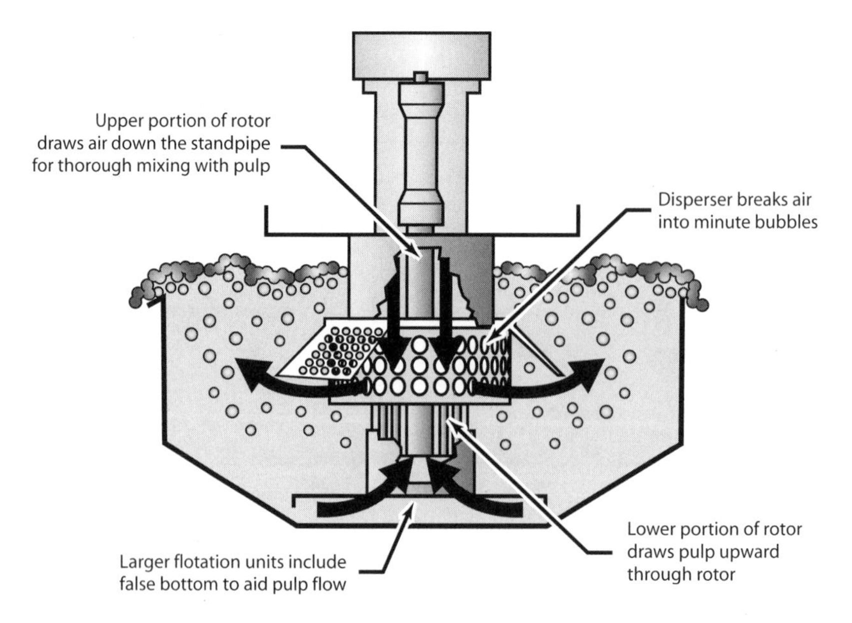

FIGURE 14–14. Induced-air flotation unit.

Efficiency of contaminant removal in induced-air devices is often improved with chemical aids injected in the water, upstream in the flotation cell. In addition to breaking oil-water emulsions, they also make the air bubbles more stable and promote formation of froth on the surface of the water. Properly conditioned wastes leave the device nearly 100% oil-free, and the suspended solid load is also significantly reduced.

Filtration. Granular-media filtration is a liquid–solids separation method that uses flow through porous media, such as sand, to remove particulate matter. To be readily filterable, the suspended solids must either be naturally flocculent, or be made so by chemical coagulation. Granular media filters are used for removal of solids (and oil) from refinery waste waters, for effluents from activated-sludge treatment plants (see next section) and for effluents from pulp and paper plants. Heavy metal precipitates may be recovered in granular filters, and process streams are clarified by similar units.

The heart of any granular-media filter is the filter bed. The size and depth of the filter medium are the most important design parameters. As an example of granular-media filtration, the operation of a shallow-bed, gravity, granular-media filter is shown in Figure 14–15. The filter is completely automatic on a controlled cycle. Several filters are customarily used in parallel to avoid interruption of the flow stream when the filter backwashes. During filtration, waste

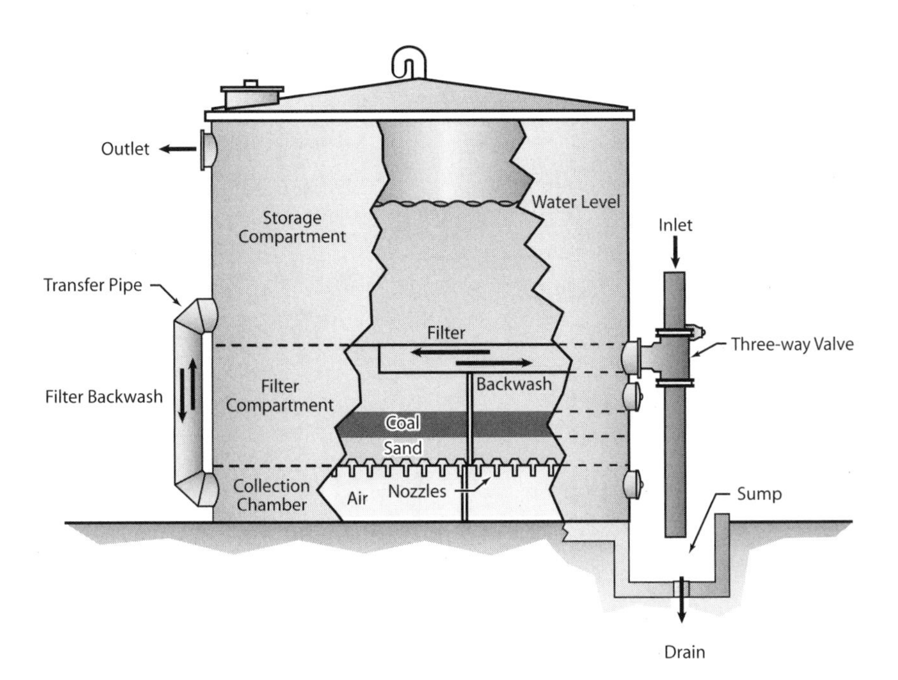

FIGURE 14–15. Granular-media filter (shallow bed, gravity type).

water is passed through the media, and solids are removed. As the cycle progresses, the pressure drop across the filter increases to a preset maximum, indicating that the bed is full of suspended solids, and a backwash-cycle controller is energized. Alternately, a timed cycle or monitoring of the suspended solids may be used to terminate filtration.

Backwash water flows by gravity through the collection chamber and the filter compartment to remove the suspended solids that were fluidized by the air wash. The backwash discharges by gravity to settling basins, where all of the suspended solids settle out and water is recovered. The addition of polymers to the backwash water accelerates the settling rate of the solids.

Biological Treatment

Biological oxidation is the major process for the removal of oxygen demand in sewage wastes; it also finds extensive use for the treatment of industrial wastes containing biodegradable organics. In biological oxidative processes, concentrated masses of microorganisms break down organic matter. These microorganisms are broadly classified as aerobic, facultative, or anaerobic. Aerobic organisms require oxygen for metabolism, anaerobes function in the absence of oxygen, and facultative microbes may function in either an aerobic or anaerobic environment. Where land is relatively stable and inexpensive, cost-effective treatment can be done in simple ponds. Figure 14–16 shows the general characteristics of such ponds.

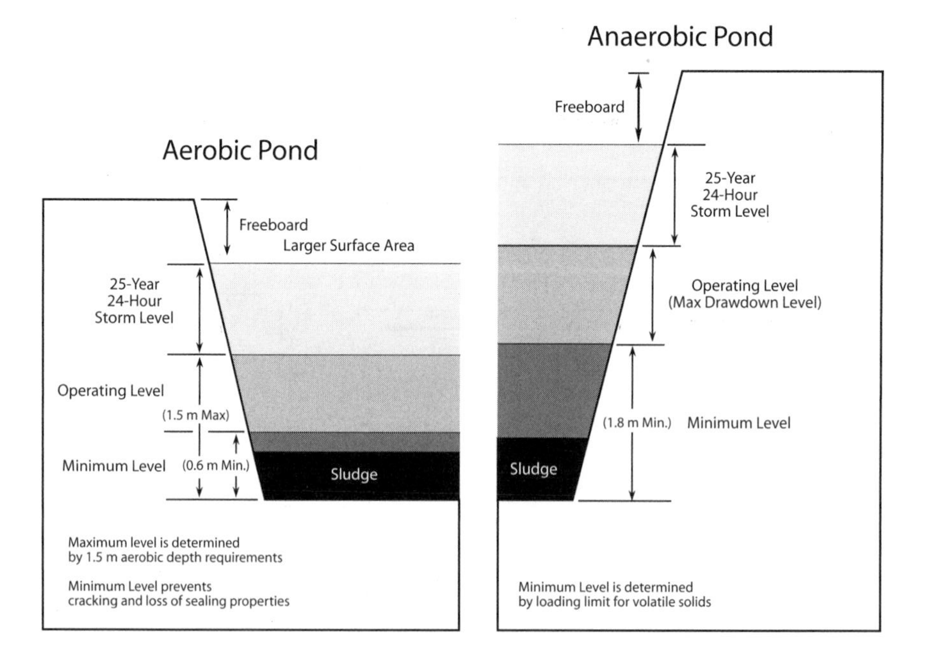

FIGURE 14–16. Basic characteristics of ponds for biological treatment of waste waters.

The predominant species used in biological systems are known as heterotrophic microorganisms; these require an organic carbon source for both energy and cell synthesis. Autotrophic organisms, in contrast, use an inorganic carbon source, such as carbon dioxide or carbonate. The autotrophs may derive energy for cell synthesis from the oxidation of inorganic compounds of nitrogen or sulfur (chemosynthetic bacteria), or from the sun (photosynthetic bacteria).

Basically, biological oxidative processes involve either of two mechanisms to accumulate and store the microbes: *(1)* as a flocculated suspension of biological growth known as activated sludge, which is mixed with the waste waters; or *(2)* as a biological film fixed to an inert medium, over which the waste waters pass.

Biological processes may not be applicable to many specific industrial waste waters. For example, cyclic organics, especially if halogenated, are resistant to biological degradation. Organochlorine pesticides may prove toxic to a biosystem if discharged in high concentrations. Slightly soluble components, such as PCB's or heavy metals, can accumulate in a biological system through adsorption and bioconcentration and may, thereby, reach levels inhibitory to the process.

Microbial populations may be specifically adapted to certain chemicals to successfully achieve oxidation. Examples of materials that are biodegradable under acclimated conditions are cyanide, phenol, formaldehyde, acrylonitrile, and hydroquinone. However, some cyanide compounds, such as the metallic-cyanide complexes, are highly resistant to degradation, even under strongly acclimated conditions.

The activated-sludge process is a continuous system in which aerobic bacteria are mixed with waste water and then physically separated by gravity clarification or by air flotation. As shown in Figure 14–17, the concentrated sludge is recycled to the reactor to mix with the incoming waste. Oxygen is provided in a variety of ways, for example, by diffused aeration, surface aeration, or static mixers, and may be introduced either as air, pure oxygen, or oxygen-enriched air. The waste product from the activated-sludge process is excess sludge, which must ultimately be disposed of, generally after partial reduction by anaerobic digestion.

As the concentration of organics in the remaining waste waters decreases, the rate of biological removal also decreases, since the remaining organics are progressively more difficult to remove. In the treatment of industrial wastes, a significant fraction of the organics may prove nonbiodegradable. Thus, although the BOD removal may be excellent, the removal of COD may be quite low.

The activated-sludge process is broadly applicable. It is used in the treatment of soluble organic wastes from many industries, including food processing, meat packing, pulp and paper, oil refining, leather tanning, textiles, organic chemical, and petrochemical.

A major modification to the conventional air-aerated activated sludge process has been the use of high purity oxygen. Some advantages of this compared to the conventional system are lower land requirements, the ability to supply oxy-

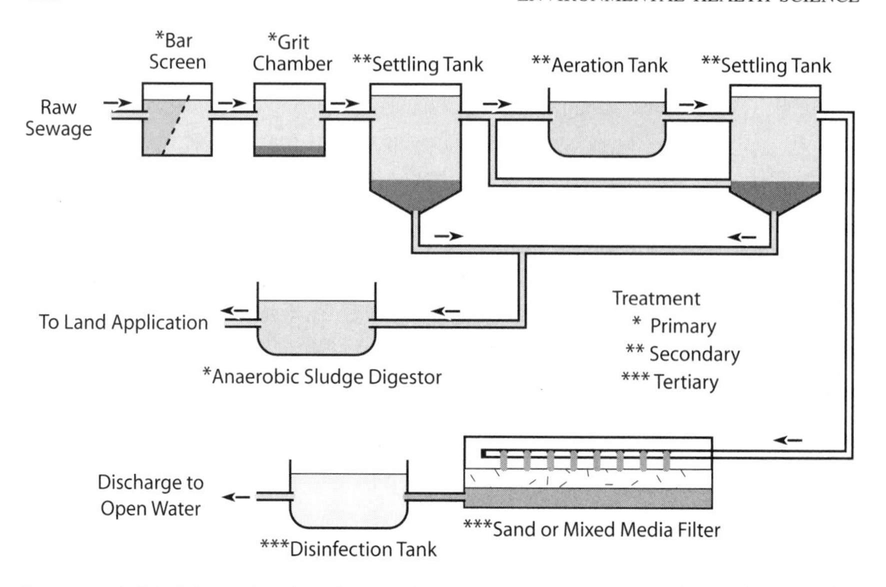

FIGURE 14–17. Schematic of typical modern waste water treatment plant using aeration tank digestion.

gen at high rates (making it amenable to high-strength wastes), and increased self-neutralization of highly alkaline wastes.

Increasingly stringent effluent criteria require the removal of inorganic nutrients, such as nitrogen, prior to stream discharge into a natural receiving water. Activated-sludge systems have been successfully operated for nitrogen removal, via the processes of nitrification and denitrification.

Nitrification is achieved by autotrophic nitrite bacteria, organisms that convert reduced nitrogen (as NH_3) to nitrite and nitrate bacteria that further oxidize the nitrite to nitrate. Sufficient alkalinity must be available to offset the production of nitrous and nitric acids.

The growth rate of the nitrifiers is significantly lower than that of the heterotrophic bacteria used in the breakdown of carbonaceous organic matter. Thus, in the presence of significant amounts of carbonaceous organic material, the nitrifiers are unable to compete successfully with the heterotrophs and cannot accumulate as significant populations. The process may, therefore, have to be a two-stage system, where carbonaceous removal is achieved in the first stage, and nitrification is performed in the second. Interstage clarification allows segregation of the two types of bacteria.

Denitrification is a biological process by which nitrite and nitrate are reduced to nitrogen gas. Facultative, heterotrophic bacteria found in activated sludges are capable of performing denitrification. Since these organisms require an organic-carbon source for cell growth, and because this process generally follows secondary treatment, some form of organic compound must be present or added.

Approximately 4.5 lb of COD (typically as methanol) per lb of nitrate are required to reduce the nitrate to nitrogen.

The predominant fixed-film biological process is the trickling filter. This is a packed bed of some medium (such as stones) covered with a biological slime, over which waste water is passed. Oxygen and organic matter diffuse into the slime film, where degradation reactions occur. End products such as CO_2, NO_3^-, etc., counter-diffuse back out of the film and appear in the filter effluent.

Trickling filters have found limited application for industrial waste waters. Removal rates for soluble industrial wastes are typically low, making filters unattractive for high BOD-removal efficiency. The process is, however, capable of accepting highly variable loadings, and, thus, may be used as a roughing filter to provide partial treatment.

Another type of fixed-film biological reactor is the rotating disk process.

Plastic disks are mounted on a shaft and placed in a tank conforming to the general shape of the disks. The disks are slowly rotated while approximately half immersed in the waste water. Rotation brings the attached bacteria culture into contact with the waste water for removal of organic matter. Rotation also provides a means of aeration, by exposing a thin film of waste water on the disk surface to the air.

Biological oxidation may be achieved in ponds, lagoons, and basins, or in soil after land application of waste water. The land requirements for oxygen demand removal are greater in these systems than those required for fixed-film processes, and are much greater than those for activated-sludge processes.

In aerated stabilization basins, air is pumped into the water or the water is sprayed through the air to increase the oxygen-demand removal capacity. In ordinary stabilization and oxidation ponds and in land irrigation, natural aeration rates are the limiting factor in determining the capacity for oxygen-demand removal.

Combined Biological and Chemical Treatment

The continuous addition of powdered activated carbon to aeration tanks of suspended-bacterial systems can improve the operation and performance of the activated sludge. The activated carbon gives the system the capability of adsorbing nonbiodegradable organic matter present in the waste waters, thereby providing a degree of tertiary treatment, and resistance to shock-loading (i.e., sudden input of a large amount of a chemical). The carbon is regenerated by pyrolysis.

Chemical Oxidation

The chemical oxidants widely used today are chlorine, ozone, and hydrogen peroxide. Their historical use, particularly for chlorine and ozone, has been for disinfection of water and waste waters. They are, however, receiving increased consideration for removing, from waste waters, organic materials that are resistant to biological or other treatment processes.

Ozone is found to be effective in many applications: for color removal, disinfection, taste and odor removal, iron and manganese removal, and in the oxidation of many complex organics, including lindane, aldrin, surfactants, cyanides, phenols, and organometal complexes. With the latter, the metal ion is released, and can be removed by precipitation.

Chlorine (and its more readily storable form, hypochlorite ion, or bleach) has long been used to purify water, destroy organisms in waste water and swimming pools, and oxidize chemicals in aqueous solutions. The destruction of cyanide and phenols by chlorine oxidation is well known in waste treatment technology. The continued use of chlorine for these applications is, however, uncertain, because of concern about the toxicity and carcinogenicity of chlorine oxidation products.

Advanced Waste Water Treatment Processes

Most conventional waste water–treatment facilities use primary and secondary-treatment stages. Table 14–8 shows typical removal efficiencies for BOD, suspended solids, and dissolved solids by these processes; dissolved solids, which may include many toxic chemicals, are not effectively removed by this treatment. Some emerging technologies for bioremediation are described in Table 14–9.

Various physical and chemical processes are used in tertiary or advanced treatment to bring the water to a higher quality level than that achievable by conventional primary and secondary treatment. The methods include air (ammonia) stripping, electrodialysis, activated carbon adsorption, reverse osmosis, distillation, and ion exchange.

Ammonia can be removed from waste water by the technique of air stripping, which involves pH control of the water. Ammonium ions in the water exist in equilibrium with ammonia and hydrogen ions. As the pH increases (usually by the addition of lime), the equilibrium shifts to the right, and above a pH of 9,

Table 14–8. Approximate Removal Efficiencies of Waste Water Treatment Stages

	Percentage Reduction from Original Waste Water		
Contaminant Category	Primary Treatment	Secondary Treatment	Tertiary Treatment
BOD	30	90	99.8
Suspended solids	60	90	100
Dissolved inorganic solids	0	5	99.5

BOD, biochemical oxygen demand.

TABLE 14–9. Current Feasibility of Bioremediation

CHEMICAL CLASS	FREQUENCY OF OCCURRENCE	STATUS OF BIOREMEDIATION	EVIDENCE OF FUTURE SUCCESS	LIMITATIONS
Hydrocarbons and derivatives				
Gasoline, fuel oil	Very frequent	Established		Forms nonaqueous-phase liquid
Polycyclic aromatic hydrocarbons	Common	Emerging	Aerobically biodegradable under a narrow range of conditions	Sorbs strongly to subsurface solids
Creosote	Infrequent	Emerging	Readily biodegradable under aerobic conditions	Sorbs strongly to subsurface solids; forms nonaqueous-phase liquid
Alcohols, ketones, esters	Common	Established		
Ethers	Common	Emerging	Biodegradable under a narrow range of conditions using aerobic or nitrate-reducing microbes	
Halogenated aliphatics				
Highly chlorinated	Very frequent	Emerging	Cometabolized by anaerobic microbes; cometabolized by aerobes in special cases	Forms nonaqueous-phase liquid
Less chlorinated	Very frequent	Emerging	Aerobically biodegradable under a narrow range of conditions; cometabolized by anaerobic microbes	Forms nonaqueous-phase liquid

(*continued*)

TABLE 14–9. Current Feasibility of Bioremediation (*continued*)

CHEMICAL CLASS	FREQUENCY OF OCCURRENCE	STATUS OF BIOREMEDIATION	EVIDENCE OF FUTURE SUCCESS	LIMITATIONS
Halogenated aromatics				
Highly chlorinated	Common	Emerging	Aerobically biodegradable under a narrow range of conditions; cometabolized by anaerobic microbes	Sorbs strongly to subsurface solids; forms nonaqueous phase-solid or liquid
Less chlorinated	Common	Emerging	Readily biodegradable under aerobic conditions	Forms nonaqueous phase-solid or liquid
Polychlorinated biphenyls				
Highly chlorinated	Infrequent	Emerging	Cometabolized by anaerobic microbes	Sorbs strongly to subsurface solids
Less chlorinated	Infrequent	Emerging	Aerobically biodegradable under a narrow range of conditions	Sorbs strongly to subsurface solids
Nitroaromatics	Common	Emerging	Aerobically biodegradable; converted to innocuous volatile organic acids under anaerobic conditions	
Metals (Cr, Du, Ni, Pb, Hg, Cd, Zn, etc.)	Common	Possible	Solubility and reactivity can be changed by a variety of microbial processes	Availability highly variable and controlled by solution- and solid-phase chemistry

ammonia may be liberated as a gas by agitating the waste water in the presence of air.

Electrodialysis uses an induced electric current to separate the cationic and anionic components of a solution. It relies on membranes, which are at right angles to the line of electric current flow, that permit ions to pass from a dilute solution on one side to a concentrated solution on the other.

Activated carbon adsorption is used for the removal of soluble organic matter not removed by conventional methods. Water passes through granular activated carbon, where organic molecules attach to the carbon surface. When the carbon reaches its adsorptive capacity, it is regenerated by pyrolysis. Large particles are removed by filtration or coagulation–sedimentation prior to carbon adsorption.

Reverse osmosis forces water at high pressures through cellulose acetate membranes against the natural osmotic pressure. The mechanisms responsible for the action of the membranes in reverse osmosis include sieving, surface tension, and hydrogen bonding. The technique removes dissolved solids.

Distillation is a vapor–liquid transfer operation for removal of dissolved solids, in which vapor is driven from waste water by heat. Because of its high cost, distillation has limited application in waste water reclamation.

Ion exchange is a very effective technique for the removal of ions from waste water. Various natural materials and synthetic ion-exchange resins may be used. Some common applications are for Cl^-, $NH_4{}^+$, $PO_4{}^{-3}$ and metal ion removal.

Control of Chemical Contamination from Diffuse Sources

Adequate control of discharges into surface waters from sewage treatment plants and industrial operations is technically feasible, even if not always achieved. It is more difficult to control the discharge of chemical contaminants associated with diffuse sources, such as the drainage from agricultural land. Such drainage contains a variety of pesticides and nutrients which can adversely affect aquatic organisms and stream productivity.

Some agricultural operations use oxidation lagoons to reduce the oxygen demand of animal wastes. However, the best prospects for reducing the fertilizer and pesticide burdens in runoff water appear to lie in educating farm operators about the problem, with the hope that they will apply these chemicals in quantities and by procedures that will minimize adverse environmental effects. Some of the problems have been, and will continue to be, resolved by the removal of the more toxic pesticides from the market.

Control of Drinking Water Quality

The provision of bacteriologically pure drinking water is one of the more notable public health success stories in this country. Disease transmission via public drinking water supplies is, fortunately, a rare event.

There are two ways to accomplish the delivery of high-quality drinking water. One is to have an adequate volume supply of clean natural water. The other is to purify and disinfect available water to the point that it is safe to use. A typical modern treatment plant system for the supply of drinking water is illustrated schematically in Figure 14–18. Another key factor is continual monitoring of the purity of the water, not only at central distributing points, but also at various points within the distribution system where it is used, to make sure that clean water is delivered to the consumer.

Selection of clean natural water sources

Natural waters, with little or no treatment other than light disinfection with chlorine, are used as drinking-water supplies by a large proportion of the people in this country. Some cities, most notably New York and Boston, maintain protected watershed areas and reservoirs that collect and distribute rainwater. Many other cities and smaller towns use groundwater from deep wells for drinking purposes. Such groundwater may be "hard," but is usually of very good quality in terms of bacterial content. Water from shallow wells in urban areas can readily by contaminated, and must be monitored carefully.

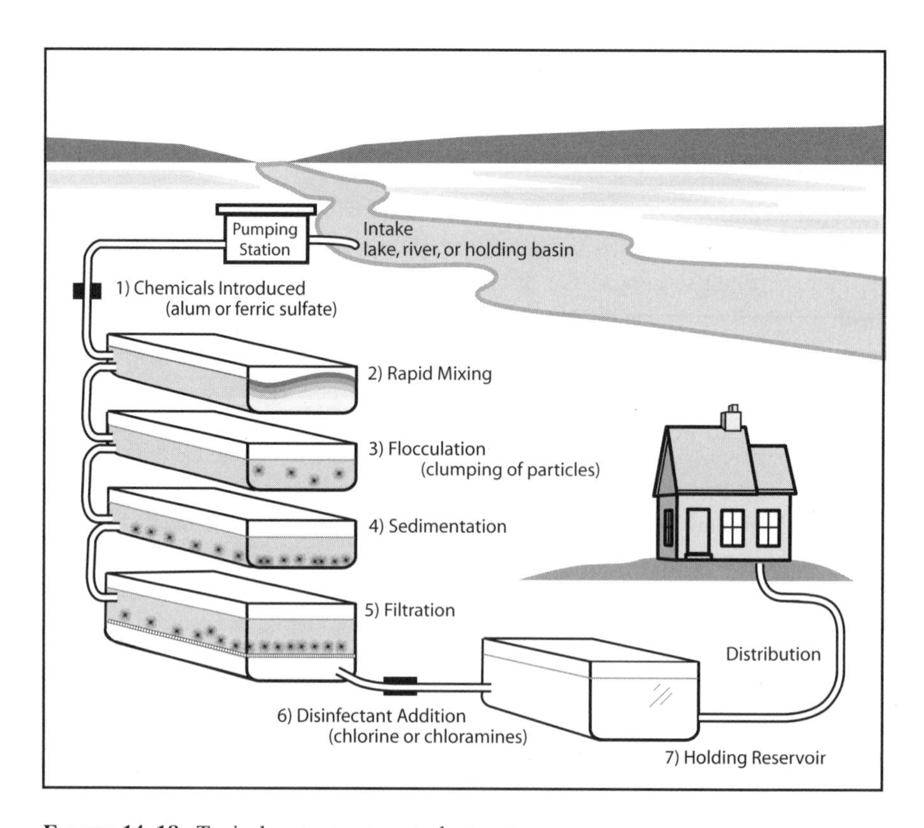

FIGURE 14–18. Typical water treatment plant system.

Little attention was paid to the chemical purity of drinking water until the mid-1900s. The extent of the problem arising from the increasing content of organic compounds and trace elements in drinking water has not yet been adequately defined.

Purification of contaminated ground water

When ground water is used as a potable water supply, it must either not be contaminated by surface sources of toxic chemicals, or it must be pretreated as are surface water supplies. Techniques are being developed to clean up locally contaminated ground water supplies. An example is shown in Figure 14–19.

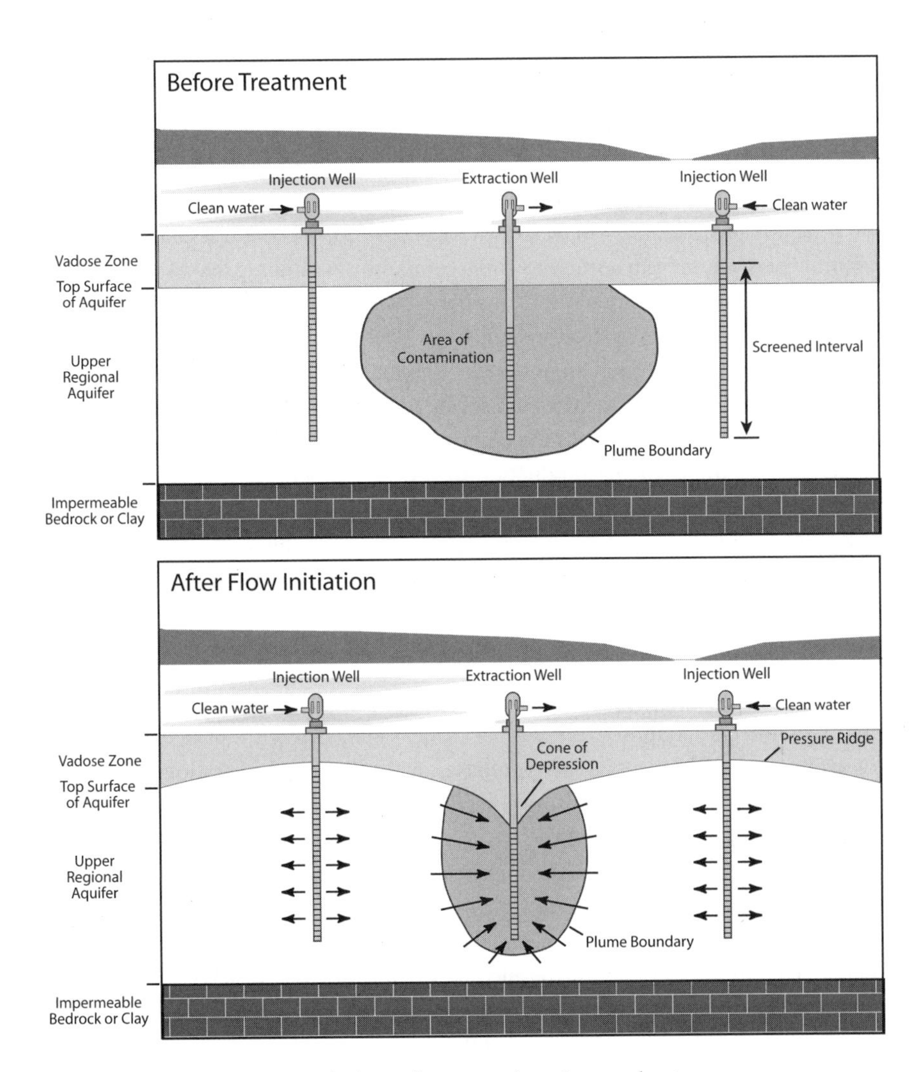

FIGURE 14–19. Treatment techniques for contaminated groundwater.

IMPACT OF AIR AND WATER CONTROLS ON ENVIRONMENTAL QUALITY

The intended effect of controls, and generally their main impact, is to reduce or eliminate releases of toxic or otherwise harmful chemicals to the workroom air or general environment. To the extent that controls are successful, they are beneficial. However, the instillation and operation of control devices does not ensure that all problems will be totally eliminated or that others will fail to develop.

Controls as Contaminant Sources

Control devices may actually be sources of contaminants. For example, if the collection efficiency for a given contaminant is not high enough, the control device may release some of the contaminant into the environment. A collector may be the source of a highly concentrated toxic material, or of a large volume of material. In many cases, the collected materials represent significant problems with respect to their handling and ultimate disposal in an environmentally acceptable manner.

There are several other ways in which controls may serve as significant sources of contaminants. Controls may consist of a network of conduits that prevent or control the releases from numerous small sources by combining them into one large source. This may solve some problems but create a new larger one. Problems may also develop when the control procedure involves chemical reactions for the purpose of contaminant degradation or neutralization. The by-products and secondary products of these reactions may themselves be harmful, for example, organochlorine compounds resulting from the chlorination of drinking water.

Another example of the production of a new problem by a control device is the release of excessive moisture, forming fogs, by some types of cooling towers used to remove heat from cooling waters. They may also release into the ambient air some of the chemicals used to prevent algae growth on the tower walls.

Incomplete Capture

The design efficiency of a contaminant-control device is generally selected on the basis of: *(1)* its ability to meet an effluent standard with an assured margin of safety; and *(2)* the cost of its purchase, instillation, and operation. These two considerations become increasingly difficult to reconcile as the desired collection efficiency approaches 100%.

When very high collection efficiencies are needed, it is generally more constructive to consider penetration rather than efficiency; the percent penetration (P) is the complement of the percent efficiency (E), i.e., $P = 100 - E$. There may not seem to be a great difference between efficiencies of 90%, 95%, 98%, 99%, and 99.5%, but their significance becomes clearer when considered as a penetration of 10%, 5%, 2%, 1%, and 0.5% respectively. Each now differs from the other by a factor of approximately 2, and the increased cost of achieving each increment may be quite large.

The strengths of collection devices as contaminant sources vary directly as their penetration efficiencies. Thus, for example, a new power-plant electrostatic precipitator having a 99% collection efficiency, which replaces one having a 90% efficiency, will discharge ten times less fly ash. While this may have a large effect on airborne total suspended particulate and some trace-metal concentrations, it will have relatively little impact on the ash-disposal problem. There would be only a 10% increase in collected fly ash, and less than that for the combined fly-ash and bottom-ash mass.

Formation of Secondary Contaminants and Release of Trace Contaminants in Effluents

In collectors that act as simple traps, where contaminants are removed from the effluent stream by physical processes such as filtration, electrostatic precipitation, scrubbing, adsorption, and condensation, the collected materials are not changed chemically, although in wet collectors they may be dissolved or suspended in water. On the other hand, in collectors utilizing chemical reactions to capture, oxidize, or neutralize the waste, the residual reaction products will differ in composition from the original materials. The major reaction products will usually be innocuous or relatively easy to handle. If this was not the case, the process would not have been selected in the first place. Problems may arise, however, from the presence of trace contaminants in the waste.

The problem of the release of trace contaminants may be exemplified by considering incineration, which is an effective means of reducing the weight and bulk of household refuse and waste paper and, to an increasing degree, may be favored as a means of resource recovery in terms of its heating value. However, mixed refuse may contain, for example, chemically treated papers, halogenated plastics, discarded batteries containing lead, mercury, nickel, and cadmium, and a host of other chemicals; these constituents may be vaporized and injected into the atmosphere along with the waste gases.

A classic example of the formation of a secondary contaminant in a control device involves the adoption of catalytic converters in motor vehicle exhaust systems. As discussed in Chapter 3, no consideration was initially given to the oxidation of the SO_2 in the exhaust to SO_3, and the hydrolysis of the latter in the exhaust stream to sulfuric acid mist.

DISPOSAL OF COLLECTED MATERIALS AND PROCESS SLUDGES

A first consideration in disposing of waste materials is to reduce the volume of materials needing disposal. The first consideration should always be waste minimization through process changes that reduce waste generation. A second consideration is the option for recycling the waste materials to recover the economic values for productive usages.

The technology of resource recovery has advanced greatly in recent years. This is illustrated for materials recovery in Figure 14–20, and for energy recovery in Figure 14–21.

The ultimate and safe disposal of liquid and solid wastes and treatment plant residues (see Fig. 14–9) is one of the most important current concerns of environmental protection and public health authorities. There are no easy, foolproof, or inexpensive solutions to most of the current problems.

Control devices such as incinerators, which destroy chemical contaminants, will produce relatively little residue material requiring disposal. On the other hand, most control devices that extract chemicals from air or liquid streams, or react them to form secondary chemicals, create difficult disposal problems. The wastes may be dry solids, concentrated suspensions of solids in water (slurries and sludges), or concentrated organic or aqueous solutions. These wastes may require further treatment or degradation before they can be disposed of in an environmentally acceptable manner.

Incineration

For combustible wastes, incineration has the advantages of relatively low cost and possibilities for heat recovery. The residual ash occupies less than 10% of the volume of the original waste, and is usually a relatively innocuous, soil-like material. However incineration can create smoke and odor nuisances. Even with nominally complete combustion, there will be unburned and noncombustible volatile contaminants in the exhaust, as previously discussed. Exhaust gas cleaners, when installed, reduce the cost advantages of incinerators, and may not collect some of the materials of interest, for example, mercury vapor. Contaminants that escape into the atmosphere will eventually be deposited on land or surface waters, becoming available for uptake into the biosphere.

Land Disposal

Most solid refuse is disposed of in sanitary landfills. The basic construction of a modern landfill is illustrated in Figure 14–22. Each layer of refuse is compacted and covered with a layer of earth or clean fill. The earth cover absorbs odorous gases of decomposition and acts as a barrier to pests and vermin. Filled land gradually settles as the waste decomposes. Thus, these areas should not be used for residential or commercial purposes without special precautions, not only because of the settlement problem, but because explosive concentrations of methane gas can build up in basement areas. Landfills in urban

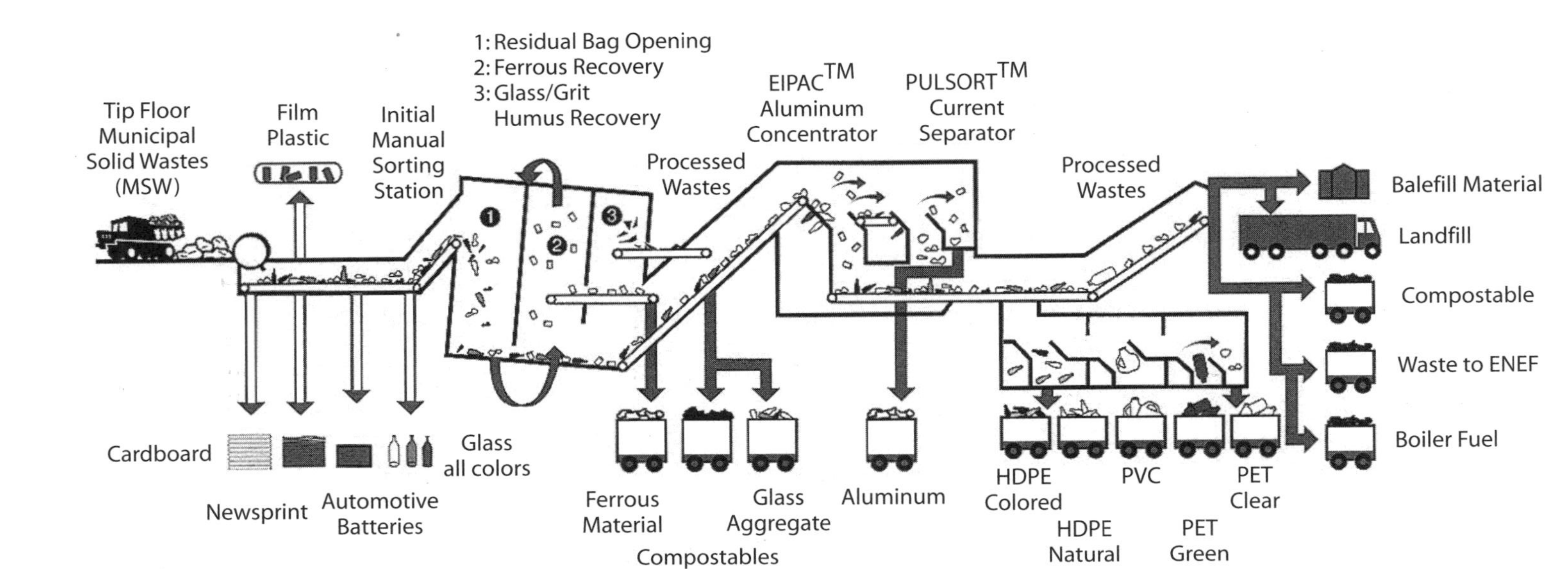

FIGURE 14–20. Schematic diagram of advanced technology for separation and recovery of materials in municipal solid wastes.

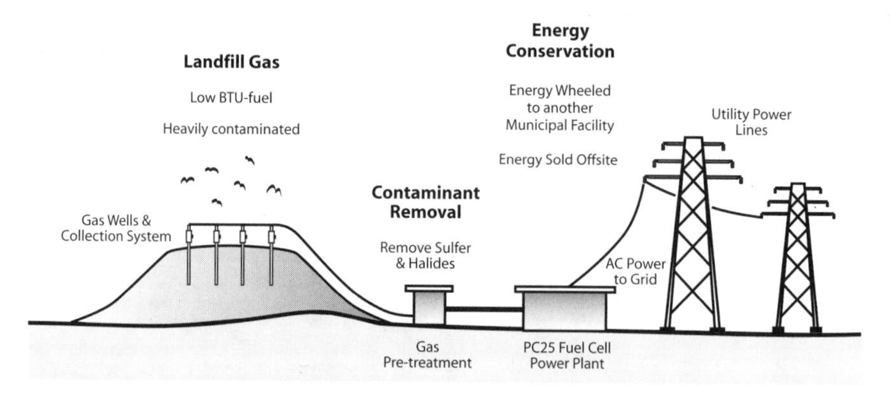

FIGURE 14–21. Schematic diagram of recovery and use of landfill gases. (*Source*: Adapted from EPA 600-R-97-008.)

areas have usually been used for recreational purposes, such as parks and golf courses.

A major problem in the selection of suitable areas for landfill, and their successful operation, is the isolation from groundwater of the leachate solutions that form in the wastes. It is generally necessary to line the bottom of the landfill with an impervious layer of clay to control the drainage patterns, and to pump out the leachate for subsequent biological treatment.

Underground Disposal

Some highly toxic and radioactive solid and liquid wastes are stored in natural underground caverns or in chambers excavated in selected geological strata such as salt domes. The sites are selected for their inaccessibility and isolation from groundwater and for their supposed geologic stability.

Large volumes of liquid wastes are disposed of by deep-well injection into underground strata. Wells are drilled into suitable permeable strata that are isolated from groundwater sources by impermeable strata and the well casing. A schematic diagram of a waste-liquid injection well is shown in Figure 14–23. Strata suitable for deep-well disposal are located in many parts of the United States, primarily in the western parts of the country.

Problems occasionally develop due to the instability of the underground rock strata. Liquids pumped into certain strata at high pressures can act as lubricants, causing slippage of contact surfaces; this effect is manifested as earthquakes at the surface. The close correlation between the times of active pumping of wastes by the U. S. Army Rocky Mountain Arsenal near Denver and the occurrence of earthquakes in the Denver region in the mid-1960s led to discontinuance of deep-well disposal there.

Old-Style Sanitary Landfall

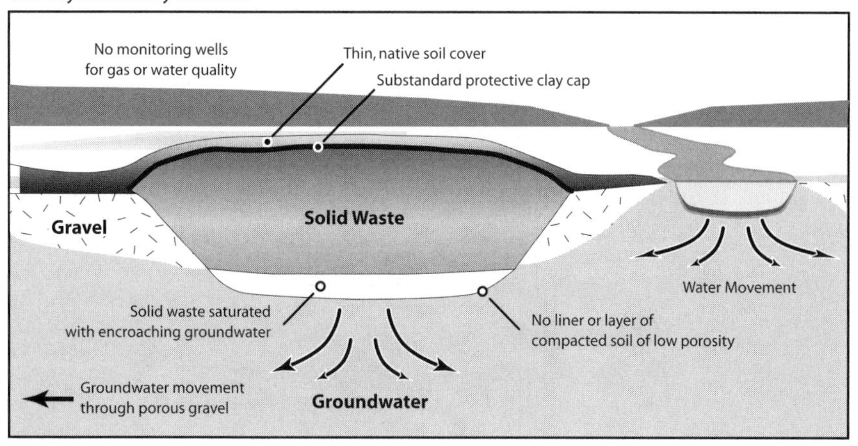

Modern Sanitary Landfall

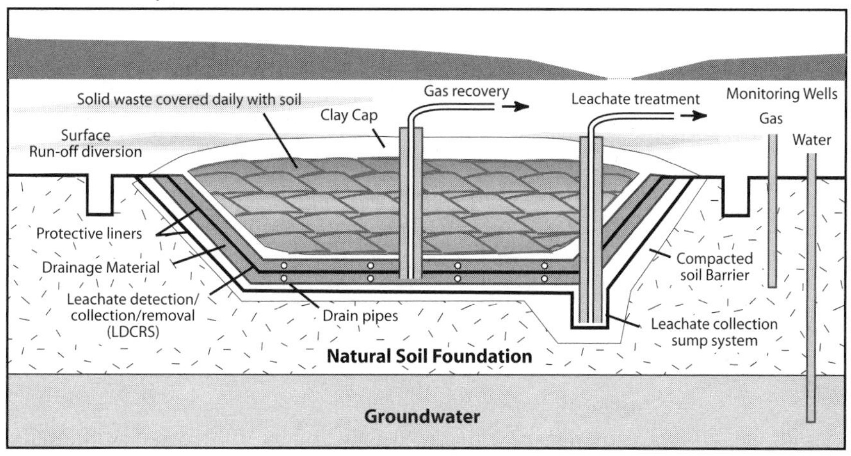

Figure 14–22. Schematic diagram of convential and more modern sanitary landfills.

Disposal in the Oceans

There are several different kinds of ocean disposal, and it is important not to confuse them. One is the disposal of waste liquid or slurries into surface waters relatively close to shore. Huge volumes of sewage sludge and industrial acid wastes have been disposed of in this manner, with the implicit rationalization that the wastes were degraded and/or neutralized within the ocean and did not accumulate excessively or do permanent damage to marine life.

Near-shoreline marine disposal is also done using pipelines that extend for distances up to several miles out to sea. In this case, the discharge is at the lower, rather than the upper, surface of the water. Such systems have been used for dis-

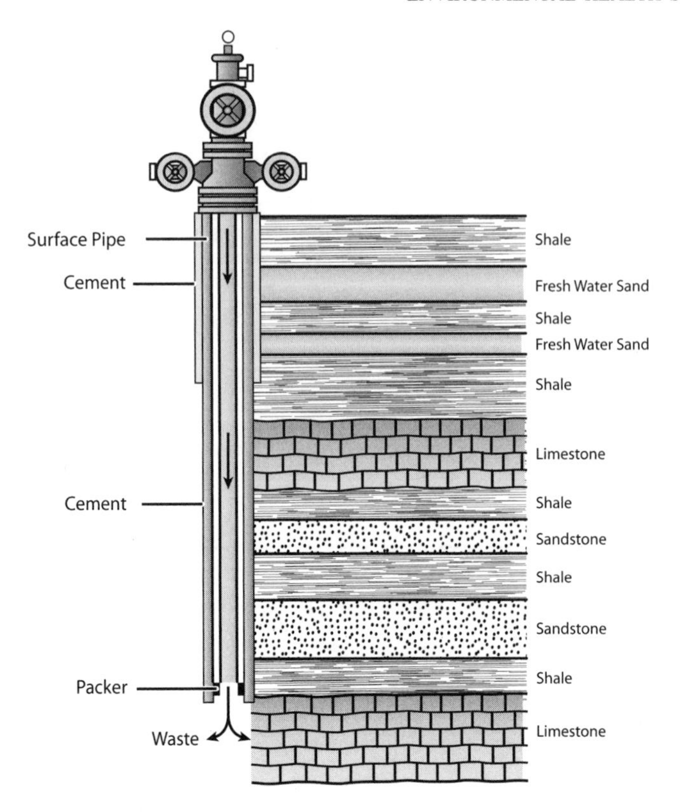

FIGURE 14–23. Deep-well disposal system. The well casing must be cemented in place to protect ground water.

posal of raw sewage by coastal cities, and may appear to be adequate initially. However, they are usually found wanting as population and sewage volume increase, especially when on-shore winds deposit floating sewage solids on the beaches. Problems may also arise when the pipe develops leaks, since inspection and maintenance are difficult and expensive.

Deep-ocean dumping is theoretically a safe and effective means of disposal for dangerous wastes. As discussed in Chapter 4, vertical diffusivity in ocean water is extremely low, and should provide an effective barrier against transfer to the surface water for periods of hundreds to thousands of years. However, diffusivity is the controlling factor only for dissolved materials; for particulate matter, their effective density would be controlling. Materials with low density, or particles of high-density materials with attached gas bubbles, could rise rapidly through the water. In addition, if the materials are ingested by marine organisms that migrate vertically or are consumed by predators who do, these chemicals can be readily transported toward the surface.

RISK REDUCTION OPTIONS

This chapter has emphasized the technical aspects of risk reduction, which is a major component of risk management. However, it should be remembered that risk management decisions will always also be influenced by other valid considerations. Figure 14–2, from a recent EPA Science Advisory Board (SAB) report[2] illustrates the iterative nature of risk management at EPA.

In practice, there are major information gap differences in risk management priorities within the political and federal agency cultures that make it quite difficult to allocate political and economic resources when making choices among the various risk reduction options.

To illustrate the issues facing the leadership at EPA, let us consider ambient air pollution. When they attempt to determine the extent of any health risk existing among the members of the population of concern resulting from the inhalation of airborne chemicals they need to know: *(1)* the distribution of the concentration of the agent in the air and, for airborne PM, the distribution of particle sizes; and *(2)* the unit risk factor, i.e., the number of cases and/or the extent of the adverse effects associated with a unit of exposure. For more sophisticated analyses, we may also need to know more about the population of concern, such as the distribution of ages, preexisting diseases, predisposing factors for illness, such as cigarette smoking, dietary deficiencies or excesses, etc. These factors were discussed in some detail in Chapter 13.

When basic information on ambient levels and unit risks is available, it is relatively straightforward to compute, tabulate, and compare the risks associated with the different chemicals in community air. However, such direct comparisons can, in practice, only be made with any quantitative reality for a handful of chemicals, i.e., the so-called criteria pollutants, whose ambient air levels are routinely monitored and for which directly measured human exposure-response relationships have been developed. For hundreds of other airborne chemicals, known collectively as hazardous air pollutants (HAPs) or air toxics, there are neither extensive ambient air concentration data nor unit risk factors that do not intentionally err on the side of safety. This disparity has resulted from the different control philosophies built into the CAA and maintained by the EPA as a part of its regulatory strategy. The rationale for the distinction is that criteria pollutants come from numerous and widespread sources, have relatively uniform concentrations across an airshed, require statewide and/or regional air inventories and control strategies for source categories (motor vehicles, space heating, power production, etc.) focused on the attainment of air quality standards (concentration limits) whose attainment provides protection to the public health with an adequate margin of safety. There is also a long history of routine, mostly daily measurements of criteria pollutant concentrations throughout the country.

By contrast, HAPs sources are far fewer in number and are considered to be definable point sources at fixed locations. Downwind concentrations are highly variable, and generally drop rapidly with distance from the source due to dilution into cleaner, background air. The national emission standards for hazardous air pollutants (NESHAPs) are based on technologically based source controls and are intended to limit facility fenceline air concentrations to those that would not cause an adverse health effect to the (most exposed) individual living at the fenceline. Also, until quite recently, there has been no program for routine measurements of air toxics in our communities.

Most of the unit risk factors for air toxics are based on cancer as the health effect of primary concern. In these studies, and in studies to assess noncancer effects, the data are most often derived from controlled exposures in laboratory animals at maximally tolerated levels of exposure. The translation of the results of these studies to unit risk factors relevant to humans exposed at much, much lower levels in the environment is inherently uncertain, and is approached conservatively, following the model pioneered for food and drug safety beginning in the 1930s by the FDA. The resulting unit risk factors are generally based on an assumption of no threshold and a linear extrapolation to zero risk at zero dose. They are generally described in terms of being 95% upperbound confidence limits, but this descriptor is undoubtedly conservative in itself.

When these conservative unit risk factors are used for the prediction of the consequences of human exposures, they are multiplied by estimates of predicted ambient air concentrations which are, themselves, in the almost universal absence of air concentration measurements, almost certainly upper bound estimates from pollutant dispersion models that apply to the most highly exposed individuals in the community.

The resulting estimates of health risk are therefore highly conservative upper bound levels. Thus, they are inherently incompatible with population impacts estimated for the more widely dispersed criteria pollutants. The margins of safety for criteria pollutants are generally less than a factor of two, rather than the multiple orders of magnitude of safety factors built into the risk assessments for air toxics.

Comparative risk analysis, as currently practiced, has other inherent limitations as well. Even when we can reasonably and reliably estimate the exposure-related numbers of cases of premature mortality, hospital admissions, other uses of medical, clinical and pharmaceutical drug resources, lost time from work or school, reduced physiological and functional capacities, we face daunting societal equity and valuation challenges in intercomparing numbers of incident cases of quite variable clinical severity and psychological impacts. For carcinogenic agents, it has become customary to expect regulations to be effective in limiting the risks of lifetime exposures to no more than one-in-ten thousand and often to less than one-in-a-million. For less dreaded diseases that also reduce lifespan, such as chronic obstructive pulmonary disease and heart attack, which also are exacerbated by air pollutant exposures, a much higher risk level has been considered acceptable by regulators and the public.

In summary, our current abilities to determine residual risks of air toxics and/or to compare risks quantitatively are quite limited by key gaps in knowledge, and by reliance on unvalidated predictive models for exposure and for dose–response. A major part of the problem is the existence of two very different cultures of risk assessment: *(1)* for carcinogens; and *(2)* for other toxicants. Carcinogen risk assessments seldom have been based on relevant data on either low-dose exposure on human exposure–response data at concentrations anywhere near ambient levels. They require high dose to low dose extrapolations and generally animal to human extrapolations as well, using unvalidated predictive models. In the face of such a high degree of uncertainty in the output of the models, conservative assumptions are used to ensure that potency and exposures are not underestimated. Thus, yields of risk estimates are almost always far higher than the real risks. Such risk estimates cannot be fairly compared to the risks associated with criteria air pollutants, which are determined largely from the product of measured air pollutant concentrations and measured responses among humans exposed to either ambient air or to controlled exposures in chambers. Fair comparisons can only be done within the separate categories of pollutants.

Comparative risk assessment is an idea whose time is coming, and if EPA is provided with appropriate research resources to harness the new technical approaches and sophisticated research tools now emerging to fill in key knowledge gaps, it can make comparative risk assessment more useful and feasible in the not-too-distant future.

Options for reducing environmental risks to human health may include measures for intervening at any point in the sequence of steps typically involved in the process by which a potentially hazardous agent is produced, is released, is transported through the environment, reaches a susceptible individual, is taken up by the individual, and subsequently gives rise to a reaction adversely affecting the health of the individual and/or his/her offspring (Fig. 14–24). Some options are not possible without action at the community level, whereas others lie within the power of the individual, acting alone. All options, however, depend to varying degrees on understanding each of the risks in question and on having the skills needed to reduce them. Research and education in the relevant aspects of environmental health and safety are, therefore, essential for arriving at sound policies for risk reduction at the individual and the community levels.[3]

At the community level, the options for risk reduction encompass a broad range of activities, including: *(1)* support of research for identifying potentially hazardous agents, elucidating their toxicity and modes of action, and defining their relevant dose–effect relationships; *(2)* systematic monitoring of the extent to which individuals or populations may be exposed to harmful agents via air, water, soil, food, or other media, and proper assessment of the magnitude of any

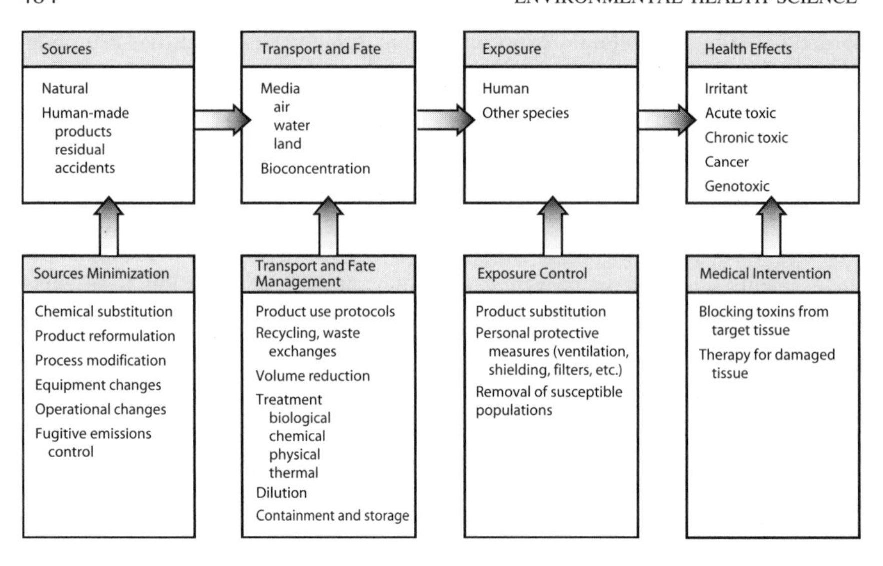

FIGURE 14–24. Summary of options for reducing environmental risks to human health.

risks that may result from such exposures; *(3)* identification of individuals or groups at unusually increased risk because of heightened susceptibility and/or level of exposure; *(4)* formulation and enforcement of standards and regulations for limiting the exposure of individuals or populations to potentially harmful agents, along with engineering measures for controlling the production and/or release of potentially toxic agents, as discussed in Chapter 15; *(5)* planning ahead to cope with emergencies that may result from the accidental release of hazardous agents; *(6)* maintaining in readiness the organizational capability needed to cope with environmental emergencies; *(7)* mounting programs of public and professional education in environmental risk reduction (including information clearinghouses, workshops, telephone hot lines, internet web pages, etc.).[4–7]

At the individual level, the options for risk reduction include: *(1)* staying abreast of relevant information received via the media and/or communications from health authorities, environmental protection agencies, and other sources; *(2)* modifying one's own behavior, diet, and lifestyle to minimize risks to oneself and to others; *(3)* carefully observing any special precautions that may be called for to protect oneself and one's fellow workers against hazardous agents in the workplace; and *(4)* joining with others in efforts to promote collective awareness of environmental risks and to reduce such risks.[5]

REFERENCES

1. ACGIH. Industrial Ventilation—A Manual of Recommended Practice, 23rd Ed. Am. Conf. Of Governmental Industrial Hygienists, Cincinnati, OH, 1998.

2. Science Advisory Board (SAB). Toward Integrated Environmental Decision Making. EPA-SAB-EC-00-011, United States Environmental Protection Agency, Aug. 2000.
3. Tones, K. Health education, behaviour change, and the public health. In: R. Detels, W. Holland, J. McEwen, and G.S. Omenn (eds.), Oxford Textbook of Public Health. New York: Oxford University Press, 1997, pp. 783–814.
4. Science Advisory Board (SAB). Reducing Risk: Setting Priorities and Strategies for Environmental Protection, SAB-EC-90-021, United States Environmental Protection Agency, Washington, DC, Sept. 1990.
5. Griffith, R. and Saunders, P. Reducing environmental risk. In: R. Detels, W. Holland, J. McEwen, and G.S. Omenn (eds.), Oxford Textbook of Public Health. New York: Oxford University Press, 1997, pp. 1601–1620.
6. Presidential/Congressional Commission on Risk Assessment and Risk Management. 1997. Risk Assessment and Risk Management in Regulatory Decision Making. Washington, DC.
7. Omenn, G.S. and Faustman, E.M. Risk assessment, risk communication, and risk management. In: R. Detels, W. Holland, J. McEwen, and G.S. Omenn (eds.), Oxford Textbook of Public Health. New York: Oxford University Press, 1997, pp. 969–986.

15

Our Environmental Future

The environment that we inhabit is ever changing, and the only thing that is reasonably certain is that it will continue to change. Furthermore, it is most likely to change at an ever increasing rate. Affluence allows some of us to directly control many aspects of our personal environments (within our homes and property boundaries). However, as we consider our neighborhoods, villages and cities, states, countries, and global communities, our individual capacity to influence factors affecting our collective environments diminishes, and we become more dependent on political and judicial processes for the protection and/or enhancement of our collective environments, through legislation, enforcement of environmental regulations, and through public information and educational programs.

In the United States, most people look to the EPA, the DHHS, and their state and local counterpart agencies to take the lead roles in the anticipation, recognition, evaluation, and control of the environmental factors and forces that could or do affect human health. While these agencies can, should, and sometimes do greatly influence our environmental quality and health status, they cannot and do not do so alone. Regulatory and control actions taken by governmental departments responsible for transportation, energy, agriculture, defense, commerce, and labor can also play significant and sometimes dominant roles in shaping our collective environments. Furthermore, two of the most important factors influencing our environmental futures are not directly influenced by regulation in most countries, i.e., human population growth and the concentration of people and economic activity within urban areas.

SCANNING THE HORIZON AT THE ENVIRONMENTAL PROTECTION AGENCY

In the United States, the EPA, an agency with large but limited resources and many complex legislative mandates to enforce, has frequently been confronted with crises and pressures for rapid responses to environmental surprises, such as high concentrations of dioxins in soil at Times Beach, MO, a leaking waste dump in Niagara Falls (Love Canal), high concentrations of mercury in fish in the Great Lakes, acid rain in the Adirondack mountains of New York, cryptosporidium in the public water supply of Milwaukee, WI, etc. In 1993, the EPA Administrator asked its SAB, an independent group of external advisors, to conduct a study of ways that the Agency could look ahead, and be better prepared to anticipate and deal with emerging environmental challenges. The resulting SAB report, entitled: "Beyond the Horizon: Using Foresight to Protect the Environmental Future" outlined a recommended approach for dealing with issues not yet on the Agency's agenda.[1] The report focussed on the time frame between 5 and 30 years in the future. For anything occurring sooner, EPA can be expected to recognize the early signs of emerging issues of some importance and to have its staff work up options and approaches for dealing with them. Beyond 30 years, the uncertainties become so large as to defy rational planning.

The SAB's report first dealt with an examination of the forces of change. The first hypothesis that was adopted by the SAB Futures Committee was that large social, economic, technological, and institutional forces will cause future environmental risks that are potentially greater than those currently recognized and managed. The forces that drive change, so-called "drivers," suggest how change will manifest itself in the future, and how the environmental effects of such change can be altered by action in the present.

These drivers are interdependent, and the changes they drive could have both positive and negative effects on the environment. For example, population growth and higher per capita income will most likely create increased demands for energy, natural resources, and manufactured goods. At the same time, higher per capita income, combined with improved education and an expanded range of personal choices, tend to reduce population growth and its pressures, while cleaner fuels and higher end-use efficiencies could reduce the local and global environmental effects of increased energy use. Thus, technological changes could either exacerbate or ameliorate environmental pressures.

The drivers of future change are the consequences of personal, community, and national choices, and are themselves subject to change. Viewed separately, they suggest the range, significance, and complexity of the forces that will affect environmental quality.

Driver #1: Population Growth and Urbanization

The continuing growth in human population, and the concentration of growing populations in large urban areas, pose enormous environmental challenges. The United Nations (UN) has projected that the global population will increase to between 7.9 and 12 billion by the year 2050. Urban areas will grow even faster, thus increasing the number of megacites with populations numbering from 10 to 20 million or more. As populations become more concentrated, environmental problems generally intensify. Providing safe drinking water, waste water and solid waste disposal systems, as well as environmentally sustainable transportation systems, will pose a daunting challenge in urban areas worldwide.

Driver #2: Economic Expansion and Resource Consumption

Over the next several decades, per capita income in many developing countries is likely to increase. This development, coupled with population growth, can be expected to result in greater consumption of energy, natural resources, and consumer goods.

Although recent U.S. and Western European experience indicates that energy use does not necessarily grow in direct proportion to economic growth, there is little doubt that energy use will rise dramatically in the developing world. According to Department of Energy (DOE) projections, energy demand in developing nations is likely to reach 240 quadrillion BTUs (quads) by the year 2010, an increase of over 40% in 20 years. During the same period, U.S. energy demand is projected to reach 105 quads, a 26% increase. By 2010, developing nations could account for more than half of the world's total energy demand. This level of growth is likely, even if per capita energy consumption in developing countries remains at much lower levels than in the industrialized world.

The fuels used to provide energy could have a profound impact on the environment. If countries such as China and India choose to generate electricity with conventional coal technologies and minimum pollution controls, the local, regional, and global environmental impacts could be substantial. On the other hand, alternative fuels and higher energy efficiency could help to reduce those effects.

Some potentially devastating effects of population growth, economic expansion, and individual behavior on natural resources already are evident in many parts of the world. All major ocean fishing areas presently are being fished at or beyond capacity, and according to the UN, global per capita seafood supplies have already declined. Approximately 5%–10% of the world's living reefs, the rainforests of the oceans, have died because of economic activity along coastlines and in coastal waters. Continuation of such trends, especially in light of expected population growth, would have adverse environmental and economic consequences for people everywhere.

Driver #3: Technological Development

Throughout history, technological change has been one of the most important factors driving economic and environmental change. Technology is likely to play an even greater role in the future, as technological development proceeds at a faster pace and has a more pervasive impact on societies and individuals.

In the past, the adverse environmental effects of growing populations and expanding economies have been ameliorated by the development of new technologies, centralized waste water treatment systems, for example. Technological advances in the future (e.g., cleaner fuels, more energy efficient transportation and power distribution systems, less wasteful manufacturing processes) are likely to yield similar environmental benefits.

At the same time, new products (e.g., alternative transportation fuels) and materials (e.g., in photovoltaic cells or next-generation batteries) may result in new exposures and increased risks to human health and ecosystems. In this sense, the future will be much like the past: technological change will bring with it both environmental improvements and environmental problems. Thus, one of the central challenges facing society today is anticipating the likely environmental effects of future technological development, and including a concern for environmental quality in the design of future technologies and products.

Driver #4: Environmental Attitudes and Institutions

Environmental quality is not determined solely by the actions of governments, regulated industries, or nongovernment organizations (NGOs). It is largely a function of the decisions and behavior of individuals, families, businesses, and communities everywhere. Consequently, the extent of environmental awareness and the strength of environmental institutions will be two critical factors driving changes in environmental quality in the future.

Concerned, educated publics, acting through responsive local, national, and international institutions, can serve as effective agents for avoiding future environmental problems, no matter what they are.

Uses of Foresight

Foresight, or futures research and analysis, has been used by government, private business, and NGOs to anticipate future change. Some government agencies, private businesses, and NGOs have used foresight in planning, goal setting, and policy shaping. The participation of management in the foresight process has been essential to its success.

While most futures studies have focussed on the nearer term (less than five years), some have reached considerably further. The Energy Information Administration within the DOE develops detailed energy use projections as far as 20 years into the future. With a shorter-term focus, the Internal Revenue Service (IRS), the Department of Defense (DOD), and the intelligence community employ scanning systems and trend analysis as part of institutional planning. The DOD uses "gaming" exercises to anticipate the possible circumstances of future warfare and prepare a range of options in response. In recent years, many regional, state, and local governments have also applied the tools of foresight.

Some foresight activities have been supported by the governments of other countries and by international organizations (e.g., the OECD, the World Bank). The Dutch government, in particular, has been a leading advocate for national level foresight and long-range planning. Five Dutch ministries have sponsored a research program to identify new technologies or technical systems that will support economic growth and environmental quality 50 years in the future.

In the private sector, foresight generally is used in relatively short-term business planning in several ways: to anticipate changing circumstances that can affect markets or competitive forces. The techniques used in the private sector include demographic and geographic analyses, statistical consumer polling, formalized environmental scanning, scenario construction, expert panels, econometrics, and other forms of computer modeling. Underlying these corporate activities is the central assumption that opportunities can be discovered and problems avoided by thinking about what lies ahead.

The Environmental Protection Agency has worked with other government agencies to anticipate and respond to the possibility of global climate change, since measurements of CO_2 buildup in the atmosphere have provided an early warning of possible global warming. In order to avoid potential environmental problems in the future, the EPA is working with other federal and state agencies to encourage energy conservation and thus reduce or limit CO_2 emissions.

Foresight Methodologies

In general, there are three basic techniques widely used to identify possible future conditions. One is a top-down approach; it involves the use of "scenarios" that postulate certain circumstances about the future and then draw some likely implications from those circumstances. The second is a bottom-up approach; it draws future implications from early warning signals, which are based either on the extrapolation of current data and trends, or on the observations of knowledgeable individuals, so-called "look-out panels." The third is scanning, which involves a continual, planned, deliberate, and thorough review of selected published information, and contacts with other "futures watching" organizations. All three approaches individually—and particularly in combination—can provide valuable insights into the possible emergence of environmental problems in the future.

In the top-down approach, scenarios are constructed to study the environmental implications of assumed future developments in "drivers" like energy use, population growth and density, technological advances, waste generation, and demand for natural resources like potable water. These images of possible futures can be studied systematically to estimate when and where environmental problems could emerge, and to assess different types of policies that could be used to forestall them.

Within a given scenario, assumptions concerning the future can be varied to reflect different rates of change (e.g., in energy use, population growth). Postulated conditions about the future also can be changed to reflect a future that is possible (exploratory scenarios), or a future that is desirable (normative scenarios). As long as these scenarios display changes in important variables over time within a consistent analytical framework, they can be useful tools for anticipating environmental problems in the future, and analyzing the range of possible responses to them.

In the bottom-up approach, a specialized "look-out panel" can provide perceptions, observations, and information about important environmental changes on, or just beyond, the horizon. Look-out panels, which can include laboratory scientists, professional field data collectors, or neighborhood volunteers, function continuously. Through systematic questioning and feedback, panelists can provide observations about the environment than can serve as early warnings of environmental changes, and they can assess the implications of these changes to human health and ecosystem viability.

In the scanning approach, information related to emerging environmental problems can be gleaned from scholarly journals, newspapers, newsletters, business plans, and science-oriented computer bulletin boards. Such sources of information include literature and academic disciplines well beyond the bounds of traditional environmental science. Scanning also can be part of the foresight activities of look-out panels.

All three approaches are independently useful in identifying the first weak signals that warn of emerging environmental problems. In addition, the techniques reinforce one another by providing early warnings from different perspectives. Scenario analyses tend to raise top-down issues generated by the assumptions used in the scenarios (e.g., CO_2 buildup as a result of the energy strategies of large countries like China and India). The look-out panels call attention to specific emerging issues (e.g., the introduction of new toxic chemicals). Scanning cuts across both approaches.

All three techniques can help identify potential environmental issues that could be subjected to in-depth risk analysis. All three, if used continuously and interactively, could serve as a first line of defense in protecting future environmental quality.

Emerging Problem Areas

Because of large-scale social, economic, technological, and institutional changes already underway, future environmental issues may emerge in at least five different problem areas. In preparing its report, the SAB applied one of the issue-identification methodologies (i.e., the bottom-up, look-out panel approach) to test the methodology and, in the process, to compile a list of possible future environmental issues that could emerge within the next 5 to 30 years. The SAB then compiled and consolidated the information into a list of 50 specific possible issues.

After compiling the list, the SAB applied six criteria that it considered useful in selecting issues to be further analyzed. Based on the results of its selection process and the inherent similarities among some potential issues, the SAB consolidated them under five large, overarching problem areas: sustainability of terrestrial ecosystems; noncancer human health effects; total air pollutant loadings; nontraditional environmental stressors; and health of the oceans.

All of these broad problem areas are affected by the major drivers of change discussed earlier in this chapter. Because they encompass a number of specific environmental issues, they merit more detailed discussion.

Sustainability of terrestrial ecosystems

In the future, the health of biosystems and the sustainable use of natural resources will be stressed by a growing human population, expanding energy use, natural resource consumption, and land development. As the stresses on biosystems intensify, the preservation of biodiversity will become increasingly important for both economic and environmental reasons. As populations grow and urban areas expand, heightened competition for the use of land will put new strains on natural habitats. In the years ahead, failure to maintain healthy terrestrial ecosystems could lead to natural resource damage, irreversible losses of species, and fragmentation of habitats, thus endangering both economic and environmental sustainability and seriously threatening human and ecological wellbeing.

Noncancer human health effects

The human health effects that can result from environmental pollution include many endpoints in addition to cancer. The loss of fertility and birth defects, for example, have been linked to certain organic chemicals. Developmental problems in children, neurological deficits, faster aging of the lung, and increased rates of mortality and morbidity have been associated with lead, mercury, ozone, and ambient particulate matter, respectively. Management of human health risks in the future will have to consider the full range of health effects under conditions of both single and multiple exposures.

Total air pollutant loadings

In the future, total loadings of pollutants in and from the atmosphere may pose environmental problems not seen before, or intensify familiar problems beyond the point where conventional controls will solve them. For example, aggregate increases in the use of fossil fuels, combined with long-range transport and local conditions, can lead to regional or global air quality problems (e.g., acid rain and global warming). Deposition of airborne contaminants could exacerbate problems on land or in the water, problems that demand new kinds of responses.

Nontraditional environmental stressors

In the future, previously unrecognized environmental stressors, and recognized stressors that are not adequately monitored or regulated, may be found to pose serious risks to human health or ecosystems. Many unregulated chemicals present in complex mixtures have been linked to such problems as sick building syndrome, multiple chemical sensitivity, and excess morbidity and mortality rates related to airborne fine particles. Control-resistant microbes, plants, and insects; new kinds of waterborne pathogens; the accidental or misguided introduction of an exotic species into susceptible ecosystems: any of these factors could lead to human health or ecological problems in the future. Moreover, relatively well-understood stressors could begin to cause new kinds of problems through the slow building of cumulative effects, or the subtle effects of well-understood stressors (e.g., developmental defects in children exposed to low levels of lead) can be expected to cause new public concerns.

Health of the oceans

The oceans, their complex biosystems, and their related food webs are likely to come under increasing stress from the worldwide activities of a growing global population. The adverse effects of overfishing, air and waterborne pollutants, and coastal development on the health and abundance of marine life, including the ecologically critical coral reefs, already are causing concerns in coastal areas. The migration of coastal stressors far from shore threatens the future health of the deep, open ocean as well. Pollutants like PCBs, pesticides, and lead have been found not only in the tissues of fish and marine mammals, but also in bottom sediments and in the seawater itself. Solid waste can be found throughout the open ocean. Moreover, future exploitation of minerals and oceanic plant life could degrade the ocean environment even further, as similar activities on land have done.

THE ENVIRONMENT: A STRATEGIC NATIONAL INTEREST

National and international environmental issues are rapidly becoming a matter of strategic national interest. The United States is part of a single global ecosystem. Political, economic, and environmental trends and events in other countries affect the United States; pollution generated in each country affects the rest of the world as well. Because of international environmental and economic linkages, environmental issues affect strategic national interests.

In recent years, the links between the environment and national security have become apparent. Nations have gone to war to protect their access to vital natural resources. Others have used environmental destruction in combat as a major instrument of war. Terrorism, a nuclear reactor accident (Chernobyl), and nuclear weapons proliferation all have major implications for public and ecosystem health around the world. Possible natural resource shortages, competition for scarce resources like potable water, and the transborder movement of refugees driven by deteriorating environmental conditions could lead to destabilized governments, international disagreements, and regional warfare. Overfishing, acid rain, and raw waste water discharges along and across national borders also are examples of how environmental and natural resource issues can lead to contentious relations among countries, and necessitate international negotiations and agreements related to environmental quality.

Moreover, the future quality of the global environment will be a factor in determining how economic activities are conducted in all countries, including the United States. Based on present trends, the future growth of the economies in regions such as Asia and Latin America, for example, with an attendant increase in energy use, could contribute to global atmospheric pollution that today is caused primarily by economically developed nations. The loss of biodiversity through the clearing of rain forests in South America and South Asia would be felt by everyone on earth. The stripfishing of marine life in the open ocean is diminishing the foodstocks available to global populations over the long term.

As can be seen from these examples, many future environmental issues, and their relationship to economic development, are likely to be matters of strategic national interest, both to the United States and to other countries, at the dawn of a new century. Environmental and natural resource-related issues almost certainly will be linked to national security concerns and to a range of bilateral and multilateral relationships.

As the Federal agency primarily responsible for protecting the environment, EPA has been charged with implementing environmental laws that have been, in large part, reactive. Just as those laws were enacted in response to existing problems, EPA spends most of its time and budget cleaning up, or remediating, pollution problems that already are relatively serious, or that already are causing public concern because of real or perceived environmental impacts. This approach has achieved considerable success.

However, nations will not be able to limit or prevent future environmental problems with the same regulatory tools and reactive approaches that they have used in the past. The future that will be as challenging as it is uncertain, and we must develop new analytical tools, new approaches to decisionmaking, and new partnerships. We must develop a capacity to anticipate problems and respond to them long before their adverse effects are widely felt. Increasing cooperative efforts among federal agencies, state governments, NGOs, international groups, and the private sector will be needed in order to solve existing environmental problems. Regulators will need to work more closely with business communities to anticipate the future environmental implications of technological innovation, as well as with other agencies, international organizations, and the agencies of other nations to identify the drivers of emerging regional or global problems, and then help define possible responses to them. The environmental problems of the future undoubtedly will be facets of large-scale economic, demographic, and technological change. Other organizations, government and nongovernment, will have major responsibilities responding to that change.

MEGATRENDS IN SOCIETY—A LONGER TIME FRAME

While EPA and other governmental agencies have critical roles and responsibilities for influencing and controlling sources and activities that influence environmental changes, there are other, sometimes overwhelming forces at work as well, and many of them have been at work far longer than EPA. A longer, and mostly positive view of some of these forces and trends was reported by Ausubel.[2] The following section summarizes some of his perspectives on our environmental future in terms of environmental foresight, with special emphasis on the implications of long-term trends. They can be grouped in terms of energy, land, water, and materials.

Energy

Figure 15–1 summarizes historic changes and trend projections for human usage of energy since 1860. It shows usage in fractional, not absolute usage, which has greatly increased over time. In 1860, wood was still the dominant source of purposely generated thermal energy. However, wood could not satisfy the energy demands of a growing population, especially in urban and industrial areas. By 1880, it was supplanted by coal, which was a fuel that could be extracted from the ground and delivered to consumers at a relatively low cost. However, burning coal efficiently and completely is technologically challenging, and incom-

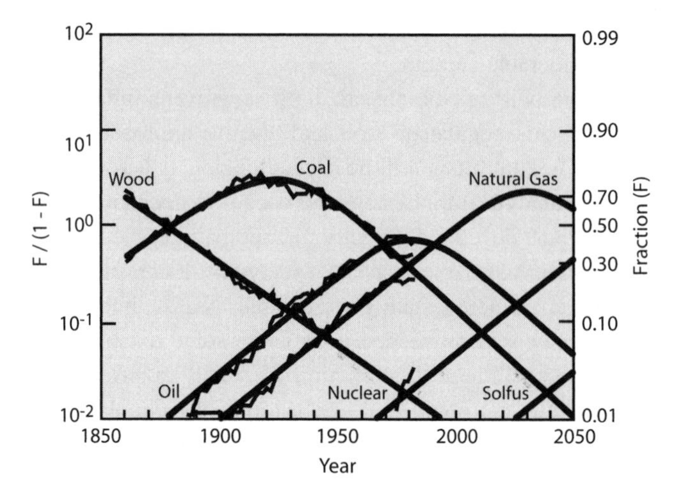

FIGURE 15–1. Global primary energy substitution from 1860 to 1982 and projections for the future, expressed in fractional market shares (F). Smooth lines represent model calculations and jagged lines are historical data. Solfus is a term employed to describe a major new energy technology, for example, solar or fusion.

plete combustion has had significant impacts on human health and the environment. Thus, coal was gradually supplanted by fuels that were easier to transport and burn, i.e., petroleum and natural gas. Coal, long our most dominant source, was succeeded in that role by oil by 1970, and by natural gas by 1995. Coal usage, in terms of absolute tonnage, has not actually declined since the 1930s. Much of it was then used for space heating, railroad locomotives, and steel production, but its current usage in developed countries is confined largely to electric power generation in large facilities.

The shift over time from wood to coal to oil to natural gas has had major implications to environmental quality. There have been reductions in the emissions of products of incomplete combustion, as well as of SO_2, NO_x, and CO_2, a major greenhouse gas. This is well illustrated in Figure 15–2, which shows the changing ratio of hydrogen (H) to carbon (C) in fuels since 1860. The increasing H/C ratio reduces the impact of fossil fuel usage on global climate change associated with the secular rise in CO_2 in the atmosphere. There are other factors limiting the emissions of CO_2. As noted by Ausubel[2] "Several factors dispose nations toward convergent, clean energy development. One is the changing composition of economic activity away from primary industry and manufacturing to services. End users in office buildings and homes do not want smoking coals. America has pared its carbon intensity of gross domestic product per capita per constant dollar from about three kilograms in 1800 to about 0.3 in 1990."

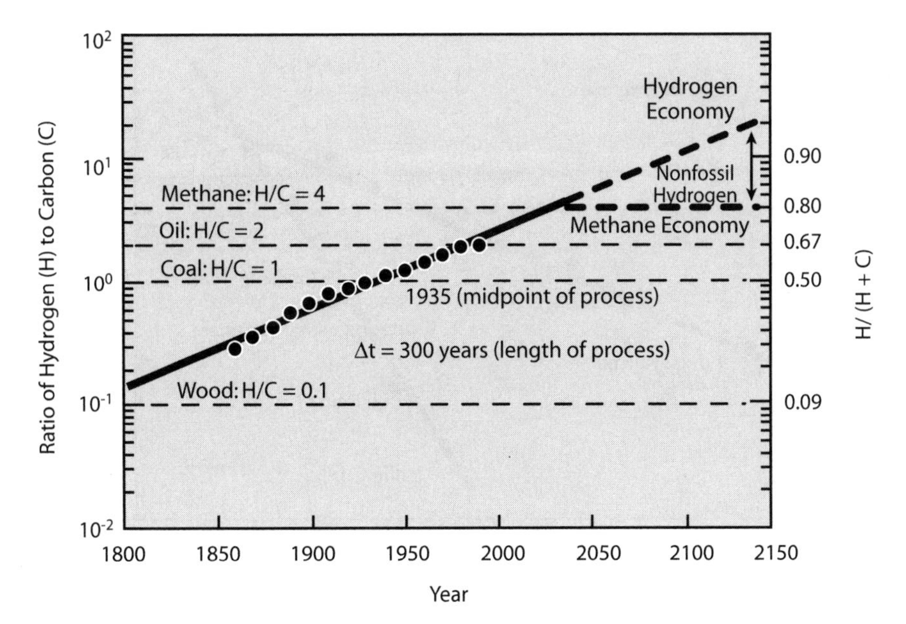

FIGURE 15–2. Ratio of hydrogen (H) to carbon (C) for global primary energy consumption since 1860 and projections for the future, expressed as a ratio of hydrogen to carbon (H/C).

Parts of the gain in overall efficiency have been attributable to gains in: *(1)* the efficiency of combustion; *(2)* conversion of heat into useful power; *(3)* delivery of power to users; and *(4)* the increasing efficiencies of devices using the power. The production of a good or service in the U.S. has, since 1800, required 1% less energy on average than it did the previous year.[2] As shown in Figure 15–3, in the 300 years since the invention of the steam engine, engine efficiencies have grown from approximately 1% to approximately 50%. In terms of illumination, Edison's first electric light in 1879 was 15× more efficient than a paraffin candle. The first fluorescent lamp in 1942 was 30× more efficient than the first incandescent lamp. The progress in illumination efficiency is also shown in Figure 15–3.

Land

At the end of the twentieth century, population growth in most economically developed countries had virtually ceased, and there were indications of reduced rates of population growth in many less well developed countries. However, the global population is expected to grow by approximately 50% to 100% by 2050, mostly in the less developed countries. At the same time, the standard of living and food consumption rates can also be expected to grow. The question then

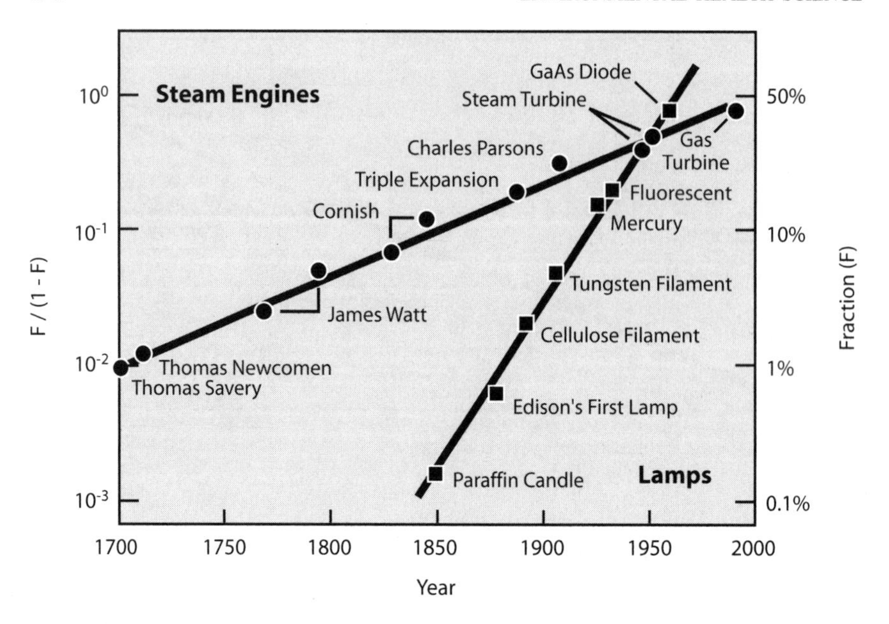

Figure 15–3. Improvement in the efficiency of motors and lamps analyzed as a sigmoid (logistic) growth process.

arises, can the food supply meet the demand. Available evidence suggests that it can. During the second half of the twentieth century, the amount of land devoted globally to agriculture remained stable while the population doubled.

Since 1940, U.S. wheat yields have tripled and corn yields have quintupled.[2] Despite these accomplishments, the potential to increase yields everywhere remains astonishing, even without invoking such new technologies as the genetic engineering of plants. The world on average grows only about half the corn per hectare of the average Iowa farmer, who in turn grows only about half the corn of the top Iowa farmer. Importantly, while all yields have risen steadily for decades, the production ratio of these performers has not changed much. Even in Iowa the average performer lags more than thirty years behind the state of the art. While cautious habits and other factors properly moderate the pace of diffusion of innovations, the effects still accumulate dramatically. By raising wheat yields fivefold during the past four decades, farmers in India have, in practice, spared for other purposes an area of cropland roughly equal to the area of the state of California.

Future caloric intake per person will likely range between the 3000 per day of an ample vegetarian diet and the 6000 that includes meat. If farmers fail to raise global average yields, people will have to reduce their portions to keep cropland to its current extent. If the farmers can lift the global average yield approximately

1.5% per year over the next six or seven decades to the level of today's European wheat, 10 billion people can enjoy a 6000 calorie diet and still spare close to a quarter of the present 1.4 billion hectares of cropland. The quarter spared, fully 300 million hectares, would equal the area of India. Reaching the level of today's average U.S. corn grower would spare for ten billion people half of today's cropland for nature, an area larger than the Amazon basin—even with the calorie intake of today's American as the diet (See Fig. 15–4).

Water

With its vast oceans, the earth suffers no overall shortage of water. However, supplies of domestic fresh water for drinking, cooking, and washing, as well as fresh water for the agricultural and industrial users vary greatly in availability and cost. Also, quality standards vary greatly with intended usage. Total per capita water withdrawals in the U.S. quadrupled between 1900 and 1970.[2] However, since 1975, per capita water use has fallen appreciably, at an annual rate of 1.3%.[3] Absolute U.S. water withdrawals peaked about 1980. Total industrial water withdrawals plateaued a decade earlier than total U.S. withdrawals, and have dropped by one-third, more steeply than the total. Notably, industrial withdrawals per unit of gross national product (GNP) have dropped steadily since

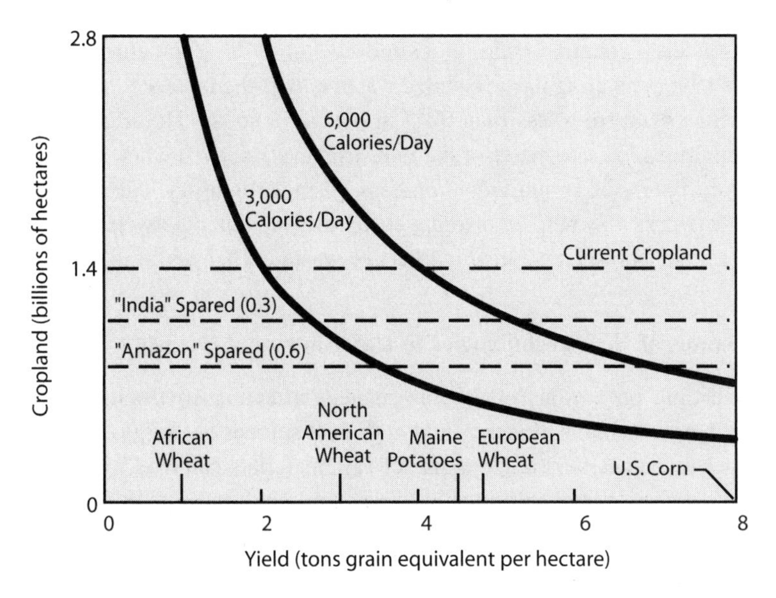

FIGURE 15–4. The sparing for nature of a reference area of 2.8 billion hectares of cropland by farmers raising yields for ten billion people consuming 3000 or 6000 calories daily.

1940, from 14 gallons per constant dollar to 3 gallons in 1990. Not only intake, but discharge per unit of production are perhaps one-fifth of what they were 50 years ago.

Law and economics as well as technology have favored frugal water use. Legislation, such as the U.S. Clean Water Act of 1972, encouraged the reduction of discharges, recycling, and conservation, as well as shifts in relative prices. Water withdrawals for all users in the industrialized countries span a 10-fold range, with the United States and Canada at the highest end.[4] In the long run, with much higher thermodynamic efficiency for processes, removing impurities to recycle water will require small amounts of energy.

Materials

The intensity of use of diverse primary materials has also plummeted during the twentieth century.[2] Lumber, steel, lead, and copper have lost relative importance, while plastics and aluminum have expanded. Many products, for example, cars, computers, and beverage cans, have become lighter, and often smaller. Although the soaring numbers of products and objects, accelerated by economic growth, raised municipal waste in the United States annually by approximately 1.6% per person in the last couple of decades, trash per unit of GNP dropped slightly. Over time new materials replace old, and theoretically each replacement should improve material properties per unit, thus lowering the intensity of use. Furthermore, as countries develop, the intensity of use of a given material (or system) declines as each country arrives at a similar level of development.

Since 1990, recycling has accounted for over half the metals consumed in the United States, up from less than 30% in the mid 1960s.[5] The trick is to make waste minimization a property of the industrial system, even when it is not completely a property of an individual process, plant, or industry. Advancing information networks may help by offering cheap ways to link otherwise unconnected buyers and sellers to create new markets or waste exchanges.

Implications of New Technologies to Environmental Quality

The preceding projections of secular changes affecting environmental quality suggest that the benefits of increasingly efficient sources of energy, usage of land and water resources, and reduced use of raw materials can lead to reduced impacts of anthropological activities on the natural environment. With a stabilization of population size, a more hydrogen-based energy system, further increases in agricultural productivity, more efficient utilization of water supplies, and a reduced dependence on natural raw materials, it should be possible to preserve more of our remaining natural ecosystems and ensure the benefits of the services that they supply to all of the earth's inhabitants.

COSTS AND BENEFITS OF ENVIRONMENTAL MANAGEMENT

Willingness to Pay

The environmental future will, to a major extent, be determined by our individual and collective willingness to bear the costs of pollution prevention, clean up and/or isolation of previously discarded wastes, protection and creation of parklands and nature preserves, and enforcement of statutory regulations and of international treaties and commitments related to environmental protection. In economic terms, willingness to pay is expressed in hard currency, as determined from appropriately designed survey data of a stratified sample of the public. In practice, the elicitation of results can be expected to vary with the ways in which the questions are constructed, and with the extent and reliability of the background information presented to or previously available to the members of the public who respond to the survey's questions. For example, by including information on both the direct and indirect effects of expenditures for environmental protection, including intangible and/or nonmonetizable benefits, an individual's willingness to pay could vary substantially.

At the national level in the United States, the willingness of Congress to commit public funds for environmental protection, and to impose control costs on individuals, on state and local governmental agencies, and on individuals has changed over time. For example, the CAA of 1970 mandated that primary standards for criteria air pollutants be set to protect the pubic health with an adequate margin of safety and without consideration of costs. However, by executive order, every proposed federal regulation submitted to the Office of Management and Budget (OMB) for review prior to promulgation must now be accompanied by a Regulatory Impact Analysis (RIA), which includes a cost-benefit analysis. Furthermore, in the CAA amendments of 1990, the Congress specifically directed the EPA to report on the benefits and costs of the CAA retrospectively from 1970 to 1990, and to prospectively analyze the benefits and costs of the additional requirements in the 1990 amendments out to 2000 and to 2010. It also directed EPA to establish an Advisory Council on Clean Air Act Compliance Analysis to assist EPA with guidance on the conduct of these analyses and to provide peer review of the reports before their submission to the Congress. Most of the Council members have been prominent economists with strong interests in environmental issues, and it functions as a component of the EPA's SAB. The Council has two subcommittees, one on air quality modelling, and the other on health and environmental effects. Both subcommittees draw heavily on SAB members for technical expertise. The balance of this chapter is largely devoted to a review of the findings of the Council's first two reports to Congress. They involved a considerably more intensive effort than any of the previous cost–benefit analyses previously submitted to OMB with proposed regulations, and the capabilities developed in the preparation of these reports will enable EPA to conduct more thorough cost–benefit analyses for its other regulatory programs that will be needed to meet the mandates imposed for such analyses by an amendment to the federal budget reconciliation act for the 1999 fiscal year that was inserted by Senator Fred Thompson of Tennessee.

Summary of Environmental Protection Agency's Retrospective Report on the Benefits and Costs of the Clean Air Act, 1970 to 1990

Study design

Estimates of the benefits and costs of the CAA and its amendments were derived by examining the differences in economic, human health, and environmental outcomes under two alternative scenarios: a "control scenario" and a "no-control scenario."[6] The control scenario reflects actual historical implementation of clean air programs, and is based largely on historical data. The no-control scenario is hypothetical, and reflects the assumption that no air pollution controls were established beyond those in place prior to enactment of the 1970 CAA Amendments. Each of the two scenarios was evaluated by a sequence of economic, emissions, air quality, physical effect, economic valuation, and uncertainty models to measure the differences between the two scenarios in economic, human health, and environmental outcomes.

Direct costs

To comply with the provisions of the CAA, businesses, consumers, and government entities all incurred higher costs for many goods and services. The higher costs were due primarily to requirements to install, operate, and maintain pollution abatement equipment. In addition, costs were incurred to design and implement regulations, monitor and report regulatory compliance, and in conducting research and development programs. Ultimately, these higher costs of production were borne by stockholders, business owners, consumers, and taxpayers.

The historical data on CAA compliance costs by year were adjusted both for inflation and for the value of long-term investments in equipment. After further adjustments were made in the direct costs incurred each year to reflect their equivalent worth in the year 1990, the annual results yielded an estimate of approximately $523 billion for the total value of 1970 to 1990 direct expenditures.

Emissions

Emissions were substantially lower by 1990 under the control scenario than under the no-control scenario. Sulfur dioxide (SO_2) emissions were 40% lower, primarily due to utilities installing scrubbers and/or switching to lower sulfur fuels. Nitrogen oxides (NO_x) emissions were 30% lower by 1990, mostly because of the installation of catalytic converters on highway vehicles. Volatile organic compound emissions were 45 percent lower and carbon monoxide (CO) emissions were 50% lower, also primarily due to motor vehicle emission controls.

For PM, changes in air quality depend both on changes in emissions of primary particles and on changes in emissions of gaseous pollutants, such as SO_2 and NO_x, which can be converted to PM through chemical transformations in the atmosphere. Emissions of PM were 75% lower under the control scenario by 1990 than under the no-control scenario. This substantial difference was due primarily to vigorous efforts in the 1970s to reduce visible emissions from utility and industrial smokestacks.

Lead (Pb) emissions for 1990 were reduced by about 99% from a no-control level of 237,000 tons to approximately 3000 tons under the control scenario. The vast majority of the difference in Pb emissions under the two scenarios was attributable to drastic reductions in the use of leaded gasoline.

These reductions were achieved during a period in which population grew by 22.3% and the national economy grew by 70%.

Air quality

The substantial reductions in air pollutant emissions attributable to the CAA translated into significantly improved air quality throughout the U.S. For SO_2, NO_x, and CO, the improvements under the control scenario were assumed to be proportional to the estimated reduction in emissions. Reductions in ground-level ozone (O_3) were achieved through reductions in emissions of its precursor pollutants, particularly VOCs and NO_x. The differences in ambient O_3 concentrations estimated under the control scenario varied significantly by location, primarily because of local differences in the relative proportion of VOCs and NO_x, weather conditions, and specific precursor emissions reductions. On a national average basis, O_3 concentrations in 1990 were approximately 15% lower under the control scenario.

There are many pollutants that contribute to ambient concentrations of PM. While some fine particles are directly emitted by sources, the most important fine particle species are formed in the atmosphere through chemical conversion of gaseous pollutants, are referred to as secondary particles. The three most important are: *(1)* sulfates, which derive primarily from SO_2 emissions; *(2)* nitrates, which derive primarily from NO_x emissions; and *(3)* organic aerosols, which can be directly emitted or can form from VOC emissions. Thus, controlling PM means controlling "air pollution" in a very broad sense. In the present analysis reductions in SO_2, NO_x, VOCs, and directly emitted primary particles achieved by the Clean Air Act resulted in a national average reduction in PM of approximately 45% by 1990.

Reductions in SO_2 and NO_x also translated into reductions in formation, transport, and deposition of secondarily formed acidic compounds. These are the principal pollutants responsible for acid precipitation, or "acid rain." Under the control scenario, sulfur and nitrogen deposition were significantly lower by 1990 than under the no-control scenario throughout the 31 eastern states covered by EPA's Regional Acid Deposition Model (RADM). Percentage decreases in sulfur deposition ranged up to more than 40% in the upper Great Lakes and Florida-Southeast Atlantic Coast areas, primarily because the no-control scenario projects significant increases in the use of high-sulfur fuels by utilities in the upper Great Lakes and Gulf Coast states. Nitrogen deposition was also significantly lower under the control scenario, with percentage decreases reaching levels of 25% or higher along the Eastern Seaboard, primarily due to higher projected emissions of motor vehicle NO_x under the no-control scenario.

Finally, decreases in ambient concentrations of light-scattering pollutants, such as sulfates and nitrates, were estimated to have led to perceptible improvements in visibility throughout the eastern states and southwestern urban areas modeled for this study.

Physical effects

The lower ambient concentrations of SO_2, NO_x, PM, CO, O_3 and Pb under the control scenario yield a substantial variety of human health, welfare and ecological benefits. For a number of these benefit categories, quantitative functions were available from the scientific literature that allowed estimation of the reduction in incidence of adverse effects. Examples of these categories include the human mortality and morbidity effects of a number of pollutants, the neurobehavioral effects among children caused by exposure to Pb, visibility impairment, and effects on yields for some agricultural products.

A number of benefit categories, however, could not be quantified and/or monetized for a variety of reasons. In some cases, substantial scientific uncertainties prevailed regarding the existence and magnitude of adverse effects (e.g., the contribution of O_3 to air pollution-related mortality). In other cases, strong scientific evidence of an effect existed, but data were too limited to support quantitative estimates of incidence reduction (e.g., changes in lung function associated with changes in long-term average exposure to O_3). Finally, there were effects for which there was sufficient information to estimate incidence reduction, but for which there were no available economic value measures; thus reductions in adverse effects could not be expressed in monetary terms. Examples of this last category include relatively small pulmonary function decrements caused by acute exposures to O_3, and reduced time to onset of angina pain caused by CO exposure.

Table 15–1 provides a summary of the key differences in quantified human health outcomes estimated under the control and no-control scenarios. Results were presented as thousands of cases avoided in 1990 due to control of the pollutants listed in the table and reflect reductions estimated for the entire U.S. population living in the 48 contiguous states. Epidemiological research alone cannot

TABLE 15–1. Criteria Pollutant Health Benefits—Estimated Distributions of 1990 Incidences of Avoided Health Effects (in thousands of incidences reduced) for 48 State Population[a]

			ANNUAL EFFECTS AVOIDED[b] (THOUSANDS)			
ENDPOINT	POLLUTANT(S)	AFFECTED POPULATION	5TH PERCENTILE	MEAN	95TH PERCENTILE	UNIT
Premature mortality	PM[c]	30 and over	112	184	257	Cases
Premature mortality	Lead	All	7	22	54	Cases
Chronic bronchitis	PM	All	498	674	886	Cases
Lost IQ points	Lead	Children	7440	10,400	13,000	Points
IQ less than 70	Lead	Children	31	45	60	Cases
Hypertension	Lead	Men 20–74	9740	12,600	15,600	Cases
Coronary heart disease	Lead	40–74	0	22	64	Cases
Atherothrombotic brain infarction	Lead	40–74	0	4	15	Cases
Initial cerebrovascular accident	Lead	40–74	0	6	19	Cases
Hospital admissions						
All respiratory	PM & ozone	All	75	89	103	Cases
Chronic obstructive pulmonary disease & pneumonia	PM & ozone	Over 65	52	62	72	Cases
Ischemic heart disease	PM	Over 65	7	19	31	Cases
Congestive heart failure	PM & CO	65 and over	28	39	50	Cases

(continued)

TABLE 15–1. Criteria Pollutant Health Benefits—Estimated Distributions of 1990 Incidences of Avoided Health Effects (in thousands of incidences reduced) for 48 State Population[a] (*continued*)

			ANNUAL EFFECTS AVOIDED[b] (THOUSANDS)			
ENDPOINT	POLLUTANT(S)	AFFECTED POPULATION	5TH PERCENTILE	MEAN	95TH PERCENTILE	UNIT
Other respiratory-related ailments						
Shortness of breath, days	PM	Children	14,800	68,000	133,000	Days
Acute bronchitis	PM	Children	0	8700	21,600	Cases
Upper and lower respiratory symptoms	PM	Children	5400	9500	13,400	Cases
Any of 19 acute symptoms	PM & ozone	18–65	15,400	130,000	244,000	Cases
Asthma attacks	PM & ozone	Asthmatics	170	850	1520	Cases
Increase in respiratory illness	NO_2	All	4840	9800	14,000	Cases
Any symptom	SO_2	Asthmatics	26	264	706	Cases
Restricted activity and work loss days						
Minor restricted activity days	PM & ozone	18–65	107,000	125,000	143,000	Days
Work loss days	PM	18–65	19,400	22,600	25,600	Days

[a]The following additional human welfare effects were quantified directly in economic terms: household soiling damage, visibility impairment, decreased worker productivity, and agricultural yield changes.

[b]The 5th and 95th percentile outcomes represent the lower and upper bounds, respectively, of the 90% credible interval for each effect as estimated by uncertainty modeling. The mean is the arithmetic average of all estimates derived by the uncertainty modeling.

[c]In this analysis, particulate matter (PM) is used as a proxy pollutant for all non-Lead (Pb) criteria pollutants which may contribute to premature mortality.

prove whether a cause–effect relationship exists between an individual pollutant and an observed health effect. This study used the epidemiological findings about correlations between pollution and observed health effects to estimate changes in the number of health effects that would occur if pollution levels change. A range was presented along with the mean estimate for each effect, reflecting uncertainties that have been quantified in the underlying health effects literature.

Adverse human health effects of the CAA "criteria pollutants", i.e., SO_2, NO_x, O_3, PM, CO, and Pb dominated the quantitative effects estimates in part because, although there were important residual uncertainties, evidence of physical consequences was greatest for these pollutants. The CAA yielded other benefits, however, which are important even though they are uncertain and/or could not be quantified. These other benefit categories include: *(1)* all benefits accruing from reductions in hazardous air pollutants (also referred to as air toxics); *(2)* reductions in damage to cultural resources, buildings, and other materials; *(3)* reductions in adverse effects on wetland, forest, and aquatic ecosystems; and *(4)* a variety of additional human health and welfare effects of criteria pollutants. A more complete list of these nonmonetized effects is presented in Table 15–2.

In addition to controlling the six criteria pollutants, the 1970 and 1977 CAA Amendments led to reductions in ambient concentrations of a number of hazardous air pollutants. Although they were not quantified in the retrospective cost–benefit report, control of these pollutants resulted both from regulatory standards set specifically to control hazardous air pollutants and from incidental reductions achieved through programs aimed at controlling criteria pollutants.

Existing scientific research suggests that reductions in both hazardous air pollutants and criteria pollutants yielded widespread improvements in the functioning and quality of aquatic and terrestrial ecosystems. In addition to any intrinsic value to be attributed to these ecological systems, human welfare is enhanced through improvements in a variety of ecological services. For example, protection of freshwater ecosystems achieved through reductions in deposition of acidic air pollutants can improve commercial and recreational fishing. Other potential ecological benefits of reduced acid deposition include improved wildlife viewing, maintenance of biodiversity, and nutrient cycling. Increased growth and productivity of U.S. forests may have resulted from reductions in ground-level O_3. More vigorous forest ecosystems in turn yield a variety of benefits, including increased timber production; improved forest aesthetics for people enjoying outdoor activities such as hunting, fishing, and camping; and improvements in ecological services such as nutrient cycling and temporary sequestration of global warming gases. These improvements in ecological structure and function were not quantified in this assessment.

Economic valuation

Estimating the reduced incidence of physical effects provided a valuable measure of health benefits for individual endpoints. However, to compare or

Table 15–2. Major Nonmonetized, Adverse Effects Reduced by the Clean Air Act (1970–1990)

POLLUTANT	NONMONETIZED ADVERSE EFFECTS
Particulate matter	Large changes in pulmonary function Other chronic respiratory diseases Inflammation of the lung Chronic asthma and bronchitis
Ozone	Changes in pulmonary function Increased in airway responsiveness to stimuli Centroacinar fibrosis Inflammation of the lung Immunological changes Chronic respiratory diseases Extrapulmonary effects (i.e., other organ systems) Forest and other ecological effects Materials damage
Carbon monoxide	Decreased time to onset of angina Behavioral effects Other cardiovascular effects Developmental effects
Sulfur dioxide	Respiratory symptoms in non-asthmatics Hospital admissions Agricultural effects Materials damage Ecological effects
Nitrogen oxides	Increased airway responsiveness to stimuli Decreased pulmonary function Inflammation of the lung Immunological changes Eye irritation Materials damage Eutrophication (e.g., Chesapeake Bay) Acid deposition
Lead	Cardiovascular diseases Reproductive effects in women Other neurobehavioral, physiological effects in children Developmental effects from maternal exposure, including IQ loss[a] Ecological effects
Air toxics	All human health effects Ecological effects

[a]IQ loss from direct, as opposed to maternal, exposure is quantified and monetized.

aggregate benefits across endpoints, the benefits had to be monetized. Assigning a monetary value to avoided incidences of each effect permits a summation, in terms of dollars, of menetized benefits realized as a result of the CAA, and allows that summation to be compared to the cost of the CAA.

It is important to recognize the substantial controversies and uncertainties that pervade attempts to characterize adverse human health and ecological effects of pollution in dollar terms. To many, dollar-based estimates of the value of avoiding outcomes such as loss of human life, pain and suffering, or ecological degradation do not capture the full and true value to society as a whole of avoiding or reducing these effects. Adherents to this view tend to favor assessment procedures that: *(1)* adopt the most technically defensible dollar-based valuation estimates for analytical purposes; but *(2)* leave the moral dimensions of policy evaluation to those who must decide whether, and how, to use a cost–benefit results in making public policy decisions. This was the paradigm adopted in this study. Given the Congressional mandate to perform a cost–benefit study of the CAA, the Project Team applied widely recognized, customary techniques of applied economics. Since social and personal values furthered by the CAA have not been effectively captured by the dollar-based measures used in this study, the Environmental Protection Agency encouraged readers to look beyond the dollar-based comparison of costs and benefits of the CAA and consider the broader value of the reductions in adverse health and environmental effects that have been achieved, as well as any additional adverse consequences of regulation that may not be reflected in the cost estimates.

For this study, unit valuation estimates were derived from the economics literature and reported in dollars per case (or, in some cases, episode or symptom-day) avoided for health effects and dollars per unit of avoided damage for human welfare effects. Similar to estimates of physical effects provided by health studies, each of the monetary values of benefits applied in this analysis can be expressed in terms of a mean value and a range around the mean estimate. This range reflects the uncertainty in the economic valuation literature associated with a given effect. The mean values of these ranges are shown in Table 15–3.

Monetized benefits and costs

The total monetized economic benefit attributable to the CAA was derived by applying the unit values (or ranges of values) to the stream of monetizable physical effects estimated for the 1970 to 1990 period. In developing these estimates, steps were taken to avoid double-counting of benefits.

The economic benefit estimation model then generated a range of economic values for the differences in physical outcomes under the control and no-control scenarios for the target years of the benefits analysis: 1975, 1980, 1985, and 1990. Linear interpolation between these target years was used to estimate benefits in intervening years. These yearly results were then adjusted to their equivalent

Table 15–3. Central Estimates of Economic Value per Unit of Avoided Effect[a]

ENDPOINT	POLLUTANT	VALUATION[b]
Mortality	PM and lead	$4,800,000 per case[c]
Chronic bronchitis	PM	$260,000 per case
IQ changes		
Lost IQ points	Lead	$3000 per IQ point
IQ less than 70	Lead	$42,000 per case
Hypertension	Lead	$680 per case
Strokes[d]	Lead	$200,000 per case-males[e] $150,000 per case-females[e]
Coronary heart disease	Lead	$52,000 per case
Hospital admissions		
Ischemic heart disease	PM	$10,300 per case
Congestive heart failure	PM	$8300 per case
Chronic obstructive pulmonary disease	PM and ozone	$8100 per case
Pneumonia	PM and ozone	$7900 per case
All respiratory	PM and ozone	$6100 per case
Respiratory illness and symptoms		
Acute bronchitis	PM	$45 per case
Acute asthma	PM and ozone	$32 per case
Acute respiratory symptoms	PM, ozone, NO_2, SO_2	$18 per case
Upper respiratory symptoms	PM	$19 per case
Lower respiratory symptoms	PM	$12 per case
Shortness of breath	PM	$5.30 per day
Work loss days	PM	$83 per day
Mild restricted activity days	PM and ozone	$38 per day
Welfare benefits		
Visibility	DeciView	$14 per unit change in DeciView
Household soiling	PM	$2.50 per household per PM-10 change
Decreased worker productivity	Ozone	$1[f]
Agriculture (net surplus)	Ozone	Change in economic surplus

[a]In 1990 dollars.

[b]Mean estimate.

[c]Alternative results, based on assigning a value of $293,000 for each life-year lost are presented.

[d]Strokes are comprised of atherothrombotic brain infarctions and cerebrovascular accidents; both are estimated to have the same monetary value.

[e]The different valuations for stroke cases reflect differences in lost earnings between males and females.

[f]Decreased productivity valued as change in daily wages: $1 per worker per 10% decrease in ozone.

PM, particulate matter.

value in the year 1990 and summed to yield a range and mean estimate for the total monetized benefits of the CAA from 1970 to 1990. These results are summarized in Table 15–4.

Combining these benefits results with the cost estimates presented earlier yielded the following analytical outcomes.

- The total monetized benefits of the CAA realized during the period from 1970 to 1990 ranged from 5.6 to 49.4 trillion dollars, with a central estimate of 22.2 trillion dollars.
- By comparison, the value of direct compliance expenditures over the same period equaled approximately 0.5 trillion dollars.
- Subtracting costs from benefits results in net, direct, monetized benefits ranging from 5.1 to 48.9 trillion dollars, with a central estimate of 21.7 trillion dollars, for the 1970 to 1990 period.
- The lower bound of this range may go down and the upper bound may go up if analytical uncertainties associated with compliance costs, macroeconomic

Table 15–4. Total Estimated Monetized Benefits by Endpoint Category for 48 State Population for 1970 to 1990 Period[a]

		Present Value		
Endpoint	Pollutant(s)	5th Percentile	Mean	95th Percentile
Mortality	PM	\$2369	\$16,632	\$40,597
Mortality	Lead	\$121	\$1339	\$3910
Chronic bronchitis	PM	\$409	\$3313	\$10,401
IQ (Lost IQ points + children with IQ < 70)	Lead	\$271	\$399	\$551
Hypertension	Lead	\$77	\$98	\$120
Hospital admissions	PM, Ozone, Lead, and CO	\$27	\$57	\$120
Respiratory related symptoms, restricted activity, and decreased productivity	PM, Ozone, NO_2, and SO_2	\$123	\$182	\$261
Soiling damage	PM	\$6	\$74	\$192
Visibility	PM	\$38	\$54	\$71
Agriculture (net surplus)	Ozone	\$11	\$23	\$35

[a]In billions of 1990 dollars.

PM, particulate matter.

effects, emissions projections, and air quality modeling could be quantified and incorporated in the uncertainty analysis. While the range already reflects many important uncertainties in the physical effects and economic valuation steps, the range might also broaden further if additional uncertainties in these two steps could be quantified.

- The central estimate of 22.2 trillion dollars in benefits may be a significant underestimate, due to the exclusion of large numbers of benefits from the monetized benefit estimate (e.g., all air toxics effects, ecosystem effects, numerous human health effects).

Clearly, even the lower bound estimate of monetized benefits substantially exceeds the costs of the historical CAA. Monetized benefits consistently and substantially exceeded costs throughout the 1970 to 1990 period.

Results of an alternative based on life-years lost

Additional analyses were needed to address an important issue raised by the Council charged with reviewing EPA's Benefit-Cost Study. Specifically, the Council requested a display of alternative premature mortality results based on an approach that estimates, and assigns a value to, the loss of statistical life-years (VSLY) (i.e., the reduction in years of remaining life expectancy) resulting from the pollution exposure. The Council's position was based on the conclusion that older individuals are more susceptible to air pollution-induced mortality.

Table 15–5 summarizes and compares the results of the mortality benefits estimates based on the value of statistical life (VSL) and VSLY approaches. Estimated 1970 to 1990 benefits from PM-related mortality alone and total mortality (i.e., PM plus Lead) benefits are reported, along with total compliance costs for the same period. Adding the VSLY-based mortality benefits estimates to the nonmortality benefits estimates from Table 15–4 yields the following results for the overall analysis.

- Alternate Result: The total monetized benefits of the CAA realized during the period from 1970 to 1990 range from 4.8 to 28.7 trillion dollars, with a central estimate of 14.3 trillion dollars.

Table 15–5. Alternative Mortality Benefits Mean Estimates for 1970 to 1990 Compared to Total 1970 to 1990 Compliance Costs[a]

	Mortality Benefits[a]	
Benefit Estimation Method	PM	PM + Pb
Statistical life method ($4.8 M/case)	16.6	18.0
Life-years lost method ($293,000/year)	9.1	10.1
Total compliance cost	—	0.5

[a]In trillions of 1990 dollars.

PM, particulate matter; Pb, lead.

- Alternate Result: Subtracting costs from benefits results in net, direct, monetized benefits ranging from 4.3 to 28.2 trillion dollars, with a central estimate of 13.7 trillion dollars, for the 1970 to 1990 period.

Conclusions and Future Directions in Cost–Benefit Analyses

First and foremost, these results indicated that the benefits of the CAA and associated control programs substantially exceeded the costs during the 1970–1990 period. Even considering the large number of important uncertainties permeating each step of the analysis, it is extremely unlikely that the converse could have been true.

A second important implication of the results of this study was that a large proportion of the monetized benefits of the historical CAA were attributed to reductions of exposures to two pollutants: lead and PM. Some may argue that, while programs to control these two pollutants may have yielded measurable benefits in excess of measurable costs, estimates of measurable benefits of many other historical CAA programs and standards considered in isolation might not have exceeded measurable costs. The historical expenditure data used in this analysis were not structured in ways that allowed attribution of control costs to specific programs or standards. On the benefit side, most control programs yielded a variety of benefits, many of which included reductions in other pollutants such as ambient particulate matter. For example, new source performance standards for SO_2 emissions from coal-fired utility plants yielded benefits beyond those associated with reducing exposures to gaseous SO_2. The reductions in SO_2 emissions also led to substantial reductions in ambient fine particle sulfates, yielding human health, ecological, and visibility benefits.

The retrospective study highlighted important areas of uncertainty associated with many of the monetized benefits included in the quantitative analysis and listed benefit categories that could not be quantified or monetized given the then current state of the science. Additional research in these areas may reduce critical uncertainties and/or improve the comprehensiveness of future assessments. Particularly important areas where further research might reduce critical uncertainties include PM-related mortality incidence, valuation of premature mortality, and valuation of PM-related chronic bronchitis and cardiovascular disease. Additional research on hazardous air pollutants and on air pollution-related changes in ecosystem structure and function might help improve the comprehensiveness of future benefit studies.

Finally, the results of the retrospective study provided useful lessons with respect to the value and the limitations of cost-benefit analysis as a tool for evaluating environmental programs. Cost–benefit analysis can provide a valuable framework for organizing and evaluating information on the effects of environmental programs. When used properly, cost–benefit analysis can help illuminate important effects of changes in policy and can help set priorities for closing information gaps and reducing uncertainty. Such proper use, however, requires that sufficient levels of time and resources be provided to permit careful, thorough, and technically and scientifically sound data-gathering and analysis. When cost–benefit analyses are presented without effective characterization of the uncertainties associated with the results, cost–benefit studies can be used in highly misleading ways. Given the substantial uncertainties that permeate cost–benefit assessment of environmental programs, as demonstrated by the broad range of estimated benefits presented, cost–benefit analysis is best used to inform, but not dictate, decisions related to environmental protection policies, programs, and research.

Summary of EPA's First Prospective Report on the Benefits and Costs of the Clean Air Act, 1990 to 2010

The Clean Air Act Amendments of 1990 built upon the significant progress made by the original CAA of 1970 and its 1977 amendments in improving the nation's air quality.[7] The amendments utilized the existing structure of the CAA, but strengthened those requirements to tighten and clarify implementation goals and timing, increase the stringency of some requirements, revamp the hazardous air pollutant regulatory program, refine and streamline permitting requirements, and introduce new programs for the control of acid rain precursors and stratospheric ozone depleting substances. Because the 1990 amendments represent an incremental improvement to the nation's clean air program, the analysis summarized in the first prospective report was designed to estimate the costs and benefits of the 1990 amendments incremental to those assessed in the retrospective analysis.

The first prospective analysis consisted of a sequence of six steps. These were:

1. Estimate air pollutant emissions in 1990, 2000, and 2010.
2. Estimate the cost of emission reductions arising from the CAA amendments.
3. Model air quality based on emissions estimates.
4. Quantify air quality related health and environmental effects.
5. Estimate the economic value of cleaner air.
6. Aggregate results and characterize uncertainties.

The methodology and results for each step are summarized below.

Air pollutant emissions

Estimation of reductions in pollutant emissions afforded by the 1990 CAA Amendments (CAAA) served as the starting point for the subsequent benefit and cost estimates. Emissions analysis focused once again on criteria pollutants and their precursors : VOCs, NO_x, SO_2, CO, thoracic particulate matter (PM_{10}), and fine particulate matter ($PM_{2.5}$). For each of these pollutants, emissions were forecast for the years 2000 and 2010 under two different scenarios: *(1)* the pre-CAAA scenario, which assumed no additional control requirements would be implemented beyond those that were in place when the 1990 CAAA were passed; and *(2)* the post-CAAA scenario, which incorporated the effects of controls that, when the scenario was formulated, were expected to occur as a result of implementing the 1990 amendments. Emissions estimates for both the pre-CAAA and post-CAAA scenarios reflected expected growth in population, transportation, electric power generation, and other economic activity by 2000 and 2010. The emissions estimates were compared under each of these scenarios to estimate the effect of the CAAA requirements on future emissions.

The results of the emissions phase of the assessment indicated that the 1990 CAAA was significantly reducing emissions of air pollutants. Substantial reductions were determined for the two major precursors of ambient ground-level O_3: VOCs and NO_x. Relative to the pre-CAAA scenario, VOC emissions under the post-CAAA were estimated to be 35% lower by 2010. This change in emissions was attributable largely to VOC reductions from motor vehicles and area sources (e.g., dry cleaners, commercial bakeries, and other widely dispersed sources).

The NO_x emission reduction under the post-CAAA scenario represents the greatest proportional emissions change estimated in the analysis. For the year 2010, the post-CAAA NO_x emissions estimate was 39% lower than the pre-CAAA estimate, representing a decrease in emissions of almost 11 million tons. Nearly half of this reduction was from utilities, largely as a result of the particular NO_x emissions cap and trading program assumed under the post-CAAA scenario. The remaining reductions were attributable to cuts in motor vehicle and non-utility point source emissions.

Carbon monoxide emissions contributed directly to concentrations of CO in the environment. The 2010 post-CAAA estimate for CO emissions was 81.9 million tons, 23% lower than the pre-CAAA projection. The reduction in CO emissions was mostly due to motor vehicle emission controls.

The CAAA were also expected to result in a substantial reduction in precursors of $PM_{2.5}$. SO_2 is an important precursor of $PM_{2.5}$. By 2010, SO_2 emissions were to be 31% lower under the post-CAAA scenario. Of the 8.2 million ton difference between pre- and post-CAAA SO_2 estimates, 96% was attributable to additional control of utility emissions through a national cap-and-trade program involving marketable SO_2 emission allowances. NO_x discussed above, was also an important fine PM precursor.

The 1990 CAAA were projected to have more modest effects on emissions of PM emitted in solid form (i.e., "primary" or "direct" PM_{10} and $PM_{2.5}$ emissions). Overall, estimated emissions of primary PM_{10} and $PM_{2.5}$ were each approximately four percent lower in 2010 under the post-CAAA scenario than under the pre-CAAA scenario. Although the incremental effects of the CAAA on primary

PM emissions was expected to be relatively small, PM in the atmosphere is comprised of both directly emitted primary particles and particles that form in the atmosphere through secondary processes as a result of emissions of SO_2, NO_x, and organic compounds. These PM species, formed by the conversion of gaseous pollutant emissions, are referred to collectively as "secondary" PM. Because, as noted above, the 1990 CAAA achieve substantial reductions in these gaseous precursor emissions, the Amendments have a much larger effect on PM_{10} and $PM_{2.5}$ levels in the atmosphere than might be apparent if only the changes in directly emitted primary particles are considered.

The emission projections for 2000 and 2010, with and without 1990 CAAA mandated controls are summarized in Table 15–6.

Compliance costs

The EPA's estimate of the costs of the CAAA provisions was based on an evaluation of the increases in expenditures incurred by various entities to meet the additional control requirements incorporated in the post-1990 CAAA case. These costs include operation and maintenance (O&M) expenditures—which includes research and development (R&D) and other similarly recurring expenditures—plus amortized capital costs (i.e., depreciation plus interest costs associated with the existing capital stock). Relative to the pre-CAAA case post-CAAA scenario total annual compliance costs were approximately $21 billion higher by the year 2000, rising to $28 billion by the year 2010.

Compliance with Title I, Provisions for Attainment and Maintenance of National Ambient Air Quality Standards (NAAQS), accounts for $14.5 billion, or over half, of the estimated increase in year 2010 compliance costs. Compliance with mobile source emissions control provisions under Title II of the CAAA accounts for an additional 30% of the total costs, or $9 billion annually by 2010. Provisions to control acid deposition and emissions of stratospheric O_3 depleting substances account for most of the remainder of the costs.

These direct compliance costs provide a good, but incomplete, measure of the total effect of the CAAA on the U.S. economy. A complete picture of the secondary impacts of these costs would include changes in employment and prices as well as impacts that might be experienced among customers of the firms that must incur these costs. While these secondary effects could be substantial, EPA believes that direct costs provide a good initial measure of the effect of the CAAA on the U.S. economy, as well as an appropriate metric for comparison with the direct benefits.

Human health and environmental benefits

To estimate benefits, the results of the emissions analysis served as the principal input to a linked series of models. The EPA used these models to estimate changes in air quality, human health effects, ecological effects, and, ultimately,

TABLE 15–6. Summary of National Annual Emissions Projections[a]

POLLUTANT	1990 BASE-YEAR	2000 PRE-CAAA	2000 POST-CAAA	2000 % CHANGE	2010 PRE-CAAA	2010 POST-CAAA	2010 % CHANGE
VOC	22,715	24,410	17,874	−27	27,559	17,877	−35
NO_x	22,747	25,021	18,414	−26	28,172	17,290	−39
SO_2	22,361	24,008	18,013	−25	26,216	18,020	−31
CO	94,385	95,572	80,919	−15	107,034	81,943	−23
Primary PM_{10}	28,289	28,768	28,082	−2	28,993	28,035	−3
Primary $PM_{2.5}$	7091	7353	7216	−2%	7742	7447	−4

Notes: The totals reflect emissions for the 48 contiguous states, excluding Alaska and Hawaii. Percent change between pre-CAAA and post-CAAA scenarios.

[a]In thousand tons.

the net economic benefits of the CAAA. The goals of these steps in the analysis were to estimate the implications of changes in emissions resulting from compliance with the CAAA on criteria pollutant air quality throughout the lower 48 states, and the impacts on human health and the environment that result from these changes. The valuations used for each monetizable effect were the same as those used in the retrospective study (see Table 15–3).

The EPA focused its air quality modeling efforts on estimating the impact of pre- and post-1990 CAAA emissions on ambient concentrations of O_3, PM_{10}, $PM_{2.5}$, SO_2, NO_x, and CO and on acid deposition and visibility in future years. It found that the majority of the total monetized benefits, however, were attributable to changes in PM concentrations and, more specifically, to the effect of these ambient air quality changes on avoidance of premature mortality. It estimated that 2010 post-CAAA PM_{10} and $PM_{2.5}$ concentrations in the eastern U.S. will average approximately 5%–10% lower than 2010 pre-CAAA concentrations, with some areas of the eastern U.S. experiencing much greater reductions (up to 30%). The air quality modeling also indicated a substantial overall reduction in future-year PM_{10} and $PM_{2.5}$ concentrations throughout the western U.S., including most population centers, following implementation of the CAAA. The projected reductions in effects incidence for 2000 and 2010 are summarized in Table 15–7.

The direct benefits of the air quality improvements estimated under the post-CAAA scenario included reduced incidence of a number of criteria pollutant related adverse human health effects, improvements in visibility, and avoided damage to agricultural crops. As summarized in Table 15–8, the estimated annual economic value of these benefits in the year 2010 ranged from \$26 billion to \$270 billion, in 1990 dollars, and had a central estimate, or mean, of \$110 billion. As in the 1970–1990 retrospective study, the estimates did not include a number of other potentially important effects that could not be readily quantified and monetized. These excluded effects include a wide range of ecosystem changes, air toxics-related human health effects, and a number of additional health effects associated with criteria pollutants. Also excluded were benefits associated with the CAAA 1990 mandated reductions in chemicals causing reductions in stratospheric O_3, which will occur long after 2010. Table 15–9 summarizes the benefits of these Title VI controls on stratospheric O_3, which exceed costs by a factor that varies considerably with discount rates (76:1 for a 2% discount rate to 8:1 for a 7% discount rate).

One particularly important assumption of EPA's primary analysis was that correlations between increased air pollution exposures and adverse health outcomes found by epidemiological studies indicate causal relationships between the pollutant exposures and the adverse health effects. Future research may lead to revisions in this assumption, as well as other key assumptions, data, and models used to estimate the benefits and costs of the CAA. Such revisions may in turn

TABLE 15–7. Changes in Incidence of Adverse Health Effects Associated with Criteria Pollutants in 2010 (Pre-CAAA minus Post-CAAA)—48 State U.S. Population (avoided cases per year)

		2010[B]			% OF BASELINE INCIDENCES FOR THE MEAN ESTIMATES[a]
ENDPOINT	POLLUTANT	5TH PERCENTILE	MEAN	95TH PERCENTILE	2010
Mortality					
Ages 30 and older	PM	14,000	23,000	32,000	1.00
Chronic illness					
Chronic bronchitis	PM	5000	20,000	34,000	3.14
Chronic asthma	O_3	1800	7200	12,000	3.83
Hospitalization					
Respiratory admissions	PM, CO, NO_2, SO_2 O_3	13,000	22,000	34,000	0.62
Cardiovascular admissions	PM, CO, NO_2, SO_2, O_3	10,000	42,000	100,000	0.86
Emergency room visits for asthma	PM, O_3	430	4800	14,000	0.55
Minor illness					
Acute bronchitis	PM	0	47,000	94,000	5.06
Upper respiratory symptoms	PM	280,000	950,000	1,600,000	0.86

(continued)

TABLE 15–7. Changes in Incidence of Adverse Health Effects Associated with Criteria Pollutants in 2010 (Pre-CAAA minus Post-CAAA)—48 State U.S. Population (avoided cases per year) (*continued*)

ENDPOINT	POLLUTANT	2010[B]			% OF BASELINE INCIDENCES FOR THE MEAN ESTIMATES[a]
		5TH PERCENTILE	MEAN	95TH PERCENTILE	2010
Lower respiratory symptoms	PM	240,000	520,000	770,000	3.57
Respiratory illness	NO_2	76,000	330,000	550,000	10.44
Moderate or worse asthma[c]	PM	80,000	400,000	720,000	0.24
Asthma attacks[c]	O_3, PM	920,000	1,700,000	2,500,000	1.04
Chest tightness, shortness of breath, or wheeze	SO_2	290	110,000	520,000	0.003
Shortness of breath	PM	26,000	91,000	150,000	1.69
Work loss days	PM	3,600,000	4,100,000	4,600,000	0.94
Minor restricted activity days/any of 19 respiratory symptoms[d]	O_3, PM	25,000,000	31,000,000	37,000,000	2.15
Restricted activity days[d]	PM	10,000,000	12,000,000	13,000,000	1.00

[a]The baseline incidence generally is the same as that used in the C-R function for a particular health effect. However, there are a few exceptions. To calculate the baseline incidence rate for respiratory-related hospital admissions, admissions for persons of all ages for International Classification of Disease (ICD) codes 460–519 were used; for cardiovascular admissions, admissions for persons of all ages for ICD codes 390–429 were used; for emergency room visits for asthma, the estimated ER visit rate for persons of all ages were used; for chronic bronchitis the incidence rate for individuals 27 and older were used; for the pooled estimate of minor restricted activity days and any-of-19 respiratory symptoms, the incidence rate for minor restricted activity days were used.

[b]Percentage was calculated as the ratio of avoided mortality to the projected baseline annual nonaccidental mortality for adults aged 30 and over. Nonaccidental mortality was approximately 95% of total mortality for this subpopulation in 2010.

[c]These health endpoints overlap with the "any-of-19 respiratory symptoms" category. As a result, although estimates for each endpoint individually were present, these results were not aggregated into the total benefits estimates.

[d]Minor restricted activity days and any-of-19 respiratory symptoms have overlapping definitions and were pooled.

TABLE 15–8. Criteria Pollutant Health and Welfare Benefits in 2010

BENEFIT CATEGORY	MONETARY BENEFITS (IN MILLIONS 1990$)[a]		
	PRIMARY LOW	PRIMARY CONTROL	PRIMARY HIGH
Mortality			
Ages 30+	14,000	100,000	250,000
Chronic Illness			
Chronic bronchitis	360	5600	18,000
Chronic asthma	40	180	300
Hospitalization			
All respiratory	76	130	200
Total cardiovascular	93	390	960
Asthma-related ER visits	0.1	1.0	2.8
Minor Illness			
Acute bronchitis	0.0	2.1	5.2
URS	4.2	19	39
LRS	2.2	6.2	12
Respiratory illness	0.9	6.3	15
Mod: worse asthma[b]	1.9	13	29
Asthma attacks[b]	20	55	100
Chest tightness, shortness of breath, or wheeze	0.0	0.6	3.1
Shortness of breath	0.0	0.5	1.2
Work loss days	300	340	380
MRAD/any-of-19	680	1200	1800
Welfare			
Decreased worker productivity	710	710	710
Visibility—recreational	2500	2900	3300
Agriculture (net surplus)	7.1	550	1100
Acidification	12	50	76
Commercial timber	180	600	1000
Aggregate Range of Benefits[c]	26,000	110,000	270,000

[a]The estimates reflect air quality results for the entire population in the U.S.

[b]Moderate to worse asthma, asthma attacks, and shortness of breath are endpoints included in the definition of MRAD/any-of-19 respiratory effects. Although valuation estimates are presented for these categories, the values are not included in total benefits to avoid the potential for double-counting.

[c]The Aggregate Range reflects the 5th, mean, and 95th percentile of the estimated credible range of monetary benefits based on quantified uncertainty.

URS, upper respiratory symptoms

LRS, lower respiratory symptoms

ER, emergency room

MRAD, minor restricted activity days

Table 15–9. Benefits of Title 6 Sections 604, 606, and 609 Related to Stratospheric Ozone

HEALTH EFFECTS-QUANTIFIED	ESTIMATE
Melanoma and nonmelanoma skin cancer (fatal)	6.3 million lives saved from skin cancer in the U.S. between 1990 and 2165
Melanoma and nonmelanoma skin cancer (nonfatal)	299 million avoided cases of nonfatal skin cancers in the U.S. between 1990 and 2165
Cataracts	27.5 million avoided cases in the U.S. between 1990 and 2165
ECOLOGICAL EFFECTS-QUANTIFIED	ESTIMATE
American crop harvests	Avoided 7.5% decrease from UV-B radiation by 2075
American crops	Avoided decrease from tropospheric ozone
Polymers	Avoided damage to materials from UV-B radiation

HEALTH EFFECTS-UNQUANTIFIED

Skin cancer: reduced pain and suffering
Reduced morbidity effects of increased UV. For example:
 Reduced actinic keratosis (pre-cancerous lesions resulting from excessive sun exposure)
 Reduced immune system suppresion

ECOLOGICAL EFFECTS-UNQUANTIFIED

Ecological effects of UV. For example, benefits relating to the following:
 Recreational fishing
 Forests
 Overall marine ecosystem
 Avoided sea level rise, including avoided beach erosion, loss of coastal wetlands, salinity of estuaries and aquifers
 Other crops
 Other plant species
 Fish harvests
Ecological benefits of reduced tropospheric ozone relating to the overall marine ecosystem, forests, man-made materials, crops, other plant species, and fish harvests
Benefits to people and the environment outside the U.S.
Effects, both ecological and human health, associated with global warming

imply significant changes in the estimates of CAA costs and benefits presented in past and future assessments. In EPA's judgment, however, the primary results reflect the best currently available science and the most up-to-date tools and data it had at its disposal, and the most reasonable assumptions that could be adopted, as each step of the analysis was implemented.

Cleaner air also yields benefits to ecological systems. This first prospective analysis devoted a great deal of effort to characterizing and, where possible, quantifying and monetizing the impacts of air pollutants on natural systems. The findings of the retrospective analysis identified a better understanding of ecological effects as an important research direction for the first prospective and subsequent analyses. Quantified benefits of CAAA programs reflected in the overall monetized benefits include: increased agricultural and timber yields; reduced effects of acid rain on aquatic ecosystems; and reduced effects of nitrogen deposited to coastal estuaries. Many other ecological benefits, however, remain difficult or impossible to quantify, or can only be quantified for a limited geographic area. The magnitude of quantified benefits and the wide range of unquantified benefits nonetheless suggest that as more is learned about ecological systems more comprehensive ecological benefits assessments, estimates of these benefits could be conducted, increasing the benefits.

Comparing costs to benefits

Based on the specific tools and techniques that were employed, EPA's primary estimate of the net benefit (benefits minus costs) over the entire 1990 to 2010 period of the additional criteria pollutant control programs incorporated in the post-CAAA case was $510 billion. These results, summarized in Table 15–10, indicate that the monetizable benefits alone exceeded the direct compliance costs by about four to one. For many of the factors contributing to this net benefit estimate (especially physical effects and economic valuation estimates), EPA was able to generate quantitative estimates of uncertainty. By statistically combining these uncertain estimates, it was able to develop a range of net benefit estimates which provided a partial indication of the overall uncertainty surrounding the central estimate of net benefits. This range, reflecting a 90% probability range around the mean, or central estimate, for 2010 was $30 to $260 billion.

The estimates for Title VI (strospheric O_3 controls) also indicate that cumulative benefits ($500 billion) well exceed cumulative costs ($27 billion). The time period of EPA's Title VI analysis (175 years) suggests that these estimates are very uncertain. Nonetheless, the conclusion that benefits well exceed costs holds even at EPA's Primary Low estimate of benefits (the low end of the 90% probability range, or $100 billion), and regardless of discount rate used to generate the cumulative estimates from the perspective of the present.

The assumptions necessitated by data limitations, by the current state of the art in each phase of the analytical approach, by the need to predict future conditions, and by the state of current research on air pollution's effects imply that both the mean estimate and the 90% probability range around the central estimate are uncertain. While alternative choices for data, models, modeling assumptions, and valuation paradigms may yield results outside the range projected in EPA's primary analysis, it believes, based on the magnitude of the difference

TABLE 15–10. Summary Comparison of Benefits and Costs[a,b]

	TITLES I THROUGH V			TITLE VI	ALL TITLES
	ANNUAL ESTIMATES 2000	2010	PRESENT VALUE ESTIMATE 1990–2010	PRESENT VALUE ESTIMATE 1990–2165	TOTAL PRESENT VALUE
Monetized Direct Costs					
Central	$19,000	$27,000	$180,000	$27,000	$210,000
Monetized Direct Benefits					
Low[c]	$16,000	$26,000	$160,000	$100,000	$260,000
Central	$71,000	$110,000	$690,000	$530,000	$1,200,000
High[c]	$160,000	$270,000	$1,600,000	$900,000	$2,500,000
Benefit/Cost Ratio					
Low[d]	Less than 1/1	Less than 1/1	Less than 1/1	Less than 4/1	1/1
Central	4/1	4/1	4/1	20/1	6/1
High[d]	More than 8/1	More than 10/1	More than 9/1	More than 33/1	12/1

[a]Estimates in millions of 1990 dollars.

[b]The cost estimates for this analysis are based on assumptions about future changes in factors such as consumption patterns, input costs, and technological innovation. We recognize that these assumptions introduce significant uncertainty into the cost results; however, the degree of uncertainty or bias associated with many of the key factors cannot be readily quantified. Thus, EPA was unable to present specific low and high cost estimates.

[c]Low and high benefits estimates are based on primary results and correspond to 5th and 95th percentile results from statistical uncertainty analysis, incorporating uncertainties in physical effects and valuation steps of benefits analysis. Other significant sources of uncertainty not reflected include the value of unquantified or unmonetized benefits that are not captured in the primary estimates and uncertainties in emissions and air quality modeling.

[d]The low benefit/cost ratio reflects the ratio of the low benefits estimate to the central costs estimate, while the high ratio reflects the ratio of the high benefits estimate to the central costs estimate. Because we were unable to reliably quantify the uncertainty in cost estimates, we present the low estimate as "less than X," and the high estimate as "more than Y," where X and Y are the low and high benefit/cost ratios, respectively.

between the estimated benefits and costs, that it is unlikely that eliminating uncertainties or adopting reasonable alternative assumptions would change the fundamental conclusion of this study: The CAAA's total benefits to society exceed its costs.

The uncertainties in the primary estimates and the controversies that persist regarding model choices and valuation paradigms nonetheless highlight the need for a variety of new and continued research efforts. Based on the findings of this study, the highest priority research needs are:

- Improved emissions inventories and inventory management systems
- A more geographically comprehensive air quality monitoring network, particularly for fine particles and hazardous air pollutants
- Development of integrated air quality modeling tools based on an open, consistent model architecture
- Development of tools and data to assess the significance of wetland, aquatic, and terrestrial ecosystem changes associated with air pollution
- Increased basic and targeted research on the health effects of air pollution, especially particulate matter
- Continued development of economic valuation methods and data, particularly valuation of changes in risks of premature mortality associated with air pollution

Properly directed and funded, such research would improve the results of future analyses of the benefits and costs of the Clean Air Act.

Need for further benefits and cost valuations

While the benefits attributed to the CAA overall were quite substantial in EPA's reports to Congress, as summarized above, and greatly exceeded the costs of the implementation of the CAA, it must be recognized that a dominant role in determining the benefits was played by PM, with most of that related to criteria pollutant-associated excess mortality as indexed by PM. The magnitude of the net benefit can dramatically change by using a valuation based on life-years lost instead of a $\$4.8 \times 10^6$ valuation on a premature death (See Table 15–5), or by using some other point valuation.

On both the benefit and cost sides of the comparisons, it must also be noted that EPA was unable to disaggregate the totals into those attributable to specific pollutants or titles in the act relating separately to individual criteria pollutants, air toxics, and ecological impacts of air pollution. Thus, the benefits of criteria air pollutant controls were, in effect, compared to all of the costs of air pollution control. In terms of the criteria pollutant control program, the subtraction of costs associated with the control of air toxics and acidic deposition would increase the benefit–cost ratio for the criteria pollutants. It would also, in all likelihood, result in a very low benefit–cost ratio for air toxics and acidic deposition control expenditures.

The Council has strongly recommended that EPA expand its analyses for its next prospective study of benefits and costs of the 1990 CAAA with respect to disaggregation of both costs and benefits. The major issue with respect to air toxics valuation is the current virtual absence of credible exposure-response relationships for carcinogenic chemicals. EPA could not rely on the reference concentrations and unit risk factors in its Integrated Risk Information System (IRIS) database for central estimates of exposure-response because of their highly conservative bases, generally involving multiple layers of relatively large safety factors. On the ecological and welfare issues, there is an extreme paucity of relevant peer reviewed literature on either exposure-response relationships or economic valuation for damages or losses caused directly or indirectly by pollutant exposures.

Other air pollution benefit and cost studies in recent years have produced findings that are generally consistent with those reported by EPA to Congress on the CAA. These include studies in the state of California, the city of Houston, TX. A study of benefits and costs of air pollution in Canada has recently been completed under the auspices of the Royal Society of Canada.[8]

OTHER FUTURES ISSUES AND SUMMARY

A number of potentially serious drivers of our environmental future have not been discussed in any detail in this chapter, including: global climate change and the major population displacements and ecological disruptions that it may cause; sudden catastrophic events, such as an asteroid impact, major earthquakes, or volcanic eruptions in heavily populated areas; nuclear or biological warfare on more than a limited, local scale; or a major pandemic of disease not amenable to public health controls. Rather, this chapter has discussed a number of factors than can broadly affect our environmental future, and are more amenable to reasonably informed speculation.

The Beyond the Horizon report[1] shows us how we can apply foresight tools in order to stay ahead of new environmental challenges and deal with them effectively and efficiently before they become crises demanding immediate actions that can be expected to be either ineffective or inefficient. Ausubels' essay shows that our ever advancing technological capabilities can provide a means of improving the standard of living of an expanding population while simultaneously enhancing environmental quality. Recognizing these possibilities and consciously planning to utilize them is our challenge. Finally, the Benefits and Cost studies provide a framework for demonstrating that improvements in environmental quality do not necessarily impose net burdens on society, and that the costs of regulations can be viewed more as productive investments than lost opportunities for social and economic improvements. These analyses provide a basis for an outreach program to the public and to legislative bodies that could lead to a more positive reception to investments in environmental cleanup and protection that can accelerate our progress toward environmental and public health improvements.

REFERENCES

1. EPA-SAB. Beyond the Horizon: Using Foresight to Predict the Environmental Future. EPA-SAB-EC-95-007. US Environmental Protection Agency, Washington, DC 20460, Jan. 1995.
2. Ausubel, J.H. The liberation of the environment. *Daedalus* 125(3):1–17, 1996.
3. USGS. U.S. Geological Survey, "Estimated Use of Water in the United States in 1990," Circular 1081. Washington, DC: U.S. Government Printing Office, 1993.
4. OECD. Organization for Economic Cooperation and Development, The State of the Environment. Paris: OECD, 1991.
5. Wernick, I.K. and Ausubel, J.H. National materials metrics for industrial ecology. *Resources Policy* 21(3):189–198, 1995.
6. EPA. The Benefits and Costs of the Clean Air Act, 1970 to 1990. US Environmental Protection Agency, Washington, DC 20460, Oct. 1997.
7. EPA. The Benefits and Costs of the Clean Air Act, 1990–2010. EPA-410-R-99-001. US Environmental Protection Agency, Washington, DC 20460, Nov. 1999.
8. RSC. The Royal Society of Canada Expert Panel Review of the Socio-Economic Modes and Related Components Supporting the Development of Canada-Wide Standards for Particulate Matter and Ozone. Royal Society of Canada, Ottawa, 2001.

Supplementary Bibliography

This bibliography lists selected references, most of which have not been previously cited, that the reader may consult for more detailed information on the various topics discussed in the text.

Historical Perspective

Bowler, P. J. The Earth Encompassed: A History of the Environmental Sciences. New York: Norton, 1992.

Atmospheric Dispersion

Lyons, T. and Scott, B. Principles of Air Pollution Meteorology. London: Bellhaven Press, 1990.

Aerosol Science

Baron, P. A. and Willeke, K. (Eds.) Aerosol Measurement: Principles, Techniques, and Applications, 2nd Ed. New York: John Wiley & Sons, 2001.
Friedlander, S. K. Smoke, Dust and Haze: Fundamental of Aerosol Dynamics, 2nd Ed. New York: Oxford University Press, 2000.

Hinds, W. C. Aerosol Technology: Properties, Behavior, and Measurement of Airborne Particles, 2nd Ed. New York: Wiley, 1999.

Chemicals in the Environment

Manahan, S. E. Environmental Chemistry. Boca Raton, FL: CRC Press, 2000.

The Biosphere

Stiling, P. Ecology: Theories and Applications. Upper Saddle River, NY: Prentice-Hall, 1999.

Toxicology

Bingham, E., Cohrssen, B., and Powell, C.H. (Eds.) Patty's Toxicology, 5th Ed., Vol. 1. New York: Wiley, 2001.

Hayes, A. W. (Ed.) Principles and Methods of Toxicology. Philadelphia: Taylor and Francis, 2001.

Klaassen, C. D. (Ed.) Casarett and Doull's Toxicology: The Basic Science of Poisons. New York: McGraw-Hill, 2001.

Wexler, P. (Ed.) Encyclopedia of Toxicology. San Diego: Academic Press, 1998.

Industrial Hygiene

Harris, R. L. (Ed.) Patty's Industrial Hygiene, 5th Ed., Vol. 1. New York: Wiley, 2000.

Occupational Medicine

Rom, W. N. (Ed.) Environmental and Occupational Medicine. Philadelphia: Lippincott-Raven, 1998.

Air Pollution

Holgate, S. T., Samet, J. M., Koren, H. S., and Maynard, R. L. Air Pollution and Health. London: Academic Press, 1999.

Hazardous Waste

Johnson, B. L. Impact of Hazardous Waste on Human Health, 1st Ed. Boca Raton, FL: CRC Press, 1999.

Exposure Assessment

APCA. Recognition of Air Pollution Injury to Vegetation: A Pictorial Atlas. Pittsburgh: Air Pollution Control Association, 1972.

Cal Tox. A Multimedia Total Exposure Model for Hazardous Waste Sites (Draft). Sacramento, CA: California Environmental Protection Agency, 1993.
McKone, T. Estimating human exposure through multiple pathways from air, water, and soil. *Regul. Toxicol. Pharmacol.* 13:36–60, 1991.
NRC. Human Exposure Assessment for Airborne Pollutants: Advances and Opportunities. Washington, DC: National Academy Press, 1991.

Noise

Cowan, J. P. Handbook of Environmental Acoustics. New York, John Wiley & Sons, 1993.

Radiation

Cohen, B.S. Radon and Its short-lived decay product aerosols. In: K. Willeke and P.A. Baron, (Eds.) Aerosol Measurement: Principles, Techniques, and Applications. New York: J. Wiley and Sons, 2001, pp. 799–815.
Firestone, R.B., Shirley, V.S., Baglin, C.M., Chu, S.Y.F., Zipkin, J., (Eds.) Table of Isotopes. New York: John Wiley and Sons, Inc., 1996.
Knoll, G.F.: Radiation Detection and Measurement, 2nd Ed. New York: John Wiley and Sons, Inc., 1989.
Mauro, J.J. and Cohen, N. Human-made ionizing radiation and radioactivity: Sources, levels, and effects. In: M. Lippmann (ed.), Environmental Toxicants: Human Exposures and Their Health Effects, 2nd Ed. New York: Wiley-Interscience, 2000, pp. 523–561.
National Council on Radiation Protection and Measurements: A Handbook of Radioactivity Measurement Procedures, 2nd Ed. NCRP Report No. 58. Bethesda, MD: NCRP, 1985.

Risk Assessment, Management, Etc.

Buchholz, R. A. Principles of Environmental Management. Upper Saddle River, NJ: Prentice-Hall, 1998.
Kammen, D. M. and Hassenzahl, D. H. Should We Risk It? Exploring Environmental, Health, and Technological Problem Solving. Princeton, NJ: Princeton University Press, 1999.
Paustenbach, D. J. Human and Ecological Risk Assessment: Theory and Practice. NY: Wiley, 2002.

Index